MECHANICAL VENTILATION

MECHANICAL VENTILATION

Neil R. MacIntyre, MD

Professor of Medicine
Duke University Medical Center
Durham, North Carolina

Richard D. Branson, BA, RRT

Associate Professor
Department of Surgery
Division of Trauma/Critical Care
University of Cincinnati Medical Center
Cincinnati, Ohio

W.B. SAUNDERS COMPANY

A Harcourt Health Sciences Company
Philadelphia   London   New York   St. Louis   Sydney   Toronto

FEB 0 8 2001

W.B. SAUNDERS COMPANY
A Harcourt Health Sciences Company

The Curtis Center
Independence Square West
Philadelphia, Pennsylvania 19106

Library of Congress Cataloging-in-Publication Data

Mechanical ventilation / [edited by] Neil R. MacIntyre, Richard D. Branson.

p. cm.

ISBN 0–7216–7361–9

1. Artificial respiration.   2. Respiratory therapy.   3. Critical care medicine.
   4. Respirators (Medical equipment).   I. MacIntyre, Neil R.   II. Branson,
   Richard D.

RC87.9.M432 2000

615.8′36—dc21   99–25457

Acquisitions Editor: Andrew Allen
Project Manager: Edna Dick
Production Manager: Shelley Hampton
Illustration Specialist: Fran Moriarty

MECHANICAL VENTILATION   ISBN 0–7216–7361–9

Printed in the United States of America

Last digit is the print number: 9   8   7   6   5   4   3   2   1

To my wife Suzanne and my children for all their support

NEIL R. MACINTYRE, MD

To Patty, my partner in all things

RICHARD D. BRANSON, BA, RRT

Contributors

Richard D. Branson, BA, RRT
Associate Professor, Department of
Surgery, Division of Trauma/Critical Care,
University of Cincinnati Medical Center,
Cincinnati, Ohio
*Classification of Mechanical Ventilators;
Modes of Ventilator Operation; The
Patient–Ventilator Interface: Ventilator
Circuit, Airway Care, and Suctioning;
Humidification and Aerosol Therapy
During Mechanical Ventilation; Mechanical
Ventilation During Transport and
Cardiopulmonary Resuscitation*

Leslie Campbell, BA
*Nutrition in the Patient on Mechanical
Ventilation*

Robert B. Campbell, MBA, RRT
Clinical Educator, Respiratory Care
Services, Duke University Medical Center,
Durham, North Carolina
Long-Term Mechanical Ventilation

Robert S. Campbell, RRT
Senior Research Associate, Volunteer
Instructor, Department of Surgery, Division
of Trauma/Critical Care, University of
Cincinnati Medical Center, Cincinnati,
Ohio
*Modes of Ventilator Operation; Mechanical
Ventilation During Transport and
Cardiopulmonary Resuscitation*

Robert L. Chatburn, BS, RRT, FAARC
Associate Professor, Department of
Pediatric Medicine, Case Western Reserve
University; Director, Respiratory Care

Department, University Hospitals of
Cleveland, Cleveland, Ohio
Classification of Mechanical Ventilators

Ira M. Cheifetz, MD
Assistant Professor of Pediatrics, Duke
University Medical Center, Durham, North
Carolina
*Extracorporeal Techniques for
Cardiopulmonary Support*

Paul M. Dorinsky, MD
Assistant Clinical Professor of Medicine,
Division of Pulmonary and Critical Care
Medicine, University of North Carolina at
Chapel Hill School of Medicine, Chapel
Hill; Principal Clinical Research Physician,
Glaxo Wellcome, Research Triangle Park,
North Carolina
*Pharmacology of Respiratory Drugs
Administered by Aerosol During
Mechanical Ventilation*

Larry G. Dukes, RPh
Staff Pharmacist, Veterans Affairs Medical
Center, Louisville, Kentucky
*Nutrition in the Patient on Mechanical
Ventilation*

David S. Foley, MD
ECMO Fellow, University of Michigan
Medical Center, Ann Arbor, Michigan
Liquid Ventilation

William J. Fulkerson, MD
Professor of Medicine, Duke University
School of Medicine, Durham, North
Carolina
Lung Injury from Mechanical Ventilation

Michael A. Gentile, RRT
Associate Director, Respiratory Care
Services, Duke University Medical Center,
Durham, North Carolina
*Extracorporeal Techniques for
Cardiopulmonary Support*

Michael S. Gorback, MD
Former Assistant Professor of
Anesthesiology and Surgery, Duke
University Medical Center, Durham, North
Carolina
Airway Management

Joseph A. Govert, MD
Assistant Professor of Medicine, Duke
University School of Medicine; Director,
Medical Intensive Care Unit, Duke
University Medical Center, Durham, North
Carolina
Positioning of the Patient

Karen L. Gunther, RN, BSN
Associate Director, Department of Clinical
Research–Respiratory, Boehringer
Ingelheim Pharmaceuticals, Inc.,
Ridgefield, Connecticut
*Pharmacology of Respiratory Drugs
Administered by Aerosol During
Mechanical Ventilation*

Dean Hess, PhD, RRT
Assistant Professor of Anesthesia, Harvard
Medical School; Assistant Director of
Respiratory Care, Massachusetts General
Hospital, Boston, Massachusetts
Heliox and Inhaled Nitric Oxide

Ronald B. Hirschl, MD, FACS
Associate Professor, Department of
Pediatric Surgery, University of Michigan
School of Medicine, Ann Arbor, Michigan
Liquid Ventilation

Yuh-Chin T. Huang, MD
Assistant Professor, Division of Pulmonary
and Critical Care Medicine, Department of
Medicine, Duke University Medical Center,
Durham, North Carolina
Supplemental Oxygen

S. Gregory Jennings, MD
Research Associate, Mid-South Pulmonary
and Critical Care Research Foundation,
Memphis, Tennessee
Noninvasive Ventilation

Jay A. Johannigman, MD
Assistant Professor of Surgery, University
of Cincinnati Medical Center, Cincinnati,
Ohio
*Mechanical Ventilation During Transport
and Cardiopulmonary Resuscitation*

Nancy W. Knudsen, MD
Assistant Professor of Anesthesiology,
Duke University School of Medicine,
Durham, North Carolina
Lung Injury from Mechanical Ventilation

Neil R. MacIntyre, MD
Professor of Medicine, Duke University
Medical Center, Durham, North Carolina
*Ventilator Monitors, Displays, and Alarms;
Respiratory System Mechanics; Alveolar
Capillary Gas Transport; Patient–
Ventilator Interactions; Mechanical
Ventilation Strategies for Parenchymal
Lung Injury; Mechanical Ventilation
Strategies for Obstructive Airway Disease;
Weaning Mechanical Ventilatory Support;
Long-Term Mechanical Ventilation;
Assessing Innovations in Mechanical
Ventilation; High-Frequency Ventilation*

Stephen A. McClave, MD
Professor of Gastroenterology/Hepatology,
Division of Gastroenterology/Hepatology,
University of Louisville School of Medicine,
Louisville, Kentucky
*Nutrition in the Patient on Mechanical
Ventilation*

Robert R. McConnell, Jr., BA, RRT
Clinical Trials Specialist/Research
Assistant, Duke University Medical Center,
Durham, North Carolina
*Modifications on Conventional Ventilation
Techniques*

Jon N. Meliones, MD, MS, FCCM
Associate Professor of Pediatrics and
Anesthesia, Duke University Medical
Center; Chief, Critical Care Medicine,
Duke Children's Hospital, Durham, North
Carolina
*The Effects of Respiratory Support on the
Cardiovascular System*

Clyde I. Miyagawa, PharmD
Assistant Professor of Clinical Pharmacy
Practice, University of Cincinnati, College
of Pharmacy; Clinical Pharmacy
Specialist–Critical Care, The University
Hospital, Cincinnati, Ohio
*Sedation and Paralysis in the Mechanically
Ventilated Patient*

Steven E. Pass, PharmD
Assistant Professor of Clinical Pharmacy
Practice, University of Cincinnati College
of Pharmacy; Clinical Pharmacy
Practitioner–Critical Care, University
Hospital, Cincinnati, Ohio
*Sedation and Paralysis in the Mechanically
Ventilated Patient*

Harvy L. Snider, MD
Associate Professor of Medicine, University
of Louisville School of Medicine, Louisville,
Kentucky
*Nutrition in the Patient on Mechanical
Ventilation*

Janice Thalman, BS, RRT
Associate Director, Respiratory Care
Services, Duke University Medical Center,
Durham, North Carolina
Long-Term Mechanical Ventilation

Karen Welty-Wolf, MD
Assistant Professor, Division of Pulmonary
and Critical Care Medicine, Division of
Infectious Diseases, Duke University
Medical Center; Staff Physician, Durham
Veterans Administration Medical Center,
Durham, North Carolina
Ventilator-Associated Pneumonia

Theodore J. Witek, Jr., Dr PH
Research Associate Professor, Department
of Pulmonary Medicine, Mount Sinai
School of Medicine, New York, New York;
Therapeutic Area Director, Respiratory and
Immunology, Clinical Research, Boehringer
Ingelheim Pharmaceuticals, Inc.,
Ridgefield, Connecticut
*Pharmacology of Respiratory Drugs
Administered by Aerosol During
Mechanical Ventilation*

Richard G. Wunderink, MD
Associate Clinical Professor, University of
Tennessee School of Medicine; Associate
Director, Clinical Research, Methodist
Healthcare Foundation, Memphis,
Tennessee
Noninvasive Ventilation

Preface

Mechanical ventilation is a mainstay of life support in care venues ranging from intensive care units to the home. Currently, an estimated 100,000 positive-pressure ventilators are in use worldwide, approximately half of them in North America. It is also estimated that approximately 1.5 million patients in the United States receive mechanical ventilation outside of operating rooms and recovery rooms each year and that the average length of stay on a ventilator in a hospital is in the neighborhood of 1 to 1.5 weeks.

There are two important trends that are occurring in the use of positive-pressure mechanical ventilation as we begin the 21st century. First, the number of patients being intubated and requiring positive-pressure mechanical ventilation is rising. There are several reasons for this. One is that the aging population presents the health care delivery system with more chronic diseases and more acute flares of those chronic diseases. In addition, aggressive surgical procedures are being carried out on older and more seriously ill patients. Similarly, more aggressive chemotherapy is being given to patients with malignancies, resulting in more immunocompromised patients and thus a higher incidence of sepsis and respiratory failure.

A second major trend in mechanical ventilation is that as the acute phase of respiratory failure is resolved, patients often enter a more chronic phase of ventilator dependence, resulting in increasing pressure to move them to more cost-effective venues of care. This means that step-down units, sub-acute hospitals, and long-term ventilator facilities are growing in number and in complexity of services provided. Both of these trends mean that the need for mechanical ventilation will only increase over the foreseeable future.

The outcome of mechanical ventilation obviously depends on the underlying disease state. Generally, in patients with rapidly reversing lung diseases and underlying good health (for example, those with asthma, drug overdose, or anesthesia recovery) mortality rates of less than 5% can be expected. On the other hand, acute respiratory distress syndrome (ARDS) and chronic obstructive pulmonary disease (COPD) may involve mortality rates approaching 40 to 50%. Moreover, in patients on mechanical ventilators who have severe multi-organ failure and the sepsis syndrome, mortality rates may approach 100%.

How mechanical ventilation is delivered can have significant impact on this outcome. For example, so-called "lung protective strategies" designed to limit overdistention injury have recently been shown to limit mortality in ARDS. Similarly, weaning protocols aimed at aggressive support reductions have been shown to reduce the days of ventilator use. Mechanical ventilation strategies can also affect cardiac function, patient comfort (and thus sedation use), infection risks, and other forms of lung injury (oxygen toxicity and airway injuries). Because the mechanical ventilator can have such profound effect on patient outcome, we have written this book for the clinicians who care for patients requiring this technology.

Our hope is that by providing a comprehensive reference work that addresses engineering issues, physiologic principles, and patient management strategies, the outcome in patients receiving mechanical ventilation will continue to improve.

NEIL R. MacINTYRE
RICHARD D. BRANSON

Acknowledgments

I would like to thank Theresa Stewart and Janet Johns for their secretarial assistance, and the Duke University Medical Center Respiratory Care Department for sound advice, technical expertise, and continuous encouragement.

NEIL R. MacINTYRE, MD

Considerable effort and sacrifice are involved in every page of a text. Much of it is borne by people other than the editors. I would like to express my appreciation to my family and my colleagues for their sacrifices, allowing me the time to complete this project. I would also like to thank the many contributors who lent their talent and expertise to this text. Finally, I want to thank my mentors, students, and patients who have taught me so much over these past 20 years.

RICHARD D. BRANSON, BA, RRT

Contents

SECTION I
Technical Aspects of Mechanical Ventilation

1 Classification of Mechanical
Ventilators   2
*Robert L. Chatburn, BS, RRT, FAARC, and
Richard D. Branson, BA, RRT*

2 Modes of Ventilator
Operation   51
*Richard D. Branson, BA, RRT,
and Robert S. Campbell, RRT*

3 The Patient–Ventilator Interface:
Ventilator Circuit, Airway Care,
and Suctioning   85
Richard D. Branson, BA, RRT

4 Humidification and Aerosol
Therapy During Mechanical
Ventilation   103
Richard D. Branson, BA, RRT

5 Ventilator Monitors, Displays, and
Alarms   131
Neil R. MacIntyre, MD

SECTION II
Physiology of Positive Pressure Ventilation

6 Respiratory System
Mechanics   146
Neil R. MacIntyre, MD

7 Alveolar Capillary Gas
Transport   161
Neil R. MacIntyre, MD

8 Supplemental Oxygen   173
Yuh-Chin T. Huang, MD

9 Patient–Ventilator
Interactions   189
Neil R. MacIntyre, MD

10 The Effects of Respiratory Support
on the Cardiovascular
System   204
Jon N. Meliones, MD, MS, FCCM

11 Lung Injury from Mechanical
Ventilation   212
*Nancy W. Knudsen, MD,
and William J. Fulkerson, MD*

SECTION III
Adjunctive Therapy During Mechanical Ventilation

12 Nutrition in the Patient on
Mechanical Ventilation   224
*Stephen A. McClave, MD, Harvy L. Snider, MD,
Larry G. Dukes, RPh, and Leslie Campbell, BA*

13 Airway Management   239
Michael S. Gorback, MD

14 Sedation and Paralysis in the
Mechanically Ventilated
Patient   257
*Clyde I. Miyagawa, PharmD,
and Steven E. Pass, PharmD*

15 Pharmacology of Respiratory Drugs Administered by Aerosol During Mechanical Ventilation   269
Karen L. Gunther, RN, BSN, Paul M. Dorinsky, MD, and Theodore J. Witek, Jr., Dr PH

16 Positioning of the Patient   283
Joseph A. Govert, MD

17 Ventilator-Associated Pneumonia   296
Karen Welty-Wolf, MD

SECTION IV

Specific Clinical Applications of Mechanical Ventilation

18 Mechanical Ventilation Strategies for Parenchymal Lung Injury   330
Neil R. MacIntyre, MD

19 Mechanical Ventilation Strategies for Obstructive Airway Disease   340
Neil R. MacIntyre, MD

20 Weaning Mechanical Ventilatory Support   348
Neil R. MacIntyre, MD

21 Long-Term Mechanical Ventilation   357
Neil R. MacIntyre, MD, Janice Thalman, BS, RRT, and Robert B. Campbell, MBA, RRT

22 Mechanical Ventilation During Transport and Cardiopulmonary Resuscitation   365

Richard D. Branson, BA, RRT, Jay A. Johannigman, MD, and Robert S. Campbell, RRT

SECTION V

Specialized Techniques and Future Therapies

23 Assessing Innovations in Mechanical Ventilation   394
Neil R. MacIntyre, MD

24 Modifications on Conventional Ventilation Techniques   400
Robert R. McConnell, Jr., BA, RRT

25 High-Frequency Ventilation   415
Neil R. MacIntyre, MD

26 Extracorporeal Techniques for Cardiopulmonary Support   425
Michael A. Gentile, RRT, and Ira M. Cheifetz, MD

27 Liquid Ventilation   433
David S. Foley, MD, and Ronald B. Hirschl, MD, FACS

28 Heliox and Inhaled Nitric Oxide   454
Dean Hess, PhD, RRT

29 Noninvasive Ventilation   481
Richard G. Wunderink, MD, and S. Gregory Jennings, MD

Case Studies   493
Neil R. MacIntyre, MD

Glossary   507

Index   517

Technical Aspects of Mechanical Ventilation

CHAPTER 1

Classification of Mechanical Ventilators

Robert L. Chatburn, BS, RRT, FAARC
Richard D. Branson, BA, RRT

BASIC CONCEPTS
INPUT POWER
Electric
Pneumatic
CONTROL SCHEME
Control Variables
Phase Variables
Conditional Variables
Modes of Ventilation
Output Waveforms

VENTILATOR ALARM SYSTEMS
Input Power Alarms
Control Circuit Alarms
Output Alarms
REFERENCES

KEY WORDS

active expiration
alarm event
closed-loop control
compressor
constant airway pressure
control circuit
control variables
cycle
cycle time
demand valve
dual control
end-expiratory pressure
external compressor

expiratory phase (expiration)
expiratory flow time
expiratory pause time
expiratory time
gauge pressure
inspiratory phase
    (inspiration)
inspiratory flow time
inspiratory pause time
inspiratory time
internal compressor
limit
mandatory breath

mean airway pressure
open-loop control
passive expiration
percent cycle time
percent pause time
phase
phase variable
phase variable value
spontaneous breaths
transrespiratory pressure
trigger

Ventilators have evolved into highly complex, microprocessor-controlled devices with a wide range of operating characteristics. Unfortunately, our language and conceptual models, which we use to understand how ventilators work, have not kept pace with the technologic development. Mushin's classic text,[1] based on ventilators common in the 1960s, provides a theoretical frame work for understanding ventilators but cannot adequately describe all the characteristics of current ventilators. This is not meant as criticism but simply reflects the fact that Mushin did not anticipate these advancements in technology.

When Mushin developed his framework, the ventilator output was dictated by the mechanical driving system. For instance, a piston ventilator provided a quasisinusoidal flow waveform, whereas early pneumatic ventilators (Bird Mark 14) provided a rectangular pressure pattern. These patterns were not able to be altered without some external modification. The advent of microprocessor technology allows a single ventilator to produce any number of output waveforms, some as limitless as the operator's imagination. This chapter presents an updated classfication scheme that effectively deals with new technology that has been accepted by leading members of the pulmonary medicine community[2-4] and most authors of respiratory care textbooks.

BASIC CONCEPTS

A ventilator is simply a machine—a system of related elements designed to alter, transmit, and direct applied energy in a predetermined manner to perform useful work.[5] Energy enters the ventilator in the form of electricity (energy = volts $\times$ amperes $\times$ time) or compressed gas (energy = pressure $\times$ volume). That energy is transmitted or transformed (by the ventilator's drive mechanism) in a predetermined manner (by the control circuit) to augment or replace the patient's muscles in performing the work of breathing (the desired output). Therefore, to understand mechanical ventilators in general, we first must understand their basic functions of

- Power input
- Control scheme (including power transmission or conversion)
- Output (pressure, volume, and flow waveforms)

This simple outline format can be ex-

panded to add as much detail about a given ventilator as desired (Table 1–1).

INPUT POWER

All ventilators require a source of power that can be used to perform the work of ventilating the respiratory system. In effect, ventilators convert input power in a readily available form to a form that is more convenient for the delicate and exacting task of supporting ventilation. The most common forms of input power for ventilators are electric and pneumatic (compressed gas). Input power should not be confused with the power for the control circuit. For example, many ventilators use pneumatic input power to drive inspiration but electric power for the control circuit. As an example, com-

TABLE 1–1. Outline of Ventilator Classification System

Input
   Electric
   Pneumatic
Control Scheme
   Control Variables
     Pressure
     Volume
     Flow
     Time
   Phase Variables
     Trigger
     Limit
     Cycle
     Baseline
   Conditional Variables
   Modes of Ventilation
   Control Subsystems
     Control Circuit
     Drive Mechanism
     Output Control Valve
Output
   Waveforms
     Pressure
     Volume
     Flow
   Displays
   Alarm Systems
     Input Power Alarms
     Control Circuit Alarms
     Output Alarms

pressed oxygen at 50 pounds per square inch gauge (psig) can be delivered to a ventilator that uses a solenoid valve to control respiratory frequency and inspiratory:expiratory (I:E) ratio. The compressed gas delivers the energy (input power) to ventilate the lungs, whereas the solenoid uses electric power to operate the control circuit.

Electric

Most ventilators in the United States use 110 to 115 volts alternating current (AC) (60 Hz) from common electrical outlets to power drive mechanisms. The AC voltage also is reduced and converted to direct current (DC) to power electronic control circuits. Some current ventilators, notably infant and transport ventilators, are designed to use rechargeable batteries as alternative sources of power when the usual AC current is not available. This capability makes them useful for transferring ventilator-dependent patients from one place to another within the hospital as well as for external transport. In the home care setting, a battery backup can be a life-saving feature in the event of a power outage. Common ventilator batteries are the lead-acid type, which supply approximately 2.5 amp-hours of energy. This usually powers a ventilator for up to 1 hour. This type of battery normally requires 8 to 12 hours to recharge. Nickel-cadmium (NiCad) batteries can be used, but because the batteries develop memory and require complete discharge before recharging, careful monitoring must be done.

Pneumatic

Because compressed air and oxygen are in abundant supply in most hospital intensive care units, many ventilators are designed to use the energy stored in pressurized gas. We usually think of pressure as a force per unit area, but pressure also has the units of energy density—thus, the more pressure available, the more useful work that can be generated. Besides being used to inflate the lungs, the input pressure often is used as the source of power for the control circuit,

as in the case of fluidic logic circuits. Ventilators operated by pressurized gas typically have internal pressure-reducing regulators, so that the normal operating pressure is lower than the source pressure. This allows uninterrupted operation from piped gas sources in hospitals, which usually are regulated to 50 psig but are subject to periodic fluctuations. The use of compressed gas as a power source makes a ventilator useful in environments in which no electrical power is available, such as during transport, or where it is undesirable, such as near magnetic resonance imaging (MRI) equipment.

CONTROL SCHEME

To understand how a machine can be controlled to replace or augment the natural function of breathing, a basic understanding of the mechanics of breathing is required. The study of mechanics deals with forces, displacements, and the rate of change of displacement. In physiology, force is measured as pressure (pressure = force × area), displacement is measured as volume (volume = area × displacement), and the relevant rate of change is measured as flow (e.g., average flow = change in volume/ change in time; instantaneous flow = dv/ dt, the derivative of volume with respect to time). Specifically, we are interested in the pressure necessary to cause a flow of gas to flow through the airways and increase the volume of the lungs.

The study of respiratory mechanics is essentially the search for simple but useful models of respiratory system mechanical behavior. Conceptually, the relatively complex respiratory system can be represented by a simple graphic model (e.g., a straw connected to a balloon). The simple graphic model is analogous to simple electrical circuits in which compliance is analogous to capacitance, flow resistance is analogous to electrical resistance, and pressure is analogous to a voltage source. The similarity of the physical and electrical model makes it possible to borrow mathematical models from electrical engineering, substituting pressure, volume, and flow for voltage, charge, and current, respectively (Fig. 1–1).

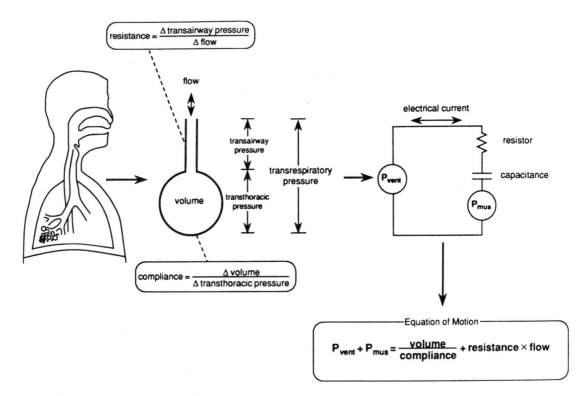

FIGURE 1–1

The study of respiratory system mechanics is based on graphic and mathematical models. The respiratory system can be modeled as a single-flow conducting tube connected to a single elastic compartment. This physical model is analogous to a simple electrical circuit consisting of a resistor and a capacitor. Two voltage sources in the circuit represent pressures generated by the muscles and the ventilator; electrical current represents airflow. The electrical circuit can be modeled by a mathematical model called the equation of motion for the respiratory system. In this model, pressure, volume, and flow are variables (i.e., functions of time), whereas resistance and compliance are constants.

The result is known as the equation of motion for the respiratory system (a simplified version)[6, 7]:

$$\text{Muscle pressure} + \text{ventilator pressure}$$
$$= \text{elastance} \times \text{volume} + \text{resistance}$$
$$\times \text{flow} \qquad (1)$$

$$\text{Muscle pressure} + \text{ventilator pressure}$$
$$= \text{elastic load} + \text{resistive load} \qquad (2)$$

In this simplified form muscle pressure is the imaginary **transrespiratory pressure** (i.e., airway pressure minus body surface pressure) generated by the ventilatory muscles to expand the thoracic cage and lungs. Muscle pressure said to be imaginary because it is not directly measurable. Ventilator pressure is the transrespiratory pres-

sure generated by the ventilator during inspiration. The combined muscle and ventilator pressure causes volume and flow to be delivered to the patient. More imply, the patient's muscle effort increases lung volume by decreasing pressure relative to atmospheric pressure while the ventilator increases lung volume by increasing pressure relative to atmospheric pressure. The total pressure results from the patient pulling gas into the lung and the ventilator pushing gas into the lung. Pressure, volume, and flow, change with time and hence are variables. Elastance and resistance are assumed to rei iain constant and are called parameters, and their combined effect constitute the load experienced by the ventilator and ventilatory muscles. *Elastance* is defined as the ratio of pressure change to volume change (i.e., the reciprocal of compliance), and *resistance* is defined the ratio of pressure change to flow change. The elastic load is the pressure necessary to overcome the elastance (or compliance) of the respiratory system, the resistive load is the pressure necessary to overcome the flow resistance of the airways (including endotracheal tube) along with lung and chest wall tissue resistance. The term *parameter* also may refer to a particular aspect of a variable, such as the peak or mean value.

Note that pressure, volume, and flow all are measured relative to their baseline values (i.e., their values at end-expiration). This means that the pressure to cause inspiration is measured as the change in airway pressure above positive end = expiratory pressure (PEEP). This is the reason, for example, that pressure support levels are measure relative to PEEP. Thinking of ventilator pressure as simply airway pressure (i.e., pressure measured at one point in space, the airway) limits our understanding of the mechanics involved in breathing. Volume is measured as the change in lung volume above functional residual capacity, and the change in lung volume during the inspiratory period is defined as the tidal volume. Flow is measured relative to its end-expiratory value (usually zero). When pressure, volume, and flow are plotted as functions of time, characteristic waveforms for volume-controlled ventilation and pressure-controlled ventilation are produced (Fig. 1–2).

Notice that if the patient's ventilatory muscles are not functioning, muscle pressure is 0 and the ventilator must generate all of the pressure required to deliver the tidal volume and inspiratory flow. Conversely, if ventilator pressure is 0 (i.e., airway pressure does not rise above baseline during inspiration) and the patient is not breathing, there is no ventilatory support. In between these two extremes, there is an infinite variety of combinations of muscle pressure (i.e., patient effort) and ventilator support that are theoretically possible for partial ventilatory support.

The concept of muscle pressure is important for another reason. There are many ventilators and bedside pulmonary function monitors that provide the clinician with estimates of respiratory system compliance and resistance based on transrespiratory system pressure (i.e., ventilator pressure), volume, and flow. All of them make calculations on the basis of this version of the equation of motion:

$$\text{Ventilator pressure} = \text{elastance} \times \text{volume} + \text{resistance} \times \text{flow} \quad (3)$$

which does not contain a term for muscle pressure. This implies that any measurement of respiratory system mechanics is valid only if the ventilatory muscles are inactive. If the patient makes an inspiratory effort during an assisted breath, he or she adds an unmeasured amount of driving pressure to that generated by the ventilator. Thus, elastance and resistance based only on the ventilator's airway pressure sensor measurements underestimate the true values.

Analysis of ventilator–patient interaction on the basis of a mathematical model suggests the proper use of the word "assist," which is another frequently confused concept. Webster's Dictionary defines assist as "to help; to aid; to give support." From the perspective of the equation of motion, whenever airway pressure (i.e., ventilator pressure) rises above baseline during inspiration, the ventilator does work on the patient. Thus, the breath is said to be assisted, independent of other breath characteristics (i.e., whether the breath is classified as spontaneous or mandatory). Do not confuse this meaning of the word "assist" with specific names of modes of ventilation (e.g., ASSIST/CONTROL). Ventilator manufacturers often coin terms for modes without regard to consistency or theoretical relevance.

In the equation of motion (3), the form of any one of the three variables (i.e., pressure, volume, or flow expressed as functions of time) can be predetermined, making it the independent variable and making the other two dependent variables. This is precisely analogous to the way in which ventilators operate. Thus, during pressure-controlled ventilation, pressure is the independent variable, and the shape of the volume and flow waveforms depends on the shape of the

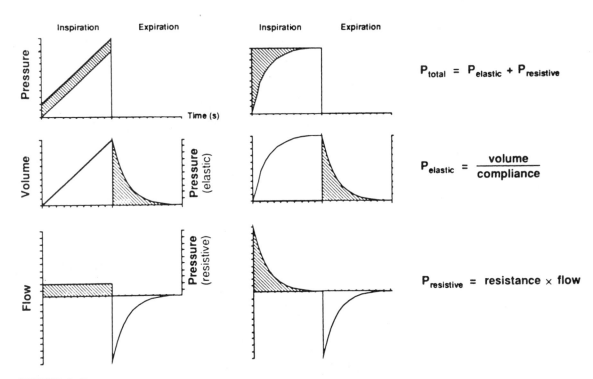

FIGURE 1–2

Some conventions for the presentation of graphic data are illustrated. The theoretical output waveforms for flow-controlled inspiration with a rectangular (i.e., pulse) flow waveform on the left compared with pressure-controlled inspiration with a rectangular pressure waveform are shown. The order of presentation is pressure, volume, and flow, according to the order specified by the equation of motion. Note that the volume waveform has the same shape as the transthoracic or lung pressure waveform (i.e., pressure caused by elastic recoil). The flow waveform has the same shape as the transairway pressure waveform (i.e., pressure caused by airway resistance). If all the pressure scales are the same, then the height of the airway pressure waveform at any instant is the sum of the heights of the other two waveforms. The origin of the airway pressure waveform is the end-expiratory pressure; the origins of the volume and flow waveforms are both zero. The shaded areas represent pressures caused by flow resistance; the open areas represent pressure caused by elastic recoil.

pressure waveform and also on the resistance and compliance of the respiratory system. Conversely, during flow-controlled ventilation, we can specify the shape of the flow waveform. This makes flow the independent variable and the shape of the volume waveform depends on the shape of the flow waveform. The shape of the pressure waveform depends on the flow waveform as well as on resistance and compliance.

Thus, we have a theoretical basis for classifying ventilators as either pressure, volume, or flow controllers. The necessary and sufficient criteria for determining which variable is controlled (i.e., which variable is the independent variable) are illustrated in

Figure 1–3. If the waveforms for all three variables are not predetermined (i.e., none of the variables can be considered independent), then the ventilator is considered to control only the timing of the inspiratory and expiratory phase and is called a time controller. From a practical standpoint, the only time controllers are some types of high-frequency ventilators.

This theoretical framework is more than just an intellectual exercise. It is essential for the understanding and interpretation of bedside pulmonary mechanics values (e.g., resistance, compliance, time constant, and the like) calculated by many ventilators. It is the very basis of a new mode of ventila-

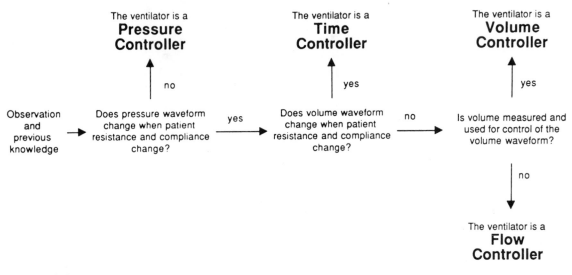

FIGURE 1-3
Criteria for determining the control variable during a ventilator-assisted inspiration.

tory support known as "proportional assist."[8] The idea of this mode of ventilation is to allow the clinician to support—and essentially cancel—the specific effects of pulmonary pathology. Thus, the ventilator can be set to support either the extra elastance or the extra resistance caused by lung disease, or both. To understand this, we start with the equation describing spontaneous breathing:

$$\text{Muscle pressure} = \text{normal elastance} \times \text{volume} + \text{normal resistance} \times \text{flow} \quad (4)$$

When pathology increases elastance and/or resistance, we have:

$$\text{Muscle pressure} = (\text{normal elastance} + \text{abnormal elastance}) \times \text{volume} + (\text{normal resistance} + \text{abnormal resistance}) \times \text{flow} \quad (5)$$

Equation 5 can be rearranged to show the normal and abnormal loads. Recall that load, in this context, is the pressure to overcome either elastance or resistance (i.e., elastance × volume = pressure; resistance × flow = pressure).

$$\text{Muscle pressure} = (\text{normal elastance} \times \text{volume}) + (\text{normal resistance} \times \text{flow}) + (\text{abnormal elastance} \times \text{volume}) + (\text{abnormal resistance} \times \text{flow}) \quad (6a)$$

$$\text{Muscle pressure} = (\text{normal elastance} \times \text{volume}) + (\text{normal resistance} \times \text{flow}) + \text{abnormal load} \quad (6b)$$

Because both the abnormal elastic load and the abnormal resistive load have units of pressure, we can add them together. This shows that in the presence of increased load, the muscle pressure must increase to provide the same (i.e., normal) tidal volume and flow. If we want to mechanically support the abnormal load(s) and allow muscle pressure to return to normal levels, all we have to do is set the ventilator to generate a sufficiently large inspiratory pressure. This can be seen by equating load to ventilator pressure and adding it to the left side of equation 6b:

$$\text{Muscle pressure} + \text{ventilator pressure} = (\text{normal elastance} \times \text{volume}) + (\text{normal resistance} \times \text{flow}) + \text{abnormal load} \quad (7)$$

In this case, the muscle pressure generates the force to overcome normal elastance and resistance while the ventilator pressure generates the force to overcome abnormal elastance and resistance so that normal tidal volume and inspiratory flow result. This analysis shows that proportional assist is a form of pressure control ventilation. Furthermore, we can see that it differs from the pressure support mode because the ventilator pressure does not necessarily generate a rectangular pressure waveform. On the contrary, the ventilator pressure varies continuously throughout inspiration.

To understand how this works, look at equations 6 and 7. We see that ventilator pressure has two components. One is elastance × volume and the other is resistance × flow. Elastance and resistance are assumed to be constant throughout inspiration, whereas volume and flow change with the continuously varying muscle pressure. Because of the requirement for muscle pressure, proportional assist works only with spontaneous breaths. Ventilator pressure is proportional to the volume and flow signals (hence the name "proportional assist") where the constants of proportionality are the abnormal elastance and resistance. In engineering terms, these constants are gain (or amplification) factors set on the volume and flow signals. The ventilator measures airway pressure and flow. The flow signal is integrated to get a volume signal. The flow and volume signals are fed through two amplifiers, through a mixer (that combines the amplified signals). The mixed signal is fed to a pressure generator (e.g., a piston) connected to the patient's airway.

The ventilator's control circuit is programmed with the equation of motion so that each moment, airway pressure is controlled to be equal to the amplified volume signal plus the amplified flow signal. The gain of the flow amplifier is set to the abnormal resistance, and the gain of the volume amplifier is set to the abnormal elastance, assuming these values have been measured or estimated. Thus, the specific mechanical abnormality of the patient is supported. In effect, the abnormal load is eliminated and the patient perceives only normal ventilatory load. It is analogous to power steering on an automobile, making driving easier while maintaining complete responsiveness to the operator's motions. No ventilator power is wasted, forcing the patient to breathe in an unnatural pattern, as can happen with pressure support. This makes proportional assist (at this writing still in the experimental phases) potentially the most comfortable mode of ventilation yet designed. Of course, there are some practical problems, such as how to continually monitor and reset the abnormal elastance and resistance levels, but these issues should be resolved soon.

The most significant revelation provided by the equation of motion, however, is that any conceivable ventilator can directly control only one variable at a time: pressure, volume, or flow. Therefore, we can think of a ventilator as simply a machine that controls either the airway pressure waveform, the inspired volume waveform, or the inspiratory flow waveform. Thus, pressure, volume, and flow are referred to in this context as **control variables**. Time is a variable that is implicit in the equation of motion. As shown in the following examples, in some cases time is viewed as a control variable. This concept allows us to understand any mode, no matter how complex, by simply observing how control switches from one variable to the next.

Having said what is controlled, we can explore how it is controlled. In discussing respiratory mechanics, we have used the term *system* without definition. Formally, a *system* is defined as a collection of elements that interact according to some particular process or function. A model is a simplified version of a real world system used to help us understand the relationships among system elements (e.g., the equation of motion is a model of the respiratory system). Specifically, we are interested in understanding the relationship between the input and the output of the system (e.g., we need to create a model). This understanding then may help us to control the system behavior.

A system can be controlled in two different ways to achieve the desired output[9]:

1. Select an input and wait for an output with no interference during the waiting period.
2. Select an input, observe the trend in the output, and modify the input accordingly to get as close as possible to the desired output.

For example, when a helmsman steers a boat toward the dock, he may do it in one of the two ways described previously:

1. Point the boat in the direction of the dock and retire to his cabin.

2. Continuously steer the boat toward the dock, by observing the direction of the dock, observing the direction the boat is moving, and making adjustments as necessary.

In this example, the system is the boat (motor, propeller, steering mechanism, etc.), the input is the position of the boat's steering wheel, and the output is the direction of the boat's motion. In both cases a change in the input causes a change in the output. However, in the first case, there is no flow of information from the output to generate a new input to "close the loop." Hence, this type of control scheme is called **open-loop control**. In the second case, the helmsman uses information about the output to modify the input, which in turn improves the output. This control scheme is called **closed-loop control** or feedback control. Feedback control is also called servo control. Figure 1–4 illustrates block diagrams (i.e., models) of open- and closed-loop control systems.

To perform closed-loop control, the output must be measured and compared with a reference value. In the aforementioned ex-

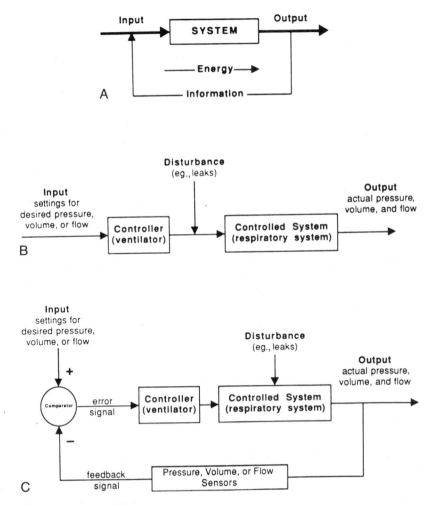

FIGURE 1–4

A, A simple block diagram of an unspecified system having one input and one output. Energy flows from input to output, and information flows from output to input. *B*, Block diagram for a ventilator using open-loop control. For example, the Newport Breeze ventilator controls airway pressure using open-loop control. *C*, Block diagram for a ventilator using closed-loop control. This is also called feedback or servo control. For example, the Infant Star ventilator uses closed-loop control of airway pressure.

ample, a human performed the measuring and comparing functions. But in ventilators, pressure and flow transducers and electronic circuitry are necessary to perform automatic closed-loop control. Closed-loop control provides the advantage of a more consistent output in the presence of unanticipated disturbances. In the previous example, disturbances that affect the direction of that the boat might include wind and water currents. In the case of ventilators, disturbances that might affect the delivery of pressure, volume, and flow include pooled condensation or leaks in the patient circuit, endotracheal tube obstructions, and changes in respiratory system resistance and compliance.

Ventilators use closed-loop control to maintain consistent inspiratory pressure, volume, or flow waveforms in the presence of changing loads. The load presented by the respiratory system changes frequently as a result of lung pathology. Ventilator design has evolved from simple open-loop control of pressure to closed-loop control of pressure, volume, and flow within a breath, to the current double–closed-loop or **dual control**. This scheme was developed to obtain the advantages of both pressure-controlled and volume-controlled ventilation while avoiding each of their disadvantages. Dual control provides the advantage of pressure control (i.e., limiting peak inspiratory pressure, at least within a given range, to avoid overdistending the lungs) while maintaining the advantage of volume control (i.e., delivering a constant minute ventilation even if lung mechanics change).

There are currently two basic approaches to dual control. The first method is to adjust the pressure waveform between breaths. This scheme was introduced by Siemens with the VOLUME SUPPORT mode on the Siemens Servo 300 (Siemens, Danvers, MA). Inspiration is pressure controlled within a breath, but the pressure limit is automatically adjusted up or down to achieve a preset target tidal volume (Fig. 1–5, *top*). The initial pressure limit (i.e., change in airway pressure above PEEP) is set automatically based on the calculated value for respiratory system compliance (also automatically derived from a test breath):

$$\text{initial pressure limit} = \text{set tidal volume/compliance.}$$

If the actual tidal volume based on the initial pressure limit is different from the set tidal volume, the pressure limit is adjusted up or down (no more than 3 cm H_2O per breath) to get closer to the set tidal volume. This process is repeated over several breaths until the delivered tidal volume equals the set tidal volume. A similar approach is used in the PRESSURE REGULATED VOLUME CONTROL mode on the Siemens 300, in the AUTOFLOW mode on the Drager Evita 4 (Drager, Telford, PA), and in the ADAPTIVE PRESSURE VENTILATION mode on the Hamilton Galileo (Hamilton, Reno, NV).

The other basic approach is to make adjustments within a breath to achieve the target volume. This is demonstrated in the PRESSURE AUGMENT mode on the Bear 1000 (Bear, Riverside, CA) and the Volume Assured Pressure Support (VAPS) mode on the Bird 8400 Sti or Tbird (Bird, Palm Springs, CA). Here, the ventilator may switch between pressure control and flow control within a breath depending on whether a preset tidal volume has been met (Fig. 1–5, *bottom*). Typical pressure and flow waveforms with this form of dual control are illustrated in Figure 1–6. Another variation of this theme is illustrated by the P_{max} feature on the Drager Evita 4, in which the ventilator begins inspiration in flow control at the set flow limit. When airway pressure reaches the set P_{max} value, the ventilator switches to pressure control at the set pressure limit while tidal volume is monitored. The ventilator attempts to increase the **inspiratory flow time** (i.e., the period from the beginning of inspiratory flow to the end of inspiratory flow) until the set tidal volume is delivered, provided that the set inspiratory time (i.e., the period from the beginning of inspiratory flow to the beginning of expiratory flow) is long enough. If the set tidal volume is not delivered in the set inspiratory time, an alarm is activated.

Control Variables

A ventilator may be classfied as a pressure, volume, or flow controller. In some cases, it

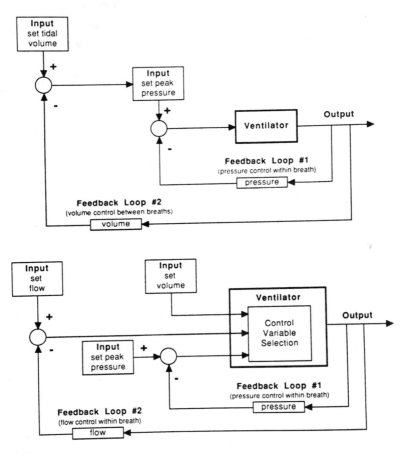

FIGURE 1–5

Double-loop or dual control. *Top,* dual control between breaths. The ventilator controls pressure during inspiration and then looks at the resultant tidal volume. The initial pressure limit is based on the set tidal volume and the value for respiratory system compliance the ventilator has calculated from a test breath (e.g., Volume Support on the Siemens 300). If the volume delivered with the initial pressure limit is different from the preset target value, the pressure waveform is changed for the next breath (either higher pressure limit or longer inspiratory flow time). *Bottom,* dual control within a breath. The ventilator starts inspiration in the pressure-controlled mode. If the set target volume has not been delivered by the time inspiratory flow has decayed to the preset inspiratory flow, the ventilator switches to flow control.

is logical to classify a ventilator as a time controller (i.e., it controls only inspiratory and expiratory times).

Ventilators can combine control schemes to create complex modes. For example, the NPB 7200a ventilator (NPB, Carlsbad, CA) can mix flow-controlled breaths with pressure-controlled breaths in the SIMV + PRESSURE SUPPORT mode. The Bear 1000 can mix pressure control with flow control within a single breath in its PRESSURE AUGMENT mode. The Siemens

Servo 300 can adjust the level of pressure control automatically to achieve a preset target volume. The Hamilton Galileo can automatically adjust the number of mandatory breaths and the pressure limit on both mandatory and spontaneous breaths along with manipulating inspiratory and expiratory times based on the measurement of expiratory time constants. The great flexibility of current ventilators is achieved at the expense of added complexity. Thus, when evaluating ventilator performance,

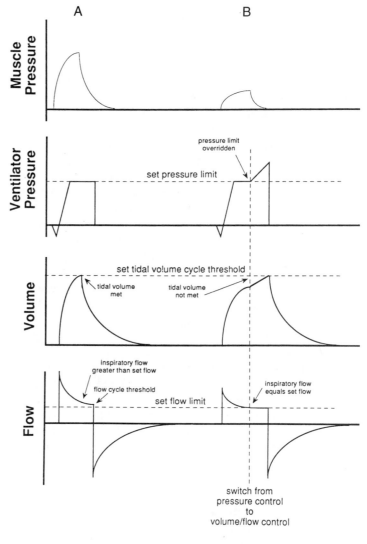

FIGURE 1–6
Pressure and flow waveforms showing the effects of dual control within breaths. *A,* Pressure controlled breath with large patient effort (muscle pressure). The set tidal volume has been reached before flow has decayed to the set flow limit so the breath continues in pressure control until the flow cycle threshold value is reached. This value may be an arbitrary percentage of the peak value for the pressure controlled portion of the breath (e.g., Pressure Augment in the Bear 1000) or the set flow rate (e.g., VAPS in the Bird 8400ST). The breath is essentially a pressure support breath. *B,* Switch from pressure control to flow control because flow decayed to the set flow before the set tidal volume was reached. This was due to a smaller patient inspiratory effort. Inspiration continues at the set flow and pressure rises as expected for a volume/flow-controlled breath.

simple and unambiguous criteria must be used for deciding which control variables are operational.

Pressure

The equation of motion tells us that if the ventilator is an ideal pressure controller, then the left side of the equation (i.e., ventilator pressure as a function of time) is determined by the ventilator settings and is unaffected by changes in parameter values on the right side (i.e., compliance and resistance).

If the control variable is pressure, then the ventilator can control either the airway pressure (causing it to rise above body surface pressure for inspiration) or the pressure on the body surface (causing it to fall below airway opening pressure for inspiration). This is the basis for classifying ventilators as being either positive or negative pressure types. For example, the Newport Wave ventilator (Newport, Newport Beach, CA) would be classified as a positive-pressure controller that generates a rectangular pressure waveform, and the Emerson Iron Lung (Emerson, Cambridge, MA) is a negative-pressure controller that produces a quasisinusoidal pressure waveform.

Volume

If the pressure waveform varies as the load imposed by the patient's respiratory system changes, we then examine the volume waveform. However, the observation that the volume waveform remains unchanged is a necessary but insufficient condition to warrant the classification of volume controller because the same holds true for a flow controller. The reason is that once the volume waveform is specified, the flow waveform is determined because they are inverse functions of each other (i.e., volume is the integral of flow and flow is the derivative of volume). Therefore, if changes in compliance and resistance do not change the volume waveform, they will not affect the flow waveform, and vice versa.

To qualify as a volume controller, a ventilator must (1) maintain a consistent volume waveform in the presence of a varying load and (2) measure volume and use the signal to control the volume waveform. Volume can be measured directly only by the displacement of a piston or bellows or similar device. With a piston or bellows, controlling the excursion of the device automatically controls the volume waveform. Alternatively, a volume signal could be derived by integrating a flow signal. Note that although some ventilators such as the Siemens Servo 900C, the NPB 7200, the Bear 5, and the Hamilton Veolar display volume readings, they all actually measure and control flow and calculate volume for displays. Thus, they all are flow controllers unless they are operated in a pressure-controlled mode (e.g., during pressure support ventilation). An examination of a ventilator's schematic diagrams and an operator's manual should provide the information necessary to decide whether volume or flow is being measured. This distinction is important in the engineering evaluation of a ventilator and in understanding ventilator performance. However, at the bedside, the difference between flow and volume control is not necessarily important. Although not correct in the engineering sense, referring to a flow-controlled breath as a volume-controlled breath is considered clinically acceptable.

Flow

If the volume change (i.e., tidal volume) remains consistent when compliance and resistance are varied and if volume change

is not measured and used for control, the ventilator is classified as a flow controller. The simplest example of open-loop flow control in a ventilator consists of a pressure regulator supplying gas to a flowmeter, such as found in infant ventilators. An infant ventilator becomes a flow controller rather than a pressure controller if the airway pressure does not reach the set pressure limit.[10] (However, the flowmeter is usually not back-pressure compensated and will vary its output slightly in the presence of a changing load.) In contrast, the Siemens Servo 900C (so-called because it uses servo control) measures flow and adjusts the output control valve (i.e., the inspiratory scissors valve) accordingly. It can maintain a more consistent inspiratory flow waveform as the load changes.

Time

Suppose that both pressure and volume are affected substantially by changes in lung mechanics. Then the only form of control is that of defining the ventilatory cycle, or alternating between inspiration and expiration. Therefore, the only variables being controlled are the **inspiratory** and **expiratory** times. This situation arises in some forms of high-frequency ventilation, when even the designation of an inspiratory and expiratory phase becomes somewhat obscure.

Phase Variables

Once the control variables and the associated waveforms are identified, more detail can be obtained by examining the events that take place during a ventilatory cycle, that is, the period of time between the beginning of one breath and the beginning of the next. Mushin and colleagues[1] proposed that this time span be divided into four **phases:** (1) the change from expiration to inspiration, (2) inspiration, (3) the change from inspiration to expiration, and (4) expiration. This convention is useful for examining how a ventilator starts, sustains, and stops an inspiration and what it does between inspirations. In each phase, a particular variable is measured and used to start, sustain, and end the phase. In this context, pressure, volume, flow, and time are referred to as **phase variables**.[11] The criteria for determining phase variables are defined in Figure 1–7.

Trigger

All ventilators measure one or more of the variables associated with the equation of motion (i.e., pressure, volume, flow, or time). Inspiration is started when one of these variables reaches a preset value. Thus, the variable of interest is considered an initiating or **trigger** variable. The most common trigger variables are time (the ventilator initiates a breath according to a set frequency, independent of the patient's spontaneous efforts), pressure (the ventilator senses the patient's inspiratory effort in the form of a decrease in baseline pressure and starts inspiration independent of the set frequency), and flow (the ventilator senses the patient's inspiratory effort as a decrease in the baseline flow through the patient circuit or senses inspiratory flow directly with a sensor at the patient's airway opening). Any variable that can be measured can potentially be used to trigger inspiration. For example, the Star Sync module allows triggering of the Infant Star (Infrasonics, San Diego, CA) ventilator by chest wall movement, the Sechrist SAVI system senses inspiration as a change in chest impedance. Of course, it is relatively simple to manually trigger inspiration.

Triggering based on a change in flow has been shown to reduce the work the patient must perform to trigger inspiration.[12] This is because work is proportional to the volume the patient inspires times the change in baseline pressure necessary to trigger. Pressure triggering requires some pressure change and hence an irreducible amount of work to trigger. But with flow or volume triggering, baseline pressure need not change, and theoretically, the patient need

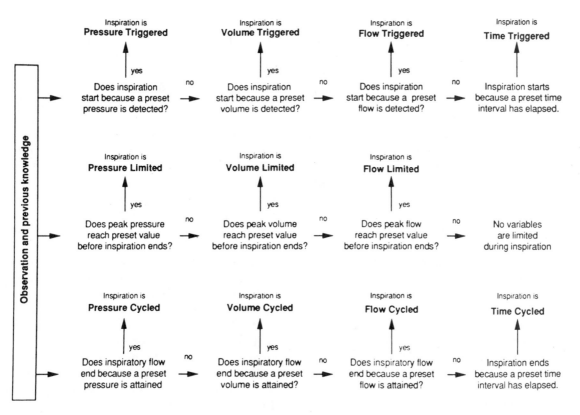

FIGURE 1–7

Criteria for determining the phase variables during a ventilator-assisted breath.

do no work on the ventilator to trigger. At least one ventilator, the Drager Babylog, may be volume triggered. The possible advantage of volume triggering over flow triggering is that when flow signal is integrated to get volume, much of the noise in the signal (e.g., from condensate in the patient circuit) is removed and the chance of false triggering is reduced. A possible disadvantage of this is the increased delay from signal processing and the phase lag between flow and volume signals.

The patient effort required to trigger inspiration is determined by the ventilator's sensitivity. Sensitivity generally is defined as the ratio of output signal amplitude to input signal amplitude. In the case of a ventilator, the output is the triggering of inspiration and the input is the change in the trigger signal required to trigger. The smaller the change in trigger signal (e.g., pressure change below baseline) required to trigger, the larger the mathematical ratio and the greater the sensitivity. Many ventilators indicate sensitivity adjustments qualitatively ("min" or "max"). Alternatively, a ventilator may specify a trigger threshold quantitatively (e.g., so many cm H_2O below baseline). For example, to make a pressure-triggered ventilator more sensitive, the trigger threshold might be adjusted from 5 to 1 cm H_2O below the baseline pressure. Sometimes the ventilator has a readout called "sensitivity" with units of pressure or flow. This confuses the issue because the readout is only half of the sensitivity ratio and a higher number in the readout is really a lower sensitivity. In such a case, the label should be "trigger threshold."

Triggering the ventilator has been studied intensively. Because the ability of the ventilator to sense patient effort and respond quickly and with sufficient flow to meet patient demands is so crucial to patient/ventilator synchrony, a technical review is in order. Time and manual triggering of the ventilator do not depend on patient effort and as such, are not described in the same detail.

MANUAL TRIGGERING

A breath can be triggered by activating the manual breath control on the ventilator. This is usually accomplished by means of a push button or membrane keypad. Manual triggering generally takes one of two forms. The first uses electronic control of the breath, and when the function is activated, a breath at the set tidal volume or pressure is delivered at the set inspiratory flow or time. The second type is often a mechanical control, and when the function is activated, inspiration continues until the operator disengages from the control. The flow is typically controlled using this method, and the high-pressure relief valve remains activated. In some instances, a maximum inspiratory time of 3 seconds automatically ends the manual breath even if the operator fails to disengage the function.

TIME TRIGGERING

A breath is time triggered when the set respiratory rate on the ventilator requires that a breath be delivered.

PRESSURE TRIGGERING

Pressure triggering is the oldest and simplest technique for detecting patient effort. The sensitivity or trigger threshold is set in centimeters of H_2O relative to the baseline pressure. As an example, if baseline pressure is 5 cm H_2O and the trigger threshold is 2 cm H_2O, then when patient effort causes pressure in the circuit to fall to 3 cm H_2O, the breath is triggered. If the baseline pressure is changed—for instance, to 10 cm H_2O—and trigger threshold remains the same (2 cm H_2O), the ventilator is triggered when circuit pressure decreases to less than 8 cm H_2O. The ability to maintain the trigger threshold constant regardless of alterations in baseline pressure is frequently referred to as PEEP (positive end-expiratory pressure) compensation." Modern intensive care unit (ICU) ventilators all have this ability, but in many simpler devices such as transport ventilators, PEEP compensation may not be available. In this instance, the trigger threshold is referenced to atmosphere. If baseline pressure is 5 cm H_2O and trigger threshold is 2 cm H_2O, then triggering will not occur until circuit pressure is -2 cm H_2O (2 cm H_2O below atmo-

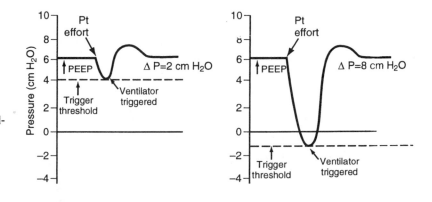

PEEP= 6 cm H_2O
SENSITIVITY = 2 cm H_2O

FIGURE 1-8
Schematic demonstrating pressure triggering. On the left, pressure triggering is compensated by positive end-expiratory pressure (PEEP). On the right, pressure triggering is not PEEP compensated.

spheric pressure). This requires that the patient create a pressure change in the circuit of 7 cm H_2O (5 cm H_2O baseline pressure +2 cm H_2O trigger threshold) to trigger inspiration. Figure 1–8 illustrates these pressure relationships.

Pressure triggering performance of a ventilator also can be influenced by accuracy and speed of the pressure transducer.[12–14] Factors leading to delay include errors due to the speed of the pressure signal propagation through sensor tubing, errors due to the polling interval of the pressure transducer, errors in the pressure transducer, errors due to differences in set and actual PEEP, errors due to circuit noise, and position of the pressure transducer in the venti-

lator circuit. This initial delay is typically less that 150 msec and represents only a small amount of the work of breathing imposed during triggering.

Position of the pressure transducer in the circuit may also effect triggering (Fig. 1–9). Ventilators sense pressure in the inspiratory portion of the ventilator, at the proximal airway, and in the expiratory side of the ventilator. Transducers in the inspiratory limb are adversely effected by the presence of any source of resistance between the patient and the transducer. This includes the ventilator circuit, filters, and humidifiers. Expiratory limb placement avoids the humidifier but still must contend with filters and circuit resistance. Proximal pres-

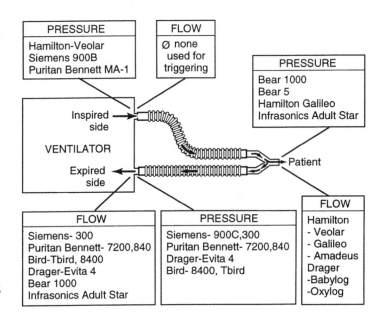

FIGURE 1-9
Position of flow (V̇) and pressure (P) sensors used for triggering in current ventilators.

sure monitoring at the Y-piece of the ventilator eliminates most circuit issues except the use of filters and passive humidifiers connected to the endotracheal tube. The endotracheal tube is typically the greatest source of resistance in the patient ventilator system, and several authors have suggested placement of the pressure transducer at the distal tip of the tube.[15, 16] This eliminates the additional work needed to overcome endotracheal tube resistance. Unfortunately, this also places the transducer in a humid, contaminated environment in which secretions may create new problems. As of June 1999, use of pressure triggering at the distal tip of the endotracheal tube has not been commercialized.

FLOW TRIGGERING

Flow triggering was introduced by Engstrom in the early 1980s but did not become popular until it was reintroduced by Puritan-Bennett in 1988. Since then, flow triggering has become standard on current ventilators. Like so much of ventilator technology, the methods of flow triggering vary from manufacturer to manufacturer. Flow-triggering systems vary in placement of the flow transducer, presence or absence of a continuous (bias) flow, and the ability to adjust bias flow and flow sensitivity.[17, 18]

Generically, flow triggering occurs when a flow transducer in the patient/ventilator system detects a change in flow (i.e., flow moves into the airway opening). This is similar to the pressure-triggering concept. The implementation of flow triggering however, has taken on several versions. Flow triggering is implemented using one of three methods. The first simply measures a change in flow caused by the patient's inspiratory effort. There is no continuous flow in the circuit, and at end-expiration flow is zero. The second provides a preset, nonadjustable level of continuous flow in the circuit, from which a change in flow (the flow sensitivity) is detected. The third allows the clinician to set the continuous flow and the flow sensitivity. In this case, a change in flow through the circuit caused by the patient's inspiratory effort reduces the flow below the flow trigger threshold setting and

a breath is triggered. In the presence of a leak, this system can be tailored to overcome the leak while maintaining appropriate triggering.

As an example, the Puritan-Bennett 7200ae uses a flow-triggering system known as FlowBy. The clinician selects a level of continuous flow, called the "base flow," between 5 and 20 L/min. This flow traverses the inspiratory and expiratory flow transducers, and the two values are compared every 20 msec. The clinician then sets the flow sensitivity between 1 and 10 L/min. With the 7200ae, the flow sensitivity cannot exceed one-half the continuous flow. Using this system at a continuous flow of 5 L/min and flow sensitivity of 2 L/min, when the patient's inspiratory effort causes flow traversing the expiratory flow transducer to fall to 3 L/min, a breath is triggered. Continuing to use the 7200ae as an example, once a spontaneous breath is triggered, flow up to 180 L/min is available. The limit and cycle variables with flow triggering are different from pressure triggering for a spontaneous breath. Once the flow-triggered breath is initiated, the ventilator attempts to maintain airway pressure at 1.0 cm H_2O above the end-expiratory pressure, and the breath is cycled when flow through the expiratory flow transducer is 2 L/min greater than the set continuous flow. As mentioned in the section on pressure triggering, this demonstrates that the operation of the 7200ae is quite different for pressure- and flow-triggered spontaneous breaths.

Another example of differences between a ventilator's pressure-triggering and flow-triggering system can be seen in the Hamilton Veolar ventilator. With this system, the limit and cycle variables for the two triggering methods are identical. However, during pressure triggering, the site of pressure measurement is inside the inspiratory side of the ventilator. As such, any resistance in the ventilator circuit (heated humidifiers, artificial noses, and so on) represents an imposed workload to triggering. In the flow-triggering mode, the ventilator is triggered from a variable orifice flow transducer placed at the Y-piece of the ventilator circuit. In this instance, the reduction in the work of breathing with flow triggering re sults from improved sensor placement.[19] The Veolar allows the clinician to set the flow sensitivity (2–10 L/min) and the continuous flow is automatically twice that value, with a minimum continuous flow of 4 L/min.

The Siemens 300 ventilator uses a combination of flow and pressure triggering, with flow triggering selected by decreasing the pressure sensitivity control into an uncalibrated range on the dial. The Siemens 300 uses set continuous flows of 2 L/min, 1 L/min, and 0.5 L/min during flow triggering during adult, pediatric, and neonatal operation, respectively. Because the sensitivity dial is uncalibrated, the actual flow sensitivity setting is unknown. The site of pressure and flow measurement are located on the expiratory side of the ventilator, and the limit and cycle variables are identical.

The Bird ventilators (8400 Sti and Tbird) use a nonadjustable continuous flow of 10 L/min and allow flow sensitivity to be set from 1 to 9 L/min. Flow is measured by the expiratory flow transducer, and when the flow sensitivity threshold is exceeded, a breath is triggered. The breath then is pressure-limited and flow-cycled (when flow through the expiratory flow transducer is >10 L/min). A comparison of flow-triggering systems is shown in Table 1–2. Schematic ex-

amples of the types of flow triggering are shown in Figure 1–10.

In some instances, manufacturers have provided a combination of continuous flow and pressure triggering. Conceptually, the continuous flow meets the patient's initial demand for flow, and when circuit pressure is reduced, the breath is triggered. This system has not been shown to have advantages compared with traditional flow or pressure triggering. Only the Newport ventilators continue to use this technique.

Potential problems with flow triggering include auto-triggering resulting from system leaks or the presence of condensate in the ventilator circuit. Devices that measure flow at the airway opening reduce problems associated with circuit condensate. Flow-triggering systems with an adjustable continuous flow can be used to compensate for leaks. In systems with a constant continuous flow, particularly at low levels, leaks may preclude the system from triggering appropriately.

VOLUME TRIGGERING

Volume triggering has been used infrequently in adults. However, the Drager Babylog ventilator uses a hot wire anemome-

TABLE 1–2. Comparison of Pressure- and Flow-Triggering Systems for Certain Ventilators

VENTILATOR	TRIGGER	SENSITIVITY	CONTINUOUS FLOW	LIMIT	CYCLE	SENSOR LOCATION
PB 7200ae	Pressure	0.5–20 cm H$_2$O	NA	PEEP-sensitivity	1 cm H$_2$O above PEEP	Expiratory side
	Flow	1–10 L/min	5–20 L/min	PEEP + 1 cm H$_2$O	Expiratory flow 2 L/min > inspiratory flow	Expiratory side
Hamilton Veolar	Pressure	0.5–10 cm H$_2$O	NA	PEEP + 1.5 cm H$_2$O	37% of initial peak flow	Inspiratory side
	Flow	3–15 L/min	6–30 L/min (twice the sensitivity)	PEEP + 1.5 cm H$_2$O	37% of initial peak flow	Proximal airway
Siemens 300	Pressure	0–17 cm H$_2$O	Adults—2 L/min Children—1 L/min Neonates 0.5 L/min	PEEP + 3 cm H$_2$O	5% of initial peak flow	Expiratory side
	Flow	Uncalibrated	Adults—2 L/min Children—1 L/min Neonates—0.5 L/min	PEEP + 3 cm H$_2$O	5% of initial peak flow	Expiratory side
Bird 8400 STi	Pressure	1–20 cm H$_2$O	NA	PEEP	PEEP + 1.0 cm H$_2$O	Expiratory side
	Flow	1–9 L/min	10 L/min	PEEP	Flow returns to 10 L/min	Expiratory side

PEEP, positive end-expiratory pressure.

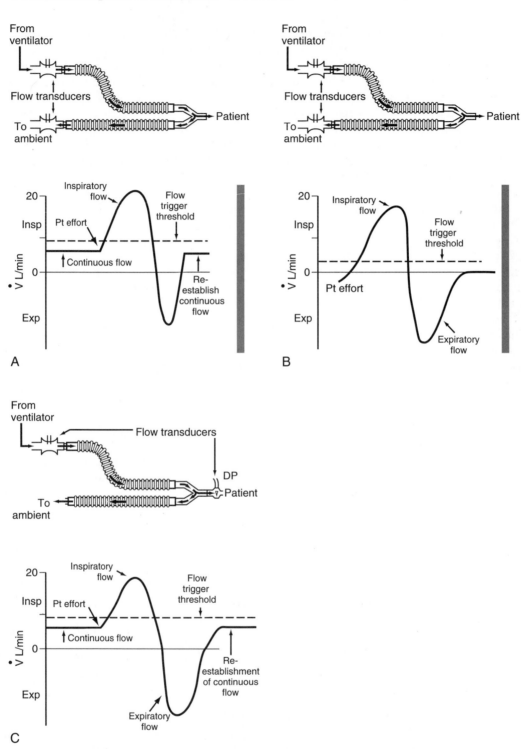

FIGURE 1–10

Schematic of three flow triggering systems *A,* Flow triggering using inspiratory and
expiratory flow sensors (e.g., 7200ae). *B,* Flow triggering using the expiratory sensor and
no continuous flow (e.g., Bird Tbird). *C,* Flow triggering using a flow sensor at the
proximal airway and an adjustable continuous flow (e.g., Hamilton Galileo).

ter at the proximal airway to volume-trigger breaths. This device is also capable of calculating leaks around the uncuffed endotracheal tube. The use of volume as a trigger signal has not been studied. Conceptually, by integrating measured flow to calculate volume, signal noise is reduced. Evaluations of this technique need to be accomplished.

IMPEDANCE TRIGGERING

Because of the difficulties associated with measuring respiratory efforts in neonates and the small endotracheal tubes required, several investigators have searched for alternate trigger signals to initiate patient effort. The first of these introduced is chest wall impedance triggering. This technique was introduced by Sechrist and is known as the SAVI system (Sechrist Industries, Anaheim, CA).[20] Standard electrocardiogram (ECG) electrodes are used, and as the chest wall expands, the change in impedance initiates inspiration. Using this technique, once inspiratory effort is detected, the control of the ventilator limit and the cycling variable returns to airway pressure.

MOTION TRIGGERING

The Infrasonics Infant Star ventilator (Nellcor Puritan-Bennett, Carlsbad, CA) has introduced a motion sensor for triggering the neonatal ventilator. This device (Star Sync) uses an abdominal sensor to detect inspiration. The sensor is a small, air-filled flexible capsule. This device is taped to the infant's abdomen (Fig. 1–11) midway between the umbilicus and the xiphisternum. As the abdomen rises, the capsule is compressed, generating a small pressure signal that is transmitted to the device which generates an electrical signal that triggers the ventilator. Pressure in the sensor is sampled eight times every 5 msec and the response time from the onset of patient effort to breath delivery is 47 msec. From a technical standpoint, this is pressure-triggered ventilation. This may require improved definitions of triggering. Pressure triggering might be considered airway pressure triggered (citing the pressure measurement site) or abdominal pressure triggered. We prefer to refer

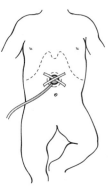

FIGURE 1–11
Placement of the abdominal sensor for motion triggering (Infrasonics Star-Sync).

to this method as motion triggered because although pressure is the measured signal, abdominal motion is the cause of the pressure change.

Limit

During the inspiratory phase, pressure, volume, and flow increase above their end-expiratory values. The **inspiratory phase** is quantitated by specifying the inspiratory time, defined as the time interval from the start of inspiratory flow to the start of expiratory flow. Note that any inspiratory hold (or pause) time is included in the inspiratory time. It is sometimes helpful to distinguish **inspiratory flow time** as the interval from the start of inspiratory flow to the end of inspiratory flow and the **inspiratory pause time** as the interval from the end of inspiratory flow to the start of expiratory flow. This distinction is useful because there is no standardized way to set these intervals on ventilators and the terminology that manufacturers use may be confusing. For example, on one ventilator, inspiratoy flow time may be set indirectly by setting tidal volume and flow, whereas pause time may be set directly (in seconds), thus indirectly increasing inspiratory time. On another ventilator, inspiratory time may be set directly with no provision for directly setting inspiratory pause time. On yet another ventilator, inspiratory time may be set using the rate and "% cycle time" controls and then changing inspiratory flow time by changing a "% inspiration" control. Finally, inspiratory flow time must be distinguished from inspiratory time to understand the way that P_{max} works on the Evita 4 ventilator (see previous description of dual control between breaths).

Cycle time (or total cycle time) is another name for ventilatory period, the reciprocal of ventilatory frequency (i.e., 60 seconds per minute/number of breaths per minute). The **percent cycle time** is the ratio of inspiratory time to total cycle time expressed as a percentage. The percent inspiratory time is the inspiratory flow time expressed as a percentage of total cycle time. The **percent pause time** is the pause time expressed as a percentage of total cycle time. An inspiratory pause is important in estimating lung pressures and calculating respiratory system mechanics.

If one (or more) of the inspiratory variables rises no higher than some preset value, we refer to the variable as a limit variable. But we must distinguish the limit variable from the variable that is used to end inspiration (called a cycle variable). Therefore, we impose the additional criterion that inspiration is not terminated because a variable has met its preset limit value. In other words, a variable is "limited" if it increases to a preset value before inspiration ends. These criteria are illustrated in Figure 1–12.

Clinicians commonly misuse the terms limit and cycle by using them interchangeably. This is encouraged by some ventilator manufacturers who use the term limit to describe what happens when a pressure alarm threshold is met (i.e., inspiration is terminated and an alarm is activated). The term **cycle** is more appropriate in this situation.

Another potentially confusing issue is that, by convention, peak inspiratory pressure (PIP) and baseline pressure are measured relative to atmospheric pressure, whereas the pressure limit sometimes is measured relative to baseline pressure (e.g., Siemens Servo 900C) and sometimes relative to atmospheric pressure (e.g., Bird V.I.P.). On the Bird V.I.P., the high pressure limit control sets the PIP limit (above ambient pressure) during pressure-controlled ventilation but cycles the breath off and activates a high-pressure alarm during volume-controlled ventilation. Hence the term *pressure limit*, in common usage, can indicate several different clinically significant situations depending on both the mode of ventilation and the manufacturer! Thus, the lack of standardization among ventilator manufacturers makes it especially important that clinicians use terminology properly.

Cycle

Inspiration always ends (i.e., is cycled off) because some variable has reached a preset value. The variable that is measured and used to terminate inspiratory time and begin expiratory time is called the *cycle variable*. Deciding which variable is used to cycle off inspiration for a given ventilator can be confusing. For a variable to be used as a feedback signal (in this case, a cycling signal), it first must be measured. Most current-generation adult ventilators allow the

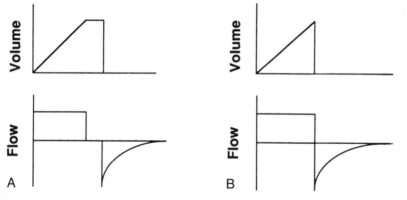

FIGURE 1–12
The importance of distinguishing between the terms limit and cycle is shown. In *A*, both volume and flow are limited (because they reach preset values before end inspiration), and inspiration is time cycled (after the preset inspiratory pause time). In *B*, flow is limited, but volume is not and inspiration is volume cycled.

operator to set a tidal volume and inspiratory flow, which would lead one to believe that the ventilator could be volume cycled. However, closer inspection reveals that these ventilators do not measure volume (which is consistent with the fact that all current-generation ventilators are flow controllers). Rather, they set the inspiratory time necessary to achieve the set tidal volume with the set inspiratory flow rate, making them time cycled. The tidal volume dial can be thought of as an inspiratory time dial calibrated in units of volume rather than time.

As mentioned earlier, the term *limit* often is substituted incorrectly for cycle in common usage. But the distinction also is ignored by ventilator designers. An example of the difficulty created by improper terminology is illustrated by the Bear Cub 750vs. This ventilator is designed to be used primarily as a pressure controller for infants. The operator typically sets both inspiratory time and inspiratory pressure limit (the knob is labeled "Inspiratory Pressure" and the ventilator is designed to maintain the pressure until the cycle mechanism is activated). Inspiration is normally time cycled. However, there is a control knob that is labeled "Volume Limit," so it would seem that inspiration could be both pressure and volume limited at the same time. However, this is not true. First, the equation of motion shows that you cannot control both volume and pressure to some preset value at the same time. This is not an example of dual control (which does not control two things at the same time but rather switches back and forth). If you try to set a pressure limit, the delivered volume will depend on lung mechanics, and if you try to set a volume limit, the pressure will vary with lung mechanics. Second, the operator's manual says that "When the set threshold is reached, the ventilator will cycle into expiration." Thus, the ventilator does one thing when the pressure limit is met (namely, stay at that level until inspiration ends) and it does another thing when the volume "limit" is met (terminate inspiration). The "Volume Limit" is really a "Volume Cycle Threshold." Calling both functions by the same name is confusing and may obscure one's understanding of the ventilator's unique ability to volume cycle in a pressure-controlled mode.

Some investigators think that a ventilator can have "mixed" cycling, which is contrary to the idea presented here that a ventilator can control only one variable at a time. The most common example given by these authors is a ventilator drive mechanism composed of a piston connected to a rod and a rotating crank. It is argued that one cannot distinguish time (i.e., inspiratory time set by the frequency at which the crank rotates) or volume (i.e., the stroke volume of the piston) as the cycling variable. However, if the inspiratory time is set low enough and the volume and patient load are high enough, a point can be reached when a piston-driven ventilator "sacrifices" (i.e., extends) the set inspiratory time as the motor struggles against the load to deliver the volume. This unmasks its true volume-cycled nature.

Baseline

The variable that is controlled during the expiratory time is the baseline variable. Expiratory time is defined as the time interval from the start of expiratory flow to the start of inspiratory flow. As with inspiratory time, it is helpful to distinguish the components of expiratory time: **expiratory flow time**, defined as the interval from the start of expiratory flow to the end of expiratory flow, and **expiratory pause time**, defined as the interval from the end of expiratory flow to the start of inspiratory flow. Expiratory pause time often is initiated to measure autoPEEP.

Note that in the equation of motion, pressure, volume, and flow are measured relative to end-expiratory or baseline values and are thus initially all zero. Although the baseline value of any of these variables theoretically could be controlled, pressure control is the most practical and is implemented by all commonly used ventilators.

Conditional Variables

Figure 1–13 illustrates that, for each breath, the ventilator creates a specific pat-

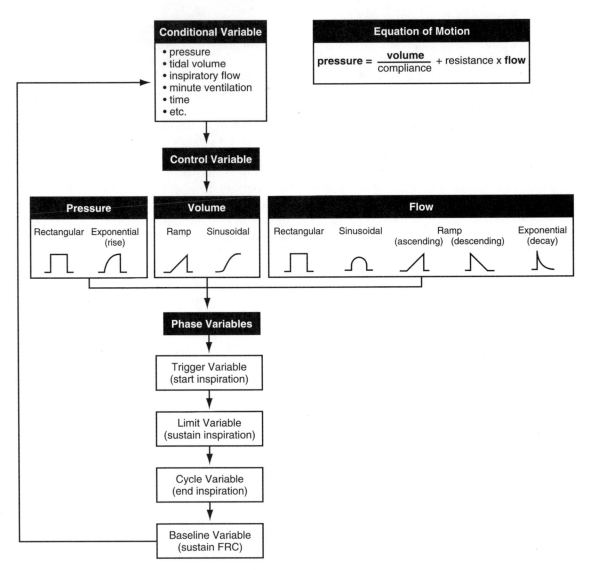

FIGURE 1–13

A ventilator classification scheme based on a mathematical model known as the "equation of motion" for the respiratory system is shown. This model indicates that during inspiration, the ventilator is able to control directly one and only one variable at time (i.e., pressure, volume, or flow). Some common waveforms provided by current ventilators are shown for each control variable. Pressure, volume, flow, and time are also used as phase variables that determine the parameters of each ventilatory cycle (e.g., trigger sensitivity, peak inspiratory flow rate or pressure, inspiratory time, and baseline pressure). FRC, functional residual capacity.

tern of control and phase variables. The ventilator either may keep this pattern constant for each breath or it may introduce other patterns (e.g., one for mandatory and one for spontaneous breaths). In essence, the ventilator must decide which pattern of control and which phase variables to implement before each breath, depending on the

value of some preset conditional variables. Conditional variables can be thought of as initiating conditional logic in the form of "if–then" statements. That is, if the value of a conditional variable reaches some preset threshold, some action occurs to change the ventilatory pattern.

A simple example would be the NPB MA-

1 in the control mode. Each breath is time triggered, flow limited, and volume cycled. The trigger, limit, and cycle variables have preset values (e.g., trigger at frequency = 20 cycles/min, limit inspiratory flow at 60 L/min, and cycle at tidal volume = 750 ml). However, every few minutes a sigh breath is introduced that has a different set of **phase variable values** (e.g., trigger at frequency = 2 sighs every 15 minutes; cycle at tidal volume = 1500 ml). How did the ventilator know to do this? Conceptually, we can say that before each breath pattern is selected, the ventilator examines the value of some conditional variable to see whether it has reached a preset threshold value. If the threshold value has been met, then one pattern is selected; if not, another pattern is selected. In the case of the NPB MA-1, the conditional variable was time: if a preset time interval has elapsed (i.e., the sigh interval), then the ventilator switches to the sigh pattern. Other examples include switching from patient-triggered to machine-triggered breaths in the SIMV and mandatory minute ventilation (MMV) modes.

So far in this discussion, we have used the terms mandatory and spontaneous without explanation. Clinicians have an intuitive understanding of the meanings of these terms. But because they play a central role in defining and understanding modes of ventilation, formal definitions must be provided. **Spontaneous breaths** are those that are both initiated and terminated by the patient. That is, the patient triggers the breath and participates in cycling of the breath. If the ventilator determines either the start or end of inspiration, then the breath is considered to be **mandatory**. A breath that is time triggered always is considered a mandatory breath. A breath that is patient triggered, but time or volume-cycled (i.e., the patient does not play a role in the cycle criteria) is also a mandatory breath.

The naming of breath types is crucial to understanding ventilator modes but is also an area of confusion as well as disagreement. The current classification system requires that breaths simply be distinguished only as *mandatory* or *spontaneous*. A consensus conference of experts (which did not exactly achieve consensus) thought that four breath types were necessary to describe the types of breaths. The consensus group added the terms *assisted* breath and *supported* breath. An *assisted breath* is a *mandatory breath* that is patient triggered. A *supported breath* is a *spontaneous breath* that has an inspiratory pressure greater than baseline pressure. We prefer to think of assisted breath as a type of mandatory breath and supported as a type of spontaneous breath. Table 1–3 describes the differences between these breaths. Although the two new breath types are certainly different in clinical application and clinical effect, from an engineering perspective they are

TABLE 1–3. Comparison of Breath Types

TYPE OF BREATH	TRIGGER	LIMIT	CYCLE
Mandatory	Ventilator (time)	Ventilator (pressure or flow)	Ventilator (time, flow, volume)
Assisted	Patient (pressure, flow, volume, impedance, motion)	Ventilator (pressure or flow)	Ventilator (time, flow, volume)
Spontaneous	Patient (pressure, flow, volume, impedance, motion)	Ventilator (pressure or flow) Inspiratory pressure = Baseline pressure	Patient
Supported	Patient (pressure, flow, volume, impedance, motion)	Ventilator (pressure or flow) Inspiratory pressure > Baseline pressure	Patient

not different. This is the origin of the lack of consensus. From a clinical perspective, a breath that is time-triggered is significantly different from one that is patient-triggered. Issues related to measurement of pressures, flow demand, and work of breathing are all different in the triggered breath. However, to the ventilator, the breath was just initiated for a different reason. It is problematic when we attempt to incorporate the patient into the equation. Ventilator classification is a study of the ventilator, not the patient.

Figure 1–14 illustrates these definitions with an algorithm. Note that if the ventilator either time or volume cycles an inspiration, the breath is considered mandatory because it is terminated by the ventilator. If, however, the ventilator flow cycles after being patient triggered, as in the pressure support mode, the breath is considered to be (supported) spontaneous. The rate of decay of inspiratory flow is determined by the patient's lung mechanics and ventilatory muscle activity. Hence, during the PRESSURE SUPPORT mode, pressure-limiting inspiration does not constrain inspiratory flow rate, and flow cycling does not necessarily dictate either the inspiratory time or the tidal volume if the ventilatory muscles are active. In other words, the ventilator attempts to match the patient's inspiratory demand and it is really the patient who

terminates the breath. If the ventilator is pressure cycled (usually an alarm condition) after being patient triggered, the breath is also spontaneous. Again, the patient's lung mechanics or ventilatory muscle activity has caused airway pressure to go above the preset threshold (in the absence of ventilator malfunction).

Modes of Ventilation

There are two general approaches to supporting the patient's inspiration: volume/flow control and pressure control. Figure 1–15 is a simplified influence diagram[21-23] that illustrates the important variables for ventilators that are either volume or flow controllers. Figure 1–16 is the influence diagram for ventilators that are pressure controllers. The equations relating these variables[24] are given in Table 1–4. For pressure-controlled ventilation, with a rectangular pressure wavefrom, peak inspiratory flow is equal to the set pressure difference (inspiratory pressure limit − PEEP) divided by the respiratory system resistance. Many ventilators (especially infant ventilators) provide the user with a control knob labeled "flow" (e.g., Bear Cub, Nellcor Puritan-Bennett Infant Star). The meaning of this flow can be confusing. If flow is set

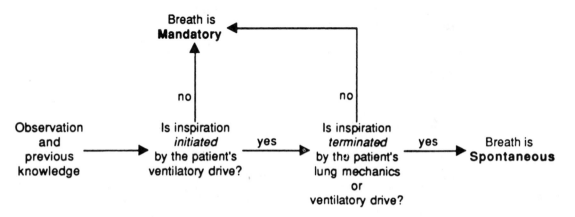

FIGURE 1–14
Algorithm defining spontaneous and mandatory breaths. In terms of current technology, if the breath is triggered according to a preset frequency or minimum minute ventilation or cycled according to a preset frequency or tidal volume, the breath is mandatory. A patient-triggered mandatory breath is an assisted breath. Spontaneous breaths are patient triggered and cycled. A spontaneous breath with an inspiratory pressure greater than expiratory pressure is a supported breath.

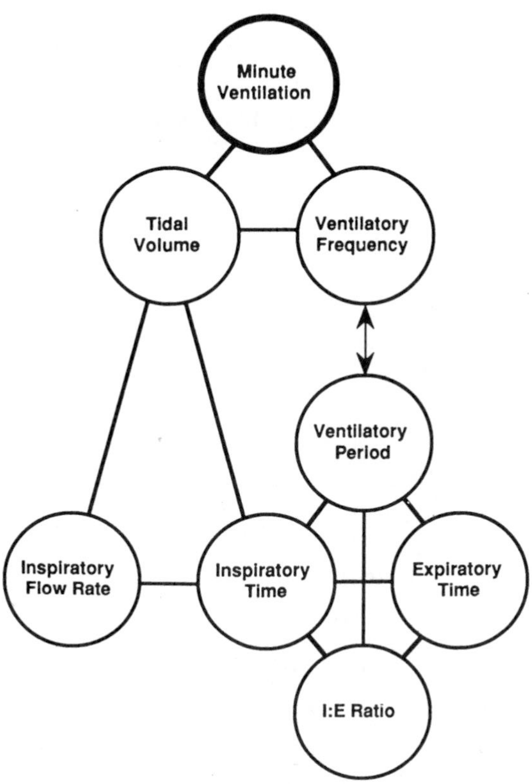

are important to the clinician. Specifically, a mode of ventilation is defined as a particular set of control variables, phase variables, and conditional variables.

Classification of Ventilation Modes

The task of understanding mechanical ventilators has become increasingly difficult in the past few years. Manufacturers try to achieve product differential by creating new and different names for ventilator features that may be fundamentally the same. However, as we already have discussed, they

FIGURE 1-15
Influence diagram for volume-controlled ventilation. Variables are connected by straight lines so that if any two are known, the third can be calculated using standard equations (see Table 1-4). The double arrow indicates that ventilatory period is the reciprocal of ventilatory frequency.

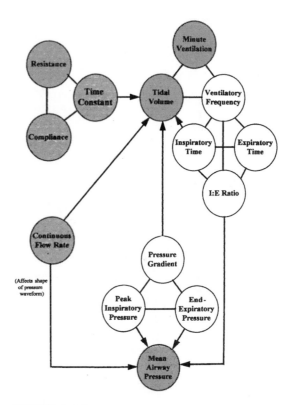

FIGURE 1-16
Influence diagram for pressure-controlled ventilation. Variables are connected by straight lines so that if any two are known, the third can be calculated using standard equations (see Table 1-4). Arrows represent relations that are either more complex or less predictable. Open circles represent variables that can be controlled directly by the ventilator; shaded circles are controlled indirectly. (Adapted from Chatburn RL, Lough MD: Mechanical ventilation. In: Lough MD, Doershuk CF, Stern RC [eds]: Pediatric Respiratory Therapy. Chicago: Year Book Medical Publishers, 1985, 148–191.)

relatively low, the set pressure limit is never reached. In this case indeed the set flow is the peak inspiratory flow. However, if flow is set relatively high, the pressure limit is reached almost immediately. Then peak inspiratory flow is determined by the pressure difference and resistance, as explained previously. If an intermediate flow is set, it has the effect of shaping the airway pressure waveform and generally decreasing the peak inspiratory flow. Compare the figures for rectangular and exponential pressure waveforms in the following section describing ventilator output.

Beyond these two general approaches to ventilatory support, it is possible to create a variety of breathing patterns or "modes" of ventilation. A mode of ventilation represents a set of breath characteristics that

TABLE 1–4. Pressure, Volume, and Flow Functions of Time During Mechanical Ventilation

	PRESSURE CONTROL	VOLUME/FLOW CONTROL
Inspiration		
Pressure	$\Delta P_{AW} = PIP - PEEP$	$P_{AW} = \left(\dfrac{V_T}{C}\right) + (R)(\dot{V})$
	$\overline{P}_{AW} \approx (PIP - PEEP)\left(\dfrac{I}{I + E}\right) + PEEP$	$\overline{P}_{AW} \approx (0.5)(PIP - PEEP)\left(\dfrac{I}{I + E}\right) + PEEP$
	$P_A \approx (\Delta P_{AW})(1 - e^{-t/\tau})$	$P_A = \left(\dfrac{V_T}{C}\right)$
Volume	$V_T = (\Delta P_{AW})(C)(1 - e^{-t/\tau})$	$V_T = \displaystyle\int_{t=0}^{t=T_I} \dot{V}dt$ (any flow waveform)
		$V_T = (\dot{V})(T_I)$ (constant flow)
Flow	$\dot{V} = \left(\dfrac{\Delta P}{R}\right)(e^{-t/\tau})$	$\dot{V} = $ constant
Expiration		
Pressure	$P_A = \left(\dfrac{V_T}{C}\right)(e^{-t/\tau})$	$P_A = \left(\dfrac{V_T}{C}\right)(e^{-t/\tau})$
Volume	$V_A = (V_T)(e^{-t/\tau})$	$V_A = (V_T)(e^{-t/\tau})$
Flow	$\dot{V} = -\left(\dfrac{P_A}{R}\right)(e^{-t/\tau})$	$\dot{V} = -\left(\dfrac{P_A}{R}\right)(e^{-t/\tau})$

General Equations Applicable to Any Mode of Ventilation

$\dot{V}_E = (f)(V_T)$ $T_I = \dfrac{(I)(60)}{(I + E)(f)}$ $T_E = \dfrac{(E)(60)}{(I + E)(f)}$

$I : E = \dfrac{T_I}{T_E}$ $f = \dfrac{(I)(60)}{(I + E)(T_I)} = \dfrac{(E)(60)}{(I + E)(T_E)}$ $period = \dfrac{f}{60} = T_I + T_E$

PAW, airway pressure; $\overline{P}_{AW}$, mean airway pressure; VT, tidal volume; $\dot{V}$, flow; $\dot{V}_E$, minute ventilation; R, respiratory system resistance; C, respiratory system compliance; t, time from beginning of inspiration; τ, respiratory system time constant; f, ventilatory frequency (cycles/min); T_I, inspiratory time; T_E, expiratory time; I, numerator of I:E; E, denominator of I:E; e, base of natural logarithm ≈ 2.72; PIP, peak inspiratory pressure; PEEP, positive end-expiratory pressure; ΔP, pressure gradient. (From Chatburn RL: Classification of mechanical ventilators. Respir Care 37:1009–1025, 1992.)

may use the same word for fundamentally different features. Our goals in clarifying terminology should be to:

- Avoid promotion of new terms that do not add to our ability to understand ventilator operating fundamentals
- When possible, use words and concepts that are widely used and presumably understood
- Maintain logical consistency among terms and, when possible, link to an underlying theoretical structure consistent with classical physiology
- Create simple terms that can be combined

to create varying degrees of complexity, such as using letters of the alphabet to create words and sentences rather than separate icons for each idea. This promotes the concept that it is easier to memorize a small number of terms and the rules for combining them (governed by the profession) rather than a never-ending list of unrelated jargon (generated by marketing interests). We cannot compel manufacturers to adopt a consistent classification scheme, but we can develop one that clearly explains what ventilators do, independent of what the manufacturers call it. Our only alternative is to memorize the manufacturers' descriptions for all the different ventilators we use and try to ignore the contradictions.

The first step in creating a unified and consistent mode classification scheme is to set up some definitions. The following terms represent a minimum set of concepts needed to construct a convenient lexicon of mechanical ventilation modes:

- Mandatory breath: inspiration is machine triggered and/or machine cycled
- Spontaneous breath: inspiration is patient triggered and patient cycled
- CMV: continuous mandatory ventilation—every breath is mandatory
- IMV: intermittent (machine-triggered) mandatory ventilation (breaths) with spontaneous breaths allowed in between
- SIMV: synchronized intermittent (patient or machine triggered) mandatory ventilation (breaths) with spontaneous breaths allowed in between
- CSV (commonly called pressure support ventilation or PSV): continuous spontaneous ventilation—every breath is spontaneous
- Pressure control: the ventilator attempts to maintain a preset airway pressure waveform during inspiration
- Volume/flow control: the ventilator attempts to maintain a preset volume or flow waveform during inspiration; direct control of flow implies indirect control of volume and vice versa
- Dual control: two variables are controlled by independent but synergistic feedback loops. Current examples are: (1) inspiration is pressure controlled within breaths, but the pressure limit is adjusted automatically between breaths to achieve a target tidal volume; and (2) inspiration switches between pressure control and flow control within a breath depending on the level of patient effort relative to machine settings
- Assist, assisted inspiration: inspiratory flow associated with a rise in transrespiratory pressure above baseline caused by an external agent (e.g., a ventilator assists the patient to breathe)

The next step in classifying modes is to

realize that simple deductive reasoning, from general to specific, can be applied to the characteristics of mandatory and spontaneous breaths. This order is analogous to the taxonomy applied in biology, in which family, genus, and species characteristics take on a hierarchical order of increasing detail. Figure 1–17 illustrates this concept. It shows that at the "family" level, we have the categories of mandatory and spontaneous breaths. At the "genus" level, we add detail by describing the possible control variables. Finally, at the "species" level, we have the smallest group to which distinctive characteristics (i.e., phase variables) can be assigned.

General Modes of Ventilation

There are many reasons that we need to describe ventilator function. Sometimes we need only to convey the most general information. At other times, we need to be quite specific about the nature of the ventilator–patient interaction. Our classification system should provide this flexibility as a logical progression of detail. One practical way to do this is to base the classification system on the pattern of mandatory breaths. The format is to specify the following characteristics: (1) the control variable (i.e., pressure, volume, or dual control); (2) the pattern of mandatory versus spontaneous breaths (i.e., CMV, SIMV and CSV); (3) the phase variables for mandatory breaths, in particular the trigger and cycle variables; (4) whether spontaneous breaths are assisted, and (5) conditional variables. Modes are discussed in detail in Chapter 2.

At this point we should say something about the potential conflict between the concepts described previously and the terms and concepts in common usage. Much common terminology is driven by manufacturers. They, in turn, are driven by manufacturing standards. For example, the American Society for Testing and Materials (ASTM) published *Standard Specifications for Ventilators Intended for Use in Critical Care* (designation: F 1100-90) in 1990. There is a section on ventilator classification that references Mushin and coworkers' text,[1] which was published in 1980. Thus,

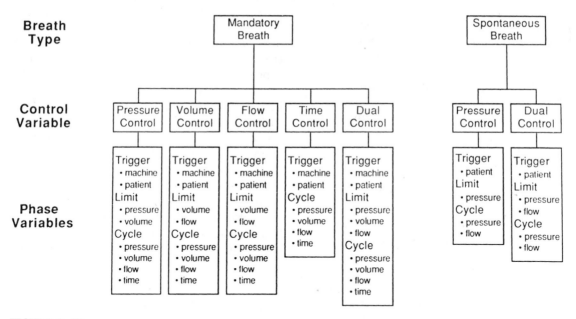

FIGURE 1–17

A hierarchical order of characteristics applied to mandatory and spontaneous breath. Once you understand the way that breath types are described, you can combine breath types to describe modes of ventilation.

ideas that were relevant almost 20 years ago, but which are largely irrelevant today, still are influencing the understanding of current clinicians. The aforementioned ASTM standard states that there are four types of ventilators:

- Controller: a device or mode of operation of a device that inflates the lungs independently of the patient's inspiratory effort.
- Assister: a device designed to augment the patient's breathing synchronously with his or her inspiratory effort.
- Assister/controller: an apparatus that is designed to function as an assister, or in the absence of the patient's inspiratory effort, a controller.
- Assister/controller/spontaneous breathing: those devices that incorporate various modes of operation that allow the patient to breathe spontaneously at or above ambient pressure levels or with or without supplemental mandatory positive pressure breaths.

The deficiencies in this classification system should be clear, despite its widespread use. The term "control," although not defined explicitly, centers on whether the

mode responds to the patient's inspiratory effort. It implies that the machine is controlling the ventilatory rate. However, when the ventilator triggers in response to the patient's effort, it is called an "assister." That was a big deal 20 years ago, but currently the ability to respond to patient effort is only one of many features that shape a breathing pattern. It seems relatively insignificant compared with the complexity of, for example, dual-control pressure and flow patterns. The term "control" is much more useful when it is broadened to its true engineering meaning, in the sense of feedback control, as described previously. In the same way, the term "assist" should not be limited to the patient-triggering feature but should be seen in the broader sense of adding force to the patient's inspiratory effort throughout inspiration (e.g., see the description of the "proportional assist" mode). Thus, inspiratory assistance can be achieved by controlling either the pressure, volume, or flow pattern generated by the ventilator. Another problem is that the terms "mandatory" and "spontaneous" are not defined. The reader evidently is supposed to "intuit" the meaning. However, if the terms are not defined explicitly, as we have done, much contradiction and confusion result when the detailed workings of modern ventilators are examined.

Once you understand this system, you can easily grasp the meaning of the jargon you hear on the job. For example, if you understand the concept of volume-controlled CMV, you can see that it is what many call "Assist/Control" or "A/C." But you also can see that Assist/Control implies only that there is both patient and machine triggering of breaths, whereas VC-CMV conveys more information. It tells about the control variable (volume) and the phase variables (patient or machine triggered, flow limited, machine cycled, due to the fact that each breath is mandatory).

The most general way of describing a mode is to state the control variable and the pattern, as in pressure-controlled intermittent mandatory ventilation (PC-IMV). This tells us that both mandatory and spontaneous breaths are allowed and that pressure, rather than volume or flow, is predetermined for mandatory breaths. If more detail is needed, we can say that mandatory breaths are either patient- or time-triggered and time-cycled. Further detail can include the fact that spontaneous breaths are pressure-supported. Finally, we can add that conditional variables determine that spontaneous inspiratory efforts can only trigger a mandatory breath within a particular trigger window as determined by the set mandatory breath frequency.

This system can be applied to even the most complex ventilator control schemes. For example, on the Siemens Servo 300, we can set a mode called "Volume Support." This term must be memorized, regardless of how any other mode on the machine works (e.g., Pressure Support) and independent of how other ventilators work. Translated, this mode becomes Dual-Controlled Continuous Spontaneous Ventilation. We could add that every breath is pressure or flow triggered, pressure limited, and flow cycled and that conditional logic adjusts the pressure limit between breaths in an attempt to achieve a preset tidal volume.

Consider another example: Using the terminology of the Bear 1000 ventilator, we can set a mode called "Assist CMV plus Pressure Augment." Translated, this would be Dual-Control SIMV. Each breath begins as patient triggered and pressure limited. If the conditional logic detects that the tidal volume has been delivered by the time flow decays to 30% of the peak flow, the breath is flow cycled (and therefore classified as spontaneous or supported). If, however, this condition is not met, then the breath switches to flow limited (i.e., volume controlled) and volume cycled (and therefore classified as a mandatory or assisted breath). Because a breath can be either mandatory or spontaneous depending on the relative value of patient effort and ventilator settings, the mode is a form of IMV rather than CMV or CSV.

By now, the reader should be able to discern three things: (1) there is a logical way to explain ventilator performance and with increasing detail to meet any communication need; (2) there are a great number of possible "modes", and (3) if you are responsible for using several brands of ventilators, you can become confused by the operator's manuals if you do not have a good general, theoretical understanding independent of their terminology.

This brings us to perhaps the most compelling reason to use the general mode classification scheme presented in this chapter. It is the increasing use of computerized hospital information systems to automate physician orders and patient notes. For example, at University Hospitals of Cleveland, we recently needed to design a system that allowed computer entry of orders for specific modes of ventilation. The basic software allowed selection of various menu items presented on different screens. The problem was that the same system would be used in seven different ICUs spanning neonatal, pediatric, and adult practices plus a variety of acute care divisions that might use home care ventilators. In addition to the wide range of possible modes for ventilation, we had to accommodate the capabilities of more than half a dozen different ventilator brands. In addition, we had the following goals:

• Orders could be written at various levels of detail.

The most commonly changed parameters should appear in earlier screens to save time looking for them.

Higher level-of-order detail means longer chain-of-order screens, encouraging brief orders that rely on external care paths and practice guidelines.

The user could not exit until minimum set of order details are entered.

• Consistency should be maintained between neonatal, pediatric, and adult areas.

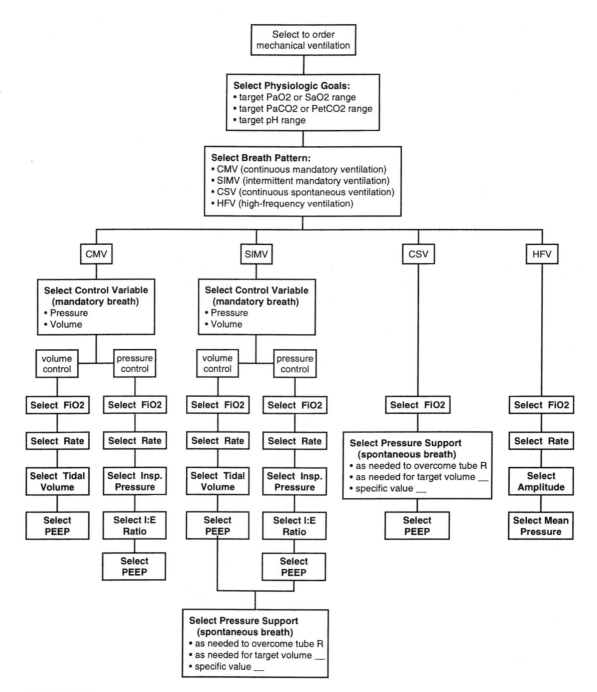

FIGURE 1-18

Schematic diagram of computerized physician order entry screens for mechanical ventilation on a hospital-wide information system.

By applying the general mode classification system in this chapter, we were able to create a logical system of entry screens, as illustrated in Figure 1–18. The general flow of information is to first select the breath pattern (CMV, SIMV, CSV, or HFV [high-frequency ventilation]), then select the control variable (for mandatory breaths), the phase variables (for mandatory breaths) and lastly the pressure support level (for spontaneous breaths). It would be easy to modify this system to include dual control.

Control Subsystems

Control Circuit. The **control circuit** is the subsystem responsible for controlling the drive mechanism and/or the output control valve. A ventilator may have more than one control circuit and more than one type.

Mechanical. Mechanical control circuits use levers, pulleys, cams, and so on. These types of circuits were used in the early manually operated ventilators illustrated in history books.[25]

Pneumatic. Pneumatic control circuits use gas pressure to operate diaphragms, jet entrainment devices, pistons, and so on. The original Bird and Bennett PR series ventilators used pneumatic control. A simple ventilator can be constructed with just two poppet valves and three flow resistors (Fig. 1–19).

Fluidic. Fluidic circuits are analogs of electronic logic circuits (Fig. 1–20).[26] They use minute gas flows to generate signals that operate timing systems and pressure switches. This makes them immune to failure from electromagnetic interference (such as around MRI equipment). Fluidic circuits can be constructed with discrete components such as comparators and flip-flops, or they can be combined in the form of integrated circuits, analogous to electronic integrated circuits. Examples of ventilators using fluidic logic control circuits are the Sechrist IV-100B and the Bio-Med MVP-10. A simple fluidic ventilator is shown in Figure 1–21.

Electric. Electric control circuits use only simple switches, rheostats (or potentiometers), and magnets to control ventilator operation. An example of a completely electri-

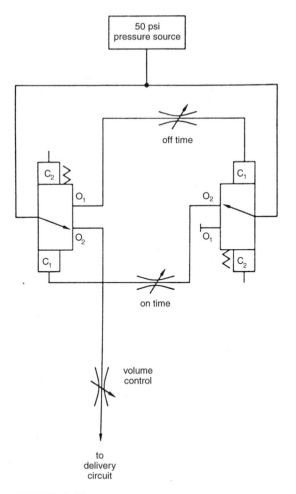

FIGURE 1–19
A simple ventilator control circuit composed of pneumatic components. Two poppet valves are connected to form a simple oscillator circuit. The on and off times (i.e., inspiratory and expiratory times) are controlled by two flow resistors. O_1 and O_2 are pneumatic signal outputs. C_1 ports are pneumatic signal inputs. The C_2 ports are spring loaded.

cally controlled ventilator is the Emerson Iron Lung.

Electronic. Electronic control circuits use devices such as resistors, capacitors, diodes, and transistors as well as combinations of these components in the form of integrated circuits. Integrated circuits can range in complexity from simple logic gates and operational amplifiers to microprocessors.

Drive Mechanism

The power transmission and conversion system, sometimes referred to as the *drive*

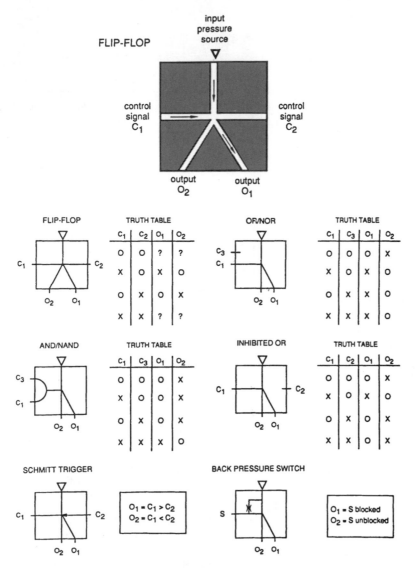

FIGURE 1–20
Basic fluidic components along with their associated input-output relations in the form of "truth tables."

mechanism, generates the force necessary to deliver gas to the patient. In general terms, this system is composed of either a compressor external to the ventilator in conjunction with a regulator inside the ventilator or an internal compressor linked to a motor. A complete description of all possible systems is beyond the scope of this chapter but may be found elsewhere.[27]

COMPRESSOR

A **compressor** is a device whose internal volume can be changed to increase the pressure of the gas it contains. Large, water-cooled, piston-type compressors often are used to supply gas under pressure to outlets near patient beds in hospitals. When a ventilator uses compressed gas from wall outlets as its only source of power to drive inspiration, the ventilator is considered to have an **external compressor**. Alternatively, a small compressor designed for use with a single ventilator may be employed. There are three types of compressors commonly used inside ventilators:

- Piston and cylinder (e.g., Emerson IMV)
- Bellows (e.g., Siemens Servo 900C)
- Turbine (e.g., Bird Tbird)

MOTOR AND LINKAGE

A motor is anything that produces motion. In a mechanical ventilator, the motor is the

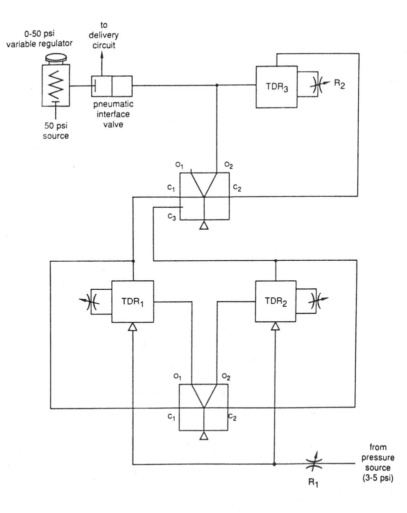

FIGURE 1-21
A simple ventilator control circuit composed of fluidic logic components. TDR, time delay relay.

device used to drive the compressor. For ventilators with **internal compressors**, the characteristics of interest are the type of motor and the linkage between the compressor and motor because these influence the waveforms that the ventilator can produce.

ELECTRIC MOTOR/ROTATING CRANK AND PISTON ROD

This sometimes is referred to as an "eccentric wheel" (Fig. 1-22). It produces a quasi-sinusoidal motion at the distal end of the piston rod (e.g., Emerson IMV). A true sinusoidal is generated only by a rotating crank in combination with a Scotch yoke.[28]

ELECTRIC MOTOR/RACK AND PINION

This produces a linear motion of the rack, driving the piston forward at either a con-

stant (e.g., Bourns LS 104-150) or variable rate, depending on the control circuit (Fig. 1-23).

ELECTRIC MOTOR/DIRECT

This can produce either a rotary motion of the output shaft, such as on a rotating vane air compressor (e.g., Bear 2), or a linear motion, as in the case of a linear drive motor. The linear drive motor is particularly versatile because it can produce a wide variety of easily controllable output waveforms.

COMPRESSED GAS REGULATOR/DIRECT

When compressed gas is used as the motor, its force often is adjusted by a pressure regulator (pressure reducing valve). The compressed gas either directly inflates the lungs (e.g., Bennet 7200) or stores energy in a

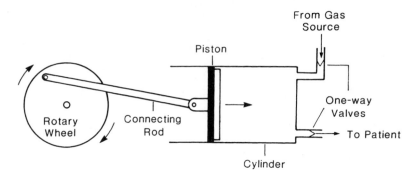

FIGURE 1-22
Drive mechanism consisting of eccentric wheel, piston rod, and piston.

spring (e.g., Siemens Servo 900C) mechanism, shown in Figure 1–24).

Output Control Valve

This valve is used to regulate the flow of gas to the patient. It may be a simple on/off valve (also called an *exhalation valve*), as in the NPB MA-1, or it may be used to shape the output waveform, as in the Siemens Servo 900C. Discussions of the most commonly used types follow.

ELECTROMAGNETIC POPPET VALVE

This type of device (also called a solenoid valve) uses magnetic force caused by an electric current to allow a small voltage to control a large pneumatic pressure in an on/off manner. Examples include the electronic interface valve (e.g., Infant Star, which uses a set of valves to approximate various pres-

sure or flow waveforms), the plunger (e.g., Bear Cub), and the pinch valve (e.g., Bunnell Life Pulse Jet Ventilator).

PNEUMATIC POPPET VALVE

This type of valve is similar to a solenoid valve except that it uses a small pneumatic pressure (e.g., a fluidic signal) to control a larger pneumatic pressure. These valves are particularly useful when electronic signals are inconvenient or hazardous.

PROPORTIONAL VALVE

Also known in industrial settings as a mass flow control valve, this device is similar to the solenoid valve because it is operated by an electromagnet, perhaps in the form of a stepper motor (i.e., an electric motor whose rotation can be controlled in discrete arcs or "steps"). The major difference is that rather

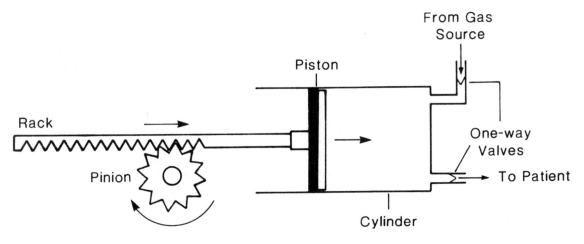

FIGURE 1-23
Drive mechanism consisting of a rack and pinion, piston rod, and piston.

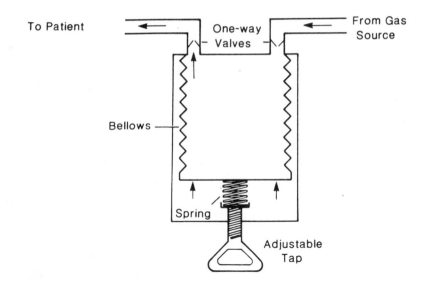

FIGURE 1–24
Drive mechanism consisting of a bellows under spring tension.

than simply turning flow on and off, this type of valve can shape the flow waveform during inspiration by changing the diameter of its outflow port and can be used to create a variety of waveforms. Proportional valves are used in the Bennett 7200 and the Hamilton Veolar ventilators and in the form of scissors valves in the Siemens Servo 900C or stepper motors in the Bear 5.

PNEUMATIC DIAPHRAGM

Usually an on/off type of valve, this device uses a flexible diaphragm or membrane (e.g., a "mushroom" valve) to divert gas from one pathway to another (Fig. 1–25). These are commonly referred to as "exhalation valves," which is a misnomer because they are primarily responsible for diverting gas

into the patient's lungs during inspiration. However, they are also responsible for slowing exhalation ("expiratory retard") and maintaining PEEP. Pneumatic diaphragms are commonly used, such as in the Newport ventilators.

Many ventilators use more than one output control valve. In particular, one valve often is used to direct flow into the patient's airway (e.g., a mushroom valve) whereas another may be used to shape the waveform (e.g., a proportional valve).

Output Waveforms

Just as the study of heart physiology involves the use of ECGs and blood pressure waveforms, the study of ventilator operation

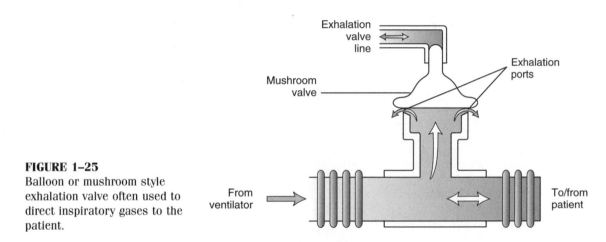

FIGURE 1–25
Balloon or mushroom style exhalation valve often used to direct inspiratory gases to the patient.

requires the examination of output waveforms. The waveforms of interest, of course, are the pressure, volume, and flow waveforms we have used throughout this discussion.

For each control variable, there are a limited number of waveforms that commonly are used by current ventilators. These waveforms can be idealized and have been grouped into four basic categories: rectangular (pulse), exponential, ramp, and sinusoidal. (Note that a rectangular volume waveform is theoretically impossible because volume cannot change instantaneously from zero to some preset value as pressure and flow can.)

Output waveforms are graphed in groups of three (Fig. 1–26). The horizontal axes of all graphs are the same and have the units of time. The vertical axes are in units of the measured variables (e.g., cm H_2O for pressure). For the purpose of identifying waveforms, the specific baseline values of each variable are irrelevant. Therefore, the origin of the vertical axis is labeled zero. The relative magnitude of each of the variables

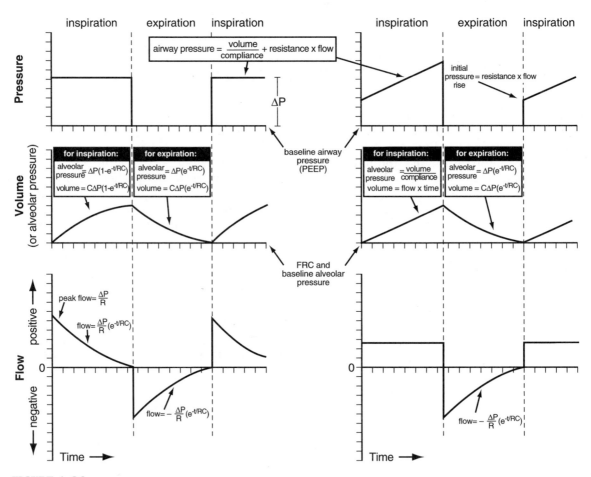

FIGURE 1–26

Typical pressure, volume, and flow waveforms for pressure-controlled (rectangular pressure waveform) and volume-controlled (rectangular flow waveform) ventilation. The curves show pressure, volume, and flow as functions of time in accordance with the equation of motion (where muscle pressure = 0). Note that all variables are measured relative to their baseline, or end-expiratory, values. ΔP, change in airway pressure; R, resistance, C, compliance; t, time; e, base of natural logarithm (<2.72); FRC, functional residual (lung) capacity.

and how the value of one affects or is affected by the value of the others are important.

Characteristic ventilator output waveforms are shown in Figures 1–27 through 1–33. They are idealized—that is, they are defined precisely by mathematical equations and are meant to characterize the operation of the ventilator's control system. As such, they do not show the minor deviations or "noise" often seen in waveforms recorded during actual ventilator use. These waveform imperfections can be caused by a variety of extraneous variables, such as vibration and turbulence, and the appearance of the waveform is affected by the scaling of the time axis. The waveforms also do not show the effects of the resistance of the expiratory side of the patient circuit because this varies depending on the ventilator and type of circuit.

No ventilator is an ideal controller, and ventilators are designed only to approximate a particular waveform. Idealized or standard waveforms are nevertheless helpful because they are common in other fields (e.g., electrical engineering), which makes it possible to use mathematical procedures and terminology that already have been developed. For example, a standard mathematical equation is used to describe the most common waveforms for each control variable. This known equation may be substituted into the equation of motion, which then is solved to get the equations of the other two variables. Once the equations for pressure, volume, and flow are known, they are graphed easily. This is the process used to generate the graphs in Figures 1–27 through 1–33.

As mentioned previously, most ventilator waveforms can be classified as one of four general types: rectangular, exponential, ramp, or sinusoidal (including sigmoidal and oscillating). Although many subtypes are possible, only the most common are described. Waveforms are listed according to the shape of the control variable waveform. Any new waveforms produced by future ventilators can be accommodated easily by this system.

Pressure

RECTANGULAR

Mathematically, a rectangular waveform is referred to as a step or instantaneous change in transrespiratory pressure from one constant value to another (Fig. 1–27). In response, volume rises exponentially from zero to a steady-state value equal to compliance times the change in airway pressure (i.e., PIP − PEEP). Inspiratory flow falls exponentially from a peak value (at the start of inspiration) equal to (PIP − PEEP) times resistance.

EXPONENTIAL

Exponential pressure waveforms are used most commonly during neonatal ventilation

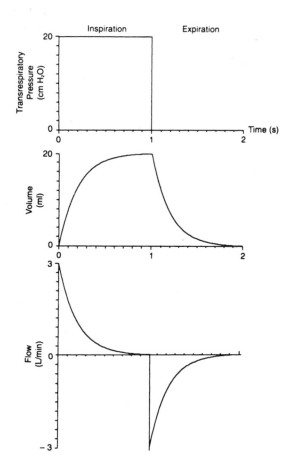

FIGURE 1–27
Characteristic waveforms for pressure-controlled ventilation with a rectangular pressure waveform. C = 0.001 L/cm H_2O; R = 200 cm H_2O/L/s.

(Fig. 1–28). Ventilators such as the Bear Cub are designed to deliver a modified rectangular waveform that typically results in a gradual rather than an instantaneous change in pressure at the start of inspiration. Depending on the specific ventilator settings (e.g., short inspiratory time, low flow rate, and high PIP), the pressure waveform may never attain a constant value and may resemble an exponential curve instead. In response, the volume and flow waveforms are also exponential, but their peak values are less than with a rectangular pressure waveform. Newer ventilators sometimes have a "slope" control that adjusts the rate of airway pressure rise (e.g. Drager Evita 4).

SINUSOIDAL

A sinusoidal pressure waveform can be created by attaching a piston to either a rotat-

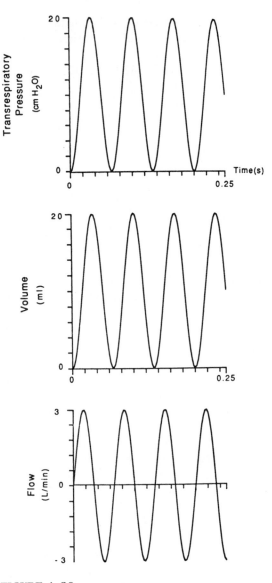

FIGURE 1–29
Characteristic waveforms for pressure-controlled ventilation with a sinusoidal pressure waveform. $C = 0.001$ L/cm H_2O; $R = 200$ cm H_2O/L/s.

ing crank or to a linear drive motor driven by an oscillating signal generator (Fig. 1–29). In response, the volume and flow waveforms are also sinusoidal, but they attain their peak values at different times (i.e., they are out of phase with each other).

OSCILLATING

Oscillating pressure waveforms can take on a variety of shapes from sinusoidal to ramp (e.g., SensorMedics 3100 oscillator) to

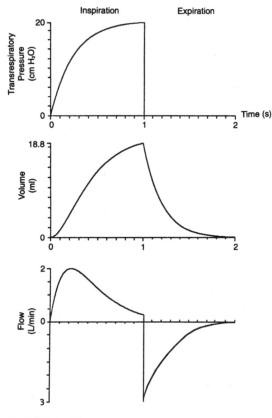

FIGURE 1–28
Characteristic waveforms for pressure-controlled ventilation with an exponential pressure waveform. $C = 0.001$ L/cm H_2O; $R = 200$ cm H_2O/L/s.

roughly triangular (e.g., Nellcor Puritan-Bennett Adult Star 1010 high-frequency jet ventilator). The distinguishing feature of a ventilator classified as an oscillator is that it can generate negative transrespiratory pressure. Thus, if the mean airway pressure is set equal to atmospheric pressure, then the airway pressure waveform oscillates above and below zero. If the pressure waveform is sinusoidal, volume and flow will also be sinusoidal but out of phase with each other. Other waveforms produce more complex volume and flow waveforms.

Volume

RAMP

Volume controllers that produce an ascending ramp waveform (e.g., the Bennett MA-1) produce a linear rise in volume from zero at the start of inspiration to the peak value (i.e., the set tidal volume) at end inspiration (Fig. 1–30). In response, the flow waveform is rectangular. The pressure waveform rises instantaneously from zero to a value equal to resistance times flow at the start of inspiration. From here, it rises linearly to its peak value (PIP) equal to (tidal volume/compliance) + (flow × resistance).

SINUSOIDAL

This waveform is produced most often by ventilators whose drive mechanism is a piston attached to a rotating crank (e.g., Emerson ventilators). The output waveform of this type of ventilator can be approximated by the first half of a cosine curve, whose shape in this case is sometimes referred to as a sigmoidal curve (Fig. 1–31). Because volume is sinusoidal during inspiration, pressure and flow are also sinusoidal.

Flow

RECTANGULAR

A rectangular flow waveform is perhaps the most common output (see Fig. 1–30). When the flow waveform is rectangular, volume is a ramp waveform and pressure is a step

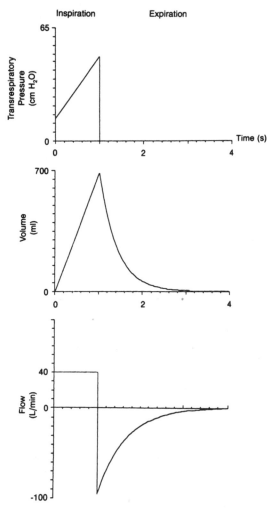

FIGURE 1–30
Characteristic waveforms for volume-controlled ventilation with an ascending ramp volume waveform. Identical to flow-controlled ventilation with a rectangular flow waveform. C = 0.02 L/cm H_2O; R = 20 cm H_2O/L/s.

followed by a ramp, as described for the ramp volume waveform.

RAMP

The ramp waveform is what many respiratory care practitioners (and ventilator manufacturers) call an "accelerating" or "decelerating" flow waveform. The term ramp is borrowed from electronic engineering and is preferred for three reasons. First, the name "ramp" gives a more obvious visual image of actual shape of the waveform. Second, the term ramp has been described mathe-

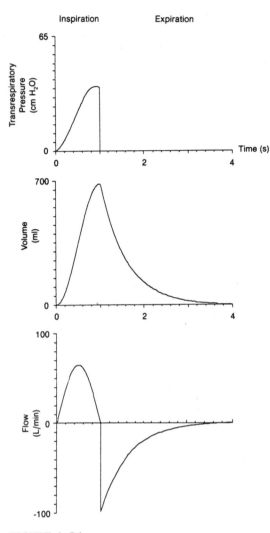

FIGURE 1–31
Characteristic waveforms for volume-controlled ventilation with a sinusoidal volume waveform. Identical to flow-controlled ventilation with a sinusoidal flow waveform. C = 0.02 L/cm H_2O; R = 20 cm H_2O/L/s.

matically and used universally for much longer than mechanical ventilators have been in existence. Third, the analogy of something accelerating or decelerating is misapplied. For example, when a car is moving, we say it has a certain speed (speed = change in distance/change in time). If the speed increases with time, we say that the car accelerates (acceleration = change in speed/change in time), not that the speed accelerates. The speed of moving gas is expressed as a flow rate (flow rate = area of tube x change in distance/change in time).

If the flow rate increases, we would properly say that the gas accelerates (acceleration = change in flow rate/change in time), not that the flow accelerates. In scientific terms, the acceleration of a particle is the rate of change of its velocity with time.[29]

Ascending Ramp. A true ascending ramp waveform starts at zero and increases linearly to the peak value (Fig. 1–32). Ventilator flow waveforms sometimes are truncated; inspiration starts with an initial instantaneous flow (e.g., the Bear 5 ventilator starts inspiration at 50% of the set peak flow). Flow then increases linearly to the set peak flow rate. In response to an ascending

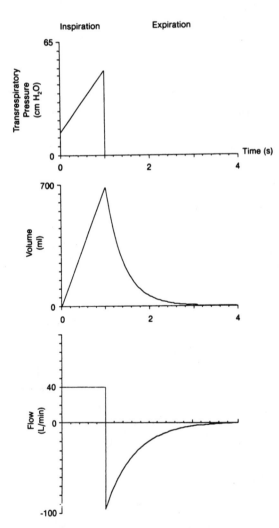

FIGURE 1–32
Characteristic waveforms for volume-controlled ventilation with an ascending ramp flow waveform. C = 0.02 L/cm H_2O; R = 20 cm H_2O/L/s.

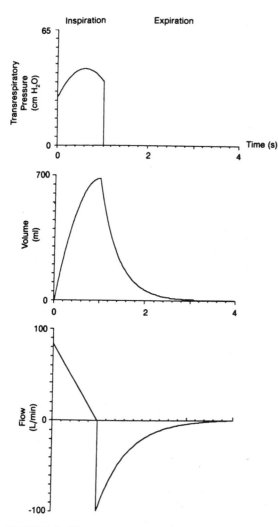

FIGURE 1–33
Characteristic waveforms for volume-controlled ventilation with a descending ramp flow waveform. C = 0.02 L/cm H_2O; R = 20 cm H_2O/L/s.

ramp flow waveform, the pressure and volume waveforms are exponential with a concave upward shape.

Descending Ramp. A true descending ramp waveform starts at the peak value and decreases linearly to zero (Fig. 1–33). Ventilator flow waveforms sometimes are truncated; inspiratory flow rate decreases linearly from the set peak flow until it reaches some arbitrary threshold at which flow drops immediately to zero (e.g., the Bennett 7200a ends inspiration when the flow rate drops to 5 L/min). In response to a descending ramp flow waveform, the pressure and volume waveforms are exponential

with a concave downward shape. Like many other topics we discuss, manufacturers may give the same technique different names, occasionally using a different technique and the same terminology. The descending ramp waveform is a good example of this problem. Depending on the manufacturer, the descending ramp may begin at a maximum flow and decelerate to 0 L/min or to a percentage of the initial flow. This is illustrated in Figure 1–34.

SINUSOIDAL

Some ventilators offer a mode in which the inspiratory flow waveform approximates the shape of the first half of a sine wave (see Fig. 1–31). As with the ramp waveform, ventilators often truncate the sine waveform by starting and ending flow at some percentage of the set peak flow rather than start and end at zero flow. In response to a sinusoidal flow waveform, the pressure and volume waveforms also will be sinusoidal but out of phase with each other.

Effects of the Patient Circuit

Thus far, we have implied that what comes out of the ventilator is the same as what goes into the patient. However, pressure, volume, and flow measured inside the ventilator are never the same as pressure, volume, and flow measured at the patient's airway opening. This is because the patient circuit has its own compliance (actually, the compliance of the tubing material plus the compressibility of the inspired gas) and resistance. Therefore, the pressure measured inside the ventilator on the inspiratory side (e.g., on a NPB MA-1) is always higher than the pressure at the airway opening because of the elastic and flow-resistive pressure decreases created by the patient circuit. Volume and flow coming out of the ventilator are always more than that delivered to the patient because of the effective compliance of the patient circuit. Patient circuit compliance includes not only the compliance of the material from which the circuit is made but also the compressibility of the gas within the circuit. This compliance effect absorbs both volume and flow.

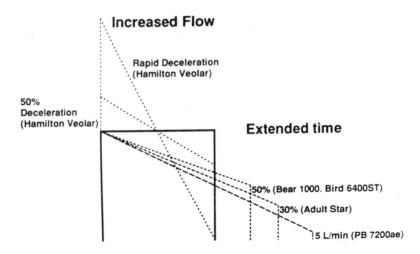

FIGURE 1-34

Differences in the flow profiles provided by different ventilators delivering the same tidal volume. The solid line represents the initial rectangular flow waveform. The Hamilton Veolar increases peak flow and decreases to 50% or 0% of the peak flow. Other ventilators maintain peak flow and decrease to 50% of peak flow to 5 L/min. In these ventilators, inspiratory time is extended and expiratory time is shortened. (From Nahum A, Shapiro R: Adjuncts to mechanical ventilation. Clin Chest Med 17:491–511, 1996.)

It can be shown by analogy to electrical circuits that the compliance of the delivery circuit is connected in parallel with the compliance of the respiratory system (i.e., both elements share the same driving pressure). Pneumatic compliance is analogous to electrical capacitance, and pneumatic resistance is analogous to electrical resistance.[7] Therefore, the total compliance of the ventilator–patient system is simply the sum of the two compliances. In a similar manner, the resistance of the delivery circuit is shown to be connected in series with the respiratory system resistance (i.e., both elements share the same flow) so that the total resistance is the sum of the two. From these assumptions, it can be shown that the relationship between the volume input to the patient (at the point of connection to the patient's airway opening) and the volume output from the ventilator (at the point of connection to the patient circuit) is described by:

$$\text{Volume input to patient} = [1/(1 + C_{PC}/C_{RS})] \times \text{volume output from ventilator} \quad (8)$$

where C_{PC} is the compliance of the patient circuit and C_{RS} is the total compliance of the

patient's respiratory system. The equation shows that the larger the patient circuit compliance, compared with the patient's respiratory system, the larger the denominator on the right-hand side of the equation. Hence, the smaller the delivered tidal volume is compared with the volume coming out of the ventilator's drive mechanism.

Assuming that the volume exiting the ventilator is the set tidal volume, the patient circuit compliance is calculated as:

$$C_{PC} = \text{set tidal volume}/(\text{Pplt} - \text{PEEP}) \quad (9)$$

where Pplt is the pressure measured during an inspiratory hold maneuver with the Y-adapter of the patient circuit occluded (patient is not connected) and PEEP is end-expiratory pressure (i.e., baseline pressure). Most authors recommend the use of peak inspiratory pressure (PIP) for Pplt in the aforementioned equation. This is acceptable, but it may lead to a slight underestimation of patient circuit compliance. Pplt is slightly lower than PIP because of the flow-resistive pressure drop of the patient circuit if pressure is not measured at the Y-adapter. This difference is greatest in small-bore, corrugated patient circuit tubing but is probably insignificant.

The effects of patient circuit compliance are most troublesome during volume-controlled ventilation. For example, when ventilating neonates, the patient circuit compliance can be as much as three times that of the respiratory system, even with small-bore tubing and a small-volume humidifier. Thus, when trying to deliver a preset tidal volume, the volume delivered to the patient may be as little as 25% of that coming from the ventilator, whereas 75% is compressed in the patient circuit. An example using adult values is shown in Figure 1–35.

Another area in which patient circuit compliance causes trouble is in the determination of autoPEEP. AutoPEEP is pressure in the lung at end-expiration caused by either insufficient expiratory time or early closure of small airways secondary to lung disease. The result is unintended positive pressure, which can result in a number of clinical problems. The patient's airway opening is occluded at end-expiration until static conditions prevail throughout the lungs. The pressure at this time is auto-PEEP ($PEEP_A$) and is an index of the volume of gas trapped in the lungs:

$$\text{True } PEEP_A = V_{RS}/C_{RS} \qquad (10)$$

where V_{RS} is the volume of the respiratory system at end-expiration and C_{RS} is respiratory system compliance.

Many ventilators allow the clinician to perform the maneuver without disconnecting the patient from the ventilator. In this case, however, the end-expiratory respiratory system volume is distributed between the lungs and the patient circuit. Thus, the autoPEEP measured under these conditions underestimates the true auto-PEEP because the patient circuit compliance is added in parallel with the compliance of the respiratory system:

$$\text{Estimated } PEEP_A = \\ V_{RS}/(C_{RS} + C_{PC}) \qquad (11)$$

The relationship between true and estimated autoPEEP is derived by solving equation 4 for volume and substituting it into equation 3:

$$\text{True } PEEP_A = [(C_{RS} + C_{PC})/C_{RS}] \times \\ \text{Estimated } PEEP_A \qquad (12)$$

Thus, true autoPEEP may be calculated from the estimated autoPEEP by multiplying by an error factor that is a function of the patient circuit compliance. This error can be substantial for small patients with stiff lungs.

You can see that the patient circuit has the same magnitude of effect on mean inspiratory flow rate by dividing both sides of equation 8 by inspiratory time. The discrepancy between the set and delivered tidal

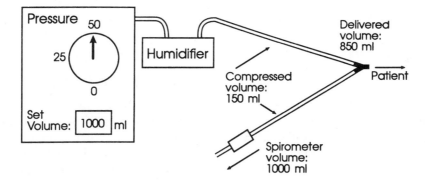

FIGURE 1–35

The concept of compressible volume is illustrated. The ventilator is set to deliver 1000 ml to the patient. If the tubing compliance is 3 ml/cm H_2O and plateau pressure is 50 cm H_2O then compressible volume is (3 ml/cm H_2O) $\times$ 50 cm H_2O = 150 ml. Actual volume delivered to the patient is 1000 ml – 150 ml = 850 ml. If the ventilator measures volume distal to the exhalation valve, tidal volume equals set volume but does not reflect the actual tidal volume delivered to the patient.

volume and flow must be taken into account when using most ventilators. However, some ventilators, such as the NPB 7200 series, automatically make the appropriate calculations and adjustments.

During pressure-controlled ventilation, the compliance of the patient circuit has the effect of rounding the leading edge of a rectangular pressure waveform which could reduce the volume delivered to the patient. This effect is avoided if the pressure limit is maintained for at least five time constants (of the respiratory system). The time constant is a measure of the time required for the passive respiratory system to respond to abrupt changes in ventilatory pressure. It has units of time (usually seconds) and is calculated as resistance times compliance.[7]

For both pressure- and volume-controlled ventilation, the patient circuit compliance and resistance, along with the resistance of the exhalation valve (in series with the patient circuit and respiratory system resistance) increase the expiratory time constant. Thus, a large circuit compliance coupled with a short expiratory time can lead to inadvertent **end-expiratory pressure.**

In summary, the "set" values for pressure, volumes and flow may be different from the "output (from ventilator)" values because of calibration errors and different from the "input (to the patient)" because of the effects of the patient circuit. Thus, there are two general sources of error that cause discrepancies between the desired and actual patient values.

VENTILATOR ALARM SYSTEMS

The ventilator classification scheme described previously centers on the basic functions of input, control, and output. If any of these functions fails, a life-threatening situation may result. Thus, ventilators are equipped with various types of alarms, which may be classified in the same manner as the other major ventilator characteristics.

Day and MacIntyre[30, 31] have stressed that the goal of ventilator alarms is to warn of events. They define an "event" as any condition or occurrence that requires clinician awareness or action. Technical events are

those involving an inadvertent change in the ventilator's performance; patient events are those involving a change in the patient's clinical status that can be detected by the ventilator.[27] A ventilator may be equipped with any conceivable vital sign monitor, but we limit the scope here to include the ventilator's mechanical/electronic operation and those variables associated with the mechanics of breathing (i.e., pressure, volume, flow, and time). Because the ventilator is in intimate contact with exhaled gas, we also include the analysis of exhaled oxygen and carbon dioxide concentrations as possible variables to monitor.

Alarms may be audible, visual, or both, depending on the seriousness of the alarm condition. Visual alarms may be as simple as colored lights or may be as complex as alphanumeric messages to the operator indicating the exact nature of the fault condition. Specifications for an *alarm event* should include (1) conditions that trigger the alarm, (2) the alarm response in the form of audible and/or visual messages, (3) any associated ventilator response, such as termination of inspiration or failure to operate, and (4) whether the alarm must be manually reset or resets itself when the alarm condition is rectified. Table 1–5 outlines the various levels of alarm priority along with alarm characteristics and appropriate alarm categories. Alarm categories are based on the ventilator classification scheme and are detailed in the following sections.

Input Power Alarms

Loss of Electric Power

Most ventilators have some sort of battery backup in case of electrical power failure, even if the batteries only power alarms. Ventilators typically have alarms that are activated if the electrical power is cut off while the machine still is switched on (e.g., if the power cord is accidentally pulled out of the wall socket).

If the ventilator is designed to operate on battery power (e.g., transport ventilators), there is usually an alarm to warn of a low-battery condition.

TABLE 1-5. Classification of Ventilator Alarms

EVENT	PRIORITY			
	Level 1	Level 2	Level 3	Level 4
	Critical ventilator malfunction*	Noncritical ventilator malfunction†	Patient status change‡	Operator alert§
ALARM CHARACTERISTICS				
Mandatory	Yes	Yes	No	Yes
Redundant‖	Yes	No	No	No
Noncancelling¶	Yes	No	No	Yes
Audible	Yes	Yes	Yes	No
Visual	Yes	Yes	Yes	Yes
AUTOMATIC BACKUP RESPONSE	Yes	No	No	No
AUTOMATIC RESET				
Audible	Yes	Yes	Yes	—
Visual	No	Yes	Yes	Yes
APPLICABLE ALARM CATEGORIES				
Input				
Electric power	Yes	No	No	No
Pneumatic power	Yes	No	No	No
Control Circuit				
Inverse I:E	Yes	Yes	No	Yes
Incompatible settings	No	No	No	Yes
Mechanical/ electronic fault	Yes	No	No	No
Output				
Pressure#	Yes	Yes	Yes	Yes
Volume**	Yes	Yes	Yes	Yes
Flow††	Yes	Yes	Yes	Yes
Minute ventilation	Yes	Yes	Yes	Yes
Time‡‡	Yes	Yes	Yes	Yes
Inspired gas (FiO$_2$, temp)§§	Yes	Yes	No	Yes
Expired gas (FeO$_2$)§§	No	No	Yes	No

*Immediately life threatening.
†Not immediately life threatening.
‡Change in neurologic ventilatory drive, respiratory system mechanics, hemodynamic, or metabolic status.
§Ventilator warns of potential danger (e.g., control variable settings high or low, alarms inappropriately set).

Specific alarm mechanisms designed in duplicate or backed up by related alarm mechanisms:
‖Operator cannot reset alarm until the alarm condition has been corrected.
¶Backup ventilator mode or patient ventilator circuit opens to atmosphere.
#High/low peak, mean, and baseline pressure.
**High/low inhaled and exhaled tidal volume. May also include alarms for leaks.
††Alarm triggered if expiratory flow does not fall below a threshold. Warns of gas trapping.
‡‡Warns that inspiratory or expiratory times are too long/short.
§§Analysis of inspired and expired gas may include other tracer gases for measurement of functional residual capacity.

Loss of Pneumatic Power

Ventilators that use pneumatic power have alarms that are activated if either the oxygen or air supply is cut off or reduced below some specified driving pressure. In some cases, the alarm is activated by an electronic pressure switch (e.g., NPB 7200), but in others the alarm is operated pneumatically as part of the blender (e.g., Siemens Servo 900C).

Control Circuit Alarms

Control circuit alarms are those that either warn the operator that the set control variable parameters are incompatible (e.g., inverse I:E ratio) or indicate that some aspect of a ventilator self-test has failed. In the latter case, there may be something wrong with the ventilator control circuitry itself (e.g., a microprocessor failure) and the ventilator generally responds with a generic message such as "Ventilator Inoperative."

Output Alarms

Output alarms are those that are activated by an unacceptable state of the ventilator's output. More specifically, an output alarm is activated when the value of a control variable (pressure, volume, flow, or time) falls outside an expected range. Some possibilities include the following.

Pressure

Pressure alarms may be available for the following conditions.

High and Low Peak Airway Pressure. These alarms occur when there is a possible endotracheal tube obstruction or leak in the patient circuit, respectively.

High and Low Mean Airway Pressure. These alarms indicate a possible leak in the patient circuit or a change in ventilatory pattern that might lead to a change in the patient's oxygenation status (i.e., within reasonable limits, oxygenation is roughly proportional to mean airway pressure).

High and Low Baseline Pressure. These alarms indicate a possible patient circuit or exhalation manifold obstruction (or inadvertent PEEP) and disconnection of the patient from the patient circuit, respectively.

Failure to Return to Baseline. Failure of airway pressure to return to baseline within a specified period indicates a possible patient circuit obstruction or exhalation manifold malfunction.

Volume

High and Low Expired Volume. These alarms indicate changes in respiratory system time constant during pressure-controlled ventilation, leaks around the endotracheal tube or from the lungs, or possible disconnection of the patient from the patient circuit.

Flow

High and Low Expired Minute Ventilation. These alarms indicate hyperventilation (or possible machine self-triggering) and possible apnea or disconnection of the patient from the patient circuit, respectively.

Time

High or Low Ventilatory Frequency. When these alarms occur, hyperventilation (or possible machine self-triggering) and possible apnea, respectively, may be occurring.

Inappropriate Inspiratory Time. Inspiratory time that is too long indicates a possible patient circuit obstruction or exhalation manifold malfunction. Inspiratory time that is too short indicates that adequate tidal volume may not be delivered (in a pressure-controlled mode) or that gas distribution in the lungs may not be optimal.

Inappropriate Expiratory Time. Expiratory time that is too long may indicate apnea. Expiratory time that is too short may warn of alveolar gas trapping (i.e., expiratory time should be greater than or equal to five time constants of the respiratory system).

Inspired Gas

Inspired gas conditions have been standard alarm parameters for some time.

- High/low inspired gas temperature
- High/low FiO_2

Expired Gas

Because ventilators are designed to control the mechanical results of exhalation, they may be adapted easily to the analysis of exhaled gas composition, and alarms may be set for specific parameters.

Exhaled Carbon Dioxide Tension. End-tidal carbon dioxide monitoring may reflect arterial carbon dioxide tension and thus indicate the level of ventilation. Calculation of mean expired carbon dioxide tension along with minute ventilation measurements could provide information about carbon dioxide production and contribute to the calculation of the respiratory exchange ratio and the tidal volume/dead space ratio.[32]

Exhaled Oxygen Tension. Analysis of end-tidal and mean expired oxygen tension may provide information about gas exchange and could be used along with carbon dioxide data to calculate the respiratory exchange ratio.

REFERENCES

1. Mushin M, Rendell-Baker W, Thompson PW, Mapelson WW: Automatic Ventilation of the Lungs. Oxford: Blackwell Scientific Publications, 1980, pp 62–166.
2. Consensus statement on the essentials of mechanical ventilators—1992. Respir Care 37:1000–1008, 1992.
3. Chatburn RL: Classification of mechanical ventilators. Respir Care 37:1009–1025, 1992.
4. Branson RD, Chatburn RL: Technical description and classification of modes of ventilator operation. Respir Care 37:1026–1044, 1992.
5. Morris W: The American Heritage Dictionary of the English Language. Boston: American Heritage Publishing Co. and Houghton Mifflin, 1975 p 780.
6. Otis AB, McKerrow CB, Bartlett RA, et al: Mechanical factors in distribution of pulmonary ventilation. J Appl Physiol 427–443, 1956.
7. Chatburn RL, Primiano FP Jr: Mathematical models of respiratory mechanics. In: Chatburn RL, Craig KC (eds): Fundamentals of Respiratory Care Research. Norwalk, CT: Appleton & Lange, 1988.
8. Younes M: Proportional assist ventilation: a new approach to ventilatory support. Am Rev Respir Dis 45:114–120, 1992.
9. Rubinstein MF: Patterns of Problem Solving. Englewood Cliffs, NJ: Prentice-Hall, 1975, pp 409–473.
10. Hess D, Lind L: Nomograms for the application of the Bourns Model BP200 as a volume-constant ventilator. Respir Care 25:248–250, 1980.
11. Desautels DA: Ventilator performance evaluation. In: Kirby RR, Smith RA, Desautels DA (eds): Mechanical Ventilation. New York: Churchill Livingstone, 1985, p 120.
12. Sassoon CSH, Giron AE, Ely EA, Light RW: Inspiratory work of breathing on flow-by and demand-flow continuous positive airway pressure. Crit Care Med 17:1108–1114, 1989.
13. Sassoon CSH, Gruer SE: Characteristics of the ventilator pressure and flow trigger variables. Intensive Care Med 21:159–168, 1995.
14. Sassoon CSH, Light RW, Lodia R, et al: Pressure-time product during continuous positive airway pressure, pressure support ventilation, and T-piece during weaning from mechanical ventilation. Am Rev Respir Dis 143:469–475, 1991.
15. Messinger G, Banner MJ, Blanch PB, Layon AJ: Using tracheal pressure to trigger the ventilator and control airway pressure during continuous positive airway pressure decreases the work of breathing. Chest 108:509–514, 1995.
16. Messinger G, Banner MJ: Tracheal pressure triggering a demand flow continuous positive airway pressure system decreases patient work of breathing. Crit Care Med 24:1829–1834, 1996.
17. Branson RD: Flow triggering systems. Respir Care 39:892–896, 1994.
18. Sassoon CSH, Del Rosario N, Fei R, et al: Influence of pressure and flow triggered synchronous intermittent mandatory ventilation on inspiratory muscle work. Crit Care Med 22:1933–1941, 1994.
19. Branson RD, Campbell RS, Davis K Jr, Johnson DJ: Comparison of pressure and flow triggering systems during continuous positive airway pressure. Chest 106:540–544, 1994.
20. Nikischin W, Gerhardt T, Everett R, et al: Patient triggered ventilation: a comparison of tidal volume and chest wall and abdominal motion as trigger signals. Pediatr Pulmonol 22:28–34, 1996.
21. Shachter RD: Evaluating influence diagrams. Operations Res 34:871–882, 1986.
22. Seiver A, Holtzman S: Decision analysis: a framework for critical care decision assistance. Int J Clin Monit Comput 6:137–156, 1989.
23. Chatburn RL, Lough MD, Primiano FP Jr: Mechanical ventilation. In: Chatburn RL, Lough MD (eds): Handbook of Respiratory Care, 2nd ed. Chicago: Year Book Medical Publishers, 1990, pp 159–223.

24. Perry DG: A simplified diagram for understanding the operation of volume-preset ventilators. Respir Care 22:42–49, 1977.
25. Morch ET: History of mechanical ventilation. In: Kirby RR, Smith RA, Desautels DA (eds): Mechanical Ventilation. New York: Churchill Livingstone, 1985, pp 1–58.
26. Russell DF, Ross DG, Manson HJ: Fluidic cycling devices for inspiratory and expiratory timing in automatic ventilators. J Biomed Eng 5:227–234, 1983.
27. Dupuis YG: Ventilators: Theory and Application. St. Louis: CV Mosby, 1986.
28. Beckwith TG, Buck NL, Marangoni RD: Mechanical Measurements, 3rd ed. Reading, MA: Addison-Wesley, 1982, p 25.
29. Halliday D, Resnick R: Fundamentals of Physics, 2nd ed. New York: John Wiley, 1981, p 29.
30. Day S, MacIntyre NR: Ventilator alarm systems. Prob Respir Care 4:118–126, 1991.
31. MacIntyre NR, Day S: Essentials for ventilator-alarm systems. Respir Care 37:1108–1112, 1992.
32. Weingarten M: Respiratory monitoring of carbon dioxide and oxygen: a ten-year perspective. J Clin Monit 217–225, 1990.

CHAPTER 2

Modes of Ventilator Operation

Richard D. Branson, BA, RRT
Robert S. Campbell, RRT

PRESSURE CONTROL
VERSUS VOLUME CONTROL

MODES
Continuous Mandatory
    Ventilation
Assist/Control Ventilation
Assisted Mechanical
    Ventilation
Intermittent Mandatory
    Ventilation
Synchronized Intermittent
    Mandatory Ventilation
Pressure Support
    Ventilation
Continuous Positive
    Airway Pressure
Airway Pressure Release
    Ventilation
Pressure Control Inverse
    Ratio Ventilation
Mandatory Minute
    Ventilation

COMBINING MODES

DUAL CONTROL MODES OF
MECHANICAL VENTILATION
Dual Control Within a
    Breath
Dual Control Breath to
    Breath—Pressure-
    Limited, Flow-Cycled
    Ventilation
Dual Control Breath to
    Breath—Pressure-
    Limited, Time-Cycled
    Ventilation

AUTOMODE

ADAPTIVE SUPPORT
VENTILATION

AUTOMATIC TUBE
COMPENSATION

PROPORTIONAL ASSIST
VENTILATION

KEY WORDS

adaptive support ventilation
proportional assist ventilation

volume-assured pressure
    support

According to the framework presented in Chapter 1, a mode is a specific combination of control, phase, and conditional variables defined for both mandatory and spontaneous breaths.[1] More simply, a mode describes whether the breaths are volume constant (volume controlled) or pressure constant (pressure controlled); whether breaths are mandatory, spontaneous, or a combination of the two; and which conditional variables determine a change in ventilator function. There are numerous names for any given mode, despite similar function. This chapter attempts to group these together whenever possible.

Unfortunately, the "names" of modes frequently are the result of a whim of the designer or are concocted by the marketing group of a manufacturer. Understanding the ventilator's function during a given mode is crucial to applying the appropriate ventilatory care to the patient. Each mode has its staunch supporters and equally determined detractors. No group seems to understand the approach of another, and most fail to realize that experience and skill with a specific mode are probably the greatest determinants of success. In subsequent chapters, when application of the modes are discussed, it should become evident that mode selection should be based on patient need, not clinician preference.

In this chapter, the modes of mechanical ventilation are described and the plethora of names for each one are listed. Important concepts related to setting ventilatory variables are included. Clinical application of these techniques, however, is not described in this chapter.

PRESSURE CONTROL VERSUS VOLUME CONTROL

As described in Chapter 1, the ventilator is capable of controlling breath delivery with any one of the variables in the equation of motion. From a practical standpoint, conventional modes of mechanical ventilation control either pressure or volume. Newer modes are capable of switching from one to the other and are called *dual control modes.* Pressure control and volume control are not modes; they indicate which variable is constant during breath delivery regardless of changes in lung mechanics. Pressure control simply means the breaths are pressure constant and volume variable. Volume control simply means that the breaths are volume constant and pressure variable.

This can be the source of some confusion.

Often, pressure control is thought to mean pressure-limited, time-cycled ventilation in the control (continuous mandatory ventilation [CMV]) mode. This may be true for a given ventilator (e.g., the 900C, Siemens, Danvers, MA); however, pressure control breaths can be delivered in the intermittent mandatory ventilation (IMV) mode as well as the CMV mode. Again, pressure control and volume control only describe the variable in the equation of motion that the ventilator is maintaining constant during breath delivery. Throughout this text, the terms *pressure control* and *volume control* may be used interchangeably with the terms *pressure targeted* and *volume targeted.*

We believe the breath delivery technique (pressure or volume) should be used as a prefix for each "mode" of ventilation—for example, volume control IMV or pressure control IMV. In these two examples, the mode is the same. That is, a certain number of ventilator breaths are delivered per minute while patients breathe spontaneously (at their own respiratory rate, tidal volume, inspiratory time, and flow) in between ventilator breaths. Pressure control IMV implies that the ventilator breaths are at a constant pressure, whereas volume control implies that the ventilator breaths are at a constant volume.

The practical aspects of pressure and volume breath delivery should be mentioned. During volume control, the clinician must set tidal volume, inspiratory flow or inspiratory time, inspiratory flow pattern, and respiratory frequency. During a volume control breath, the tidal volume, flow, and flow pattern remain constant regardless of patient effort or respiratory system impedance. The clinician may select the flow pattern during a volume control breath. Figure 2–1 demonstrates the effects of changing flow patterns during volume control ventilation on appearance of the pressure and volume waveforms.

During a pressure control breath, the clinician must set the peak inspiratory pressure, inspiratory time, and respiratory frequency. During a pressure control breath, the peak inspiratory pressure and inspiratory time remain constant. Flow during a

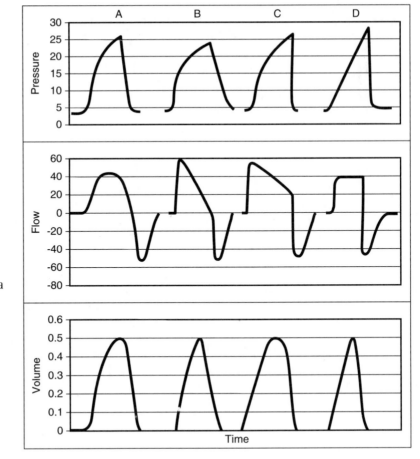

FIGURE 2-1

The effects of changing inspiratory flow pattern during volume control ventilation on pressure waveform. Breath A shows a volume control breath using a sine wave flow pattern. Breath B shows a volume control breath using a full decelerating flow pattern. Breath C shows a volume control breath using a 50% decelerating flow pattern. Breath D shows a volume control breath using a constant (square) flow waveform.

pressure control breath is variable, depending on patient effort and respiratory system impedance. Flow during a pressure control breath always takes the shape of a decelerating waveform. This is necessary to allow the set pressure to be reached early during the breath and remain constant throughout the inspiratory time. The speed at which the flow decelerates during a pressure control breath, and hence the appearance, changes with changes in respiratory system impedance. Table 2-1 compares the characteristics of pressure and volume control breaths. Figure 2-2 demonstrates pressure, volume, and flow waveforms against time for both kinds of breaths and depicts the changes caused by respiratory system impedance changes.

MODES

Continuous Mandatory Ventilation

Descriptive Definition. Continuous mandatory ventilation (CMV) is a mode of ventilator operation in which all breaths are mandatory and are delivered by the ventilator at a preset frequency (f), volume or pressure, and inspiratory time. In the proposed list of modes, CMV encompasses all modes that deliver only mandatory or a combination of mandatory and assisted breaths. The only difference between an assisted breath and a control breath is that the patient triggers the assisted breath, whereas the ventilator triggers the mandatory breath.

Other Terms. The term CMV is listed in the literature as continuous mechanical ventilation, continuous mandatory ventilation, controlled mechanical ventilation, and controlled mandatory ventilation.[2-5] Interestingly, many authors preserve the CMV acronym while choosing its meaning haphazardly. CMV also frequently is called volume-controlled ventilation (VCV) or just simply control mode.[2, 3]

Manufacturer Terms. Currently available mechanical ventilators refer to CMV as

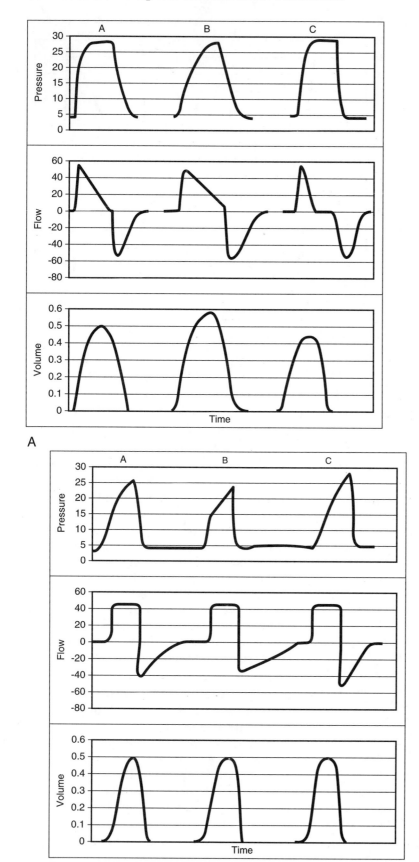

FIGURE 2–2
(A) Comparison of pressure control ventilation at a normal lung compliance (breath A) to elevated compliance (breath B) and reduced compliance (breath C). (B) Comparison of a volume control breath at normal lung compliance (breath A) to elevated (breath B) and reduced (breath C) lung compliance.

TABLE 2–1. Comparison of Pressure Control and Volume Control Breaths

VARIABLE	VOLUME CONTROL BREATH	PRESSURE CONTROL BREATH
Tidal volume	Set by clinician; remains constant	Variable with changes in patient effort and respiratory system impedance
Peak inspiratory pressure	Variable with changes in patient effort and respiratory system impedance	Set by clinician; remains constant
Inspiratory time	Set directly or as a function of respiratory frequency and inspiratory flow settings	Set by clinician; remains constant
Inspiratory flow	Set directly or as a function of respiratory frequency and inspiratory flow settings	Variable with changes in patient effort and respiratory system impedance
Inspiratory flow waveform	Set by clinician; remains constant; can use constant, sine, or decelerating flow waveform	Variable with changes in patient effort and respiratory system impedance; flow waveform always is decelerating.

CMV assist control, control, volume control, and a host of others. In some cases, this mode strictly adheres to the aforementioned definition, but in others the patient is allowed to trigger mandatory breaths by exceeding the sensitivity setting. This mode often is called assist/control. On many ventilators, CMV and assist/control are the same, the only difference being the sensitivity setting. For instance, on the Hamilton Veolar (Hamilton Medical, Reno, NV), if desired, the sensitivity setting is dialed to its least sensitive position (-20 cm H_2O).[6] Otherwise, patient triggering is possible. It would be wise to sedate and paralyze the patient in this situation.

Classification. CMV is classified as volume or pressure controlled; time triggered; volume, pressure, or flow limited; and volume, pressure, flow, or time cycled. All breaths are mandatory breaths. Figure 2–3 demonstrates volume-controlled CMV and Figure 2–4 demonstrates pressure-controlled CMV. In these examples, the modes are volume control CMV (all breaths are volume constant, and each breath is triggered by the ventilator) and pressure control CMV (all breaths are pressure constant,

and each breath is time triggered by the ventilator).

Simplifying this by substituting the more generic terms, CMV is pressure or volume controlled; machine triggered; and machine cycled (Table 2–2). It should be obvious to the reader at this point that simply conveying the message that the patient is "on CMV" hardly describes the mode of operation. Depending on the ventilator used and local practice, CMV could mean that mandatory breaths are pressure or volume controlled; patient (using any of the possible variables) and/or machine triggered; pressure, volume, or flow limited; and time, flow, volume, or pressure cycled. This requires that the mode be referred to as volume control CMV or pressure control CMV.

Assist/Control Ventilation

Descriptive Definition. Assist/control (A/C) ventilation is a mode of ventilator operation in which mandatory breaths are delivered at a set frequency, pressure or volume, and inspiratory flow. Between machine-initiated breaths, the patient can

TABLE 2-2. Breath Types for the Modes of Ventilator Operations

MODE (COMMON NAMES)	MANDATORY			ASSISTED			SUPPORTED			SPONTANEOUS			CONDITIONAL VARIABLE	ACTION
	Trigger	Limit	Cycle	Trigger	Limit	Cycle	Trigger	Limit	Cycle	Trigger	Limit	Cycle		
VC-CMV	Time	Flow	Volume or time	—	—	—	—	—	—	—	—	—	—	—
VC-A/C	Time	Flow	Volume or time	Patient	Flow	Volume or time	—	—	—	—	—	—	Patient effort and time	Mandatory or assisted breath
VC-IMV	Time	Flow	Volume or time	—	—	—	—	—	—	Patient	Pressure	Pressure or flow	—	—
VC-SIMV	Time	Flow	Volume or time	—	—	—	—	—	—	Patient	Pressure	Pressure or flow	Patient effort and time	Mandatory or assisted breath
PC-CMV	Time	Pressure	Time	—	—	—	—	—	—	—	—	—	—	—
PC-A/C	Time	Pressure	Time	Patient	Pressure	Time	—	—	—	—	—	—	Patient effort and time	Mandatory or assisted breath
PC-IMV	Time	Pressure	Time	—	—	—	—	—	—	Patient	Pressure	Pressure or flow	—	—
PC-SIMV	Time	Pressure	Time	—	—	—	—	—	—	Patient	Pressure	Pressure or flow	Patient effort and time	Mandatory or assisted breath
PSV	—	—	—	—	—	—	Patient	Pressure	Flow	Patient	Pressure	Pressure or flow	—	—
CPAP	—	—	—	—	—	—	—	—	—	Patient	Pressure	Pressure or flow	—	—
APRV	Time	Pressure	Time	—	—	—	—	—	—	Patient	Pressure	Flow or pressure	—	—
PAV	—	—	—	—	—	—	Patient	Pressure	Flow	—	—	—	Patient effort, elastance and resistance	Increase or decrease pressure to overcome resistive and elastic work
DC within a breath VAPS	Time	Pressure or flow	Flow or volume	Patient	Pressure or flow	Flow or volume	Patient	Pressure or flow	Flow or volume	—	—	—	Delivered volume vs set tidal volume	If V_T > set = PSV breath; If V_T < set V_T = volume cycled breath

Mode											
DC breath to breath volume support	—	Pressure	Time	—	Patient	Pressure	Flow	—	—	Tidal volume	Increase or decrease pressure limit to keep V_T constant
DC breath to breath AutoFlow	Time	Pressure	Time	—	Patient	Pressure	—	—	—	Tidal volume	Increase or decrease pressure limit to keep V_T constant
ATC	—	—	—	—	Patient	Pressure	Flow	—	—	Patient flow demand	Pressure increases or decreases to overcome a known resistance
ASV	Time	Pressure	Time	—	Patient	Pressure	Flow	—	—	Patient effort changes in impedance	Deliver mandatory or supported breaths; Increase or decrease pressure limit to adjust VT; Change I:E to prevent air trapping

APRV, airway pressure release ventilation; ASV, adaptive support ventilation; ATC, automatic tube compensation; CPAP, continuous positive airway pressure; DC, dual control; I:E, inspiratory:expiratory ratio; PAV, proportional assist ventilation; PC-A/C, pressure control-assist/control (ventilation); PC-CMV, pressure control-continuous mandatory ventilation; PC-IMV, pressure control-intermittent mandatory ventilation; PC-SIMV, pressure control-synchronized IMV; PSV, pressure support ventilation; VC-A/C, volume control-assist/control (ventilation); VC-CMV, volume control-continuous mandatory ventilation; VC-IMV, volume control-intermittent mandatory ventilation; VC-SIMV, volume control-synchronized IMV; V_T, tidal volume.

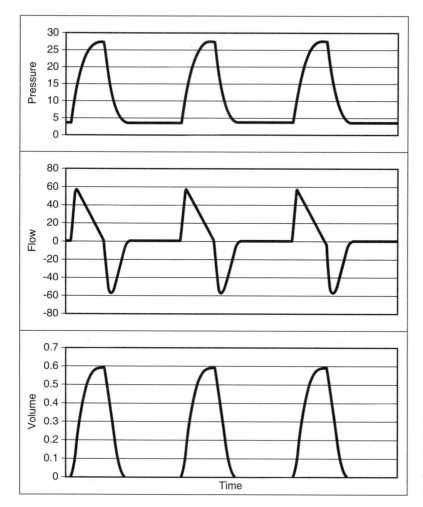

FIGURE 2–3
Pressure, flow, and volume vs. time during volume control-continuous mechanical ventilation (VC-CMV) with a decelerating flow pattern.

trigger the ventilator and receive an assisted breath at the volume or pressure set on the ventilator.[2-5] Machine- and patient-triggered breaths are delivered using the same limit and cycle variables. Technically speaking, the only difference between CMV and A/C ventilation is that during A/C ventilation, the patient also can trigger a breath. From a ventilator classification standpoint, this is a subtle difference. In fact, A/C ventilation could be considered "patient- and time-triggered CMV." However, the clinical implications of patient triggering and active respiratory muscles are clinically important. Distinguishing between breaths that are time triggered and those that are patient triggered is important to monitoring and manipulating the ventilator.

Other Terms. A/C ventilation has been described in the literature as assisted mechanical ventilation (AMV), assisted ventilation, and CMV with assist.

Manufacturer Terms. Many ventilators use the term CMV to describe assist/control, the only difference being the position of the sensitivity setting. Other terms include assist/control and volume control.

Classification. Regardless of the terminology used, A/C can be described as pressure or volume controlled; time, pressure, flow, or volume triggered; pressure, flow, or volume limited; and flow, volume, pressure, or time cycled (see Table 2–2). Again, it is quite obvious that although a group of similarly trained clinicians understand what the term A/C indicates, the term is too imprecise to allow real understanding. Using the simplified version, A/C ventilation can be

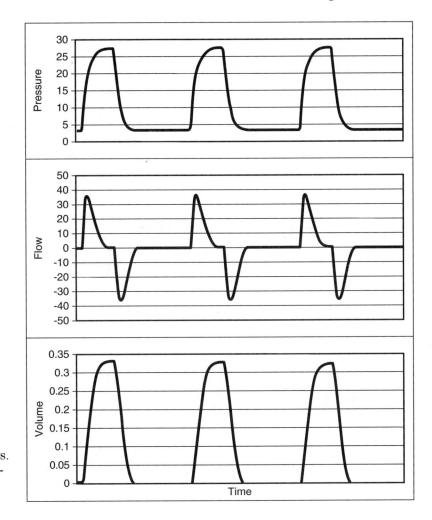

FIGURE 2–4

Pressure, flow, and volume vs. time during pressure control-continuous mechanical ventilation (PC-CMV).

described as pressure or volume controlled; machine and patient triggered; and machine cycled. Breaths would be either time triggered (based on the set rate) or patient triggered (based on patient effort and sensitivity). Thus, A/C ventilation combines mandatory and assisted breaths that can be either volume controlled (Fig. 2–5) or pressure controlled (Fig. 2–6).

Assisted Mechanical Ventilation

Descriptive Definition. Assisted mechanical ventilation (AMV) is a proposed version of A/C ventilation in which there is no set frequency.[2-5] In this case, all breaths are patient triggered and delivered at the ventilator's set tidal volume or pressure. This means that all breaths are assisted breaths.

Other Terms. The pure form of AMV, without a set backup rate, is not often discussed. The term assisted ventilation has been used but frequently alludes to A/C ventilation. MacIntyre prefers to call this mode pressure assist when the breaths are pressure controlled and volume assist when breaths are volume constant. These terms can be seen in subsequent chapters.

Manufacturer Terms. To our knowledge, no manufacturer labels a mode of operation as only assist. AMV can be produced by placing the patient in the CMV or A/C mode and turning the rate control to 0 breaths/min.

Classification. Assist mode ventilation is classified as volume or pressure controlled; pressure, flow, or volume triggered; flow, volume, or pressure limited; and time, flow, volume, or pressure cycled. The sim-

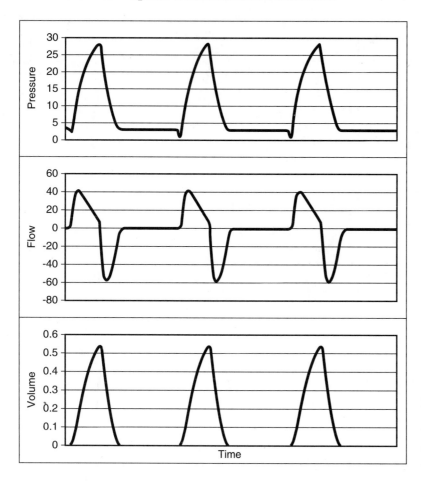

FIGURE 2–5
Pressure, flow, and volume vs. time during volume control-assist/control ventilation (VC-A/C).

pler classification system (see Table 2–2) classifies this mode as volume or pressure controlled; patient triggered; and machine cycled. Volume-controlled AMV and pressure-controlled AMV appear the same as Figures 2–5 and 2–6, except that every breath is patient triggered.

Intermittent Mandatory Ventilation

Descriptive Definition. Intermittent mandatory ventilation (IMV) is a mode of ventilator operation in which mandatory (machine) breaths are delivered at a set frequency and volume or pressure. Between machine breaths, the patient can breathe spontaneously from either a continuous flow of gas or demand system.[2–5, 7–12]

Other Terms. For the most part, IMV has survived the interchangeable name calling if not the derogatory name calling. At

one time, IMV was frequently referred to as intermittent demand ventilation (IDV) and was occasionally called "intermittent respiratory failure" by its most ardent critics.[13]

Manufacturer Terms. The terms IMV or synchronized IMV (SIMV, discussed subsequently) are used to identify this mode by most manufacturers. The term IMV sometimes is linked with continuous positive airway pressure (CPAP) on the mode selection switch, dial, or keypad.

Classification. As a mode, IMV presents the new problem of classifying both mandatory and spontaneous breaths. According to our classification system, mandatory breaths during IMV are volume or pressure controlled; time triggered; pressure, volume, or flow limited; and pressure, volume, flow, or time cycled. Spontaneous breaths are not controlled and therefore have no trigger, limit, or cycle variable if a continuous flow of gas is used. Demand systems (i.e., a sys-

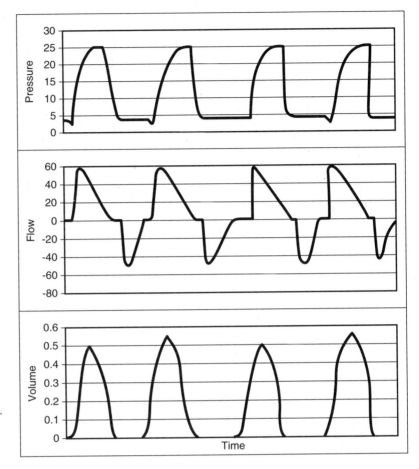

FIGURE 2–6
Pressure, flow, and volume vs. time during pressure control-assist/control ventilation (PC-A/C).

tem that responds to the patient's inspiratory effort by varying gas delivery) allow spontaneous breaths to be classified. During IMV, spontaneous breaths are pressure controlled; pressure, volume, or flow triggered; pressure limited; and pressure or flow cycled (see Table 2–2). Using the simpler system allows a more succinct description. Mandatory breaths are pressure or volume controlled; machine triggered; and machine cycled. Spontaneous breaths are pressure controlled, patient triggered, and patient cycled. Figure 2–7 demonstrates pressure, volume, and flow waveforms for pressure control IMV.

Synchronized Intermittent Mandatory Ventilation

Descriptive Definition. Synchronized intermittent mandatory ventilation (SIMV) is a version of IMV in which the ventilator creates a timing window around the scheduled delivery of the mandatory breath and attempts to deliver the breath in concert with the patient's inspiratory effort.[2–5, 13, 14] This mode uses a conditional variable to determine which type of breath to deliver. If no inspiratory effort occurs during this time, the ventilator delivers the mandatory breath at the scheduled time (time triggered). If the patient initiates an inspiration, the mandatory breath is synchronized with the patient's effort.

Other Terms. The term SIMV appears to be accepted universally, although the first description of this mode named it intermittent demand ventilation (IDV).[13]

Manufacturer Terms. All manufacturers who offer SIMV refer to it as such.

Classification. Classification of SIMV is identical to IMV, except that mandatory breaths can be machine or patient triggered. During SIMV, mandatory breaths are

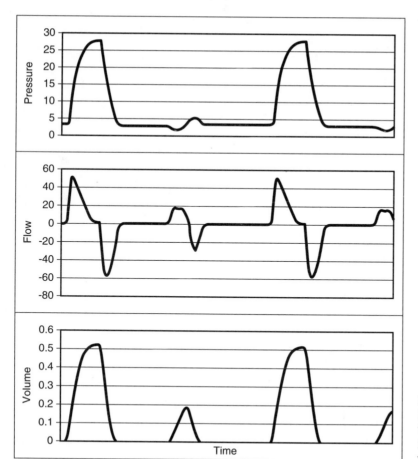

FIGURE 2–7
Pressure, flow, and volume vs. time during pressure control–intermittent mandatory ventilation (PC-IMV).

pressure or volume/flow controlled; time, pressure, flow, or volume triggered; pressure, volume, or flow limited; and pressure, volume, flow, or time cycled. Spontaneous breaths are pressure controlled; pressure, volume, or flow triggered; pressure limited; and pressure or flow cycled. The simpler classification describes mandatory breaths during SIMV as pressure or volume controlled; machine or patient triggered; and machine cycled. Spontaneous breaths are classified as pressure controlled, patient triggered, and patient cycled. Because of the synchronization process, SIMV is not possible with only a continuous flow source. Some authors describe demand flow IMV and continuous flow IMV as different modes, which clearly is not the case. Although the implications to the respiratory care practitioner are quite different, the fundamental operation is the same. Figure 2–8 demonstrates the SIMV "window" concept, which allows synchronization of the

mandatory breath with patient effort. Figure 2–9 demonstrates pressure control SIMV.

Pressure Support Ventilation

Descriptive Definition. Pressure support ventilation (PSV) is a mode of ventilator operation in which the patient's inspiratory effort is assisted by the ventilator up to a preset level of inspiratory pressure. Inspiration is terminated when peak inspiratory flow rate reaches a minimum level or a percentage of initial inspiratory flow. Quite simply, PSV is patient triggered, pressure limited, and flow cycled. This allows patients to determine their own frequency, inspiratory time, and tidal volume.[2–3, 15–17]

Other Terms. PSV has suffered a fate similar to CPAP in the variations of its name. The literature refers to PSV as inspi-

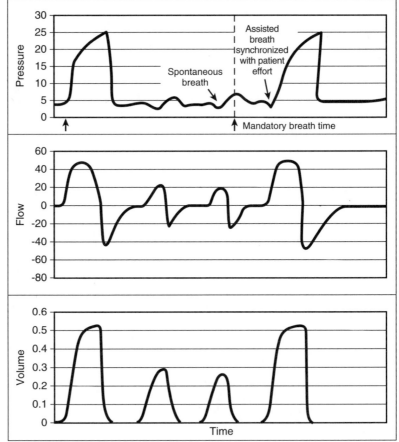

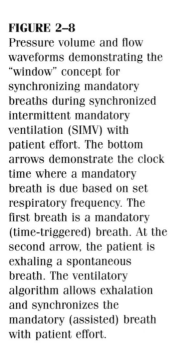

FIGURE 2–8
Pressure volume and flow waveforms demonstrating the "window" concept for synchronizing mandatory breaths during synchronized intermittent mandatory ventilation (SIMV) with patient effort. The bottom arrows demonstrate the clock time where a mandatory breath is due based on set respiratory frequency. The first breath is a mandatory (time-triggered) breath. At the second arrow, the patient is exhaling a spontaneous breath. The ventilatory algorithm allows exhalation and synchronizes the mandatory (assisted) breath with patient effort.

ratory assist (IA), inspiratory pressure support (IPS), spontaneous pressure support (SPS), and inspiratory flow assist (IFA). Ventilators used for noninvasive ventilation via a mask often are thought of as bilevel, but typically provide pressure support.

Manufacturer Terms. All manufacturers have different algorithms for the provision of pressure support, but all label it PSV. Unfortunately, the PSV mode often is invoked through the spontaneous mode control, leading some to believe that the ventilator is not providing positive pressure ventilation.

Classification. According to the definitions of spontaneous and mandatory breaths, all PSV breaths are spontaneous. However, because the inspiratory pressure is greater than the baseline pressure, breaths are considered *supported*. The difference between a spontaneous breath and a supported breath is that in the former,

inspiratory pressure equals baseline pressure, and in the latter, inspiratory pressure is greater than baseline pressure. Therefore, PSV can be classified as pressure controlled (pressure is constant); pressure, flow, or volume triggered; pressure limited; and flow cycled. The simpler classification is pressure-controlled, patient-triggered, pressure-limited, patient-cycled ventilation. Figure 2–10 depicts pressure, flow, and volume waveforms seen during pressure support ventilation.

Algorithms for delivering pressure support vary between manufacturers. The important components of the pressure support breath include the trigger, rise time to pressure, the limit, and the cycle variable. Triggering can be accomplished by ventilator detection of a change in pressure, flow, or other input. The speed at which the breath reaches the set pressure is referred to as the rise time. In many ventilators, this is preset and nonadjustable. Other ventilators

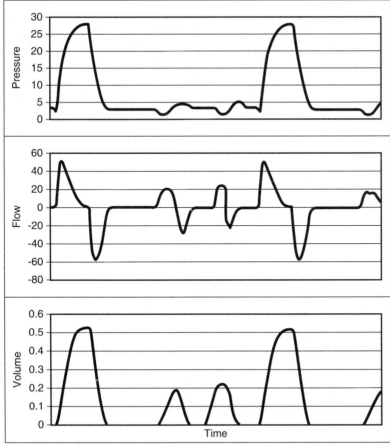

FIGURE 2–9
Pressure, flow, and volume vs. time during pressure control-intermittent mandatory ventilation (PC-SIMV).

use a clinician-set control to adjust the speed (faster or slower) at which the ventilator attempts to reach the pressure limit. If the speed is too fast, "overshoot" of the pressure limit can occur and premature cycling may result. If the speed is too slow, the patient's work of breathing increases. The limit variable demonstrates the ability of the ventilator to maintain a constant pressure.

The cycle variable of a pressure support breath typically is flow. Two schemes are commonly used, a percentage of the initial peak flow or a set terminal flow. However, there are other cycle variables implemented for safety. These typically include time and pressure. During a pressure support breath, the longest allowed inspiratory time is usually 3 seconds. This prevents prolonged inspiratory times when a low cycle flow criterion is used (i.e., 5 L/min) in the presence of an air leak. Cycling of the PSV breath also can occur if the pressure exceeds the set

pressure by a set value (1.5 cm H_2O) or the pressure alarm setting is reached. In most ventilators, these cycle variables are buried in the software. However, some ventilators (Bear 3, Bear Medical Systems, Riverside, CA, and Hamilton Galileo, Hamilton Medical, Reno, NV) allow the flow cycle variable to be set at a percentage of the initial flow. Figure 2–11 depicts the important components of a pressure support breath. Table 2–3 compares the capabilities of currently available ventilators in the pressure support mode.

Simplicity always has been a hallmark of the pressure support mode. However, these changes can allow the more sophisticated clinician to tailor the mode to the patient's needs. As examples, looking at the Puritan Bennett 7200ae (Puritan Bennett Corp., Carlsbad, CA) and Hamilton Galileo may provide some clarity.

The 7200ae uses pressure or flow triggering, has a set rise time, and cycles when

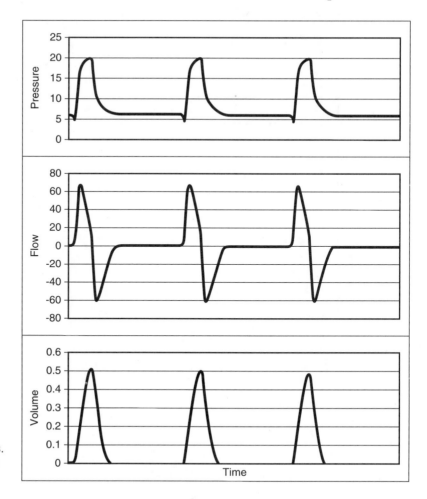

FIGURE 2–10
Pressure, flow, and volume vs. time during pressure support ventilation (PSV).

flow reaches a set flow of 5 L/min. Secondary cycle variables include an inspiratory time greater than 3.0 seconds and a pressure 1.5 cm H_2O greater than the set pressure limit. In this case, it is not unusual to

see pressure support breaths become pressure cycled, when the patient wants to exhale before the ventilator reaches the 5 L/min flow criteria (Fig. 2–12).

The Galileo can be pressure or flow trig-

FIGURE 2–11
Important components of a pressure support breath. (A) Trigger; (B) rise time; (C) pressure limit (plateau); (D) cycle. Under ideal conditions, the PSV breath appears as the solid line. Alterations in patient effort and ventilator algorithm can cause the pressure waveform to appear different. A1, inappropriate sensitivity setting or slow response time; B1, slow rise time relative to patient demand, which can result in an increased work of breathing; B2, rise time too fast, causing overshoot and contributing to premature cycling; D1, inspiratory time too long (caused by late-cycle criteria), causing the patient to exhale, creating a pressure spike; D2, breath cycles too early because of B2 or early cycle criteria.

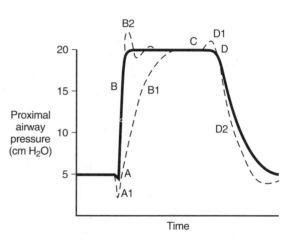

TABLE 2–3. Comparison of the Pressure Support Mode Operation of Different Ventilators

VENTILATOR	TRIGGER	RISE TIME	CYCLE VARIABLE			FLOW CYCLE (FIXED OR ADJUSTABLE)
			Flow	Pressure	Time	
Bear 1000	Flow or pressure	Adjustable	25%	Pressure alarm	3.0 s	Fixed
Bear 3	Pressure	Fixed	25%	Pressure alarm	3.0 s	Adjustable 25–50%
Bird 8400	Flow or pressure	Fixed	25%	Pressure alarm	3.0 s	Fixed
Bird Tbird (Therma Respiratory Group, Riverside, CA)	Flow or pressure	Fixed	25%	Pressure alarm	3.0 s	Fixed
Drager E4 (Drager, Telford, PA)	Flow or pressure	Adjustable	25% adult 6% pediatric	Pressure alarm	4.0 s adult 1.5 s pediatric	Fixed
Hamilton Galileo (Hamilton Medical, Reno, NV)	Flow or pressure	Adjustable	25%	Pressure alarm	25%	Adjustable 10–50%
Puritan Bennett 7200 (Mallinckrodt, Carlsbad, CA)	Flow or pressure	Fixed	5 L/min	1.5 cm above set	3.0 s	Fixed
Puritan Bennett 840 (Mallinckrodt, Carlsbad, CA)	Flow or pressure	Adjustable	25%	2 cm H_2O above set	2.0 s	Adjustable 1–45%
Puritan Bennett 740 (Mallinckrodt, Carlsbad, CA)	Flow or pressure	Fixed	25%	2 cm H_2O above set	2.0 s	Fixed
Pulmonetics LTV 1000 (Pulmonetic Systems, Inc., Colton, CA)	Flow	Adjustable	25%	High pressure	3.0 s	Adjustable Flow 10–40% Time 0.5–3.0 s
Siemens 900C	Pressure	Fixed	25%	High pressure	3.0 s	Fixed
Siemens 300 (Siemens, Danvers, MA)	Flow or pressure	Adjustable	5%	High pressure	80% of total cycle time	Fixed

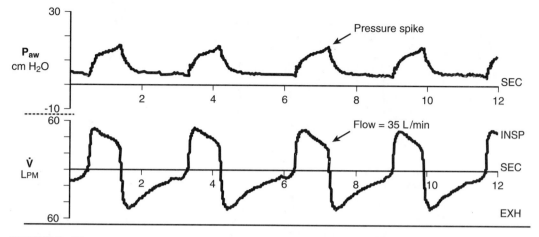

FIGURE 2-12

Pressure and flow waveforms demonstrating pressure cycling of a pressure support breath. The flow cycle criteria is 5 L/min. However, because the patient exhales before flow decelerating to this value, the breath is cycled by pressure (1.5 cm H_2O above set pressure limit). The inspiratory flow at the time the breath is terminated is 35 L/min.

gered, the rise time is adjustable between 50 and 200 msec, and the flow cycle variable is adjustable from 10% to 40% of the initial peak flow. Secondary cycle criteria include an inspiratory time greater than 3.0 seconds and a pressure exceeding the high pressure alarm setting. Figure 2-13 depicts a normal pressure support breath, with additional breaths demonstrating the effects of altering rise time and expiratory termination (cycle) criteria.

Continuous Positive Airway Pressure

Descriptive Definition. Continuous positive airway pressure (CPAP) is a mode of ventilator operation in which a clinician-set level of pressure is maintained constant while the patient is allowed to breathe spontaneously.[2-5, 18]

Other Terms. Few processes have garnered the virtual avalanche of acronyms heaped on CPAP. Although differences do exist, the following all have been used to describe or have been used interchangeably with CPAP: positive end-expiratory pressure (PEEP), end-expiratory pressure (EEP), inspiratory positive airway pressure (IPAP), expiratory positive airway pressure

(EPAP), continuous distending pressure (CDP), and continuous positive pressure breathing (CPPB). The most common explanation of the difference between PEEP and CPAP is that PEEP is elevated baseline pressure during mechanical ventilation, whereas CPAP is elevated baseline pressure during spontaneous breathing. This explanation falls short when IMV is used because an elevated baseline pressure is used after both spontaneous and mandatory breaths. Perhaps the best way to differentiate the two is that CPAP is, as we are discussing, a mode of ventilatory operation, whereas PEEP is simply control of baseline pressure during use of a separate mode of ventilation. On some occasions, CPAP has been described as IMV with a frequency of 0.

Manufacturer Terms. The term CPAP is used by all manufacturers to describe this mode. In some instances, there is a control labeled CPAP, and in others the mode is accessed via the "spontaneous" mode. In both cases, the level of end-expiratory pressure is selected using a baseline or PEEP/CPAP control.

Classification. Because CPAP is devoid of mandatory breaths, only the spontaneous breaths need to be considered. Spontaneous breaths are pressure controlled; pressure, flow, or volume triggered; pressure limited;

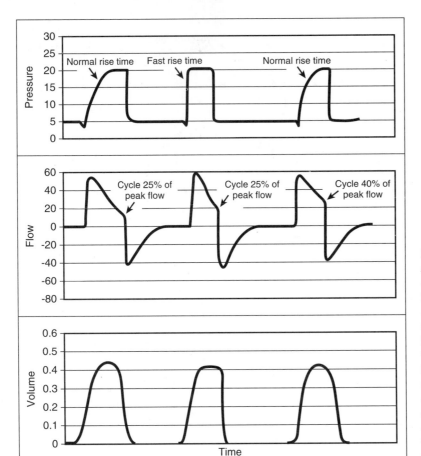

FIGURE 2–13
A pressure support breath (left) and the effects of increasing the rise time (middle) and decreasing the cycle criteria (right). As rise time increases, flow and volume increase whereas inspiratory time tends to decrease. When rise time is constant and the cycle criteria changes from 25% to 40% of peak flow, inspiratory time is shortened and tidal volume tends to diminish.

and pressure or flow cycled. More simply, CPAP is pressure-controlled, patient-triggered, patient-cycled, unsupported spontaneous breathing. Figure 2–14 depicts spontaneous breathing during CPAP.

Airway Pressure Release Ventilation

Descriptive Definition. Airway pressure release ventilation (APRV) often is described as two levels of CPAP that are applied for set periods of time, allowing spontaneous breathing to occur at both levels. This mode is said to allow the clinician to set the two CPAP levels (known as CPAP or pressure high and release pressure or pressure low) and the time spent at each level (time high or inspiratory time and time low or expiratory time).[2–5, 19–23]

Other Terms. APRV has been referred to as bilevel airway pressure (BiPAP), variable positive airway pressure (VPAP), intermittent CPAP, and CPAP with release.

Manufacturer Terms. The Drager Dura and Evita 4 (Drager Inc., Telford, PA) offer APRV and use that terminology. The Puritan Bennett 840 provides APRV and calls the mode bilevel.

Classification. Scrutiny of the APRV pressure, volume, and flow waveforms demonstrates its similarity to pressure control inverse ratio ventilation (PCIRV). In fact, if spontaneous breathing is absent, the two modes are indistinguishable. Mandatory breaths (which occur when the pressure increases from low pressure to higher pressure) are pressure controlled, time triggered, pressure limited, and time cycled. Spontaneous breaths are pressure controlled, pressure triggered, pressure limited, and pressure cycled during APRV (Fig. 2–15). In the original description by Downs

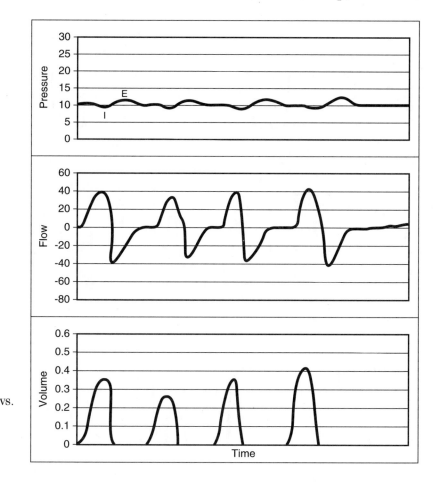

FIGURE 2–14
Pressure, flow, and volume vs. time during continuous positive airway pressure (CPAP). I, inspiration; E, expiration.

and Stock,[19] a continuous flow of gas was used; therefore, spontaneous breaths were not controlled. This mode demonstrates the strength of this classification system. Whereas proponents of APRV talk about bi-level CPAP, dropping from CPAP to release pressure, applying the classification principles unmasks the black box. Certainly, every neonatal ventilator performs what has been described as APRV and has done so for more than 20 years.

The uniqueness of APRV rests in how it is applied, not in the specific ventilator function. In a patient who is paralyzed, APRV is simply pressure control, time-triggered, pressure-limited, time-cycled ventilation. However, when the patient is breathing spontaneously, the transition of pressure from higher to lower results in tidal movement of gas and subsequent carbon dioxide elimination. The short expiratory time (time at the low pressure) prevents complete exhalation and maintains alveolar distension.

The ability of APRV to allow the patient to breathe spontaneously during any phase of the ventilator's mechanical cycle makes it a viable alternative as a partial support mode.

Pressure Control Inverse Ratio Ventilation

Descriptive Definition. Pressure control inverse ratio ventilation (PCIRV) is a particular version of pressure control-CMV (PC-CMV) in which all breaths are pressure limited and time cycled and the patient cannot initiate an inspiration.[2-5, 24-29] Additionally, as the name implies, inspiration is longer than expiration.

Other Terms. PCIRV sometimes is shortened simply to IRV; otherwise, it has few aliases.

Manufacturer Terms. No manufacturer has labeled a mode as PCIRV. In most in-

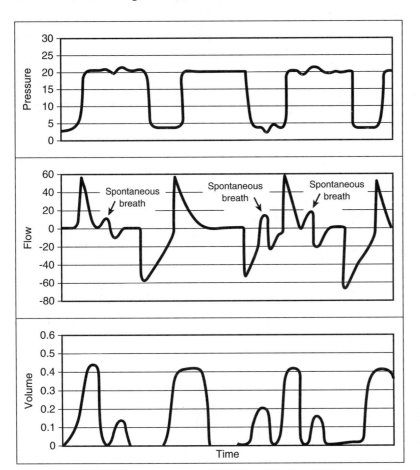

FIGURE 2–15
Pressure, flow, and volume vs. time during airway pressure release ventilation (APRV).

stances, PCIRV is initiated by selecting the PCV mode and adjusting parameters to provide the desired inspiratory:expiratory (I:E) ratio.

Classification. PCIRV can be classified as pressure controlled, time triggered, pressure limited, and time cycled. All breaths are mandatory. The simpler classification refers to PCIRV as pressure controlled, machine triggered, pressure limited, and machine cycled (Fig. 2–16). These descriptions should lead the reader to question why PCIRV is considered a separate mode because the only difference between it and PCV is the I:E ratio. Volume-oriented modes are not classified separately with respect to I:E ratio, although VCV certainly can be delivered using a prolonged inspiratory time (Fig. 2–17). This technique is not a new mode but rather is pressure control CMV in which the inspiratory time is longer than the expiratory time.

Mandatory Minute Ventilation

Descriptive Definition. Mandatory minute ventilation (MMV) is a mode of ventilator operation that allows the patient to breathe spontaneously yet ensures that a minimum level of minute ventilation (V_E), set by the clinician, always is achieved.[4, 5, 30–32] This can be accomplished by the use of increasing levels of PSV (Hamilton Veolar)[6] or by delivery of mandatory breaths (BEAR 5,[33] Drager E4[34]).

Other Terms. MMV has been called minimum minute volume, augmented minute volume (AMV), and extended mandatory minute ventilation (EMMV).

Manufacturer Terms. The initial description of MMV was termed mandatory minute volume, and ventilators use all the terms listed previously (EMMV, MMV, AMV).

Classification. MMV is one of the modes

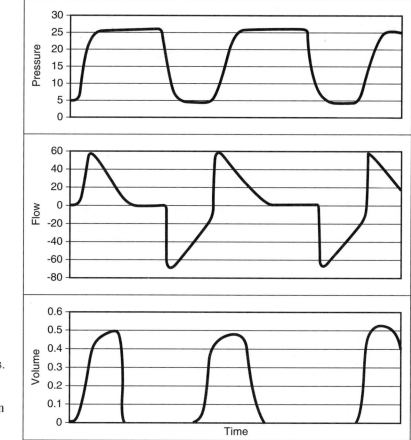

FIGURE 2–16

Pressure, flow, and volume vs. time during pressure control-continuous mandatory ventilation (PC-CMV) using an inspiratory time greater than the expiratory time.

in which the conditional variable (in this case, V_E) is critically important to classification. In fact, MMV is the first of the modes that can be considered closed loop modes. Closed loop simply means that the ventilator changes its output based on a measured input variable. If spontaneous breathing is used, breaths are pressure controlled; pressure, flow, or volume triggered; pressure limited; and flow cycled. Essentially, the patient is receiving pressure support ventilation with a varying pressure support level. As long as the conditional variable is met, this system does not change. If V_E decreases below the minimum, classification depends on the ventilator used. With the Hamilton Veolar, breaths are supported with increasing levels of PSV. In this instance, there are still no mandatory breaths. Therefore, MMV is pressure controlled; pressure, flow, or volume triggered; pressure limited; and flow cycled. The sim-

pler classification is pressure-controlled, patient-triggered, pressure-limited, patient-cycled ventilation. If the conditional variable is not met with the other ventilators, mandatory breaths are delivered. In this case, the ventilator anticipates the minute volume based on the minute volume occurring in the past 30 seconds. If the predicted minute volume is lower than the set minute volume, mandatory breaths at the volume set on the ventilator are delivered to make up the difference. This creates an IMV-like situation in which both spontaneous and mandatory breaths must be described. Spontaneous breaths are classified identically to CPAP or PSV depending on the clinician's setting of parameters, and mandatory breaths are volume/flow controlled, time triggered, flow or volume limited, and time or flow cycled. More simply, mandatory breaths are volume controlled, machine initiated, and machine cycled.

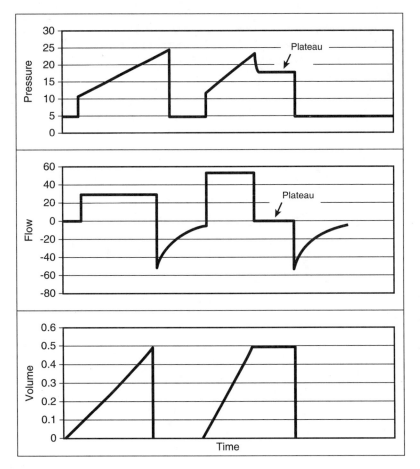

FIGURE 2-17
Pressure, flow, and volume vs. time during volume control-continuous mandatory ventilation (VC-CMV) using an inspiratory time greater than the expiratory time. On the left, this is accomplished by a low inspiratory flow, and on the right, by using normal flows with an inspiratory pause.

COMBINING MODES

Modes of ventilator operation do not have to be used in isolation. Although certain modes have to stand alone based on their function, others can be combined. We have previously discussed the combination of IMV and CPAP. Essentially, any mode that has both spontaneous breathing and mandatory breaths can be combined. For instance, PSV can be combined with IMV, but not with CMV. In these cases, creation of a new term to describe the combined modes is undesirable. It is simpler and more descriptive to acknowledge the contributions of each mode (i.e., IMV + PSV, IMV + CPAP).

DUAL CONTROL MODES OF MECHANICAL VENTILATION

Dual control modes are capable of controlling either pressure or volume based on a measured input variable. They cannot control both at the same time, but rather one or the other. There are currently two techniques for performing dual control. We prefer to think of these techniques as dual control within a breath and dual control from breath to breath. The former uses a measured input to switch from pressure control to volume control in the middle of the breath. The latter simply uses a measured input to manipulate the pressure level of a pressure-limited breath (either pressure control mandatory breath or a pressure support breath).

Dual Control Within a Breath

Descriptive Definition. These modes allow the ventilator to deliver a pressure support breath (pressure control) or switch from a pressure support breath to a volume-controlled breath within the breath. As such, two types of breaths can be delivered during **volume-assured pressure support** (VAPS). The first is a pressure-controlled, patient- or time-triggered, pressure-limited, and flow cycled breath. The second is a volume-controlled, patient- or time-triggered, flow-limited, volume-cycled breath.

Manufacturer Terms. VAPS (Bird 8400ST and Tbird, Bird Corp., Palm Springs, CA) and pressure augmentation (PA) (Bear 1000, Bear Medical, Riverside, CA) are common terms. Although both manufacturers use a different mode name, operation is the same.

Other Terms. VAPS sometimes is known as volume-assisted pressure support. Currently, no other ventilators use this mode or another name.

Classification. Both of these techniques can operate during mandatory breaths or pressure-supported breaths. Conceptually, VAPS and PA are meant to combine the high variable flow of a pressure-limited breath with the constant volume delivery of a volume-limited breath. The initial description of VAPS by Amato and associates[35] described volume-*assisted* pressure support. This initial report clearly considers VAPS a technique to be used instead of volume control-continuous mandatory ventilation (VC-CMV). During pressure support, VAPS and PA can be considered a safety net that always supplies a minimum tidal volume.

During VAPS and PA, the clinician must set the respiratory frequency, peak flow, PEEP, inspired oxygen concentration, trigger sensitivity, and minimum desired tidal volume. During VAPS or PA, the ventilator's inspiratory flow waveform is constant (square). Additionally, the pressure support setting must be set. The pressure support control is nonfunctional during VC-CMV unless the VAPS or PA mode is activated. Selecting the appropriate pressure support setting is difficult, and no studies have been accomplished that identify the best setting. Our practice has been to set the pressure support setting at a level equivalent to the plateau pressure obtained during a volume control breath at the desired tidal volume. The peak flow setting is also important dur-

ing VAPS and PA. Peak flow should be adjusted to allow for the appropriate inspiratory time and I:E ratio required by the patient.[36-38]

A VAPS or PA breath may be initiated by the patient or time triggered. Once the breath is triggered, the ventilator attempts to reach the pressure support setting as quickly as possible. This portion of the breath is the pressure control portion and is associated with a rapid variable flow, which may reduce the work of breathing. As this pressure level is reached, the ventilator's microprocessor determines the volume that has been delivered from the machine (note that this is not exhaled tidal volume), compares this measurement with the desired tidal volume, and determines whether the minimum desired tidal volume will be reached.

There are several differences in ventilator output based on the relationship between delivered and set tidal volume. These are shown in Figure 2–18. If the delivered tidal volume and set tidal volume are equivalent, the breath is a pressure support breath. That is, the breath is pressure limited at the pressure support setting and flow cycled—in this instance, at 25% of the initial peak flow. This type of breath occurring during VAPS is shown in Figure 2–18, breath A.

If the patient's inspiratory effort is diminished, the ventilator delivers a smaller volume, and when delivered and set volume are compared, the microprocessor determines that the minimum set tidal volume will not be delivered. As the flow decelerates and reaches the set peak flow, the breath changes from a pressure-limited to a volume-limited breath. The flow remains constant, increasing the inspiratory time, until the volume has been delivered. Again, remember that the volume is volume exiting the ventilator not exhaled tidal volume. During this time, the pressure increases above the set pressure support setting. Setting the high pressure alarm remains important during VAPS. If pressure increases abruptly, the high pressure alarm setting is reached and the breath is pressure cycled. This type of breath is shown in Figure 2–18, breath B.

A similar condition can occur if there is

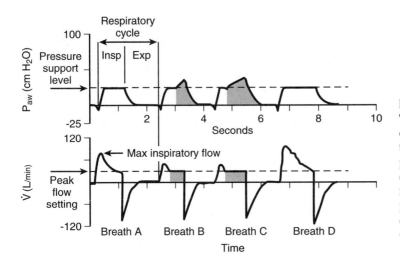

FIGURE 2–18
The possible breath delivery characteristics occurring during the use of volume-assured pressure support. See text for details. (Used with permission from Branson RD: Volume assured pressure support ventilation: a clinical manual. Bird Products Corporation, Palm Springs, CA, 1996.)

an acute decrease in lung compliance or increase in airways resistance. This is shown in Figure 2–18, breath C. The same sequence of events occurs as described for breath B. However, this breath demonstrates the possibility of prolonging inspiratory time during a VAPS breath. There are secondary cycle characteristics for these breaths, and an inspiratory time lasting longer than 3 seconds automatically is time cycled. This finding suggests that when used for patients with airflow obstruction, intrusions of the constant flow on the patient's I:E ratio should be monitored.

Lastly, and perhaps most importantly, the VAPS breath can allow the patient a tidal volume larger than the set volume. Because the pressure limit remains the same, this breath is also a pressure support breath (i.e., it is pressure limited and flow cycled). Figure 2–18, breath D demonstrates the effect of an increase in patient effort. This system allows for normal variations in patient tidal volume and sighing and increased volumes during times of hyperpnea.

VAPS then is patient or machine triggered, pressure or flow limited (depending on the relationship of set and actual tidal volume), and flow or volume cycled.

Dual Control Breath to Breath—Pressure-Limited, Flow-Cycled Ventilation

Descriptive Definition. Dual control breath to breath in the pressure support

mode quite simply is closed loop pressure support ventilation, with tidal volume as the input variable.

Manufacturer Terms. Volume support (Siemens 300, Siemens Medical Systems, Inc., Danvers, MA) and variable pressure support (Venturi, Cardiopulmonary Corporation, New Haven, CT) are commonly used terms.

Other Terms. No other terms are used.

Classification. Dual control breath to breath during the pressure support mode was introduced on the Siemens 300 ventilator. Volume support is pressure support ventilation that uses tidal volume as a feedback control for continuously adjusting the pressure support level.[39, 40] All breaths are patient triggered, pressure limited, and flow cycled. Volume support is selected with the mode selector switch, and the desired tidal volume is set. The ventilator initiates volume support by delivering a "test breath" with a peak pressure of 5 cm H_2O when a patient effort is sensed. The delivered tidal volume (again, this is not exhaled tidal volume, but volume exiting the ventilator) is measured, and total system compliance is calculated. The following three breaths are delivered at a peak inspiratory pressure of 75% of the pressure calculated to deliver the minimum tidal volume. Each subsequent breath uses the previous calculation of system compliance to manipulate peak pressure to achieve the desired tidal volume. From breath to breath, the maximum pressure change is less than 3 cm H_2O and can range from 0 cm H_2O above PEEP to 5 cm H_2O below the high-pressure alarm setting. Because all breaths are pressure support breaths, cycling normally occurs at 5% of the initial peak flow. A secondary cycling mechanism is activated if inspiratory time exceeds 80% of the set total cycle time. There is also a relationship between the set ventilator frequency and tidal volume. If the desired tidal volume is 500 ml and the respiratory frequency is set at 15 breaths per minute, the minute volume setting is 7.5 L/min. If the patient's respiratory frequency decreases below 15 breaths per minute, the tidal volume target automatically is increased by the ventilator up to 150% of the initial value (in this example, 750 ml). This is done in an effort to maintain the minute volume constant. Figure 2–19 depicts the volume support mode response to a decrease in lung compliance. If lung compliance increases, the opposite response (decreasing

pressure support and constant tidal volume) occurs.

Dual Control Breath to Breath—Pressure-Limited, Time-Cycled Ventilation

Descriptive Definition. Dual control in the pressure control mode, like volume support, is simply closed loop pressure-controlled, patient- or time-triggered, pressure-limited, time-cycled ventilation with tidal volume as the input variable.

Manufacturer Terms. Pressure-regulated volume control (PRVC) (Siemens 300), Adaptive pressure ventilation (APV) (Hamilton Galileo), Auto-flow (Evita 4), and Variable pressure control (Venturi) are commonly used terms.

Other Terms. No other terms are used.

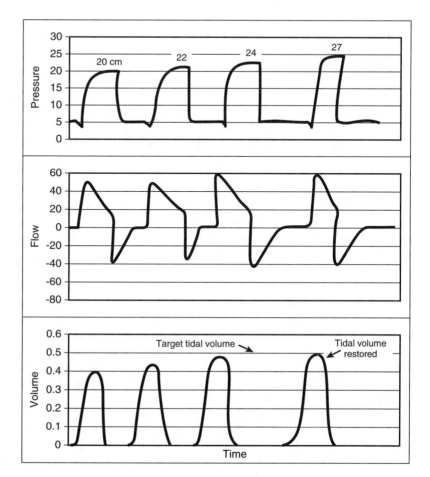

FIGURE 2–19
The effect of decreased compliance on dual control breath to breath (pressure support). The target tidal volume is 500 ml. When compliance decreases, pressure increases gradually until tidal volume is restored.

Classification. All these techniques are forms of pressure-limited, time-cycled ventilation that use tidal volume as a feedback control for continuously adjusting the pressure limit. As such, these modes are patient or machine triggered, pressure limited, and time cycled, with tidal volume as the conditional variable used to change the pressure limit.[41] As in previous examples, the volume signal used for ventilator feedback is not exhaled tidal volume, but volume exiting the ventilator. This prevents a kind of runaway effect that could occur if a leak in the circuit prevented accurate measurement of exhaled tidal volume. Despite the fact that each technique has a different name, operation is fairly consistent between devices. All breaths in these modes are time or patient triggered, pressure limited, and time cycled. One difference between devices is that the Siemens 300 only allows PRVC in the CMV mode. The other ventilators allow dual control breath to breath using CMV or SIMV. During SIMV, the mandatory breaths are the dual control breaths. Volume measurement for the feedback signal is also different between ventilators. The Siemens 300 uses the volume leaving the inspiratory flow sensor. The Hamilton Galileo uses the flow sensor at the airway and the inspiratory flow sensor to determine an average volume. This latter technique eliminates compressible volume, can detect the presence of leaks, and may be the preferred method of volume monitoring in dual control.

PRVC is selected on the mode selector switch, and the desired tidal volume is set. Like volume support, a "test breath" is delivered, and total system compliance is calculated. The next three breaths are delivered at a pressure limit 75% of that necessary to achieve the desired tidal volume based on the compliance calculation. The ensuing breaths increase or decrease the pressure limit at less than 3 cm H_2O per breath in an attempt to deliver the desired tidal volume. The pressure limit fluctuates between 0 cm H_2O above the PEEP level to 5 cm H_2O below the upper-pressure alarm setting. The ventilator sounds an alarm if the tidal volume and maximum pressure limit settings are incompatible.

Like volume support, the proposed advantage of PRVC or other dual control breath to breath modes is maintaining the minimum peak pressure, which provides a constant set tidal volume and automatic weaning of the pressure as the patient improves. Likewise, during periods of limited staffing, these modes maintain a more consistent tidal volume as compliance decreases or increases. Figure 2-20 depicts the effects of increasing compliance on the ventilator response during dual control breath to breath.

AUTOMODE

Descriptive Definition. AutoMode combines dual control breath to breath time-cycled breaths with dual control breath to breath flow-cycled breaths. AutoMode allows the ventilator to alternate between these two modes based on another input. In this instance, patient effort or the lack of patient effort determines whether the breaths are time cycled or flow cycled.

Manufacturer Terms. AutoMode is a mode available on the Siemens 300A ventilator.

Other Terms. No other terms are used.

Classification. AutoMode combines volume support and PRVC in a single mode. If the patient is paralyzed, the ventilator provides PRVC. All breaths are mandatory breaths that are time triggered, pressure limited, and time cycled. The pressure limit increases or decreases to maintain the desired tidal volume set by the clinician. If the patient breathes spontaneously for two consecutive breaths, the ventilator switches to volume support. In this case, all breaths are supported breaths that are patient triggered, pressure limited, and flow cycled. If the patient becomes apneic for 12 seconds in the adult setting, 8 seconds in the pediatric setting, or 5 seconds in the neonatal setting, the ventilator switches back to the PRVC mode. The change from PRVC to volume support is accomplished at equivalent peak pressures. This mode is simply the combination of two existing modes using the conditional variable of patient effort to decide whether the next breath is time cycled or flow cycled.

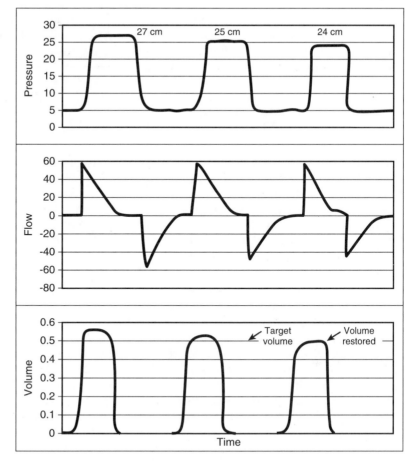

FIGURE 2–20

The effects of an improvement in compliance on dual control breath to breath (pressure control). The target tidal volume is 500 ml. As compliance improves, tidal volume exceeds the target. Pressure is decreased by 1- to 3-cm H_2O increments on a breath-to-breath basis until the tidal volume target is achieved.

AutoMode also switches between pressure control and pressure support or volume control to volume support. In the volume control to volume support switch, the volume support pressure limit is equivalent to the pause pressure during volume control. If an inspiratory plateau is not available, the pressure level is calculated as (Peak pressure − PEEP) × 50% + PEEP. AutoMode only recently has been introduced. One concern is that during the switch from time-cycled to flow-cycled ventilation, mean airway pressure will decrease. This may result in hypoxemia in the patient with acute lung injury. The ventilator's algorithm is fairly simple, and the patient is either assisting all the breaths or none of the breaths.

ADAPTIVE SUPPORT VENTILATION

Descriptive Definition. Adaptive support ventilation (ASV) is a mode that com-

bines the dual control breath to breath time-cycled and flow-cycled breaths and allows the ventilator to choose the initial ventilator settings based on the clinician input of ideal body weight and percent minute volume. This is the most sophisticated of closed loop techniques, allowing the ventilator to choose set respiratory frequency, tidal volume, pressure limit of mandatory and spontaneous breaths, inspiratory time of mandatory breaths, and, when spontaneous breathing is absent, I:E ratio.

Manufacturer Terms. Adaptive support ventilation (ASV) (Hamilton Galileo) is used.

Other Terms. No other terms are used.

Classification. ASV is based on the minimal work of breathing concept developed by Arthur B. Otis, which was published in 1950.[42] This concept suggests that the patient breathes at a tidal volume and respiratory frequency that minimizes the elastic and resistive loads while maintaining oxygenation and acid–base balance. Otis and colleagues[42] developed an equation that describes the minimal work concept shown below:

$$RR = \sqrt{\frac{1 + 4\pi^2\, RC \cdot (V'A/VD) - 1}{2\pi^2 RC}}$$

where RR = respiratory rate, RC = respiratory time constant, VA = alveolar ventilation, and VD = deadspace volume.

The ASV algorithm uses this formula along with patient weight (which determines deadspace) to adjust a number of ventilator variables. The clinician inputs the patient's ideal body weight; sets the high pressure alarm, PEEP, and inspired oxygen concentration; and adjusts the rise time and flow cycle variable for pressure support breaths from 10% to 40% of initial peak flow. The ventilator attempts to deliver 100 ml/min/kg of minute ventilation for an adult and 200 ml/min/kg for children. This can be adjusted by a setting known as the percent minute volume control. This control can be set from 20% to 200%. In the latter case, 200%, a minute volume of 200 ml/min/kg would be delivered to an adult patient. This setting allows the clinician to provide full ventilatory support or encourage spontaneous breathing and facilitate weaning.

When connected to the patient, the ventilator delivers a series of test breaths and measures system compliance, airway resistance, and intrinsic PEEP (PEEPi) using a least squares, fitting technique.[43, 44] This measurement system is important for accurate measurement of variables used in the minimal work equation. The input of body weight allows the ventilator algorithm to choose a required minute volume. The ventilator then uses the clinician input and measured respiratory mechanics to select a respiratory frequency, inspiratory time, I:E ratio, and pressure limit for mandatory and spontaneous breaths. These variables are measured on a breath-to-breath basis and are altered by the ventilator's algorithm to meet the desired targets. If the patient breathes spontaneously, the ventilator pressure supports breaths and encourages spontaneous breathing. However, spontaneous

TABLE 2–4. The Minimum and Maximum Values for Ventilator Variables

VARIABLE	MINIMUM	MAXIMUM
Peak pressure limit	PEEP + 5 cm H$_2$O	Clinician set high-pressure limit
Tidal volume	4.4 ml/kg	15.4 ml/kg
Respiratory frequency	5 bpm	60 bpm
Inspiratory time	0.5 s or 1 RC	2 × RC
Expiratory time	2 × RC	None

PEEP, positive end-expiratory pressure; RC, expiratory time constant.

and mandatory breaths can be combined to meet the minute ventilation target. The pressure limit of both the mandatory and spontaneous breaths are always being adjusted. This means that ASV continuously is employing dual control breath to breath of mandatory and spontaneous breaths.

The ventilator also can adjust the I:E ratio and inspiratory time of mandatory breaths to prevent air trapping and PEEPi. This is done by calculation of the expiratory time constant (compliance × resistance) and maintenance of sufficient expiratory time (Table 2–4).

If the patient is paralyzed, the ventilator determines the respiratory frequency, tidal volume, pressure limit required to deliver that tidal volume, inspiratory time, and I:E ratio. As the patient begins to breathe spontaneously, the number of mandatory breaths decreases and the ventilator chooses a pressure support level that maintains a tidal volume sufficient to ensure alveolar ventilation, based on a deadspace calculation of 2.2 ml/kg.

As a synopsis, ASV can provide pressure-limited, time-cycled ventilation, add dual control of those breaths on a breath-to-breath basis, allow for mandatory breaths and spontaneous breaths (a kind of dual control PC-SIMV + pressure support) and eventually switch to pressure support with dual control breath to breath (variable pressure with each pressure support breath). During mandatory breath delivery, the ventilator can set inspiratory time and I:E ratio.[45–50]

AUTOMATIC TUBE COMPENSATION

Descriptive Definition. Automatic tube compensation is a technique of ventilator operation that uses the known resistive characteristics of artificial airways to overcome the imposed work of breathing caused by those airways.[51, 52]

Manufacturer Term. Automatic tube compensation (ATC) (Evita 4, Drager Inc., Telford, PA) is the common term.

Other Terms. No other terms are used.

Classification. ATC is pressure controlled, patient triggered, pressure limited, and flow cycled. The pressure delivered is a consequence of the known resistive characteristics of the airway and the flow demand of the patient. As the airway diameter decreases, the pressure applied for any given flow increases. As the flow demand increases, the pressure increases for any given airway caliber.

According to Poiseuille's law, pressure decrease across the endotracheal tube is inversely proportional to the radius to the fourth power and is directly proportional to the length. Increasing flow through the same size endotracheal tube results in a curvilinear increase in resistance. Several investigators have advocated using pressure support ventilation to overcome the imposed work presented by the endotracheal tube.[53–55] This method requires increasing pressure support levels as endotracheal tube diameter diminishes and inspiratory flow increases. Under static conditions, pressure support can effectively eliminate endotracheal tube resistance. However, variable inspiratory flow and changing demands of the patient cannot be met by a single level of pressure support (Fig. 2–21). During periods of tachypnea, the previously chosen level of pressure support no longer eliminates work imposed by the endotracheal tube.

Additionally, the resistance of the endotracheal tube creates a condition early in the breath in which ventilator flow is high, tracheal pressure remains low, and undercompensation for imposed work occurs. Late in the breath, when pressure begins to equilibrate during the pressure plateau, pressure support tends to overcompensate, prolong inspiration, and exacerbate overinflation.

In 1993, Guttmann and associates described a technique for continuously calculating tracheal pressure in intubated, mechanically ventilated patients.[55] This system uses the known resistive component of the endotracheal tube and the measurement of flow to calculate tracheal pressure. These authors successfully validated their system in a group of mechanically ventilated pa-

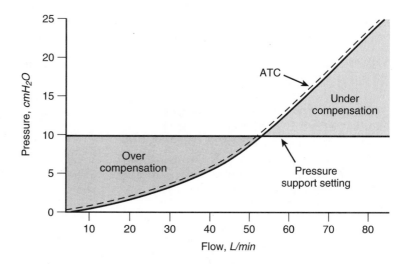

FIGURE 2–21
The capabilities of pressure support and automatic tube compensation (ATC) on overcoming the work of breathing caused by the artificial airway. Pressure support only eliminates the work precisely at a given flow. Above and below that flow, pressure support undercompensates for resistance or overcompensates. ATC compensation can overcome resistance regardless of patient flow demand.

tients, finding favorable comparisons between calculated and measured tracheal pressure.

This work has led to the introduction of ATC on the Drager Evita 4.[34] ATC attempts to compensate for endotracheal tube resistance via closed loop control of *calculated* tracheal pressure. This system uses the known resistive coefficients of the tracheal tube (tracheostomy or endotracheal) and measurement of instantaneous flow to apply pressure proportional to resistance throughout the total respiratory cycle. The equation for calculating tracheal pressure is:

$$\text{Tracheal pressure (cm } H_2O) = \text{Proximal airway pressure (cm } H_2O) - \text{Tube coefficient (cm } H_2O/L/s) \times \text{flow}^2 \text{ (L/min)}$$

The operator inputs the type of tube, endotracheal or tracheostomy, and the percentage of compensation desired (10–100%). Most of the interest in ATC revolves around eliminating the imposed work of breathing during inspiration. However, during expiration there is also a flow-dependent pressure decrease across the tube. ATC also compensates for this flow-resistive component and may reduce expiratory resistance and unintentional hyperinflation. During expiration, the calculated tracheal pressure is greater than airway pressure. Under ideal conditions, a negative pressure at the airway may help reduce expiratory resistance. Because this is not always desirable or possible, ATC can reduce PEEP to 0 cm H_2O during expiration to facilitate compensation of expiratory resistance posed by the endotracheal tube.[56–59]

PROPORTIONAL ASSIST VENTILATION

Descriptive Definition. Proportional assist ventilation (PAV) is a mode of mechanical ventilation based on the equation of motion.[60–65] This concept was presented in Chapter 1 and is reviewed briefly.

The equation of motion for the respiratory system states:

$$P_{AW} + P_{MUS} = \text{Volume} \times \text{elastance} + \text{Flow} \times \text{resistance}$$

where P_{AW} is pressure created by the ventilator and P_{MUS} is pressure created by the respiratory muscles. The larger the volume and greater the elastance, the more pressure required (either greater driving pressure by the ventilator or greater respiratory muscle effort by the patient). Similarly, as resistance or flow increases, the pressure provided by the ventilator or pressure created by the respiratory muscles must increase. This proportionality is the hallmark of PAV. Regardless of changes in patient effort, the ventilator continues to do the same percentage of work.

The design of PAV allows the ventilator to change the pressure output (pressure control) to always perform work proportionally to patient effort. Because the left side of the equation includes both ventilator pressure and patient muscle pressure, the ventilator can determine its output based on the online measurement of elastance (the reciprocal of compliance) and resistance. PAV requires only the traditional values of PEEP and inspired oxygen concentration (FiO_2) be set. The other settings are the percent volume assist (to overcome elastance) and percent flow assist (to overcome resistance). The interface for PAV remains a challenge. Another method might be to set percent work, which would control both the volume and flow assist. PAV is still new enough that we do not know whether there ever is any reason to set the assist settings at any value other than 80%.

Other Terms. Proportional assist ventilation was named by the designer, Magdy Younes. To date, no new terms for PAV have been introduced.

Manufacturer Terms. At the time of this writing, only Drager has introduced a version of PAV, which they term proportional pressure support.

Classification. PAV uses the measurement of elastance and resistance to determine ventilator output. PAV is pressure controlled, patient triggered, pressure limited, and flow cycled. The pressure delivered is not a set value, as in pressure support, but changes as a multiple of the sum of the volume and flow signals. Safety settings for high pressure and high tidal volume also can be set and cause the breaths to be pressure or volume limited (cycled if this is set as the alarm threshold). The pressure delivered changes from breath to breath depending on elastance, resistance, and flow demand. Typically, PAV is set to overcome 80% of the elastic and resistive loads. If elastance is measured at 40 cm H_2O/L the ventilator provides a pressure for that breath that overcomes 80% of that elastance value. In this example, the pressure required to overcome 80% of the work of breathing for a 1.0 L tidal volume is 32 cm H_2O.

PAV can be thought of as similar to cruise control on a car. When the cruise control is set, the accelerator changes position to maintain a constant speed regardless of terrain (uphill or downhill). With PAV, if the volume and flow assist are set at 80% (over-come 80% of the elastic and resistive load), as the patient's tidal volume increases, the pressure applied by the ventilator increases. This is shown in Figure 2–22. The percentage of patient work stays the same, regardless of the volume. In the original piston device described by Younes, as the patient demand or volume increased, the forward movement of the piston increased (larger volume delivered). If the volume remains constant but inspiratory flow increases, the ventilator increases pressure to overcome the increased resistive load. In the piston device, the stroke of the piston would be quicker, whereas the piston displacement remained constant. In essence, the ventilator attempts to maintain the percentage of work the patient performs per breath, regardless of the volume of the breath or inspiratory flow of the breath. The successful introduction of PAV requires that elastance

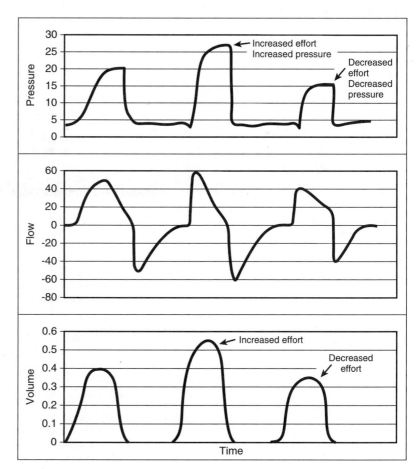

FIGURE 2–22
Pressure volume and flow waveforms during proportional assist ventilation (PAV). Note that as patient effort and volume increase, pressure applied by the ventilator increases.

and resistance be measured instantaneously breath to breath.

The major impediments to implementing PAV include the accurate breath-to-breath measurement of elastance and resistance, the confounding effects of endotracheal tube resistance and auto-PEEP, the problem of the nonlinearity of elastance and resistance, and the effect termed "runaway." Runaway is a form of overassist that occurs when the elastance improves dramatically or is measured inaccurately and the ventilator continues to provide volume after the patient has terminated inspiration. This could lead to overdistension, worsening of air trapping, and, potentially, barotrauma. This requires that high pressure and high tidal volume alarms be set appropriately. Additionally, because PAV always is patient triggered, a backup mode is necessary to take over in the event of apnea.

REFERENCES

1. Chatburn RL: A new system for understanding mechanical ventilators. Respir Care 36:1123–1155, 1992.
2. Sassoon CSH, Mahutte CK, Light RW: Ventilator modes old and new. Crit Care Clin 6:605–634, 1990.
3. Sassoon CSH: Positive pressure ventilation: alternate modes. Chest 100:1421–1429, 1991.
4. Hotchkiss RS, Wilson RS: Mechanical ventilatory support. Surg Clin North Am 63:417–438, 1983.
5. DuPuis YG: Ventilators: Theory and Clinical Application. St. Louis, CV Mosby, 1986.
6. Hamilton Veolar. Operators Manual. Reno, NV: Hamilton Medical, 1990.
7. Luce JM, Pierson DJ, Hudson LD: Intermittent mandatory ventilation. Chest 79:678–685, 1981.
8. Weisman IM, Rinaldo JE, Rogers RM, et al: Intermittent mandatory ventilation. Am Rev Respir Dis 127:641–647, 1983.
9. Downs JB, Stock MC, Tabeling B: Intermittent mandatory ventilation (IMV): a primary ventilatory support mode. Ann Chir Gynaecol 196(suppl):57–63, 1982.
10. Downs JB, Block AJ, Venum KB: Intermittent mandatory ventilation in the treatment of patients with chronic obstructive pulmonary disease. Anesth Analg 55:437–443, 1974.
11. Downs JB, Douglas ME, Sanfelippo PM, et al: Ventilatory pattern, intrapleural pressure, and cardiac output. Anesth Analg 56:88–96, 1977.
12. Downs JB, Klein EF, Desautels D, et al: Intermittent mandatory ventilation: a new approach to weaning patients from mechanical ventilators. Chest 64:331–335, 1973.
13. Shapiro BA, Harrison RA, Walton JR, Davison R: Intermittent demand ventilation: a new technique for supporting ventilation in critically ill patients. Respir Care 21:521–525, 1976.
14. Heenan TJ, Downs JB, Douglas ME, et al: Intermittent mandatory ventilation: is synchronization important? Chest 77:598–602, 1980.
15. MacIntyre NR: Respiratory function during pressure support ventilation. Chest 89:677–683, 1986.
16. Murphy DF, Dobb GD: Effect of pressure support of spontaneous breathing during intermittent mandatory ventilation. Crit Care Med 15:612–613, 1987.
17. MacIntyre NR: Weaning from mechanical ventilatory support: volume-assisting intermittent breaths versus pressure-assisting every breath. Respir Care 33:121–125, 1988.
18. Gregory GA, Kitterman JA, Phibbs RH, et al: Treatment of the idiopathic respiratory distress syndrome with continuous positive airway pressure. N Engl J Med 284:1333–1340, 1971.
19. Stock MC, Downs JB: Airway pressure release ventilation: a new approach to ventilation support during acute lung injury. Respir Care 32:517–524, 1987.
20. Stock MC, Downs JB, Frolicher DA: Airway pressure release ventilation. Crit Care Med 15:462–466, 1987.
21. Downs JB, Stock MC: Airway pressure release ventilation: a new concept in ventilatory support. Crit Care Med 15:459–461, 1987.
22. Rasanen J, Downs JB, Stock MC: Cardiovascular effect of conventional positive pressure ventilation and airway pressure release ventilation. Chest 93:911–915, 1988.
23. Garner W, Downs JB, Stock MC, et al: Airway pressure release ventilation (APRV): a human trial. Chest 94:779–781, 1988.
24. Abraham E, Yoshihara G: Cardiorespiratory effects of pressure control ventilation in severe respiratory failure. Chest 98:1445–1449, 1990.
25. Gurevitch MJ, Van Dyke J, Young ES, et al: Improved oxygenation and lower peak airway pressure in severe adult respiratory distress syndrome: treatment with inverse ratio ventilation. Chest 89:211–213, 1986.
26. Abraham E, Yoshihara G: Cardiorespiratory effects of pressure controlled inverse ratio ventilation in severe respiratory failure. Chest 96:1356–1359, 1989.
27. Lain DC, DiBenedetto R, Morris SL, et al: Pressure control inverse ratio ventilation as a method to reduce peak inspiratory pressure and provide adequate ventilation and oxygenation. Chest 95:1081–1088, 1989.
28. Marini JJ, Crooke PS III, Truwit JD: Determinants and limits of pressure-preset ventilation: a mathematical model of pressure control. J Appl Physiol 67:1081–1092, 1989.

29. Tharratt RS, Allen RP, Albertson TE: Pressure controlled inverse ratio ventilation in severe adult respiratory failure. Chest 94:755–762, 1988.

30. Hewlett AM, Platt AS, Terry VG: Mandatory minute volume. Anesthesia 32:163–169, 1977.

31. East TD, Elkhuizan PHM, Pace CL: Pressure support in mandatory minute ventilation supplied by the Ohmeda CPU-1 prevents alveolar hypoventilation due to respiratory depression in a canine model. Respir Care 34:795–800, 1989.

32. Ravenscroft PS: Simple mandatory minute volume. Anesthesia 33:246–249, 1978.

33. Operators Manual Bear 5. Riverside, CA: Bear Medical, 1990.

34. Operators Manual Drager E4. Telford, PA: Drager Inc. 1997.

35. Amato MBP, Barbos CSV, Bonassa J, et al: Volume assisted pressure support ventilation (VAPSV): a new approach for reducing muscle workload during acute respiratory failure. Chest 102:1225–1234, 1992.

36. Haas CF, Branson RD, Folk LM, et al: Patient determined inspiratory flow during assisted mechanical ventilation. Respir Care 40:716–721, 1995.

37. MacIntyre NR, Gropper C, Westfall T: Combining pressure limiting and volume cycling features in a patient-interactive mechanical ventilation. Crit Care Med 22:353–357, 1994.

38. Branson RD, MacIntyre NR: Dual control modes of mechanical ventilation. Respir Care 41:294–305, 1996.

39. Piotrowski A, Sobala W, Kawczynski P: Patient initiated, pressure regulated, volume controlled ventilation compared with intermittent mandatory ventilation in neonates: a prospective, randomised study. Intensive Care Med 23:975–981, 1997.

40. Alvarez A, Subirana M, Benito S: Decelerating flow ventilation effects in acute respiratory failure. J Crit Care 13:7–12, 1998.

41. Raneri VM: Optimization of patient ventilator interactions: closed loop technology. Intensive Care Med 23:936–939, 1997.

42. Otis AB, Fenn WO, Rahn H: Mechanics of breathing in man. J Appl Physiol 2:592–607, 1950.

43. Brunner JX, Laubscher TP, Banner MJ, et al: A simple method to measure total expiratory time constant based on the passive expiratory flow-volume curve. Crit Care Med 23:1117–1122, 1995.

44. Iotti GA, Braschi A, Brunner J, et al: Respiratory mechanics by least squares fitting in mechanically ventilated patients: applications during paralysis and during pressure support ventilation. Intensive Care Med 21:406–413, 1995.

45. Weiler N, Henrichs W, Kebler W: The AVL mode: a safe closed loop algorithm for ventilation during total intravenous anesthesia. Int J Clin Monit Comput 11:85–88, 1994.

46. Laubscher TP, Frutiger A, Fanconi S, et al: Automatic selection of tidal volume, respiratory frequency and minute volume in intubated ICU patients as startup procedure for closed-loop

controlled ventilation. Int J Clin Monit Comput 11:19–30, 1994.

47. Laubscher TP, Frutiger A, Fanconi S, Brunner JX: The automatic selection of ventilation parameters during the initial phase of mechanical ventilation. Intensive Care Med 22:199–207, 1996.

48. Linton DM, Potgieter PD, Davis S, et al: Automatic weaning from mechanical ventilation using an adaptive lung controller. Chest 106:1843–1850, 1994.

49. Weiler N, Eberle B, Latorre F, et al: Adaptive lung ventilation. Anaesthetist 45:950–956, 1996.

50. Campbell RS, Sinamban RP, Johannigman JA, et al: Clinical evaluation of a new closed loop ventilation mode: adaptive support ventilation. Respir Care 43:856, 1998 (abstract).

51. Bersten AD, Rutten AJ, Vedig AE, Skowronski GA: Additional work of breathing imposed by endotracheal tubes, breathing circuits, and intensive care ventilators. Crit Care Med 17:671–680, 1989.

52. Shapiro M, Wilson RK, Casar G, et al: Work of breathing through different sized endotracheal tubes. Crit Care Med 14:1028–1031, 1986.

53. Bersten AD, Rutten AJ, Vedig AE: Efficacy of pressure support in compensating for apparatus work. Anaesth Intensive Care 21:67–71, 1993.

54. Brochard L, Rua F, Lorini H, et al: Inspiratory pressure support compensates for the additional work of breathing caused by the endotracheal tube. Anesthesiology 75:739–745, 1991.

55. Guttmann J, Eberhard L, Fabry B, et al: Continuous calculation of intratracheal pressure in tracheally intubated patients. Anesthesiology 79:503–513, 1993.

56. Fiastro JF, Habib MP, Quan SF: Pressure support compensation for inspiratory work due to endotracheal tubes and demand continuous positive airway pressure. Chest 93:499–505, 1988.

57. Stocker R, Fabry B, Haberthur C: New modes of ventilatory support in spontaneously breathing intubated patients. In: Vincent JL (ed): Yearbook of Intensive Care and Emergency Medicine, vol 12. Berlin: Springer-Verlag, 1997, pp 514–533.

58. Fabry B, Guttman J, Eberhard L, Wolff G: Automatic compensation of endotracheal tube resistance in spontaneous breathing patients. Technol Health Care 1:281–291, 1994.

59. Guttmann J, Bernhard H, Mols G, et al: Respiratory comfort of automatic tube compensation and inspiratory pressure support in conscious humans. Intensive Care Med 23:1119–1124, 1997.

60. Fabry B, Zappe D, Guttman J, et al: Breathing pattern and additional work of breathing in spontaneously breathing patients with different ventilatory demand during inspiratory pressure support and automatic tube compensation. Intensive Care Med 23:545–552, 1997.

61. Ranieri VM, Grasso S, Mascia L, et al: Effects of proportional assist ventilation on inspiratory muscle effort in patients with chronic obstructive pulmonary disease and acute respiratory failure. Anesthesiology 86:79–81, 1997.

62. Younes M, Puddy A, Robert D, et al: Proportional

assist ventilation: results of an initial clinical trial. Am Rev Respir Dis 145:121–129, 1992.

63. Younes M: Proportional assist ventilation, a new approach to ventilatory support. Am Rev Respir Dis 145:114–120, 1992.

64. Bigatello LM, Nishimura M, Imanaka H, et al: Unloading of the work of breathing by proportional assist ventilation in a lung model. Crit Care Med 25:267–272, 1997.

65. Navalesi P, Hernandez P, Wongsa A, et al: Proportional assist ventilation in acute respiratory failure: effects of breathing pattern and inspiratory effort. Am J Respir Crit Care Med 154:1330–1338, 1996.

CHAPTER 3

The Patient–Ventilator Interface: Ventilator Circuit, Airway Care, and Suctioning

Richard D. Branson, BA, RRT

THE VENTILATOR CIRCUIT
Ventilation
Exhalation Valves
CARE OF THE ARTIFICIAL AIRWAY
Tube Position
Securing the Tube
Management of the Endotracheal Tube Cuff
Monitoring Cuff Pressure

SUCTIONING
Bronchial Suctioning
Use of Saline Instillation
Complications of Suctioning
PATIENT–VENTILATOR SYSTEM CHECK

KEY WORDS

---

closed circuit suction catheter
colorimetric CO_2 detector
compressible volume

cuff pressure
end-expiratory valve
endotracheal tube
minimal occlusive technique

minimal seal technique
suction catheter
ventilator circuit

Care of the mechanically ventilated patient includes airway maintenance, secretion clearance, proper positioning, and provision of ancillary equipment. Because many of these subjects are intertwined in the fabric of other chapters, this chapter concentrates on technical and device-related issues.

THE VENTILATOR CIRCUIT

The **ventilator circuit** is approximately 60 inches of plastic tubing that connects the mechanical ventilator to an artificial airway or mask. Circuits for adults traditionally use 22-mm tubing, whereas pediatric circuits range from 9 to 13 mm in diameter. The ventilator circuit may contain filters, humidifiers, water traps, heated wires, artificial noses, closed **suction catheters**, and devices for aerosol administration. Issues related to humidification and aerosol therapy are covered elsewhere.

Ventilator circuits are associated with certain characteristics, including compliance, resistance, and dead space. Each of these characteristics can affect the efficiency of ventilation. Ventilator circuits often are associated with the potential for nosocomial infection, and the frequency of ventilator circuit changes has recently been the subject of several investigations.[1-3] These topics are discussed relative to the pertinent literature and the effects on the mechanically ventilated patient.

Ventilation

The length, diameter, and materials used to construct a ventilator circuit all affect the circuit compliance. Typical disposable adult ventilator circuits possess a compliance of 2 to 3 ml/cm H_2O. This typically is known as the **compressible volume** of the circuit. Nondisposable circuits generally have a lower compliance because of the more rigid materials used in manufacturing (1.5–2.0 ml/cm H_2O). The initial cost of a nondisposable circuit is approximately $300. These circuits tend to improve ventilator performance because they are leak free, frequently have a smooth internal bore, and are relatively unaffected by prolonged use.[4] The cost of a disposable circuit is approximately $7.00 with water traps and $12.00 with heated wires. The cost of cleaning (washing and sterilizing) nondisposable circuits is quite high and possibly the most important reason that disposable circuits remain popular.

Compressible volume usually plays a small part in the discrepancy between actual tidal volume delivered to the patient and tidal volume measured by the ventilator. If compressible volume of the circuit is known, measurement of distending pressure (peak inspiratory pressure [PIP] − positive end-expiratory pressure [PEEP]) allows the volume trapped in the tubing to be determined.

If tidal volume is 600 ml, PIP is 40 cm H_2O, PEEP is 8 cm H_2O, and compressible volume is 3 ml/cm H_2O, then:

$$(40 \text{ cm } H_2O - 8 \text{ cm } H_2O) \times 3 \text{ ml/cm } H_2O$$
$$= \text{compressible volume}$$
$$32 \text{ cm } H_2O \times 3 \text{ ml/cm } H_2O = 96 \text{ ml}$$
$$600 \text{ ml} - 96 \text{ ml} = 504 \text{ ml actual tidal}$$
$$\text{volume}$$

The issue of compressible volume is handled in various ways by different ventilator manufacturers. In many ventilators (Siemens 900C [Siemens, Danvers, MA]; Bear 1, 2, and 3 [Bear Medical Systems, Thermo Electron Corporation, Riverside, CA]), the set tidal volume is delivered into the circuit, and the expiratory flow sensor measures the actual exhaled tidal volume plus the compressible volume. Using the aforementioned example, the ventilator is set at 600 ml, the patient receives 504 ml, and the exhaled tidal volume displays 600 ml. This represents an error in tidal volume measurement of 16%, which would invalidate measurements of compliance and resistance made using this value for tidal volume.

Several ventilators (Puritan Bennett 7200ae, 840 [Puritan Bennett, Carlsbad, CA]) measure compressible volume of the circuit during setup and "compensate" for compressible volume. Using our example, the ventilator would deliver 696 ml (set tidal volume + calculated compressible volume), actual tidal volume would be 600 ml, and measured tidal volume would read 600 ml (measured exhaled tidal volume − calculated compressible volume). In this case, PIP would increase based on the required volume increase and patient impedance (in our example, 6 cm H_2O).

Several ventilators (Hamilton Veolar [Hamilton Medical, Reno, NV], Amadeus, Galileo, Pulmonetic Systems LTV [Pulmonetic Systems Inc., Colton, CA], Drager Babylog [Drager, Telford, PA]) use a flow sensor positioned between the circuit and **endotracheal tube.** In this case, tidal volume delivered into the circuit would be 600 ml, measured actual tidal volume would be 504 ml, and the presence of compressible volume would be unmasked. The clinician then could increase the set tidal volume until measured exhaled tidal volume was 600 ml, if desired.

Compressible volume can also result in the underestimation of autoPEEP when using the expiratory hold maneuver. When both inspiratory and expiratory valves are closed, the volume trapped in the lung can redistribute throughout the entire patient/ventilator system. As the volume of the system increases, the pressure decreases. The understimation of autoPEEP in this situation is typically quite small.

The compliance of the circuit can also complicate evaluation of pressure and flow tracings. The circuit "exhales" the compressible volume more quickly than the patient, particularly the patient with dynamic hyperinflation. This gives the expiratory flow signal an initial steep deceleration followed by a gradual slope toward zero. Clinicians should be aware of the effects of the circuit on graphics (Fig. 3–1).

Resistance of the ventilator circuit is not typically a problem during mechanical ventilation. Compared with the resistance of the endotracheal tube, circuit resistance is minute. Resistance is greatest at the Y-piece and elbow. Occasionally, these areas can interfere with proximal pressure and flow measurements.[5] These components should be inspected for excessive resistance before use.

Exhalation Valves

Exhalation valves can be a considerable source of resistance in the patient circuit, increasing the work of breathing and retarding expiratory flow.[6–9] Most current-generation ventilators have internal exhalation valves, eliminating this circuit component as a point of concern. However, in many home care and transport ventilators, disposable exhalation valves remain in use.

The exhalation valve can result in an increased work of breathing because of resistance and the requirement that the valve functionally close for pressure in the circuit to fall. This is important during pressure triggering, a common triggering method in ventilators that use disposable exhalation valves. For patient effort to result in a negative pressure in the circuit, the exhalation valve must come to rest against the gas outflow port. The time required for the exhalation valve to move from an open to closed position is a measurable delay in response time of the ventilator. The resistance to gas flow of the exhalation valve also contributes to the work of breathing as a consequence of the increased work to close the valve.

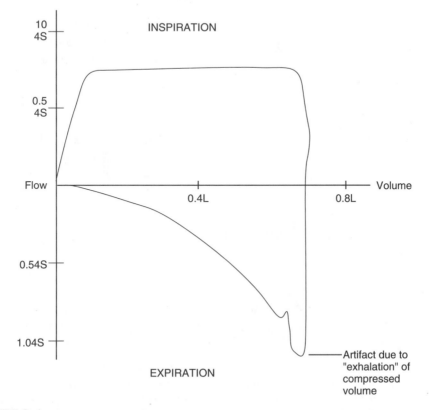

FIGURE 3–1
The effects of compressible volume on the flow volume loop during mechanical ventilation.
The initial flow spike represents the volume of gas trapped in the tubing being released.

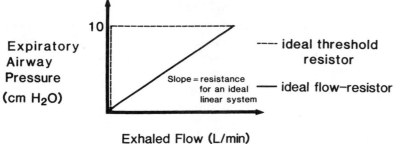

FIGURE 3–2
The effects of increasing flow on the pressure provided by flow-resistive and threshold expiratory valve devices. (From Banner MJ: Expiratory positive pressure valves and work of breathing. Respir Care 32:431–436, 1987.)

End-expiratory valves or PEEP valves commonly are used with home care and transport ventilators. These devices have been classified as flow resistors or threshold resistors on the basis of performance.[10] A flow resistor requires a constant flow to maintain a constant pressure. A decrease in flow results in a pressure lower than desired, and an increase in flow results in a pressure greater than desired (Fig. 3–2). Threshold resistors maintain a constant or nearly constant pressure regardless of gas flow. Threshold resistors are preferred to flow resistors. Examples of a flow resistor and a threshold resistor are shown in Figures 3–3 and 3–4.

CARE OF THE ARTIFICIAL AIRWAY

Not too long ago, mechanical ventilation always was associated with an artificial airway. The advent of noninvasive ventilation has changed this paradigm and required re-evaluation of our preconceptions. Masks and other devices are discussed in the chapter on noninvasive ventilation. Caring for the artificial airway includes ensuring proper tube placement, securing the tube, maintaining appropriate **cuff pressure**, and suctioning secretions. Following is a discussion of each of these.

Tube Position

Ensuring appropriate airway placement after placement and during prolonged use

FLOW RESISTOR
(P∝RV̇)
(High Flow-Resistant)

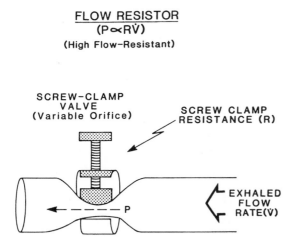

FIGURE 3–3
A flow resistor for providing PEEP. (From Banner MJ, Lampotang S: Expiratory pressure valves. In: Branson RD, Hess D, Chatburn RL [eds]: Respiratory Care Equipment. Philadelphia: JB Lippincott, 1995.)

THRESHOLD RESISTOR
(P∝F/SA)
(Low Flow-Resistant)

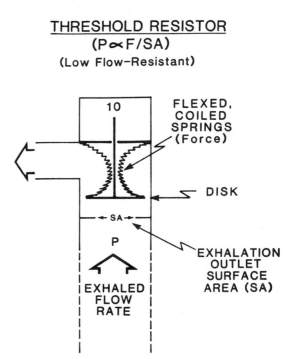

FIGURE 3–4
A threshold resistor for providing PEEP. (From Banner MJ, Lampotang S: Expiratory pressure valves. In: Branson RD, Hess D, Chatburn RL [eds]: Respiratory Care Equipment. Philadelphia: JB Lippincott, 1995.)

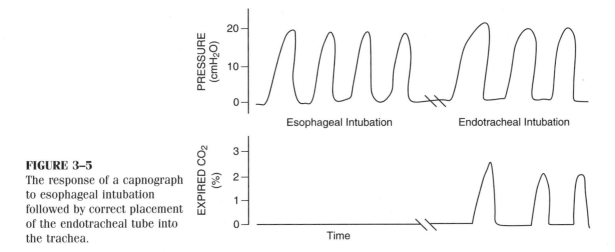

FIGURE 3–5
The response of a capnograph to esophageal intubation followed by correct placement of the endotracheal tube into the trachea.

is essential for safe mechanical ventilation. Proper placement should, of course, be verified visually, during intubation. However, because even in experienced hands esophageal intubation can occur, several techniques have been devised to detect esophageal placement of an artificial airway.[11–13]

Carbon dioxide (CO_2) monitoring generally is considered the gold standard for determining esophageal intubation.[14, 15] A tube inserted into the esophagus and connected to the ventilator or manual resuscitator does not have CO_2 in the expired gas. The measurement of expired CO_2 can be accomplished quantitatively through use of a capnometer (Fig. 3–5) or qualitatively through use of a detector. In the former, expired CO_2 is measured in percent or millimeters of mercury (mm Hg). In the latter, the presence of CO_2 is displayed by a color change.

The **colorimetric CO_2 detector** technique uses a pH-sensitive chemical, bonded to a paper element (Fig. 3–6). In the presence of CO_2, the paper changes color.[16–22] As the patient is ventilated, the detector changes color with inspiration (absence of CO_2) and expiration (presence of CO_2). This color change is typically yellow to purple. Several devices are currently available to serve this purpose. Some devices simply change one color, whereas others change through a series of shades as CO_2 concentration increases. The major limitation of CO_2 detection as a method of ensuring endotracheal tube placement is seen during cardiopulmonary resuscitation. In the absence of cardiac output and hence pulmonary blood

flow, CO_2 concentration may be very low or zero. This creates the unfavorable situation in which the tube may be placed correctly, but the absence of CO_2 in expired gas causes the clinician to remove the tube.[23–30] In these instances, the clinician should use

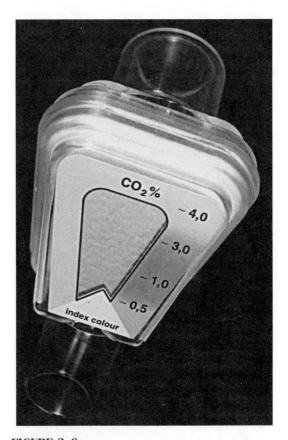

FIGURE 3–6
A colorimetric device for detecting the presence of CO_2 in expired gas.

clinical judgment along with other observations (e.g., breath sounds) before removing the tube.

Another method of determining proper tube placement involves the use of negative pressure applied to the airway. These devices are collectively known as esophageal detection devices (EDDs). The principle of operation resides in the fact that the lungs are full of air, while under normal conditions the esophagus is collapsed. The EDD is either a syringe or squeeze bulb connected to the endotracheal tube. If the tube is in the trachea, the syringe fills easily or the bulb inflates quickly. If the tube is in the esophagus, the negative pressure further collapses the esophagus, and the syringe does not fill or the bulb stays flat.

Several investigators have shown that clinicians can use the EDD in determining appropriate tube placement.[31–37] Like the CO_2 monitor, the EDD also occasionally predicts esophageal tube placement, even though the tube is in the trachea. This may result from reduced lung volume, airway secretions, airway obstruction, or bronchospasm.

Chest radiographs also can be used to determine tube placement. The chest radiograph is reliable but requires considerably more time to check placement than the other devices. Auscultation of the chest also remains an important adjunct to these techniques. Auscultation is simple and readily available but is subjective. However, the use of CO_2 monitoring or the EDD can be complemented by simple auscultation.

Once the tube is placed and proper position is confirmed, the position of the tube should be noted by recording the length of the tube at the teeth. This value then can be checked during subsequent ventilator checks. The tube should be secured to prevent migration.

Previous discussions have concentrated on verifying tube placement. During the course of intubation, these techniques also may be useful if the patient becomes extubated or if the tube migrates cephalad. Distal migration of the tube into the right mainstem bronchi is also of concern, requiring different detection techniques. Commonly, distal migration of the tube is de-tected by an increase in airway pressure during volume control ventilation, a decrease in tidal volume during pressure control ventilation, or absence of breath sounds on one side, or it is detected on routine chest radiograph.[38, 39]

The appropriate depth of endotracheal tube insertion has been determined for both endotracheal and nasotracheal tubes. Eagle[40] suggests that the distance from the teeth to the midpoint of the trachea can be predicted by the height in centimeters divided by 10, plus 2. For nasotracheal tubes, the distance from the external naris to the midpoint of the trachea is the height in centimeters divided by 10, plus 8.[40] Other studies have shown that, during orotracheal intubation, placement of the tube at the gums at 23 cm for men and 21 cm for women aids in preventing endobronchial intubation.[41, 42]

There are many causes of endobronchial intubation. Patient movement and position of the head causes the endotracheal tube to move distal with flexion and proximal with extension of the neck.[43] Turning of the patient by the nursing staff, transport, and position changes for procedures all play a role in tube misplacement. Patient activity and vigorous coughing also may result in tube movement.

Chest radiograph remains the gold standard for assessing endotracheal tube position. The incidence of tube malposition has been demonstrated to be between 15% and 30%.[38, 44] The risk of malposition is greatest immediately after intubation and in women.[45] Endobronchial intubation, predominantly of the right mainstem bronchus, occurs in approximately 5% of cases.[38, 46] Radiographic evaluation of tube placement should be accomplished with knowledge of head and neck position. Movement of the tube 2 cm either cephalad or caudad is common with flexion and extension of the head.

Current cost-cutting strategies frequently call for less frequent chest radiographs. However, in many cases, tube malposition occurs many days after the initial intubation.[44–46] In patients at risk for tube movement (frequent movement, transport) daily chest radiographs remain important for ensuring adequate position. Additional assessments, including checking position at the gums, evaluating breath sounds, and cuff palpation, may be used when chest radiographs are unavailable.

Securing the Tube

Once tube placement has been verified, the endotracheal tube should be secured to prevent accidental extubation or migration of the tube. Unplanned extubation can result from self-extubation or accidental extubation. In the former, the patient removes the tube because of anxiety or agitation. In the latter, the tube is removed inadvertently during patient movement, transport, or positioning. The incidence of unplanned extubation ranges from 2% to 13%.[47-56] Boulain and colleagues evaluated the factors associated with unplanned extubation and found the four most frequent attributes were lack of intravenous sedation, chronic respiratory failure (prolonged intubation time), oral tube placement, and use of adhesive tape to secure the tube.[48] The use of adhesive tape also generally means that no tube-securing protocol was in place. Efforts to reduce the incidence of unplanned extubations have been instituted in the form of continuous quality improvement programs. In several

cases,[47, 57, 58] the use of properly controlled sedation and an endotracheal tube fixation protocol resulted in reduced rates of unplanned extubations.

Methods for securing the endotracheal tube range from the very simple to application of specialty devices manufactured specifically for this purpose. Adhesive tape is a common, simple method for securing the endotracheal tube (Fig. 3–7). This is best accomplished using 1-inch tape of moderate strength. A length of tape twice that necessary to encircle the patient's head is cut, and a second piece 6 to 8 inches in length is placed across the midportion in opposite position. This second piece of tape prevents the original piece from sticking to the patient's hair and neck. This piece may be extended in patients with facial hair. Benzoin or another skin protective substance should be placed wherever the tape comes in direct contact with the patient's skin. Each end of the tape should be torn longitudinally, leaving four pieces of tape 2 to 3 inches in length. Each of these tape sections is wrapped around the endotracheal tube and resecured to the patient's face. If a bite block is used, it should be taped separately. The tape should be placed firmly around the patient's head, but binding of the skin should be prevented. The tape should be

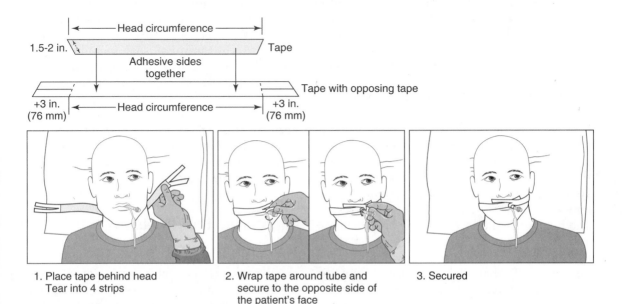

FIGURE 3–7
A method for using adhesive tape to secure an endotracheal tube.

changed when soiled or aesthetically un-pleasing, or when changing edema of the face results in the tape being either too loose or too tight.

Other techniques for securing the endo-tracheal tube include the use of cloth tape, sometimes called trach tape or twill tape. This cloth tape is wrapped around the head, looped around the tube, and tied in a bow near the patient's cheek. Other securing devices are available that use Velcro, plastic, or metal retaining devices.[59-62] These devices vary in the ability to secure the tube, prevent skin breakdown, and allow for effective mouth care. Success with any device often is predicated on clinician experience and preference.

Adequate tube fixation is crucial to prevent tube migration and unplanned extubation, facilitate mouth care, and prevent skin breakdown. Each of these should be considered when choosing a fixation device. Patient comfort also plays an important role, dictating the need for a fixation method that is as unobtrusive as possible and the judicious use of sedation in these patients.

Management of the Endotracheal Tube Cuff

The use of endotracheal tubes to facilitate mechanical ventilation is, by historical standards, a fairly modern technique. Advantages of the endotracheal tube were offset by problems associated with pressure exerted by the endotracheal tube cuff on the tracheal mucosa.[63-66] Early tubes used the so-called low-volume, high-pressure cuffs that exerted high pressures on the tracheal wall, occluding mucosal blood flow. Under normal conditions, the perfusion pressure of the tracheal mucosa (capillary pressure) is 25 to 35 mm Hg.[67] However, it should be noted that in patients with shock, sepsis, and hypotension this value may be considerably lower. Current standards suggest that the pressure in the new high-volume, low-pressure cuffs should be kept at less than 25 mm Hg to prevent mucosal damage. Lower pressures are associated with less damage but also are associated with silent aspiration around and through folds in the cuff.[68, 69] This aspiration has been shown to be more prevalent at pressures less than 20 mm Hg. Aspiration of oropharyngeal secretions is responsible for nosocomial pneumonia and should be avoided. Given this small range of function, it seems prudent to maintain cuff pressures between 20 and 25 mm Hg.

Techniques for determining the adequate volume for filling the cuff include the **minimal leak** and **minimal seal techniques.**[70] The minimal seal technique also frequently is called the **minimal occlusion technique.** Both these techniques use the auscultation of air leak during inspiration around the cuff. The minimal leak technique adjusts cuff inflation volume such that at end inspiration there is a small leak of air around the cuff. This leak is sometimes audible to the naked ear but is best heard using a stethoscope placed over the trachea. Commonly, stethoscope placement for best sound detection is just above the suprasternal notch. Minimal seal or occlusion is one step past the minimal leak technique. That is, additional volume from a syringe is added to the cuff until the leak no longer can be heard. The minimal leak technique uses the lowest cuff pressure and therefore is thought to reduce tracheal damage compared with the minimal seal method. However, the minimal seal method is conceptually superior to the minimal leak method with respect to preventing silent aspiration. The minimal seal technique also facilitates mechanical ventilation, improves monitoring of respiratory mechanics, and reduces nuisance alarms. Our preference has been to use the minimal seal technique because the risk of nosocomial pneumonia from aspiration of oropharyngeal secretions is of more immediate concern than damage to the tracheal mucosa.

Monitoring Cuff Pressure

Measuring pressure within the endotracheal tube cuff is a standard of care. Cuff pressures should be monitored routinely and the results recorded on the patient's chart. The frequency of cuff pressure measurement is not well defined. Ideally, cuff pressure should be measured and recorded at least once a day. If the tube is repositioned, if a leak occurs, or if volume is added or removed from the cuff, cuff pressure should be reassessed. The measurement of cuff pressure typically is accomplished after the minimal seal technique has been used. That is, although it is desirable to maintain cuff pressure at below tracheal mucosa perfusion pressure, higher pressure may be required to prevent air leaks and silent aspiration.

Measuring cuff pressure can be accomplished by a variety of means, and several commercial devices are available for this purpose. Cuff pressures typically are measured using a syringe, a three-way stopcock, and an aneroid pressure gauge. This method is easily accomplished with equipment commonly stocked in the intensive care unit. Figure 3–8 shows the system recommended for cuff pressure measurement. By using a three-way stopcock, the volume of the air in the cuff can be increased or decreased while pressure is measured continuously. Cuff pressure is affected by compliance of the cuff, volume of air inserted

into the cuff, and airway pressure in the ventilator circuit. In fact, increases in airway pressure during inspiration are followed closely by increases in cuff pressure. In many circumstances, elevated cuff pressures must be tolerated to ensure adequate ventilation. Careful monitoring of the cuff pressure and using the minimum volume that maintains a seal should be accomplished frequently whenever cuff pressure exceeds 25 mm Hg.[71–73]

Cuff pressures can be elevated for many reasons. One of the most common causes of elevated cuff pressure is placement of an endotracheal tube of incorrect size. When a tube that is too small is inserted into the trachea, the cuff must be expanded to its maximum volume to form a seal. Careful choice of an appropriately sized tube is paramount in avoiding this problem. The volume of an individual tracheal tube cuff is selected to maintain pressures less than 25 mm Hg. If this volume is exceeded, cuff pressures increase rapidly. The maximum volume of a cuff is easily measured by filling the cuff with air before placement in the patient and recording the volume at which

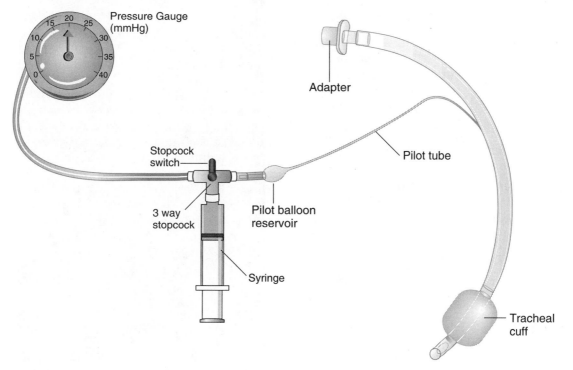

FIGURE 3–8
The system used for cuff pressure measurement.

pressure less than 25 mm Hg is maintained. This is not best accomplished during an emergency intubation.

Other causes of elevated cuff pressures include malposition of the tube, overinflation of the cuff, and tracheal malacia.[73] Tube malposition, particularly migration cephalad into the larynx, requires that a greater volume be placed in the cuff to seal the larger diameter upper airway. Despite concern over cuff pressure and the production of tubes with low-pressure, high-volume cuffs, certain surgical procedures such as laser surgery require tubes with low-volume, high-pressure cuffs. Anode tubes are used during laser surgery. When these tubes are left in postoperatively, cuff pressures are high. Replacement of the tube is typically the only remedy to this problem.

In the course of mechanical ventilation, it is not unusual for the pilot balloon or the cuff of the tube to leak, or the pilot tube to be severed or nicked.[74] The latter commonly is caused when patients are shaved and the razor lacerates the pilot tube. Cuff leaks are less common if the tube is cared for properly. Laceration of the cuff occurs most often during nasotracheal intubation. As the tube passes through the nasal turbinates, the cuff can become ruptured. If the pilot balloon develops a leak, placing a stopcock into the port and closing it to the patient can identify this problem. If the leak persists, the problem is not in the pilot balloon. In critically ill patients, incompetent pilot balloons or leaks in the pilot tube can be overcome using a host of methods. These include severing the pilot balloon, placing a blunt needle into the pilot tube, and running a continuous flow of gas through the pilot tube to maintain the cuff inflated. This latter method requires adequate humidification of the gas to prevent drying of secretions. This method should also be considered a temporizing measure until reintubation can be accomplished safely.

SUCTIONING

Removal of tracheobronchial and upper airway secretions to maintain airway patency and reduce the risk of silent aspiration is also a standard of care.[75] The use of routine suctioning should be avoided. Assessment of the patient, including auscultation, palpation, and visual inspection, should be used to determine the need for endotracheal suctioning. Endotracheal suctioning is associated with a litany of complications and should be undertaken only when necessary, keeping the potential complications in mind.[76]

Suction catheters vary greatly in design but have the same general characteristics (Fig. 3–9). Most catheters are 56 cm in length to allow the catheter to travel into the mainstem bronchi.[75] The distal tip of the catheter has several openings for secretion removal, and the proximal portion contains a thumb port that is occluded by the practitioner to activate the suction. The distal tip of the catheter should be blunt to avoid trauma to the mucosa and possible perforation of the tracheobronchial tree. The side holes in the distal tip of the catheter also serve to limit local tissue damage. If the catheter had a single opening in the distal

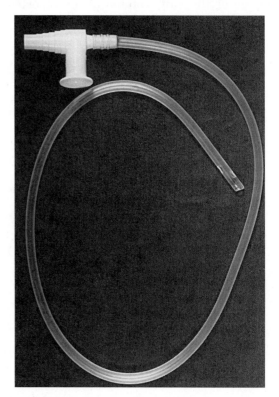

FIGURE 3–9
A standard suction catheter.

end, the mucosa could be drawn into the catheter tip and torn during withdrawl of the catheter. The addition of side holes helps eliminate this problem. Suction catheters should be transparent to allow visual inspection of secretions, rigid enough to pass through the endotracheal tube, yet pliable enough to traverse airway structures without damaging mucosa.

Recently, **closed circuit suction catheters** have become popular for a number of reasons (Fig. 3–10). These include prevention of problems associated with disconnecting the patient from the ventilator, reduced costs, and reduced exposure of caregivers to infectious materials. Comparisons of closed and open circuit suctioning techniques suggest that there is no difference in the ability of each device to evacuate secretions.[77-79] Because the patient does not need to be disconnected from the ventilator when closed circuit suctioning is used, several authors have suggested that this device reduces complications associated with the suctioning procedure.[80, 81] These investigations have produced disparate results. Taken together, however, these authors appear to suggest that closed circuit suctioning reduces the incidence of dysrhythmias and desaturation when compared with open circuit suctioning.

Manufacturers of closed circuit suction devices have often claimed that these devices reduce patient and caregiver contamination. This contention is supported by two studies that, although not conclusive, appear to favor closed circuit suctioning for reducing caregiver exposure.[82, 83] Many institutions have adopted the use of closed circuit suctioning systems for all mechanically ventilated patients. The added expense of these systems, however, suggests that the widespread use of these devices in all care settings may not be cost-effective. Additionally, the desire for caregivers to be protected from exposure to secretions also forces this issue.

We have adopted a priority system for using closed circuit suction catheters. Patients requiring frequent suctioning (> 6 times/day), those who suffer deterioration in hemodynamic performance or oxygen saturation during suctioning, and patients

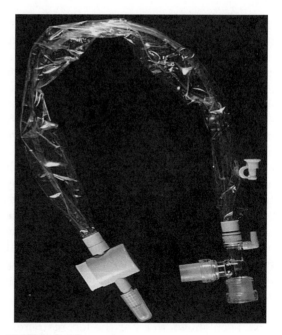

FIGURE 3–10
A closed circuit suction catheter.

with communicable diseases are considered candidates for use of closed circuit catheters. Patients at risk for complications during disconnection for open circuit suctioning are typically those requiring elevated PEEP levels (> 10 cm H_2O), elevated inspired oxygen concentration (FiO_2) (> 0.60), and pressure control ventilation. Certain patients have hemodynamic deterioration after disconnection from the ventilator, which unfortunately can be detected only though trial and error. These patients should also use closed circuit suctioning devices.

The cost of closed circuit suction devices is considerably greater than that of open circuit devices. However, this is the out-of-box cost. Prolonged use of closed circuit catheters in patients requiring frequent suctioning attempts actually can result in cost savings. As with ventilator circuit changes, conventional wisdom and several recent studies suggest that these devices need only be changed weekly. The longer the duration of use, the more cost-effective closed circuit suctioning becomes.[84, 85]

Bronchial Suctioning

During routine endotracheal suctioning, the suction catheter most likely enters the right mainstem bronchus if the catheter is advanced far enough. This is caused by the more acute angle of the left mainstem bronchus at the carina compared with the right mainstem, which is almost a direct shot. As such, the left lung is less likely to be suctioned. Attempts at suctioning the left mainstem have been described and range all the way from simple maneuvers to use of special catheters.[86-88] One simple way of suctioning the left mainstem bronchus is by turning the head to the right in an attempt to increase the likelihood of passage of the catheter into the left mainstem. The same effect may be gained by placing the patient in the left lateral position and attempting to use gravity to further the catheter's passage.

Specialized catheters using a curved tip have been shown to enter the left mainstem bronchus in up to 90% of cases (Fig. 3–11). The success of bronchial suctioning can be affected by tube position, patient body and head position, and type of tube (endotracheal tube vs. tracheostomy tube). We have not found selective endobronchial suctioning to be a necessary routine technique. Frequent changes in patient body position facilitate movement of secretions to the ca-

rina, where they can be suctioned. In patients with infectious processes confined to the left lung, selective endobronchial suctioning may prove useful.

Use of Saline Instillation

During the suctioning procedure, it is common for practitioners to instill 5 to 10 ml of normal saline in an attempt to thin tracheobronchial secretions. This practice remains a point of contention, and studies have failed to show any advantage of saline instillation.[89-91] Our own studies of humidification techniques reveal that the only correlation between saline instillation and patient care is practitioner preference. That is, our research fails to show that saline instillation is used uniformly or has any benefit in terms of liquefying secretions. Saline instillation frequently does cause the patient to cough violently, which may aid in the secretion removal process. From a conceptual standpoint, this practice makes sense, but the current literature does not support the use of saline instillation. From a mucus rheology perspective, the properties of mucus are unlikely to change with the addition of water unless some physical means of mixing the two is accomplished. There appear to be no real contraindications to using saline. However, severe coughing episodes and bronchospasm occasionally may result from the instillation of saline. Given this evidence, the use of saline to thin secretions currently is unsupported.

Complications of Suctioning

The long list of complications associated with endotracheal suctioning is frequently studied in an effort to arrive at methods that minimize patient discomfort and instability. These complications include hypoxemia, cardiac arrhythmias, trauma to the airway mucosa, and atelectasis. Contamination of the lower airway of the patient also may occur during suctioning if appropriate techniques are not used. Contamination of health care providers exposed to secretions is also of concern.[92-103]

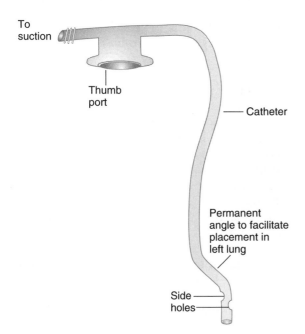

To suction

Thumb port

Catheter

Permanent angle to facilitate placement in left lung

Side holes

FIGURE 3–11
A catheter for selective suctioning of the left lung.

Hypoxemia is by far the most frequent complication of endotracheal suctioning.[92-96] The causes of hypoxemia during suctioning are multifactorial. These include the obvious, such as disconnection of mechanical ventilation and the resultant loss of PEEP, decreased FiO_2, and lack of ventilator assistance. Suctioning also reduces lung volume by evacuating gas from the lung and entrains room air into the airway. The duration of suctioning is directly related to the frequency and severity of these problems. Generally speaking, the suctioning procedure should last only 10 to 15 seconds. A rule of thumb that helps limit the duration of suctioning is for the clinician to hold his or her breath during the procedure. When the clinician begins to feel air hungry, the patient certainly is, and the procedure should be ended.[97]

Avoiding hypoxemia during suctioning typically is accomplished by hyperoxygenation before the procedure.[92] This can be accomplished by manually ventilating the patient with an FiO_2 of 1.0 before the procedure, increasing the FiO_2 on the ventilator to 1.0 before the procedure, or using the hyperoxygenation program of the ventilator (usually a preprogrammed increase in FiO_2 followed by an automatic return to the previous FiO_2 after 2–3 minutes). Manual hyperinflation or sighs from the ventilator also may be used.[94-96] This type of hyperinflation therapy has fallen out of favor recently with the improved understanding of overdistension lung injury. We believe that manual ventilation is less effective and associated with more frequent complications than the use of manually triggered breaths from the ventilator. The use of manual resuscitators results in unstable tidal volume, FiO_2, and minute volume. In fact, manual ventilation commonly is associated with a reduction in delivered tidal volume, rapid increase in respiratory rate, and elevated airway pressures. This combination can result in hemodynamic compromise during the manual hyperinflation procedure.

Arrhythmias commonly are seen with suctioning procedures and may be caused by hypoxemia, vagal stimulation, or both.[102-104] The use of hyperoxygenation before suctioning can help eliminate this problem.

Sudden disconnection of a patient from PEEP also may cause arrhythmias because venous return is suddenly unimpeded. Closed circuit suction devices should be used when this problem is identified. Mucosal trauma from suction catheters generally results from overzealous suctioning or use of a catheter that is too rigid or has a pointed tip. As previously discussed, the use of a blunt-tipped catheter with multiple side holes reduces this problem. Proper setting of the negative pressure used for suctioning is also important.

Other complications include atelectasis, coughing, bronchospasm, and, in head-injured patients, an increase in intracranial pressure.[104-107] From the patient's side of the suction catheter, suctioning is at best uncomfortable and at worst unbearable. Irritation of the airway causes coughing, and hypoxemia can promote anxiety and dyspnea. Preoxygenation, proper suctioning technique, and careful patient monitoring are important in limiting these complications.

The issue of contamination during the suctioning procedure is often an emotional one. The procedure should be performed using the sterile technique to prevent contamination of the lower respiratory tract. Contamination of the clinician should be avoided by use of universal precautions. Despite some level of concern, contamination of caregivers during suctioning procedures has never been documented to result in illness.

PATIENT–VENTILATOR SYSTEM CHECK

Checking the ventilator has long been an important role for the respiratory care practitioner. This task or procedure recently has been redefined by the American Association for Respiratory Care in a clinical practice guideline.[108] It should be remembered that the patient–ventilator system check need not always be recorded. Checks should be recorded on a regularly scheduled basis based on patient acuity. The guidelines suggest that in addition to regularly scheduled intervals, checks should be performed before obtaining blood gas values, before obtaining hemodynamic or respiratory mechanics data, after a change in settings (except FiO_2), after an acute deterioration in patient condition, or any time the performance of the ventilator is in question. This system was adopted to allow stable patients to receive documented patient–ventilator system checks every 6 hours or more. In a critically ill patient requiring numerous manipulations and frequent blood gas determinations, patient–ventilator system checks might be done every hour. It is also crucial to remember that a patient–ventilator system check is not merely a verification of ventilator settings. It also includes documentation of patient response to ventilation and evaluation of breath sounds, tube placement, cuff pressure, and results of suctioning. The term "patient–ventilator system" emphasizes that the patient is the most important component of the system. Every patient–ventilator check should include assessment of the patient.

REFERENCES

1. Hess D, Burns E, Romangnoli D, Kacmarek RM: Weekly ventilator circuit changes. Anesthesiology 82:903–911, 1995.
2. Kollef MH, Shapiro SD, Fraser VJ, et al: Mechanical ventilation with or without 7-day circuit changes. Ann Intern Med 123:168–174, 1995.
3. Dreyfuss D, Djedani K, Gros I, et al: Mechanical ventilation with heated humidifiers or heat and moisture exchangers: effects on patient colonization and incidence of nosocomial pneumonia. Am J Respir Crit Care Med 151:986–992, 1995.
4. Sanborn WG: Microprocessor based mechanical ventilation. Respir Care 38:72–109, 1993.
5. Branson RD, Campbell RS, Thompson D: Ventilator circuits: what you see may not be what you get. Respir Care 36:629–630, 1991.
6. Banner MJ, Lampotang S, Boysen PG, et al: Flow resistance of expiratory pressure valves systems. Chest 90:212–217, 1986.
7. Banner MJ: Expiratory positive pressure valves: flow resistance and the work of breathing. Respir Care 32:431–439, 1987.
8. Marini JJ, Culver BH, Kirk W: Flow resistance of exhalation valves and positive end-expiratory pressure devices used in mechanical ventilation. 131:850–854, 1985.
9. Pinsky MR, Hrehocik D, Culpepper JA, Snyder JV: Flow resistance of expiratory positive pressure systems. Chest 94:788–791, 1988.
10. Banner MJ, Lampotang S: End expiratory pressure valves. In: Branson RD, Hess D, Chatburn RL (eds): Respiratory Care Equipment. Philadelphia: JB Lippincott, 1998.
11. Birmingham PK, Cheney FW, Ward RJ: Esophageal intubation: a review of detection techniques. Anesth Analg 65:886–891, 1986.
12. Hess D: Monitoring during resuscitation. Respir Care 37:739–768, 1992.
13. Cardoso MSC, Banner MJ, Melker RJ, et al: Portable devices used to detect endotracheal intubation during emergency situations: a review. Crit Care Med 26:957–964, 1998.
14. Murray IP, Modell JH: Early detection of endotracheal tube accidents by monitoring carbon dioxide concentration in respiratory gas. Anesthesiology 59:344–346, 1983.
15. Linko K, Paloheimo M, Tammisto T: Capnography for detection of accidental oesophageal intubation. Acta Anaesthesiol Scand 27:199–202, 1983.
16. Bhende MS, Thompson AE, Howland DF: Validity of a disposable end-tidal carbon dioxide detector in verifying endotracheal tube position in piglits. Crit Care Med 19:566–568, 1991.
17. Bhende MS, Thompson AE, Orr RA: Utility of an end-tidal carbon dioxide detector during stabilization and transport of critically ill children. Pediatrics 89:1042–1044, 1992.
18. Bhende MS: Colorimetric end-tidal carbon dioxide detector. Pediatr Emerg Care 11:58–61, 1995.
19. Goldberg JS, Rawle PR, Zehnder JL, et al: Colorimetric end-tidal carbon dioxide monitoring for tracheal intubation. Anesth Analg 70:191–194, 1990.
20. Higgins DJ, Addy V: Efficacy of the FEF colorimetric end-tidal carbon dioxide detector in children. Anesth Analg 76:683–684, 1993.
21. Jones BR, Dorsey MJ: Sensitivity of a disposable end-tidal carbon dioxide detector. J Clin Monit 7:268–270, 1991.
22. O'Flaherty D, Adams AP: The end-tidal carbon dioxide detector: assessment of a new method to distinguish oesophageal from tracheal intubation. Anaesthesia 45:653–655, 1990.
23. Petroianu GA, Maleck WH, Bergler WF, et al: Preliminary observations on the Colibri CO_2-indicator. Am J Emerg Med 16:677–680, 1998.
24. Barton C, Callaham M: Lack of correlation between end-tidal carbon dioxide concentrations and $PaCO_2$ in cardiac arrest. Crit Care Med 19:108–110, 1991.
25. Garnett AR, Ornato JP, Gonzalez ER, et al: End tidal carbon dioxide monitoring during cardiopulmonary resuscitation. JAMA 257:512–515, 1987.
26. Higgins D, Hayes M, Denman W, et al: Effectiveness of using end-tidal carbon dioxide concentration to monitor cardiopulmonary resuscitation. BMJ 300:581, 1990.
27. Isserles SA, Breen PH: Can changes in end-tidal PCO_2 measure changes in cardiac output? Anesth Analg 73:808–814, 1991.
28. Ornato JP, Garnett AR, Glauser FL: Relationship between cardiac output and the end-tidal carbon dioxide tension. Ann Emerg Med 19:1104–1106, 1990.

29. Sanders AB, Kern KB, Otto CW, et al: End-tidal carbon dioxide monitoring during cardiopulmonary resuscitation: a prognostic indicator for survival. JAMA 262:1347–1351, 1989.

30. Levine RL, Wayne MA, Miller CC: End-tidal carbon dioxide and outcome of out-of-hospital cardiac arrest. N Engl J Med 337:301–306, 1997.

31. Kasper CL, Deem S: The self-inflating bulb to detect esophageal intubation during emergency airway management. Anesthesiology 88:898–902, 1998.

32. Ardagh M, Moodie K: The esophageal detector device can give false positives for tracheal intubation. J Emerg Med 16:747–779, 1998.

33. Zaleski L, Abello D, Gold M: The esophageal detector device: does it work? Anesthesiology 79:244–247, 1993.

34. Williams KN, Nunn JF: The oesophageal detector device: a prospective trial on 100 patients. Anaesthesia 44:412–414, 1989.

35. Wee M: The oesophageal detector device: assessment of a new method to distinguish oesphageal from tracheal intubation. Anaesthesia 43:27–29, 1988.

36. Pelucio M, Halligan L, Dhindsa H: Out-of-hospital experience with the syringe esophageal detector device. Acad Emerg Med 4:463–468, 1997.

37. Donahue PL: The esophageal detector device: an assessment of accuracy and ease of use by paramedics. Anaesthesia 49:863–865, 1994.

38. Gray P, Sullivan G, Ostryzniuk P, et al: Value of postprocedural chest radiographs in the adult intensive care unit. Crit Care Med 20:1513–1518, 1992.

39. Henschke CI, Yankelevitz DF, Wand A, et al: Accuracy and efficacy of chest radiography in the intensive care unit. Intensive Care Radiol 34:21–31, 1996.

40. Eagle CCP: The relationship between a person's height and appropriate endotracheal tube length. Anaesth Intens Care 20:156–160, 1992.

41. Owen RL, Cheney FW: Endobronchial intubation: a preventable complication. Anesthesiology 67:255–257, 1987.

42. Roberts JR, Spadafora M, Cone DC: Proper depth placement of oral endotracheal tubes in adults prior to radiographic confirmation. Acad Emerg Med 2:20–24, 1995.

43. Conrardy PA, Goodman LR, Lainge F, et al: Alteration of endotracheal tube position: flexion and extension of the neck. Crit Care Med 4:8–12, 1976.

44. Brunel W, Coleman DL, Schwartz DE, et al: Assessment of routine chest roentgenograms and the physical examination to confirm endotracheal tube position. Chest 96:1043–1045, 1989.

45. Kollef MH, Leagre EJ, Damiano M: Endotracheal tube misplacement: incidence, risk factors, and impact of a quality improvement program. South Med J 87:248–254, 1994.

46. Schwarts DE, Lieberman JA, Cohen NH: Women are at greater risk than men for malpositioning of the endotracheal tube after emergent intubation. Crit Care Med 22:1127–1131, 1994.

47. Tominga GT, Rudzwick H, Scannell G, et al: Decreasing unplanned extubations in the intensive care unit. Am J Surg 170:586–590, 1995.

48. Boulain T: Unplanned extubations in the adult intensive care unit: a prospective multicenter study. Am J Respir Crit Care Med 157:1131–1137, 1998.

49. Listello D, Sessler CN: Unplanned extubation: clinical predictors for reintubation. Chest 105:1496–1503, 1994.

50. Christie JM, Dethlefsen M, Cane RD: Unplanned endotracheal extubation in the intensive care unit. J Clin Anesth 8:289–293, 1996.

51. Vassal T, Anh NG, Gabillet JM, et al: Prospective evaluation of self-extubations in a medical intensive care unit. Intens Care Med 19:340–342, 1993.

52. Taggart JA, Lind MA: Evaluating unplanned endotracheal intubations. Dimens Crit Care Nurse 13:114–121, 1994.

53. Whelen J, Simpson SQ, Levy H: Unplanned extubation: predictors of successful termination of mechanical ventilatory support. Chest 105:1808–1812, 1995.

54. Coppolo DP, May JJ: Self-extubations: a 12-month experience. Chest 98:165–169, 1990.

55. Atkins PM, Mion LC, Mendelson W, et al: Characteristics and outcomes of patients who self-extubate from ventilatory support: a case-control study. Chest 112:1317–1323, 1997.

56. Betbase A, Perez M, Rialp G, et al: A prospective study of unplanned endotracheal extubation in intensive care unit patients. Crit Care Med 26:1180–1186, 1998.

57. Chiang AA, Lee KC, Lee JC, et al: Effectiveness of a continuous quality improvement program aiming to reduce unplanned extubation: a prospective study. Intensive Care Med 22:1269–1271, 1996.

58. Sessler CN: Unplanned extubations: making progress using CQI. Intensive Care Med 23:143–145, 1997.

59. Kaplow R, Bookbinder M: A comparison of four endotracheal tube holders. Heart Lung 23:59–66, 1994.

60. Levy H, Griego L: A comparative study of oral endotracheal tube securing methods. Chest 104:1537–1540, 1993.

61. Volsko TA, Chatburn RL: Comparison of two methods for securing the endotracheal tube in neonates. Respir Care 42:288–291, 1997.

62. Clarke T, Evans S, Way P, et al: A comparison of two methods of securing and endotracheal tube. Aust Crit Care 11:45–50, 1998.

63. Cooper JD, Grillo HC: The evolution of tracheal injury due to ventilatory assistance through cuffed tubes: a pathologic study. Ann Surg 169:334–348, 1969.

64. Cooper JD, Grillo HC: Experimental production and prevention of injury due to cuffed tracheal tubes. Surg Gynecol Obstet 129:1235–1241, 1969.

65. Grillo HC, Cooper JD, Geffin B, et al: A low-pressure cuff for tracheostomy tubes to minimize tracheal injury. J Thorac Cardiovasc Surg 62:898–907, 1971.

66. Knowlson GTG, Bassett HFM: The pressures exerted on the trachea by endotracheal inflatable cuffs. Br J Anaaesth 42:834–837, 1970.

67. Dobrin P, Canfield T: Cuffed endotracheal tubes: mucosal and tracheal wall blood flow. Am J Surg 133:562–568, 1977.

68. Pavlin EG, Van Mimwegan D, Hornbein TF: Failure of a high-compliance low-pressure cuff to prevent aspiration. Anesthesiology 42:216–219, 1975.

69. Bernhard WN, Cottrell JE, Sivakumaran C, et al: Adjustment of intracuff pressure to prevent aspiration. Anesthesiology 50:363–366, 1979.

70. Hess DR, Branson RD: Airway and suction equipment. In: Branson RD, Hess DR, Chatburn RL (eds): Respiratory Care Equipment. Philadelphia: Lippincott Williams and Wilkins, 1999, pp 157–186.

71. Crimlisk JT, Horn MH, Wilson DJ, et al: Artificial airway: a survey of cuff management practices. Heart Lung 25:225–235, 1996.

72. Off D, Braun SR, Tompkins B, et al: Efficacy of the minimal leak technique of cuff inflation in maintaining proper intracuff pressures for patients with cuffed artificial airways. Respir Care 28:1115–1118, 1983.

73. Cox PM, Schatz ME: Pressure measurements in endotracheal cuffs: a common error. Chest 65:84–87, 1974.

74. Ho AM, Contrardi LH: What to do when an endotracheal tube cuff leaks. J Trauma 40:486–487, 1990.

75. Branson RD, Campbell RS, Chatburn RL, et al: AARC Clinical Practice Guideline: endotracheal suctioning of mechanically ventilated adults and children with artificial airways. Respir Care 38:500–504, 1993.

76. Tarnow-Mordi W: Is routine endotracheal suction justified? Arch Dis Child 66:374–375, 1991.

77. Witmer MT, Hess D, Simmons M: An evaluation of the effectiveness of secretion removal with the Ballard closed-circuit suction catheter. Respir Care 36:844–848, 1991.

78. Craig KC, Benson MS, Pierson DJ: Prevention of arterial oxygen desaturation during closed-airway endotracheal suction: effect of ventilator mode. Respir Care 29:1013–1018, 1984.

79. Carlon GC, Fox SJ, Ackerman NJ: Evaluation of a closed-tracheal suction system. Crit Care Med 15:522–525, 1987.

80. Johnson KL, Kearney PA, Johnson SB, et al: Closed versus open tracheal suctioning: costs and physiologic consequences. Crit Care Med 22:654–666, 1994.

81. Hrashbarger SA, Hoffman LA, Zullo TG, et al: Effects of a closed tracheal suction system on ventilatory and cardiovascular parameters. Am J Respir Crit Care Med 3:57–61, 1992.

82. Deppe SA, Kelly JW, Thoi LL, et al: Incidence of colonization, nosocomial pneumonia, and morality in critically ill patients using a Trach Care closed-suction system versus an open-suction system: prospective, randomized study. Crit Care Med 18:1389–1393, 1990.

83. Cobley M, Atkins M, Jones PL: Environmental contamination during tracheal suction. Anaesthesia 46:957–961, 1991.

84. Ritz R, Scott LR, Coyle MB, et al: Contamination of a multiple-use suction catheter in a closed-circuit system compared to contamination of a disposable, single-use suction catheter. Respir Care 31:1086–1091, 1986.

85. Kollef MH, Prentice S, Shapiro SD, et al: Mechanical ventilation with or without daily changes of in-line suction catheters. Am J Respir Crit Care Med 156:466–472, 1997.

86. Anthony JS, Sieniewicz DJ: Suctioning of the left bronchial tree in critically ill patients. Crit Care Med 5:161–162, 1977.

87. Panacek EA, Albertson TE, Rutherford WF, et al: Selective left endobronchial suctioning in the intubated patient. Chest 95:885–887, 1989.

88. Haberman PB, Green JP, Archibald C, et al: Determinants of successful selective tracheobronchial suctioning. N Engl J Med 313:1060–1063, 1973.

89. Shorten DR, Byrne PJ, Jones RL: Infant responses to saline instillations and endotracheal suctioning. J Obstet Gynecol Neonatal Nurs 20:464–469, 1991.

90. Gray JE, MacIntyre NR, Kronberger WG: The effects of bolus normal-saline instillation in conjunction with endotracheal suctioning. Respir Care 35:785–790, 1990.

91. Hagler DA, Traver GA: Endotracheal saline and suction catheters: sources of lower airway contamination. Am J Crit Care 3:444–447, 1994.

92. Berman IR, Stahl WM: Prevention of hypoxic complications during endotracheal suctioning. Surgery 63:586–587, 1968.

93. Preusser BA, Stone KS, Gonyon DS, et al: Effects of two methods of preoxygenation on mean arterial pressure, cardiac output, peak airway pressure, and postsuctioning hypoxemia. Heart Lung 17:290–299, 1988.

94. Baker PO, Baker JP, Koen PA: Endotracheal suctioning techniques in hypoxemic patients. Respir Care 28:1563–1568, 1983.

95. Glass C, Grap MJ, Corley MC, et al: Nurses' ability to achieve hyperinflation and hyperoxygenation with a manual resuscitation bag during endotracheal suctioning. Heart Lung 22:158–165, 1993.

96. Singer M, Vermaat J, Hall G, et al: Hemodynamic effects of manual hyperventilation in critically ill mechanically ventilated patients. Chest 106:1182–1187, 1994.

97. George RB: Duration of suctioning: an important variable. Respir Care 28:457–459, 1983.

98. Baier H, Begin R, Sackner MA: Effect of airway diameter, suction catheters, and the bronchofiberscope on airflow in endotracheal and tracheostomy tubes. Heart Lung 5:235–238, 1976.

99. Amikam B, Landa J, West J, et al: Bronchofiberscopic observations of the tracheobronchial tree during intubation. Am Rev Respir Dis 105:747–755, 1972.

100. Landa JF, Chapman GA, Sackner MA: Effects of suctioning on mucociliary transport. Chest 77:202–207, 1980.
101. Sackner MA, Landa JF, Greeneltch N, et al: Pathogenesis and prevention of tracheobronchial damage with suction procedures. Chest 64:282–290, 1973.
102. Shim C, Fine N, Fernandez R, et al: Cardiac arrhythmias resulting from tracheal suctioning. Ann Intern Med 71:1149–1153, 1969.
103. Winston SJ, Gravelyn TR, Stirin RG: Prevention of bradycardic responses to endotracheal suctioning by prior administration of nebulized atropine. Crit Care Med 15:1009–1011, 1987.
104. Walsh JM, Vanderwarf C, Hoscheit D, et al: Unsuspected hemodynamic alterations during endotracheal suctioning. Chest 95:162–165, 1989.
105. Rudy EB, Baun M, Stone K, et al: The relationship between endotracheal suctioning and changes in intercranial pressure: a review of the literature. Heart Lung 15:488–494, 1986.
106. Dohi S, Gold I: Pulmonary mechanics during general anesthesia: the influence of mechanical irritation of the airway. Br J Anaesth 51:205–213, 1979.
107. Gugielminotti J, Desmonts J, Dureuil B: Effects of tracheal suctioning on respiratory resistances in mechanically ventilated patients. Chest 113:1335–1338, 1998.
108. AARC Clinical Practice Guideline Group. Patient/Ventilator System Check. 37:882–886, 1992.

CHAPTER 4

Humidification and Aerosol Therapy During Mechanical Ventilation

Richard D. Branson, BA, RRT

PHYSICAL PROPERTIES

PHYSIOLOGIC PRINCIPLES

HIGH-FLOW HUMIDIFIERS

Types of High-Flow
  Humidifiers

PASSIVE HUMIDIFIER

CHARACTERISTICS OF
ARTIFICIAL NOSES

Moisture Output

Resistance

Dead Space

Additives

USE OF HUMIDIFICATION
DEVICES DURING
MECHANICAL VENTILATION

ACTIVE HYGROSCOPIC
HEAT AND MOISTURE
EXCHANGERS

Heat and Moisture
  Exchanger Booster

AEROSOL THERAPY
DURING MECHANICAL
VENTILATION

Physical Properties

Types of Aerosol
  Generators

Aerosol Delivery During
  Mechanical Ventilation

Monitoring Bronchodilator
  Efficacy

Recommendations for
  Aerosol Therapy in
  Mechanically Ventilated
  Patients

REFERENCES

KEY WORDS

absolute humidity	heat and moisture exchanger	lithium chloride
active heat and moisture exchanger	heat and moisture exchanging filter	mass median aerodynamic diameter
auto-positive end-expiratory pressure (autoPEEP)	heated wire circuit	metered-dose inhaler
bubble humidifier	high-flow humidifier	moisture output
calcium chloride	hygroscopic heat and moisture exchanger	passover humidifier
cascade humidifier	hygroscopic heat and moisture exchanging filter	rainout
condensation		relative humidity
dead volume	inertial impaction	saturated
gravitational sedimentation	isothermic saturation boundary	small-volume nebulizer
heat and moisture exchanger (HME) booster		spacer

PHYSICAL PROPERTIES

Water is found in all three states of matter within a relatively small temperature range. When energy is applied to liquid water, usually in the form of heat, water molecules move independently of one another. As molecules leave the surface of the liquid, they become water vapor. The amount of water vapor present in a gas is commonly referred to as humidity. Water vapor also can be called molecular water.

The amount of water vapor in a gas can be measured and expressed in a number of ways. In medicine, the most common terms are absolute humidity and relative humidity. **Absolute humidity** is the amount of water vapor present in a gas mixture. Absolute humidity is directly proportional to gas temperature, increasing with an increasing gas temperature and decreasing with a decreasing gas temperature (Table 4–1). Absolute humidity typically is expressed in mg/L, g/cm^3, or as a partial pressure (P$_{H_2O}$). Absolute humidity can be calculated using the equation

$$AH = 16.42 - 0.73T + 0.04T^2$$

where AH is absolute humidity and 100% saturation and T is the gas temperature in °C. Alveolar gas is 37°C and contains 43.9 mg H_2O/L of gas.

A gas mixture holding all the water vapor it is capable of holding is said to be **saturated** or at the maximum capacity of water vapor. The amount of humidity in a gas that is less than saturated can be determined by comparing the absolute humidity (the water vapor present) to the maximum capacity (the maximum possible water vapor) of the gas at a given temperature. This value is known as **relative humidity.** Relative humidity is expressed as a percentage using the following equation:

Relative humidity (%) = (absolute humidity)/(maximum capacity) × 100.

These measurements are useful in determining the causes of some common clinical phenomena. For example, if gas leaves a heated humidifier outlet at a temperature of 34°C and 100% relative humidity and is heated by a heated wire circuit to 37°C at the airway, relative humidity decreases because the higher gas temperature has a greater capacity for carrying water. In the previous example, if the gas temperature were 37°C and the absolute humidity measured was 37 mg H_2O/L, then we can determine the relative humidity by comparing this value to the maximum capacity for water vapor at 37°C from Table 4–1.

$$\% \text{ Relative Humidity} = \frac{37}{43.9} \times 100 = 84.3\%$$

This explains reports of dried secretions in the endotracheal tubes of patients using

TABLE 4–1. The Relationship of Gas Temperature, Absolute Humidity, and Water Vapor Pressure

GAS TEMPERATURE (°C)	ABSOLUTE HUMIDITY (mg H₂O/L)	WATER VAPOR PRESSURE (PH₂O)
0	4.85	4.6
5	6.8	6.5
10	9.4	9.2
15	12.8	12.8
20	17.3	17.5
25	23.0	23.7
30	30.4	31.7
32	33.8	35.5
34	37.6	39.8
36	41.7	44.4
37	43.9	46.9
38	46.2	49.5
40	51.1	55.1
42	56.5	61.3
44	62.5	68.1

heated humidification and heated wire circuits. The greater the difference between temperature at the chamber and temperature at the airway, the lower the relative humidity. This temperature offset is important to keep the circuit free of rainout. Unfortunately, in certain environments (e.g., near windows, fans, heating units, and air conditioning vents) the environmental changes can affect heated wire circuit efficacy. However, clinicians should be careful to ensure that the patient receives adequate relative humidity as a priority over a circuit free from rainout. When a heated humidifier without a heated wire circuit is used, it is often necessary for the temperature of the gas in the humidification chamber to reach temperatures of 50°C for temperature delivered to the airway to approach 37°C. An example of this is shown in Figure 4–1. In this example, the maximum water vapor content of gas at 50°C is 83 mg H₂O/L and the maximum water vapor content of gas at 37°C is 43.9 mg H₂O/L. The difference in water vapor content between the two gases—83 − 43.9 = 39.1 mg H₂O/L—represents the amount of condensate or **rainout** that accumulates in the circuit. For a minute ventilation of 10 L/min, this would result in a little more than 0.5L of rainout in a 24-hour period.

If the relative humidity and temperature are known, the water vapor content also can be calculated. For example, if a heat and moisture exchanger provides 32°C and 95% relative humidity, then the water vapor content can be calculated:

$$\text{Water vapor content} = \frac{\% \text{ relative humidity} \times \text{maximum capacity}}{100}$$

$$\text{Water vapor content} = \frac{(95\% \times 33.8 \text{ mg H}_2\text{O/L})}{100\%} = 32.1 \text{ mg H}_2\text{O/L}$$

The relative humidity of a gas saturated with water vapor at any temperature is 100%. This point is also commonly known as the dew point.

PHYSIOLOGIC PRINCIPLES

During normal breathing, the upper respiratory tract warms, humidifies, and filters inspired gases. This task is accomplished primarily in the nasopharynx, where gases are exposed to the highly vascular, moist mucus membrane. Upper airway efficiency is enhanced further by the large surface area and turbulent flow afforded by the na-

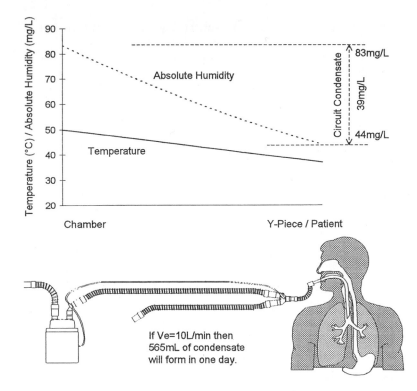

FIGURE 4–1

Gas cooling and condensate formation when a heated humidity generator and unheated delivery system are combined. Gas leaves the humidifier at more than 50°C (83 mg/L) and cools to 37°C (44 mg/L), creating 39 mg/L of condensate. (From Peterson BD: Heated humidifiers: structure and function. Respir Care Clin North Am 4:243–259, 1988.)

sal turbinates. The oropharynx and conducting airways also contribute to this process but are less efficient because they lack the exquisite architecture of the nasopharynx. During exhalation, the upper airways reclaim a large percentage of the heat and moisture added during inspiration. This function often is overlooked, but the moisture conservation properties of the upper airway rival the humidity properties as part of an extremely efficient countercurrent heat and moisture exchange. Over the course of a normal day, the respiratory tract loses approximately 1470 joules of heat and 250 ml of water.[1] This net loss of heat and moisture is predominantly the result of water vapor escaping in expired gases. Little heat actually is lost through the warming of inspired gas because the specific heat of air is very low.

The efficiency of the normal upper airway is quite remarkable. Even at extremes of inspired temperature and humidity, gas that reaches the alveolar level is 100% saturated at body temperature.[2] Measurements accomplished in patients with an intact upper airway suggest that after passing through the nasopharynx, inspired gases

are 29°C to 32°C at nearly 100% relative humidity. As the gases approach the carina, gases are 32°C to 34°C and nearly 100% relative humidity.[3, 4] These values become important as a template for deciding which level of heat and humidity to deliver to intubated patients, in whom inspired gases bypass the upper airway and are delivered directly to the lower trachea.

The point at which gases reach alveolar conditions (37°C and 100% relative humidity) is known as the **isothermic saturation boundary** (ISB). Under normal conditions, the ISB resides in the fourth to fifth generation of subsegmental bronchi. The position of the ISB is fairly constant, regardless of environmental temperature and humidity conditions. Position of the ISB also can be shifted by the presence of lung disease and patient fluid status. Above the ISB, the respiratory tract performs the function of a countercurrent **heat and moisture exchanger,** adding heat and moisture on inspiration and conserving heat and moisture during expiration. Below the ISB, temperature and water content remain relatively constant.

After intubation, the ISB is shifted down

the respiratory tract as the normal upper airway heat and moisture exchanging structures are bypassed. This places the burden of heat and moisture exchange on the lower respiratory tract, a task for which it is poorly suited. The delivery of cold, anhydrous medical gases further burdens the lower respiratory tract and plunges the ISB down the bronchial tree. The combined effects of intubation and mechanical ventilation with dry gases can result in severe losses of heat and moisture from the respiratory mucosa. In extreme cases, damage to the structure and function of the respiratory epithelium can occur, which has clinical implications.[5-8] Table 4–2 lists the known alterations caused by breathing cool, dry gas via an artificial airway.

The provision of heat and humidity during mechanical ventilation is a standard of care during mechanical ventilation around the world.[9, 10] There is little disagreement about the importance of humidification, but there exists considerable disagreement as to the best method of humidification delivery and the amount of humidification required. The methods for providing humidity include active, microprocessor-controlled, heat and humidifying systems (heated humidifiers) and simple, passive, heat and moisture exchangers (artificial noses).

HIGH-FLOW HUMIDIFIERS

High-flow humidifiers are capable of providing a wide range of temperatures and humidities.[11] High-flow humidifiers generically consist of a heating element, a water reservoir, a temperature control unit (including temperature probe and alarms), and a gas/liquid interface that increases the surface area for evaporation. Most high-flow humidifiers fit into one of the following categories: **passover humidifiers, cascade humidifiers,** or **wick humidifiers.** Because these devices are heated, they also prevent loss of body heat from the patient, which is particularly important in neonatal applications. When heated humidifiers are used, the temperature at the patient's airway should be monitored continuously with a thermometer or thermistor. Although not common, it also may be desirable to monitor the relative humidity at the proximal airway.

With high-flow humidifiers, the water level in the reservoir can be maintained manually by adding water from a bag through a fill-set attached to the humidifier or by a float-feed system that keeps the water level constant. Manual methods tend to increase the risk of reservoir contamination and pose the additional risk of spilling and overfilling. Fill-set and float-feed systems are preferable. The float-feed systems also avoid fluctuations in the temperature of gas delivered, which occurs when a volume of cold water is added to the humidifier.

Most humidifiers are servo-controlled, that is, the operator sets the desired gas temperature at the thermistor, and the sys-

TABLE 4–2. Structural and Functional Changes in the Respiratory Tract and the Physiologic Effects Caused by Breathing Cool, Dry Gases Via an Artificial Airway

STRUCTURAL	FUNCTIONAL	PHYSIOLOGIC
Loss of ciliary function	Interruption of the mucociliary escalator	Retained secretions
Destruction of cilia		Mucus plugging of airways
Desiccation of mucus glands	Increases mucus viscosity	Atelectasis
Reduction in cellular cytoplasm	Reduced pulmonary compliance	Increased work of breathing
Ulceration of mucosa	Increased airway resistance	Hypoxemia
Loss of surfactant	Intrapulmonary shunting	Hypothermia

tem maintains control of patient gas temperature despite changes in gas flow or level of water in the reservoir. These systems also are equipped with audiovisual alarms to alert the user of high temperature conditions. The temperature-monitoring devices used in these systems have a relatively slow response time and only reflect the average temperature of the inspired gas. Actual temperatures fluctuate above and below the average temperature with cyclic gas flow, as may occur in a mechanical ventilator circuit. This creates a situation in which gas in the ventilator circuit cools during inspiration while gas above the humidifier becomes superheated. The resulting gas delivered to the patient begins at a temperature below set temperature, then exceeds set temperature as gas from the humidifier reaches the patient.

Heated wire circuits contain electric wires that impart heat to the gas as it travels down the ventilator circuit. Heated wire circuits prevent a temperature decrease in the tubing, provide a more precise gas temperature delivered to the patient, and prevent **condensation** of water in the tubing. The temperature of the heated wire is controlled by the humidifier in concert with the servo temperature control system. When used with a heated humidifier, the heated wire circuit commonly increases temperature of the gas as it traverses the length of the circuit. This prevents condensate because gas arriving at the patient airway is capable of carrying more moisture then gas exiting the humidifier. This intended positive attribute also causes the relative humidity of delivered gases to decrease. This decrease in relative humidity may result in drying of secretions and endotracheal tube obstruction.[12] Conversely, if the temperature of the tubing is less than the temperature of the gas leaving the humidifier, condensation occurs in the tubing. Because heated wire circuits are commonly a single, nonjointed piece of tubing, placing a water trap in the inspiratory limb is impractical. As such, the presence of condensate in heated wire circuits is discouraged because of difficulties in removing it. However, if set properly, heated wire circuits may develop a small amount

of condensate, which requires draining only daily.

The use of servo-controlled heated wire circuits can become complex when the gas is delivered to neonates in an incubator or those under a radiant heater.[13] The problem is related to exposure of the circuit to two temperatures: room temperature and the temperature in the incubator (or under the radiant heater). In these applications, the thermistor should be placed directly outside the incubator (or out from under the radiant heater) rather than at the proximal airway of the patient.

In systems that do not use heated wire circuits, water that collects in the tubing can serve as a potential source of nosocomial infection. Water in the tubing also can result in an accidental lavage of the patient's airway during turning. Condensation in the circuit should be collected in a water trap and disposed of appropriately. The water that condenses in the tubing should be considered contaminated and never should be allowed to drain back into the humidifier.

Types of High-Flow Humidifiers[11]

Passover Humidifier (Fig. 4–2)

Gas from the ventilator is introduced into the humidifier chamber, passes over the surface of the water reservoir, and exits to the ventilator circuit. This is the simplest form of heated humidifier.

Bubble Humidifier (Fig. 4–3)

Gas from the ventilator is directed through a tube that is submerged in the water reservoir. The gas exits under the water through a diffuser or grid and travels into the ventilator circuit.

Cascade Humidifier (Fig. 4–4)

Gas from the ventilator is directed below the surface of the water reservoir and bubbles upward through a grid. The cascade humidifier is a very efficient bubble humidifier. The grid creates a froth of small bubbles that absorb water. Humidifier tempera-

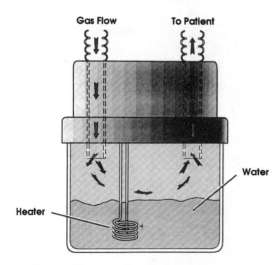

FIGURE 4–2
Passover heated humidifier. (From Branson RD, Hess DR, Chatburn RL: Respiratory Care Equipment. Philadelphia: JB Lippincott, 1996.)

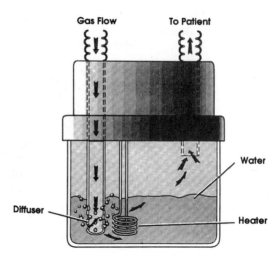

FIGURE 4–4
Cascade heated humidifier. (From Branson RD, Hess DR, Chatburn RL: Respiratory Care Equipment. Philadelphia: JB Lippincott, 1996.)

ture is maintained by a thermostat. A thermometer or thermistor is used at the patient's airway to monitor the temperature of the gas delivered. Unless the tubing leading to the patient is heated, the temperature of the gas between the humidifier and the patient decreases resulting in condensation. Although the cascade humidifier delivers water vapor, it also may deliver microaerosols to the patient, which can transmit bacteria to the patient if the reservoir becomes contaminated.[14] However, the temperature in the water reservoir of a system that does not use a heated wire circuit inhibits the growth of pathogens.[15] This is not the case for systems using heated wire circuits. The temperature of the reservoir with heated wire circuit systems approximates body temperature (34–37°C) and can support growth of bacteria.[16]

Wick Humidifier

The wick humidifier (Fig. 4–5) is a modified passover humidifier that directs gas into a cylinder, lined with a wick of blotter paper. The wick is surrounded by a heating element, and the base of the wick is immersed in water. The wick absorbs water, and as the gas contacts the moist heated wick, the relative humidity of the gas increases. This is a simple method of increasing the temperature and humidification capabilities of the device by increasing the gas/liquid interface without increasing the volume of the reservoir.

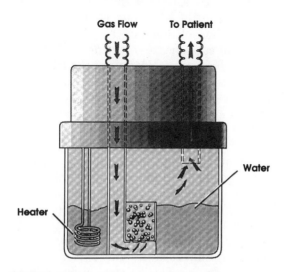

FIGURE 4–3
Bubble heated humidifier. (From Branson RD, Hess DR, Chatburn RL: Respiratory Care Equipment. Philadelphia: JB Lippincott, 1996.)

PASSIVE HUMIDIFIER

Passive humidifier is a generic term used to describe a group of similar humidification

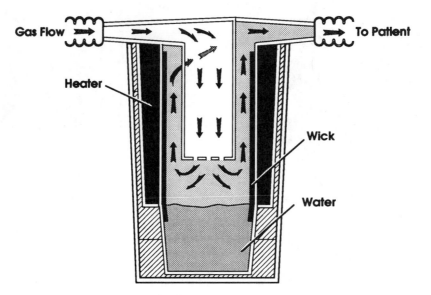

FIGURE 4–5
Heated wick humidifier. (From Branson RD, Hess DR, Chatburn RL: Respiratory Care
Equipment. Philadelphia: JB Lippincott, 1996.)

devices that operate without electricity or a supplementary water source. These devices also frequently are called "artificial noses." The name comes from the device's similarity in function to the human nose. By definition, a passive humidifier is a device that collects the patient's expired heat and moisture and returns it during the following inspiration. The term passive humidifier is preferred over artificial nose because it is more specific to function.[11]

There are several types of passive humidifiers. The differences are related to device design. Figure 4–6 depicts the types of passive humidifiers and Figure 4–7 shows an example of these devices. Devices that use only physical principles of heat and moisture exchange are known as **heat and moisture exchangers** (HMEs). The addition of a filter to an HME results in a **heat and moisture exchanging filter** (HMEF). Other devices are hygroscopically treated to improve moisture-exchanging properties by adding a chemical means of heat and moisture exchange. These devices are called **hygroscopic heat and moisture exchangers** (HHMEs), and the addition of a filter creates an HHMEF. The term hygroscopic HME is more representative of the actual function of the device and allows differentiation from the HME. These devices

frequently have been referred to as hygroscopic condenser humidifiers.

The HME is the simplest of these devices and was the first passive humidifier to be introduced. An HME usually consists of a layered aluminum insert with or without an additional fibrous element. Aluminum exchanges temperature quickly, and during expiration, condensation forms between the aluminum layers. The retained heat and moisture are returned during inspiration. The addition of a fibrous element aids in the retention of moisture and helps reduce pooling of condensate in the dependent portions of the device. HMEs are the least efficient passive humidifiers and often are not used. These devices also tend to be cheaper than other passive humidifiers and may be used in the operating room for short-term humidification. These devices have a nominal moisture output, providing 10 to 14 mg H_2O/L at tidal volumes of 1000 ml to 500 ml.[17, 18]

HMEFs have improved performance compared with HMEs secondary to either the presence of a spun filter media or an increase in the volume (increased surface area) of the media. Surface area is commonly increased by pleating the media and increasing its thickness. Laboratory evaluations of these devices demonstrate a mois-

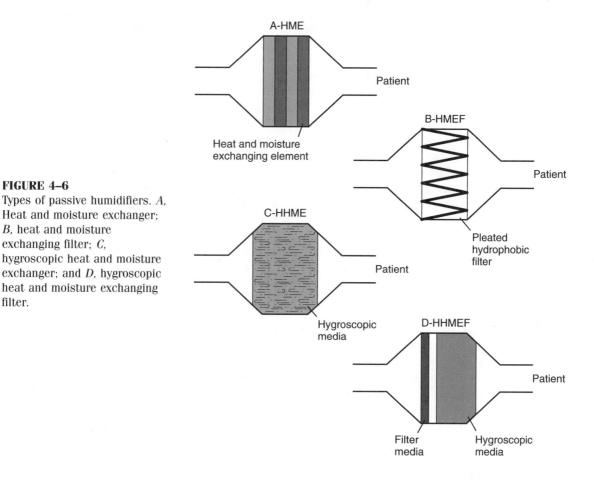

A-HME

Patient

Heat and moisture
exchanging element

B-HMEF

Patient

Pleated
hydrophobic
filter

C-HHME

Patient

Hygroscopic
media

D-HHMEF

Patient

Filter
media

Hygroscopic
media

FIGURE 4–6
Types of passive humidifiers. *A*, Heat and moisture exchanger; *B*, heat and moisture exchanging filter; *C*, hygroscopic heat and moisture exchanger; and *D*, hygroscopic heat and moisture exchanging filter.

ture output of 18 to 28 mg H_2O/L at a tidal volume of 1000 to 500 ml.[18–28]

The HHME is the most popular style of artificial nose. These devices vary widely in shape, size, and type of media insert used. Most HHMEs use a paper or polypropylene insert treated with a hygroscopic chemical, usually calcium or lithium chloride, to en-hance moisture conservation. Comparative studies have shown that HHMEs can provide a moisture output of 22 to 34 mg H_2O/L at tidal volumes from 500 to 1000 ml. The addition of a filter media to an HHME creates an HHMEF.[18–28] The filter media typically is placed between the ventilator connection and the HHMEF's media insert.

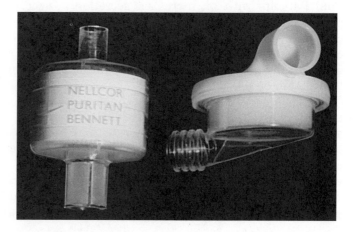

FIGURE 4–7
Typical passive humidifiers used during mechanical ventilation.

This places the hygroscopically treated material between the patient's expired gases and the filter. Typical filtration material is made from spun polypropylene that is electrostatically charged, attracting airborne materials and trapping them. The filter is poorly suited as a heat and moisture exchanging media, but when combined with the hygroscopic element appears to increase moisture output by 1 to 2 mg H_2O/L. The presence of the filter also increases resistance.

CHARACTERISTICS OF ARTIFICIAL NOSES

Moisture Output

The amount of heat and humidity provided by a passive humidifier typically is referred to as **moisture output.** Moisture output is measured under laboratory conditions and reported in milligrams per H_2O/L. There are currently no standards for the minimum moisture output of a passive humidifier. The standard for heated humidifiers suggests a minimum of 33 mg H_2O/L.[29] Application of this standard to HMEs and HHMEs is not very helpful. The AARC has recommended that the required moisture output changes with duration of use and application. For example, a patient with normal respiratory function requiring intubation for a 2-hour operation probably only requires 15 to 20 mg H_2O/L. Mechanically ventilated patients with normal secretions appear to require a minimum of 26 mg H_2O/L to prevent drying of secretions and maintain mucociliary function. Patients with an increased secretion production probably require additional heat and moisture, which a passive humidifier cannot supply. In patients with thick, copious amounts of sputum, heated humidification should be used.

The moisture output reported in the package insert is based on a certain tidal volume, inspiratory time, respiratory rate, and temperature.[30] Deviations from these values cause moisture output to change. As tidal volume increases, moisture output decreases. The amount of this decrease depends on the efficiency of the device and

the dead space. Larger devices tend to be affected less by an increase in tidal volume due to rebreathing. That is, if an HME with an internal volume of 100 ml is used, 100 ml of each inspiration contains expired gases. An increase in respiratory rate or decrease in inspiratory time also decreases moisture output. Likewise, an increase in expiratory flow due to a decrease in lung compliance causes moisture output to decrease. In each of these instances, the decrease in transit time (gas moves through the media more quickly) reduces the ability of the device to remove moisture from exhaled gas and add moisture to inspired gas. When using a passive humidifier, there is always a net heat and moisture loss from the respiratory tract.

Resistance

The resistance to gas flow of a passive humidifier increases as media density increases and as dead space decreases. This increase in resistance may adversely affect the patient's work of breathing.[31-34] However, compared with the added resistance of the endotracheal tube, this increase is small. Most currently manufactured devices have a resistance of less than 3.5 cm H_2O. During use, as the media absorbs water, resistance increases slightly. After prolonged use, the increase in resistance to expiratory flow may cause air trapping and **auto-positive end-expiratory pressure** (autoPEEP).

The greatest concern with resistance occurs when the media becomes occluded with secretions, blood, or water from a secondary source. Several reports have demonstrated an increase in resistance from water and blood accumulating in the media.[35-39] In one instance, the saline intended to aid in loosening secretions before suctioning accumulated in the HHME media.[40] Aerosolized drugs also can cause an increase in resistance as the drug or its carrier becomes trapped in the media or filter. Before delivery of aerosolized medications (delivered by up-draft nebulizer), passive humidifiers should be removed from the airway. During mechanical ventilation, the need for frequent aerosol treatments may necessitate a switch to heated humidification.

Manufacturing defects have resulted in total or partial occlusion of passive humidifiers.[41-44] In each report to date, a remnant from the plastic housing remained in the path of gas flow. Clinicians should visually inspect each device before use.

Dead Space

Placing a passive humidifier on the end of the patient's airway increases dead space. To maintain normal alveolar ventilation, the patient must increase either respiratory rate or tidal volume, or both. If the patient cannot increase alveolar ventilation, arterial carbon dioxide increases. This effect is most pronounced in spontaneously breathing patients and is related to the relationship between the patient's tidal volume and the dead space.

A 70-kg patient with a spontaneous tidal volume of 350 ml and a respiratory rate of 20 breaths/min has a minute ventilation of 7.0 L/min.

$$20 \text{ breaths/min} \times 350 \text{ ml} = 7.0 \text{ L/min.}$$

If the patient's anatomic dead space is 150 ml, then alveolar ventilation is 20 breaths/min $\times$ (350 ml $-$ 150 ml) $=$ 4.0 L/min.

If an HME with a dead space of 100 ml is added to the airway, while minute ventilation remains the same (7.0 L/min), alveolar ventilation decreases to 2.0 L/min.

$$20 \times 350 \text{ ml} - (150 \text{ ml} + 100 \text{ ml}) =$$
$$2.0 \text{ L/min.}$$

For alveolar ventilation to be restored to 4.0 L/min, minute ventilation must increase via an increase in respiratory rate, tidal volume, or both.

$$20 \times 450 \text{ ml} - 150 \text{ ml} + 100 \text{ ml}) =$$
$$4.0 \text{ L/min and minute ventilation} =$$
$$9.0 \text{ L/min.}$$

Several authors have shown the adverse effects of added dead space on respiratory mechanics.[45-48] In each study, the addition of an HME or an HHME with a dead space of 100 ml resulted in an increase in the work of breathing, an increase in the required minute ventilation, and an increase in autoPEEP. When patients were able to increase respiratory rate and/or tidal volume, arterial carbon dioxide remained constant. When patients were unable to increase minute ventilation (weak respiratory muscles) arterial carbon dioxide concentrations increased. Pressure support ventilation can be used to overcome the additional work of breathing, but this can lead to the requirement for higher airway pressures, can increase tidal volumes, and can worsen autoPEEP.

When choosing a passive humidifier, the smallest dead space possible that provides adequate humidification should be selected.

Additives

HHMEs use either **calcium chloride** or **lithium chloride** as hygroscopic additives to increase moisture output. Some manufacturers also add chlorhexidine as a bacteriostatic treatment. Lithium, delivered by mouth or injection, is used in the treatment of psychological disorders including depression and mania. It has been suggested that lithium from HHME media may be washed into the trachea and absorbed into the bloodstream, where blood levels may increase to a therapeutic level.[49, 50] This is a theoretical possibility that has never been conclusively proved. The only report of a patient seen to have elevated serum lithium levels while using an HHME had used lithium by mouth before admission to the hospital. The small amount of lithium in these devices appear to make this concern unwarranted.

Cost

Cost is an important feature of any piece of medical equipment. At the time of this writing, the average cost of an HHME is $3.25. The range of costs is extensive

($1.95–$5.75), with HHMEFs and HMEFs being the most expensive devices.

Choosing the Right Passive Humidifier

The important features of a passive humidifier were described previously. During mechanical ventilation in the intensive care unit, I believe the most important features are moisture output, dead space, resistance, and cost. In this setting, an acceptable passive humidifier should have a minimum moisture output of 28 mg H_2O/L, a dead space of less than 50 ml, a resistance of less than 2.5 cm $H_2O/L/sec$, and a cost of less than $2.50 each. Features for devices used in the operating room may be different.

USE OF HUMIDIFICATION DEVICES DURING MECHANICAL VENTILATION

Passive humidifiers function by returning a portion of the heat and moisture exhaled by the patient. As such, there always is a net loss of heat and moisture. The most efficient passive humidifiers return 70 to 80% of the patient's expired humidity. Passive humidifiers are not as efficient as heated humidification devices. We have developed an algorithm for safe and judicious use of passive humidifiers in the intensive care unit[51] (Fig. 4–8). This protocol uses contraindications to passive humidifiers use to advise practitioners when to use heated humidification. Contraindications to use of passive humidifiers include thick, copious amounts of sputum; grossly bloody secretions; and hypothermia (< 32°C).

Passive humidifiers are attractive alternatives to heated humidifiers because of their low cost, passive operation, and ease of use. Table 4–3 compares the advantages and disadvantages of heated and passive humidifiers.

Not all patients can use a passive humidifier. Patients with pre-existing pulmonary disease characterized by thick, copious secretions should receive heated humidification. The same is true for patients with grossly bloody secretions because blood can occlude the media or filter and result in excessive resistance, air trapping, hypoventilation, and possibly barotrauma. Patients with hypothermia should receive heated humidification because passive humidifiers can return only a portion of the moisture exhaled. If patient body temperature is only 32°C (absolute humidity of 32 mg H_2O/L), even a very efficient HHME (80%) can only deliver an absolute humidity of 25.6 mg H_2O/L. Patients with bronchopleural fistula or incompetent tracheal tube cuffs also should not use passive humidifiers. Because the device requires the collection of expired heat and moisture, any problem that allows expired gas to escape to atmosphere without passing through the media will reduce humidity.

Passive humidifiers should never be used in conjunction with heated humidifiers. Particulate water in the media increases resistance and prevents adequate delivery of humidity from either device. If water occludes the filter, the patient cannot be ventilated adequately and may be unable to completely exhale during positive pressure ventilation.

In the intensive care unit, passive humidifiers may be used for extended periods of time. Our experience suggests that a 5-day period is safe and effective. This recommendation is based on numerous studies that find that partial or complete obstruction of endotracheal tubes (suggesting inadequate humidity) appear to occur around this time. Patient sputum characteristics should be assessed with every suctioning attempt. If the secretions appear thick on two consecutive suctioning procedures, the patient should be switched to a heated humidifier. Judging the quality of sputum can be done using the following method, described by Suzukawa and colleagues[52]:

- Thin—The suction catheter is clear of secretions after suctioning.
- Moderate—The suction catheter has secretions adhering to the sides after suctioning, which are removed easily by aspirating water through the catheter.
- Thick—The suction catheter has secretions adhering to the sides after suctioning which are not removed by aspirating water through the catheter.

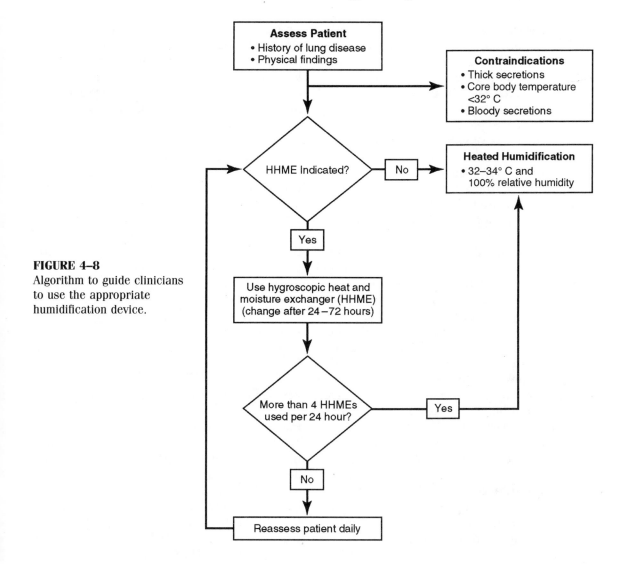

FIGURE 4–8
Algorithm to guide clinicians
to use the appropriate
humidification device.

TABLE 4–3. Comparison of the Advantages and Disadvantages of Humidification Devices Used During Mechanical Ventilation

DEVICE	ADVANTAGES	DISADVANTAGES
Heated humidifiers	Universal application (neonates to adults)	Cost
		Water usage
	Wide range of temperature and humidity	Condensation
		Risk of circuit contamination
	Alarms	Overheating
	Temperature monitoring	Small chance of electric shock/burns
	Reliability	
Artificial noses	Cost	Not applicable in all patients
	Passive operation	Increased dead space
	Simple use	Increased resistance
	Elimination of condensate	Potential for occlusion
	Portable	

Recent work has suggested that the presence of condensate in the elbow or flex tube between the HME and the patient implies adequate humidification. This makes sense because the presence of condensate suggests that gases are saturated with water vapor.[53] Using this technique should help clinicians decide on a case-by-case basis when to switch from an artificial nose to a heated humidifier, if ever. Despite this recommendation, many authors report use of artificial noses safely for up to 30 days.

We believe patients requiring mechanical ventilation for more than 5 days, by definition, are critically ill. At day 5, if lung function has not improved, heated humidification may be considered to prevent secretion retention and maximize mucociliary function. If the patient begins the weaning process at day 5, the added dead space and resistance of the passive humidifier may hinder spontaneous breathing. Although this point may be debated, we believe it to represent the best compromise between cost efficiency, humidification efficiency, and patient safety.[16] Using the clinical evaluation of humidification performance may allow this time period to be extended in some patients.

Most manufacturers suggest changing passive humidifiers every 24 hours. Recent work has shown that if the device remains free of secretions, the change interval can be increased to every 48 or 72 hours, without adverse effect.[54-56] This requires that respiratory care practitioners inspect the device frequently for the presence of secretions and change the device as required. If the device is contaminated frequently by secretions and requires more than three changes daily, the patient should be switched to heated humidification. The frequent soiling of the device suggests that the patient has a secretion problem, and the frequent changes will negate any cost savings.

Early work suggested that the use of passive humidifiers might decrease the incidence of nosocomial pneumonia. However, no reliable evidence supports this conclusion. In fact, in patients with bacteria already in the sputum, the passive humidifier is readily colonized. If there is no sputum contamination of the media, however, replication of bacteria appears controlled.[57]

Patients requiring tracheostomy and prolonged mechanical ventilation in subacute care hospitals and long-term care facilities may use artificial noses for much longer periods of time. The maximum duration has yet to be determined. The reason for this prolonged use is multifactorial. Patients requiring tracheostomy have their upper airway permanently bypassed and the morphologic structure of the lower airway may adapt to provide greater heat and moisture exchange capabilities. Additionally, many of these patients have chronic diseases and are not subject to the multitude of homeostasis problems seen in the hospital. The decision to use heated humidification in this setting should, however, be similar to that described previously.

ACTIVE HYGROSCOPIC HEAT AND MOISTURE EXCHANGERS

Passive humidifiers cannot be used in all situations as a consequence of available moisture output and patient disease. As has been discussed, there are patients who require the addition of heat and moisture to the respiratory tract. In an effort to expand the use of HHMEs, Gibeck-Dryden has introduced the active HHME. This device incorporates an HHME that fits inside a heated housing. The housing contains a paper element that acts like a wick to increase the surface area for gas/moisture transfer. A water source continuously drips water onto the wick. Figure 4–9 is a diagram of the active HME. The wick is warmed by the heated housing increasing moisture output of the device. This system works much like a wick humidifier, except the source of heat and moisture is added at the airway. This eliminates condensate in the inspiratory limb and the need for water traps. In addition, if the water source runs out, this device continues to operate as an HHME. There is never the possibility of delivering dry gas to the airway, as can occur with a traditional heated humidifier.

In a recent evaluation, we found that the

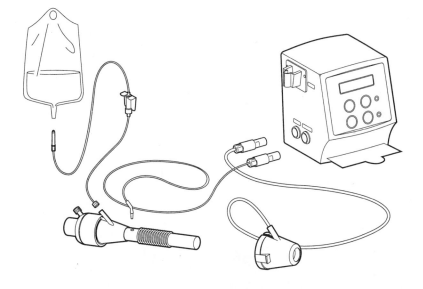

FIGURE 4–9
Schematic of the active heat and moisture exchanger (HME).

active HHME provided temperatures of 36° to 38°C and 90 to 95% relative humidity. Compared with a heated humidifier and a heated humidifier with a heated wire circuit, the active HHME provided equivalent efficiency with lower water usage. The potential disadvantages of this product are the possibility of skin burns and the increase in dead space compared with a heated humidifier of HHME alone. The external temperature of the housing is near 37°C. Under normal conditions, this temperature is safe. However, patients with peripheral edema or low cardiac output may have reduced blood flow to the skin. In these instances, heat transfer is reduced and modest temperatures can cause local burns. Experience with this device is scant at the time of this writing. Future studies can determine whether this device provides any additional benefit compared with conventional heated humidifiers.[58]

Heat and Moisture Exchanger Booster

The **HME booster** is similar in concept to an active HME, but simpler and less efficient. The booster is a small heating element placed between the passive humidifier and the patient. The heating element is covered with a Gore-Tex membrane. Water flows onto the surface of the heating ele-ment and is vaporized (Fig. 4–10). The water passes through the membrane and is delivered to the patient during inspiration. During expiration, the additional moisture is trapped in the passive humidifier, serving to "load" the media with moisture. Some moisture of course escapes through the HME. The water flow is controlled by a small pinhole-sized orifice adjacent to the heating element. This prevents pooling of excess water. Reports of the booster's use are scant. Our laboratory experience suggests that the device can add an additional 2 to 5 mg H_2O/L to inspired gases depending on the tidal volume, inspiratory:expiratory (I:E) ratio, and type of passive humidifier used. Whether this small increase in moisture output is worth the additional equipment and expense remains to be proven.[59]

AEROSOL THERAPY DURING MECHANICAL VENTILATION

Physical Properties

Delivery of medications via the respiratory tract has several advantages over systemic therapy in patients with lung disease. Compared with systemic therapy, aerosol therapy provides a more rapid onset of action and similar efficacy at lower doses. Numerous factors affect aerosol delivery to the respiratory tract. These include particle size,

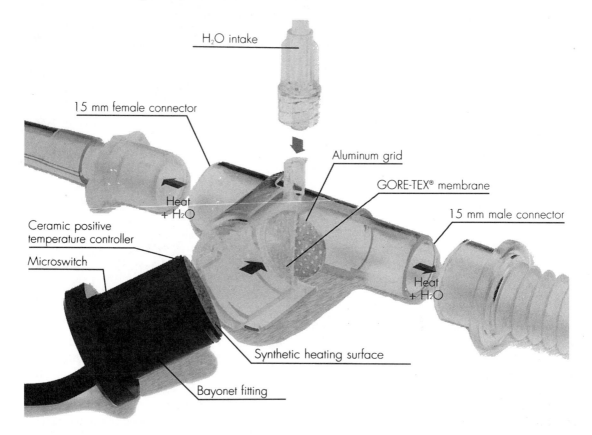

FIGURE 4-10
The heat and moisture exchanger (HME) booster.

inertial impaction, gravitational sedimentation, and diffusion.[60-64] A quick review of these subjects is in order before discussing the additional factors present in the mechanically ventilated patient.

Factors Affecting Aerosol Delivery

Aerosols delivered to the respiratory tract can produce the desired clinical effect only if the particle size is appropriate for the application. In ambulatory patients, aerosols with a **mass median aerodynamic diameter** (MMAD) greater than 5 μm are trapped in the naso- and oropharynx. Bronchodilators and drugs meant to act on the airways should have an MMAD of 2 to 5 μm. Drugs intended for peripheral distribution into the lung parenchyma, such as pentamidine, should have an MMAD of 1 to 3 μm. Particles smaller than 1 μm travel into the respiratory tree, but are commonly removed during exhalation without producing

any effect. The particles in an aerosol vary greatly in size. The MMAD of an aerosol refers to the point at which half the particles in an aerosol are larger than and half the particles are smaller than the stated value. The aerosol particle size creates a standard bell-shaped curve, which is used to determine MMAD. Bronchodilators are the most common drugs delivered by aerosol therapy in the mechanically ventilated patient. Effective delivery requires a MMAD of 3 to 5 μm.[60-64]

Deposition of aerosol particles primarily results from **inertial impaction.** Inertia is the tendency of an object in motion to remain in motion along a straight trajectory. In the continuously branching tracheobronchial tree, gas carrying an aerosol is constantly changing direction at bifurcations in the airways. The larger the mass of a particle, the greater the particle's inertia. More simply, a large particle approaching a branching airway is less likely to change trajectory with gas flow than a small particle. In essence, the inertia of the particle causes it to collide with the surface of the airway and be deposited. Other factors that affect inertia include inspiratory flow (higher flows increase inertia) and turbulent flow (turbulence increases impaction). These two factors are particularly important during mechanical ventilation.

Particles that enter deep into the respiratory tract tend to lose inertia and are deposited primarily as a result of **gravitational sedimentation.** During gravitational sedimentation, the larger the particle, the greater the effect of gravity, and the faster it is deposited. Gravitational sedimentation may be an important method of aerosol deposition during breath holding, when airflow has ceased. The role of an inspiratory hold maneuver during aerosol therapy is discussed later in this chapter. Diffusion plays an important role in deposition of small particles (1–3 μm) in the periphery of the lung. This can occur by direct deposition onto the mucosa or result from collision of aerosol particles causing coalescence and deposition.

Types of Aerosol Generators

Aerosols most commonly are delivered via a **metered-dose inhaler** (MDI) or **small-volume nebulizer** (SVN) during mechanical ventilation.[11] There are advantages and disadvantages to each device. The SVN has been the traditional device of choice, al-though increasing evidence suggests that the MDI is as efficient and less expensive.

Small-Volume Nebulizer

The SVN is typically a disposable device consisting of a reservoir, a gas inlet, a baffle, and a venturi or capillary system that creates the aerosol by combining gas flow and solution at a point of high gas velocity (Fig. 4–11). Performance of an SVN can be affected by innumerable factors. These factors include the construction of the nebulizer, the dead volume, the gas flow powering the nebulizer, the drug being nebulized, the volume of solution, the duration of nebulization, and the gas used to power the nebulizer.[65, 66]

The **dead volume** refers to the volume of solution that is trapped in the reservoir but that cannot be nebulized. Appropriate construction of the nebulizer can serve to reduce the dead volume. To minimize the effects of the dead volume, a minimum solution of 5 ml is recommended. Increasing flow to the nebulizer results in creation of a smaller particle size but also speeds the duration of nebulization and results in greater waste (nebulization during the expiratory phase). Because both too low and too high a flow may be problematic, a flow of 8 to 10 L/min is generally used.

Gases with low densities (helium) tend to improve nebulizer function by increasing velocity and creating small particle sizes.[67, 68] The low density of helium also may improve aerosol delivery by carrying particles through narrow airways. The abil-

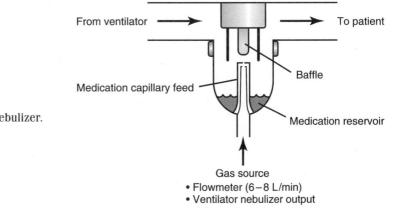

FIGURE 4–11
A typical small-volume nebulizer.

ity of helium to carry an aerosol is less than that of gases with higher densities, and nebulization times may be increased. The use of heliox mixtures to power the SVN should be reserved for patients with severe airflow obstruction (e.g., asthma).

Continuous nebulization is sometimes used to deliver large doses of bronchodilators. As nebulization progresses, evaporation of the diluent increases the drug concentration in the remaining solution. When continuous nebulization is used, the reservoir should be emptied of the dead volume between doses.

Metered-Dose Inhalers

An MDI is a simple, single-patient use, drug delivery system that consists of a pressurized, aluminum drug-filled canister and an actuator (Fig. 4–12). The device is activated by compressing the canister into the actuator, causing the pressure to release a unit dose (normally called a puff) of medication. The initial particle size of aerosol from an MDI is relatively large (> 30 μm), with particle size decreasing as the propellant evaporates. The medication released from the MDI creates a plume of aerosol traveling away from the actuator.[69–71]

The "metered" portion of MDI refers to the metering valve that controls the dose of drug delivered. Each actuation delivers a fixed volume of 25 to 100 μl and results in 15 to 20 ml of aerosol volume. This is accomplished by using a dose-metering chamber that is physically separate from the main reservoir. The metering chamber refills after each actuation and is stored, ready for the next dose.

Factors affecting MDI performance include separation of the drug and propellant, temperature, tail-off, and position. Shaking and warming the canister in the hands helps eliminate the first two problems. Tail-off refers to the lower dose delivered near the end of the canister volume.[11] This problem can be remedied by using only the number of doses specified on the canister. The MDI always should be held in an upright position during dosing.

A **spacer** or holding chamber is a device combined with an MDI to improve drug delivery. The spacer serves to reduce the velocity of the dose and reduce MMAD. Factors affecting the efficiency of a spacer include size, shape, and duration of use. Spacers frequently are used in ambulatory patients but have become popular during the use of an MDI during mechanical ventilation. Figure 4–13 depicts spacer devices used during mechanical ventilation.

Aerosol Delivery During Mechanical Ventilation

Numerous circumstances within the patient/ventilator system affect the efficiency of aerosol delivery using either an SVN or

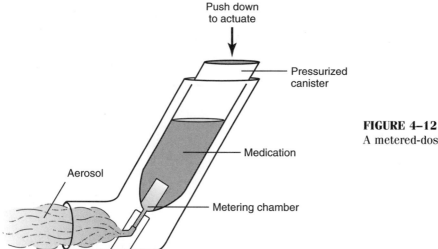

Push down to actuate

Pressurized canister

Medication

Aerosol

Metering chamber

FIGURE 4–12
A metered-dose inhaler.

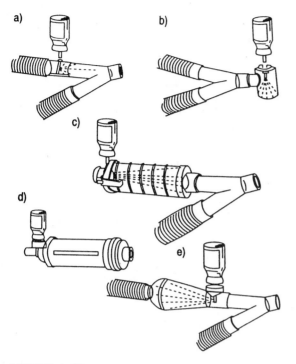

FIGURE 4–13

Different types of commercially available adapters to connect a metered-dose inhaler (MDI) to the ventilator circuit. A, in-line adapter; B, elbow adapter; C, collapsible spacer; D, noncollapsible chamber; E, chamber where actuation of the MDI delivers aerosol away from the patient. (From Dhand R, Tobin MJ: Bronchodilator delivery with metered dose inhalers in mechanically ventilated patients. Eur J Respir Dis 9:585, 1996.)

an MDI. These include the artificial airway, the ventilator circuit, humidity, humidification devices, ventilator settings, and position of the aerosol generator in the circuit.[72–85] Each of these is discussed.

The artificial airway typically is considered the major impediment to aerosol delivery to the lower respiratory tract.[82, 85] The artificial airway acts as the primary site of aerosol impaction, removing a large portion of the aerosol particles. The ventilator circuit includes the Y-piece, elbow connector, and corrugated tubing, all of which serve as areas of impaction, removing aerosol as a function of circuit length and acuity of angles.[73, 75, 77, 83] The position of the aerosol generator in the circuit also affects efficiency.[77] If the device is too far from the patient, aerosol may be lost because of impaction. If the device is too close to the pa-

tient, aerosol may be lost secondary to impaction and through the expiratory side of the breathing circuit. When the aerosol generator is placed approximately 25 to 30 cm from the Y-piece, the circuit serves as a spacer, improving aerosol delivery. The addition of a spacer only marginally improves aerosol delivery with an SVN.

When an MDI is used, the actuator adapter may be paced in-line in the inspiratory limb of the circuit, at the elbow, or directly onto the airway. The use of a spacer in the inspiratory limb significantly improves aerosol delivery with an MDI.[76, 79, 80] The MDI can be actuated during expiration such that the plume is carried to the patient on the subsequent breath or, in some cases, synchronized with breath delivery. Some authors have suggested that synchronization with inspiration improves aerosol delivery by one third.[73] Numerous methods for improving aerosol delivery during use of an MDI have been suggested.

Humidity in the ventilator circuit tends to result in an increase in particle size and diminished aerosol delivery.[75] The amount of alteration in particle size is a function of relative humidity. During heated humidification, the dose may be diminished by half. Heated humidification with a nonheated wire circuit has the highest relative humidity and greatest adverse effect on aerosol delivery. In these cases, it may be wise to bypass the heated humidifier during use of an SVN. Heated humidification with a heated wire circuit generally has a relative humidity of less than 100% and has less effect. The ventilator circuit has no humidity when a passive humidifier is used. However, the presence of a passive humidifier acts as a filter, removing aerosol particles. In the case of the SVN, nebulization of solutions into a passive humidifier may result in occlusion. When a passive humidifier is used, it must be removed during use of the SVN. If an MDI is used, it should be removed unless the actuator adapter is between the patient and the passive humidifier. Patients requiring continuous nebulization of bronchodilators never should use a passive humidifier.[11]

Ventilator settings, mode, the presence of continuous flow, and the source of gas flow all may affect aerosol delivery.[75, 77, 78] Spontaneous breaths tend to improve aerosol delivery over mandatory breaths when tidal volume is sufficient. Sufficient tidal volume means a volume greater than the volume of the ventilator circuit and artificial airway. In adults, a tidal volume of greater than 500 ml generally improves aerosol delivery. A longer inspiratory duty cycle (longer inspiratory time) also improves aerosol delivery because a greater volume from the aerosol generator is delivered with each breath. Prolonged inspiratory times also may improve aerosol delivery by enhancing deposition in the airways.

When flow-triggering systems are used, a continuous flow of gas from 2 to 20 L/min may travel through the ventilator circuit. This continuous flow of gas increases aerosol being washed through the ventilator circuit and out to the atmosphere. When using an SVN, the continuous flow should be disabled, if possible. When using an MDI, the actuation should be synchronized with inspiration.[73]

When using an SVN treatment, time can affect total aerosol deposition. Generally the longer the treatment time, the greater the dose of drug that is deposited. This concept is the pretext for using continuous nebulization of bronchodilators with an SVN in patients with severe airway obstruction.

Use of the mechanical ventilators nebulizer option also may influence SVN efficiency. McPeck and associates found that the flow-through delivered via the ventilator's nebulizer port varied considerably.[78] Lower flow can result in large particle size and prolonged nebulization times. The activation of ventilator nebulizers is also different from manufacturer to manufacturer. In some instances, only mandatory breaths result in initiation of the nebulizer. In others, every breath triggers the nebulizer flow. The duration of nebulizer flow also changes with inspiratory flow waveform (Table 4–4). Nebulization systems were designed to prevent augmentation of tidal volume during aerosol delivery using an SVN and a continuous flow of gas. Sophisticated ventilator algorithms also maintain inspired oxygen concentration (FiO_2) and tidal volume constant during nebulizer function.

TABLE 4–4. Factors Influencing the Deposition of Aerosol Delivery in Intubated, Mechanically Ventilated Patients

VENTILATOR-RELATED FACTORS
Mode of mechanical ventilation
Tidal volume
Respiratory frequency
Inspiratory time (duty cycle)
Inspiratory flow waveform
Presence of continuous flow (flow triggering)

DEVICE-RELATED FACTORS
Position of nebulizer in circuit—SVN
Position of adapter and/or spacer in the circuit—MDI
Timing of actuation—MDI
Type of nebulizer (SVN) or adapter (MDI)
Duration of operation and continuous vs. intermittent nebulization (SVN)

VENTILATOR CIRCUIT-RELATED FACTORS
Endotracheal tube size
Presence of angles in the circuit (90 degree elbow, flex tubes)
Relative humidity of inspired gases
Density of inspired gases (heliox)
Presence of a passive humidifier

DRUG-RELATED FACTORS
Dose
Aerosol particle
Duration of action

PATIENT-RELATED FACTORS
Severity of airway obstruction
Mechanism of airway obstruction (mucus, bronchospasm, mechanical)
Presence of dynamic hyperinflation
Patient–ventilator synchrony

MDI, metered-dose inhaler; SVN, small-volume nebulizer.
Modified from Dhand R, Tobin MJ: Bronchodilator delivery with metered dose inhalers in mechanically ventilated patients. Eur J Respir Dis 9:585, 1996.

Interestingly, the continuous flow of an SVN powered by an external flowmeter can complicate ventilator triggering and volume monitoring. During flow triggering, the additional external flow prevents triggering by forcing the patient to increase effort to overcome both the ventilator continuous flow and the external continuous flow.[86] This additional flow also passes through the expiratory flow transducer, causing the ventilator to overestimate actual tidal volume. In these instances, aerosol delivery affects the efficacy of mechanical ventilation, the opposite effect of our previous discussions. Additionally, the presence of aerosolized medications in the expiratory limb of the ventilator may affect the accuracy of some flow sensors. This usually is seen only when continuous nebulization using an SVN is used. Filters often are placed in the expiratory limb of the ventilator circuit to protect these devices. When this is done, it is imperative to change the filters regularly, otherwise they become partially occluded, prevent triggering, retard exhalation, and cause air trapping.

Monitoring Bronchodilator Efficacy

Determining the effect of aerosolized bronchodilators commonly is done simply by listening to breath sounds and observing patient comfort. The actual response to bronchodilator therapy depends on a multitude of factors, including the severity of airflow obstruction, the reversibility of bronchospasm, the volume of secretions, the degree of inflammation, and the use of concomitant parenteral bronchodilators.[87–96]

Monitoring the shape of the expiratory flow–volume curve may be useful in detecting a reduction in expiratory airway resistance (Fig. 4–14). Subtle improvements may not be detected in this manner, but most ventilators provide this measurement, making it readily available. When observing the expiratory flow–volume curve, both the peak expiratory flow and the shape of the curve may show signs of reduced airway resistance. When bronchodilation is successful, the peak expiratory flow commonly increases and the duration of expiratory flow may be diminished. These observations are frequently all that is necessary in routine clinical decision making.

More accurate measurements of bronchodilator response are available, although routine application may not be warranted. The equipment and expertise to measure these variables are not routinely available. Measurements of inspiratory parameters (peak inspiratory pressure, inspiratory resistance) are rarely helpful because positive pressure and lung inflation alter resistance by mechanical means. Measurements of expiratory parameters are more sensitive and are described subsequently.

Expiratory airway resistance is measured by delivering a constant flow, passive in-

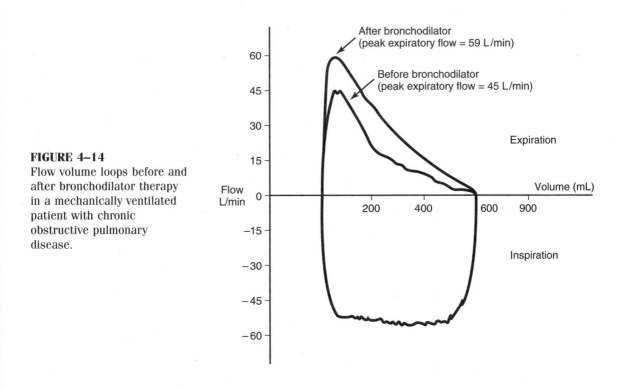

FIGURE 4–14
Flow volume loops before and after bronchodilator therapy in a mechanically ventilated patient with chronic obstructive pulmonary disease.

flation coupled with an inspiratory plateau.[90, 91] If the flow is not constant or the
patient contributes inspiratory or expiratory effort, the measurement is invalid.
The duration of the required inspiratory
pressure plateau depends on the degree of
airway obstruction. Typically, 2 to 3 seconds
are sufficient. However, in some cases, up to
5 seconds are necessary to reach a plateau.
Dhand and colleagues have proposed the
measurement of both minimal and maximal
resistance.[91] These measurements are
shown in Figure 4–15. During passive inflation, the peak inspiratory pressure is
measured as well as the initial pressure at
the beginning of the plateau pressure. This
initial pressure change (peak pressure −
initial plateau pressure/flow) represents
ohmic resistance. By use of the difference
between peak pressure and final plateau
pressure divided by flow, the maximum or
total expiratory resistance can be determined. The difference between the minimum and maximum airway resistance measurements can provide some insight into the
degree of airway obstruction. Alveolar units
with inhomogeneous time constants require
different times before reaching the steady
state plateau pressure. The greater the difference between minimum and maximum
resistance, the greater the inhomogeneties.

Changes in autoPEEP also can provide
evidence of reduced expiratory resistance as
a response to bronchodilator therapy (Fig.
4–16). As expiratory resistance diminishes,
the lung empties more rapidly, resulting in
a decrease in autoPEEP. AutoPEEP is measured more simply than expiratory resistance but is not as sensitive as the expiratory resistance measurement.

The required dose of bronchodilator to
achieve the desired effect depends on the
patient factors previously discussed. Routine administration of 2.5 mg of albuterol
by SVN or 4 puffs of albuterol by MDI provide the maximum effect with minimum

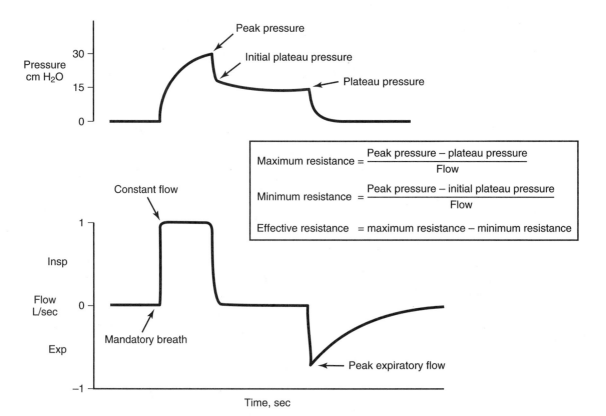

$$\text{Maximum resistance} = \frac{\text{Peak pressure} - \text{plateau pressure}}{\text{Flow}}$$

$$\text{Minimum resistance} = \frac{\text{Peak pressure} - \text{initial plateau pressure}}{\text{Flow}}$$

$$\text{Effective resistance} = \text{maximum resistance} - \text{minimum resistance}$$

FIGURE 4–15
Measurement of minimum and maximum expiratory resistance using flow and pressure
waveforms.

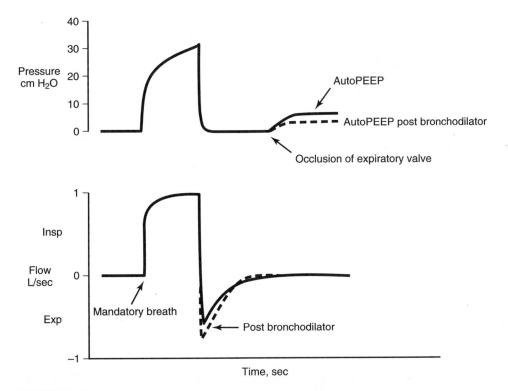

FIGURE 4–16
Measurement of auto-positive end-expiratory pressure (autoPEEP) before and after delivery of a bronchodilator.

TABLE 4–5. Recommendations for Small-Volume Nebulizer (SVN) and Metered-Dose Inhaler (MDI) Use

PROPER TECHNIQUE FOR USING SVN	PROPER TECHNIQUE FOR USING MDI
Fill nebulizer with medication and diluent to appropriate fill volume (4–6 ml)	Choose appropriate MDI adapter/spacer and place in the inspiratory limb of the ventilator circuit
Place nebulizer in the inspiratory limb of the ventilator circuit 25–35 cm from the patient (circuit acts as a spacer)	Adjust ventilation parameters for optimum drug delivery (increase tidal volume, decrease respiratory frequency, lengthen inspiratory time—reset alarms if necessary)
Establish appropriate flow for nebulizer operation (6–8 L/min)—intermittent flow from the ventilator's nebulization system is preferred	Warm MDI with hands and shake vigorously
Adjust ventilation parameters for optimum drug delivery (increase tidal volume, decrease respiratory frequency, lengthen inspiratory time—reset alarms if necessary)	Remove passive humidifier or bypass heated humidifier
If a pediatric continuous flow ventilator is used, reduce ventilator flow to maintain constant tidal volume	Actuate MDI with mandatory breath delivery (adapter)
Turn off continuous flow, if possible	Actuate MDI near end-exhalation (spacer)
Remove passive humidifier or bypass heated humidifier	Wait 30–60 sec between actuations
Observe nebulization, tap sides to reduce dead volume, and continue until all solution is delivered	Remove MDI from circuit adapter and maintain the MDI clean
Remove SVN from circuit and maintain the SVN clean	Monitor patient for signs of improvement or complications
Monitor patient for signs of improvement or complications	

side effects (tachycardia, dysrhythmias). In patients with refractory bronchospasm, continuous nebulization by SVN may be necessary. Monitoring of bronchodilator therapy for dose response using these measurements in routine cases is probably more trouble than it is worth. MDI therapy is cheap, and monitoring in routine cases can be accomplished with simple patient assessment. In severe cases, particularly when continuous nebulization is used, more intensive monitoring is justified.

Recommendations for Aerosol Therapy in Mechanically Ventilated Patients

Based on the aforementioned data, MDI should be used to deliver aerosol therapy during mechanical ventilation. There is no evidence to support the widely held belief that an SVN improves drug delivery or provides faster relief than an MDI. In fact, the MDI is cheaper and requires less time to administer. Use of the SVN is complicated by variation in device performance, dead volume, driving gas flow, and the potential for contamination. SVNs should be used to deliver drugs not available in an MDI system or when continuous nebulization is required for severe airway obstruction.

Recommendations for SVN and MDI use are shown in Table 4–5.

REFERENCES

1. Walker AKY, Bethune DW: A comparative study of condenser humidifiers. Anaesthesia 31:1086–1093, 1976.
2. Drery R: The evolution of heat and moisture in the respiratory tract during anaesthesia with a non-

rebreathing system. Can Anaest Soc J 20:269–277, 1967.
3. Ingelstedt S: Studies on conditioning of respired air in the respiratory tract. Acta Otolarygol 131(suppl):7–21, 1956.
4. Drery R, Pelletier J, Jacques A, et al: Humidity in anesthesiology III: heat and moisture exchange in the respiratory tract during anesthesia with the semi-closed system. Can Anaesth Soc J 14:287–295, 1967.
5. Burton JDK: Effects of dry anaesthetic gases on the respiratory mucous membrane. Lancet 1:235–238, 1962.
6. Chalon J, Loew DAY, Malenbranche J: Effects of dry anesthetic gases on tracheobronchial epithelium. Anesthesiology 37:338–343, 1972.
7. Fonkalsrud EW, Sanchez M, Higgashijima I, et al: A comparative study of the effects of dry vs humidified ventilation on canine lungs. Surgery 78:373–380, 1975.
8. Forbes AR: Humidification and mucus flow in the intubated trachea. Br J Anaesth 45:874–878, 1973.
9. American Association for Respiratory Care Clinical Practice Guidelines: Humidification during mechanical ventilation. Respir Care 37:887–890, 1992.
10. American Association for Respiratory Care: Consensus statement on the essentials of mechanical ventilators—1992. Respir Care 37:1000–1008, 1992.
11. Hess DR, Branson RD: Humidification: humidifiers and nebulizers. In: Branson RD, Hess DR, Chatburn RL (eds): Respiratory Care Equipment. Philadelphia: JB Lippincott, 1995.
12. Miyao H, Hirokawa T, Miyasaka K, Kawazoe T: Relative humidity, not absolute humidity, is of great importance when using a humidifier with a heating wire. Crit Care Med 20:674–679, 1992.
13. Chatburn R: Physiologic and methodologic issues regarding humidity therapy (editorial). J Pediatr 114:416–420, 1989.
14. Rhame FS, Streifel A, McComb C, Boyle M: Bubbling humidifiers produce microaerosols which can carry bacteria. Infect Control 7:403–407, 1986.
15. Goularte TA, Manning MT, Craven DE: Bacterial colonization in humidifying cascade reservoirs after 24 and 48 hours of continuous mechanical ventilation. Infect Control 8:200–203, 1987.
16. Branson RD, Davis K Jr, Brown R, et al: Comparison of three humidification techniques during mechanical ventilation: patient selection, cost, and infection considerations. Respir Care 41:809–816, 1996.
17. Shanks CA: Clinical anesthesia and the multiple gauze condenser humidifier. Br J Anaesth 46:773–777, 1974.
18. Mapelson WW, Morgan JG, Hillard ER: Assessment of condenser humidifiers with special reference to the multiple gauze model. Br Med J 1:300–305, 1963.
19. Branson RD, Davis K Jr: Evaluation of 21 passive humidifiers according to the ISO 9360 standard: moisture output, deadspace, and flow resistance. Respir Care 41:736–743, 1996.
20. Medical Devices Directorate Evaluation. Department of Health, Scottish Home and Health Department, Welsh Office and Department of Health and Social Services Northern Ireland, London, 1994.
21. Cigada M, Elena A, Solca M, Damia G: The efficiency of twelve heat and moisture exchangers: an in vitro evaluation. Intensive Care World 7:98–101, 1990.
22. Shelly M, Bethune DW, Latimer RD: A comparison of five heat and moisture exchangers. Anaesthesia 41:527–532, 1986.
23. Weeks DB, Ramsey FM: A laboratory investigation of six artificial noses for use during endotracheal anesthesia. Anesth Analg 62:758–763, 1981.
24. Mebius CA: A comparative evaluation of disposable humidifiers. Acta Anaesthesiol Scand 27:403–409, 1983.
25. Hayes B: Evaluation report: heat and moisture exchangers. J Med Eng Technol 11:117–128, 1987.
26. Ogino M, Kopotic R, Mannino FL: Moisture-conserving efficiency of condenser humidifiers. Anaesthesia 40:990–995, 1985.
27. Heat and moisture exchangers. Health Devices. 12:155–166, 1983.
28. Unal N, Pompe JC, Holland WPJ, et al: An experimental set-up to test heat-moisture exchangers. Intensive Care Med 21:142–148, 1995.
29. Annual Book of ASTM Standards: F1690-96 Standard Specification for Humidifiers for Medical Use—Part 1: General Requirements for Active Humidification Systems. Section 13: Medical Devices and Services. Volume 13.01: Medical Devices: Emergency Medical Services. West Conshohocken, PA, American Society for Testing and Materials, 1996, pp 1078–1092.
30. International Organization for Standardization 1992: ISO 9360. Anaesthetic and Respiratory Equipment—Heat and Moisture Exchangers for Use in Humidifying Respired Gases in Humans. Geneva, Switzerland, International Organization for Standardization, 1992.
31. Ploysongsang Y, Branson RD, Rashkin MC, Hurst JM: Effect of flowrate and duration of use on the pressure drop across six artificial noses. Respir Care 34:902–907, 1989.
32. Nishimura M, Nishijima MK, Okada T, et al: Comparison of flow-resistive work load due to humidifying devices. Chest 97:600–604, 1990.
33. Manthous CA, Schmidt GA: Resistive pressure of a condenser humidifier in mechanically ventilated patients. Crit Care Med 22:1792–1795, 1994.
34. Chiaranda M, Verona L, Pinamonti O, et al: Use of heat and moisture exchanging (HME) filters in mechanically ventilated ICU patients: influence on airway flow-resistance. Intensive Care Med 19:462–466, 1993.
35. McEwan AI, Dowell L, Karis JH: Bilateral tension pneumothorax caused by a blocked bacterial filter in an anesthesia breathing circuit. Anesth Analg 76:440–442, 1993.
36. Loeser EA: Water induced resistance in disposable respiratory-circuit bacterial filters. Anesth Analg 57:269–271, 1978.

37. Buckley PM: Increase in resistance of in-line breathing filters in humidified air. Br J Anaesth 56:637–643, 1984.
38. Tenaillon A, Cholley G, Boiteau R, et al: Heat and moisture exchanging bacterial filters versus heated humidifier in long term mechanical ventilation. Care Critically Ill 7:56–66, 1991.
39. Prasad KK, Chen L: Complications related to the use of a heat and moisture exchanger. Anesthesiology 72:958, 1990.
40. Martinez FJ, Pietchel S, Wise C, et al: Increased resistance of hygroscopic condenser humidifiers when using a closed circuit suction system. Crit Care Med 22:1668–1673, 1994.
41. Stacey MRW, Asai T, Wilkes A, Hodzovic I: Obstruction of a breathing system filter. Can J Anaesth 43:1276, 1996.
42. Smith CE, Otworth JR, Kaluszyk P: Bilateral tension pneumothorax due to a defective anesthesia breathing circuit filter. J Clin Anesth 3:229–234, 1991.
43. Yoga Y, Iwatsuki N, Takahashi M, Hashimoto Y: A hazardous defect in a humidifier. Anesth Analg 71:712, 1990.
44. Prados W: A dangerous defect in a heat and moisture exchanger. Anesthesiology 71:804, 1989.
45. Iotti GA, Olivei MC, Palo A, et al: Unfavorable mechanical effects of heat and moisture exchangers in ventilated patients. Intensive Care Med 23:399–405, 1997.
46. Pelosi P, Solca M, Ravagnan I, et al: Effects of heat and moisture exchangers on minute ventilation, ventilatory drive, and work of breathing during pressure-support ventilation in acute respiratory failure. Crit Care Med 24:1184–1188, 1996.
47. Conti G, De Blasi RA, Rocco M, et al: Effects of heat-moisture exchangers on dynamic hyper-inflation of mechanically ventilated COPD patients. Intensive Care Med 16:441–443, 1990.
48. Le Bourdelles G, Mier L, Fiquet B, et al: Comparison of the effects of heat and moisture exchangers and heated humidifiers on ventilation and gas exchange during weaning trials from mechanical ventilation. Chest 110:1294–1298, 1996.
49. Rathberger J, Zielman S, Kietzman D, et al: Is the use of lithium chloride coated "Heat and Moisture Exchangers" (artificial noses) dangerous for patients? Der Anaesthesist 41:204–207, 1992.
50. Rosi R, Buscalferri A, Monfregola MR, et al: Systemic lithium reabsorption from lithium chloride coated heat and moisture exchangers. Intensive Care Med 18:97–100, 1992.
51. Branson RD, Davis K, Campbell RS, Porembka DT: Humidification in the intensive care unit: prospective study of a new protocol utilizing heated humidification and a hygroscopic condenser humidifier. Chest 104:1800–1805, 1993.
52. Suzukawa M, Usuda Y, Numata K: The effects of sputum characteristics of combining an unheated humidifier with a heat-moisture exchanging filter. Respir Care 34:976–984, 1989.
53. Beydon L, Tong D, Jackson N, Dreyfuss D: Correlation between simple clinical parameters and the in vitro humidification characteristics of filter heat and moisture exchangers. Chest 112:739–744, 1997.
54. Djedaini K, Billiard M, Mier L, et al: Changing heat and moisture exchangers every 48 hours rather than 24 hours does not affect their efficacy and the incidence of nosocomial pneumonia. Am J Respir Crit Care Med 152:1562–1569, 1995.
55. Kollef MH, Shapiro SD, Boyd V, et al: A randomized clinical trial comparing an extended use hygroscopic condenser humidifier with heated water humidification in mechanically ventilated patients. Chest 113:759–767, 1998.
56. Davis K Jr, Evans SL, Campbell RS, et al. Prolonged use of heat and moisture exchangers does not effect efficiency or incidence of nosocomial pneumonia. Crit Care Med (In press).
57. Powner DJ, Sanders CS, Bailey BJ: Bacteriologic evaluation of the Servo 150 hygroscopic condenser humidifier. Crit Care Med 14:135–137, 1986.
58. Branson RD, Campbell RS, Davis K Jr, et al: Comparison of a new active heat and moisture exchanger to conventional heated humidification. Respir Care 1999 (In press).
59. Branson RD, Campbell RS, Johannigman JA, Frame SB: Laboratory evaluation of two novel methods of humidification (abstract). Crit Care Med 27(suppl):A71, 1999.
60. Newhouse MT, Dolovich MB: Control of asthma by aerosols. N Engl J Med 315:870–874, 1986.
61. Dhand R, Tobin MJ: Bronchodilator delivery with metered-dose inhalers in mechanically ventilated patients. Eur J Respir Dis 9:585–595, 1996.
62. Brain JD, Valberg PA: Deposition of aerosol in the respiratory tract. Am Rev Respir Dis 120:1325–1373, 1979.
63. Gross NJ, Jenne JW, Hess D: Bronchodilator therapy. In: Tobin MJ (ed): Principles and Practice of Mechanical Ventilation. New York: McGraw Hill, 1994, pp 1077–1123.
64. Dolovich M: Physical principles underlying aerosol therapy. J Aerosol Med 2:171–186, 1989.
65. Hess D, Horney D, Snyder T: Medication delivery performance of eight small volume, hand-held nebulizers: effects of diluent volume, nebulizer flow, and nebulizer model. Respir Care 34:717–723, 1989.
66. Hess D, Fisher D, Williams P, et al: Medication nebulizer performance: effects of diluent volume, nebulizer flow, and nebulizer brand. Chest 110:498–505, 1996.
67. Svartengren M, Anderson M, Philipson K, Camner P: Human lung deposition of particles suspended in air or in helium/oxygen mixture. Exp Lung Res 15:575–585, 1989.
68. Anderson M, Svartengren M, Bylin G, et al: Deposition in asthmatics of particles inhaled in air or in helium/oxygen. Am J Respir Crit Care Med 47:524–528, 1993.
69. Dhand R, Malik SK, Balakrishnan M, Verna SR: High speed photographic analysis of aerosols produced by metered dose inhalers. J Pharm Pharmacol 40:429–430, 1988.

70. Dolovich M, Ruffin RE, Roberts R, Newhouse MT: Optimal delivery of aerosols from metered dose inhalers. Chest 80:911–915, 1981.
71. Fuller HD, Dolovich MB, Posmituck G, et al: Pressurized aerosol versus jet aerosol delivery to mechanically ventilated patients: comparison of dose to the lungs. Am Rev Respir Dis 141:440–444, 1990.
72. Consensus Conference on Aerosols Delivery: Aerosol consensus statement. Chest 100:1106–1109, 1991.
73. Fink JB, Dhand R, Grychowski J, et al: Reconciling in vitro and in vivo measurements of aerosol delivery from a metered dose inhaler during mechanical ventilation and defining efficiency enhancing factors. Am J Respir Crit Care Med 159:63–68, 1999.
74. Fuller HD, Dolovich MB, Chambers C, Newhouse MT: Aerosol delivery during mechanical ventilation: a predictive in vitro lung model. J Aerosol Med 5:251–259, 1992.
75. O'Riordan TG, Greco MJ, Perry RJ, Smaldone GC: Nebulizer function during mechanical ventilation. Am Rev Respir Dis 145:1117–1122, 1992.
76. Rau JL, Harwood RJ, Groff JL: Evaluation of a reservoir device for metered dose bronchodilator delivery to intubated adults: an in vitro study. Chest 102:924–930, 1993.
77. Hughes JM, Saez J: Effects of nebulizer mode and position in a mechanical ventilator circuit on dose efficiency. Respir Care 32:1131–1135, 1987.
78. McPeck M, O'Riordan TG, Smaldone GC: Choice of mechanical ventilator influence on nebulizer performance. Respir Care 38:887–895, 1993.
79. Bishop MJ, Larson RP, Buschman DL: Metered dose inhaler aerosol characteristics are affected by the endotracheal tube actuator/adapter used. Anesthesiology 73:1263–1265, 1990.
80. Fuller HD, Dolovich MB, Turpie FH, Newhouse MT: Efficiency of bronchodilator aerosol delivery to the lungs from the metered dose inhaler in mechanically ventilated patients: a study comparing four different actuator devices. Chest 105:214–218, 1994.
81. Manthous CA, Hall JB, Schmidt GA, Wood LDH: Metered dose inhaler versus nebulized albuterol in mechanically ventilated patients. Am Rev Respir Dis 148:1567–1570, 1993.
82. Ahrens RC, Ries RA, Popendorf W, Wiese JA: The delivery of therapeutic aerosols through endotracheal tubes. Pediatr Pulmonol 2:19–26, 1986.
83. O'Riordan TG, Palmer LB, Smaldone GC: Aerosol deposition in mechanically ventilated patients: optimizing nebulizer delivery. Am J Respir Crit Care Med 149:214–219, 1994.
84. Thomas SHL, O'Doherty MJ, Fidler HM, et al: Pulmonary deposition of a nebulized aerosol during mechanical ventilation. Thorax 48:154–159, 1993.
85. MacIntyre NR, Silver RM, Miller CW, et al: Aerosol delivery in intubated, mechanically ventilated patients. Crit Care Med 13:81–84, 1985.
86. Beaty CD, Ritz RH, Benson MS: Continuous in-line nebulizers complicate pressure support ventilation. Chest 96:1360–1363, 1989.
87. Duarte AG, Dhand R, Reid R, et al: Serum albuterol levels in mechanically ventilated patients and healthy subjects after metered dose inhaler administration. Am J Respir Crit Care Med 54:1658–1663, 1996.
88. Fernandes A, Lazaro A, Garcia A, et al: Bronchodilators in patients with chronic obstructive pulmonary disease on mechanical ventilation: utilization of metered dose inhalers. Am Rev Respir Dis 141:164–168, 1990.
89. Manthous CA, Chatila W, Schmidt GA, Hall JB: Treatment of bronchospasm by metered dose inhaler albuterol in mechanically ventilated patients. Chest 107:210–213, 1995.
90. Dhand R, Jubran A, Tobin MJ: Bronchodilator delivery by metered dose inhaler in ventilator supported patients. Am J Respir Crit Care Med 151:1827–1833, 1995.
91. Dhand R, Duarte AG, Jubran A, et al: Dose response to bronchodilator delivered by metered dose inhaler in ventilator supported patients. Am J Respir Crit Care Med 154:388–393, 1996.
92. Gay PC, Rodarte JR, Tayyab M, Hubmayr RD: Evaluation of bronchodilator responsiveness in mechanically ventilated patients. Am Rev Respir Dis 136:880–885, 1987.
93. Gay PC, Patel HG, Nelson SB, et al: Metered dose inhalers for bronchodilator delivery in intubated, mechanically ventilated patients. Am Rev Respir Dis 99:66–71, 1991.
94. Pepe PE, Marini JJ: Occult positive end expiratory pressure in mechanically ventilated patients with airflow obstruction: the auto PEEP effect. Am Rev Respir Dis 26:166–170, 1982.
95. Turner JR, Corkery KJ, Eckman D, et al: Equivalence of continuous flow nebulizer and metered dose inhaler with reservoir bag treatment of acute airflow obstruction. Chest 93:476–481, 1988.
96. Bowton DL, Goldsmith WM, Haponik EF: Substitution of metered dose inhalers for hand held nebulizers: success and cost savings in a large, acute care hospital. Chest 101:305–308, 1992.

CHAPTER 5

Ventilator Monitors, Displays, and Alarms

Neil R. MacIntyre, MD

MONITORING AND
MONITORS
PATIENT–VENTILATOR
INTERFACE MONITORS AND
DISPLAYS
Interface Sensors and
Monitors
Flow and Volume Sensors
and Monitors
Gas Concentration
Monitors

Calculations from Pressure/
Flow/Volume Monitors
Normal and Abnormal
Pattern Recognition
VENTILATOR ALARM
SYSTEMS
Levels of Events and Alarm
Strategies
Alarm Cost-Effectiveness
REFERENCES

KEY WORDS

airway pressure
alarm
esophageal pressure

flow
inspired gas concentrations
monitor

transducer
volume

MONITORING AND MONITORS

Monitoring is the process of continued or repetitive measurement of a parameter. With mechanical ventilators, the purpose of monitoring is generally to detect patient or machine events or trends that require management changes. Monitoring patients on mechanical ventilators is usually done in one of three locations: the ventilator itself, the patient–ventilator interface (usually in the ventilator circuitry), and the patient. Typical **monitors** inside the ventilator include continuous assessments of electrical, software, and pneumatic functions. Typical

interface monitors include measurements of airway/circuit/tracheal pressures, circuit gas flow, delivered volume, and circuit gas concentrations. Typical direct patient monitors include measurements of esophageal pressure, arterial oxygenation, pulmonary vascular pressures, invasive and noninvasive assessments of cardiac output, hemoglobin content, and tissue perfusion. Direct patient monitoring also includes repetitive clinical evaluation.

Although all the aforementioned monitoring capabilities can be important, the remainder of this chapter focuses only on monitoring capabilities integral to the venti-

131

lator system. Specifically, the following sections describe the various sensors in the patient–ventilator interface, their displays of both real-time and trend data, and how these monitors can affect patient–ventilator management. A consensus conference described the importance of these ventilator integral monitors for patients receiving various levels of mechanical ventilatory support (Table 5–1).[1]

PATIENT–VENTILATOR INTERFACE MONITORS AND DISPLAYS

Interface Sensors and Monitors

Pressure Sensors and Monitors

Pressure generally is measured by either aneroid manometers or electromechanical **transducers.**[2] Aneroid manometers use an

TABLE 5–1. Ventilator Consensus Statement—1992. Essential, Recommended, and Optional Variables* to Be Monitored on Mechanical Ventilators†

VARIABLE	PRINCIPAL VENTILATOR APPLICATION		
	Critical Care	Transport	Home Care
Pressure			
P_{PEAK}	Essential	Essential	Essential
P_{MEAN}	Essential	Optional	Optional
P_{PLAT}	Essential	Optional	Optional‡
Intrinsic PEEP (auto-PEEP)	Recommended	Optional	Optional
Volume§			
V_T expired machine	Essential	Recommended	Optional
$\dot{V}_E$ machine	Essential	Optional	Optional
V_T expired spontaneous	Essential	Recommended	Optional
$\dot{V}_E$ spontaneous	Essential	Optional	Optional
V_T inspired spontaneous	Recommended	Optional	Optional
Timing			
Flow mechanical	Recommended	Optional	Optional
Flow spontaneous	Optional	Optional	Optional
I:E ratio§	Essential	Recommended	Optional
Rate mechanical	Essential	Recommended	Optional
Rate spontaneous	Essential	Recommended	Optional
Gas Concentration			
F_{DO_2}‖	Essential	Optional‡	Optional‡
Lung mechanics			
Effective compliance	Optional	Optional	Optional
Inspiratory airways resistance	Optional	Optional	Optional
Expiratory airways resistance	Optional	Optional	Optional
Maximal inspiratory pressure	Optional	Optional	Optional
Circuit characteristics			
Tubing compliance	Recommended	Optional	Optional

*Essential, considered necessary for safe and effective operation in most patients in the specified setting; recommended, considered necessary for optimal management of virtually all patients in the specified setting; optional, considered possibly useful in limited situations but not necessary for most patients in the specified setting.

†Monitors need not be integral part of ventilator.

‡Essential if feature is used on a specific patient.

‖F_{DO_2}, oxygen concentration delivered by device; FiO_2 when patient demand (inspiratory flowrate) is met.

§I:E, inspiratory:expiratory time; PEEP, positive end-expiratory pressure; V_E, minute volume; V_T, tidal volume.

From American Association for Respiratory Care Consensus Group: Essentials of mechanical ventilation. Respir Care 37:1001–1009, 1992.

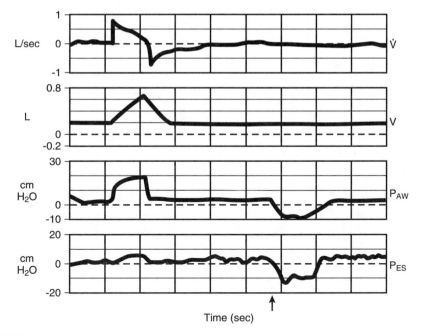

FIGURE 5–1

The "sniff" test to ensure proper placement of an esophageal balloon. Flow *(upper panel)*, tidal volume *(2nd panel)*, airway pressure *(3rd panel)*, and esophageal pressure *(bottom panel)* are plotted over time. The tracings demonstrate a positive pressure breath followed by a sniff test (a maneuver performed by an inspiratory effort against an occluded airway [i.e., no flow or volume change, *arrow*]). If the balloon is positioned properly, similar pressure swings are observed in the airway and in the esophagus.

expandable chamber that responds to pressure changes by changing its volume and moving a gear that rotates a needle around a calibrated dial. Electromechanical transducers convert pressure into an electrical current. Standard specifications for ventilator pressure monitors are of $\pm 10\%$ accuracy.[3]

Pressure can be monitored in the ventilator, the ventilator circuitry (often the patient wye connector), the distal endotracheal tube, and the esophagus **(esophageal pressure)**. The actual pressure transducer is often within the ventilator and connected to the sensing site by low-compliance, air-filled tubing. By convention, pressures measured in the ventilator or ventilator circuitry often are considered as **airway** or airway opening **pressures** (P_{AW} or P_{AO}, respectively). Pressures in the distal endotracheal tube often are considered tracheal pressures (P_{TR}), and pressures from a balloon in the esophagus (P_{ES}) generally are considered reflective of pleural pressures if

they have been positioned properly (Fig. 5–1).[4]

A number of important pressure measurements are made over the ventilatory cycle (Fig. 5–2). In the airway these include: peak pressure (the highest pressure during inspiration [P_{PEAK}]), inspiratory plateau pressure (end-inspiratory pressure under no-flow conditions [P_{PLAT}]), mean inspiratory pressure (average pressure during inspiration [inspP_{MEAN}]), positive end-expiratory pressure (pressure just before delivery of the next breath [PEEP]), and mean airway pressure (average pressure throughout the ventilatory cycle [P_{MEAN}]). In addition, a pause or hold at end expiration can allow measurement of end-expiratory alveolar pressure (intrinsic plus applied PEEP). Tracheal pressure monitoring can provide similar information, although the pressure due to flow through the endotracheal tube is eliminated. Esophageal pressures are expressed as peak (end-inspiratory), mean, and end-expiratory pressures depending on

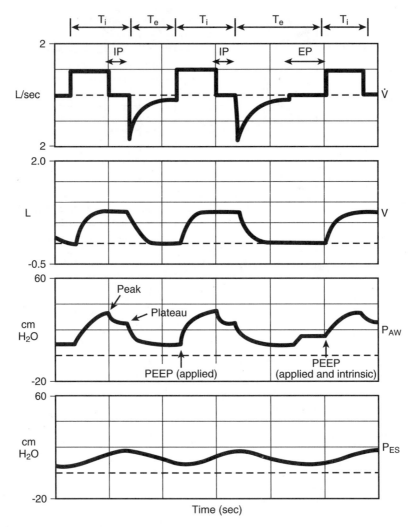

FIGURE 5–2

Ventilator circuit flow ($\dot{V}$), volume (V_T) and airway pressure (P_{AW}) over time illustrating various measurements during controlled ventilation. In this example, the inspiratory phase (T_I) has both a flow delivery phase and an inspiratory pause (IP). In addition, during expiration (T_E) of the second breath, an expiratory pause also is illustrated (EP). During inspiration, the highest pressure is the peak airway pressure, the P_{AW} during the inspiratory pause is the plateau pressure, and the mean P_{AW} during the entire inspiratory phase is the mean inspiratory pressure. During expiration, the end-expiratory P_{AW} is positive end-expiratory pressure. If the expiratory circuit is occluded before the next breath delivery (expiratory pause), this PEEP reflects both applied and intrinsic PEEP. Without such an occlusion, the measured PEEP is only the applied one. The average P_{AW} over the entire steady state inspiratory and expiratory phases is the mean airway pressure.

when they are measured during the ventilatory cycle.

Flow and Volume Sensors and Monitors

Older ventilators usually would monitor only exhaled volume by either volume-displacing spirometers or turbines. Most modern systems, however, monitor **flow** with various types of pneumotachometers and integrate flow to obtain **volume**. The most common pneumotachometers work on one of the three following principles:[2, 5]

DIFFERENTIAL PRESSURE FLOWMETERS

These devices determine flow from the pressure drop across a known resistance. The most widely used types incorporate either a screen or a series of capillary tubes (Fleisch) as the resistance element. Advantages of these flowmeters include a nearly linear bidirectional pressure–flow relationship and a high-frequency response. An important disadvantage of these types of flowmeters in the intensive care setting is that they are highly sensitive to moisture and mucus accumulation if placed in the patient's airway. Additional disadvantages are that a large housing is often necessary to produce the required laminar flow, and gas viscosity affects calibration (e.g., an error of 12% occurs if 100% O_2 is used on a flowmeter calibrated with 21% O_2). Because of these limitations, screen and Fleisch flowmeters usually are not maintained for prolonged periods in the patient's airway but rather are placed elsewhere in the ventilator circuitry. Another type of differential pressure flowmeter more applicable to patient airway application uses either a fixed or variable orifice resistor. A fixed resistor results in turbulent flow and thus is inherently nonlinear. These types of flowmeters are affected less by mucus and moisture than are Fleish or screen devices. Another alternative is the variable orifice resistor, which mechanically linearizes flow through an elastic "flap." These devices have low resistance and dead space characteristics, and they provide reasonable clinical accuracy.

"HOT-WIRE" FLOWMETERS

These flow sensors operate on the principle that cooling of a heated wire or film is proportional to gas flow past it. The rate of cooling also depends on gas viscosity and thermal conductivity. Advantages to these devices are that dead space and resistance are very small, a very high frequency response is possible, and mucus-moisture effects are lessened because the sensor is heated. Disadvantages are that only unidirectional flow can be sensed by a single sensor and that different gas mixtures can have different thermal conductivities.

ULTRASONIC FLOWMETERS

These flow sensors use an ultrasonic transmitter–receiver and function on the princi-

ple that ultrasonic transit times are proportional to gas flow. A variation of this approach is to produce small air-flow obstructions, which create vortices. The intensity of an ultrasonic signal across these vortices is proportional to flow. Advantages are low resistance to flow, little impact by viscosity or mucus-moisture, and a high frequency response to the ultrasonic transmitter–receiver system. Disadvantages are that ultrasonic signal transmission is affected by both gas composition and temperature.

When flow is measured and displayed over the ventilatory cycle (see Fig. 5–2), measurements include peak inspiratory flow, mean inspiratory flow, the inspiratory flow pattern, peak expiratory flow, and mean expiratory flow. Volume measurements over time include the delivered and the exhaled tidal volume (V_T).

Gas Concentration Monitors

Gas concentrations in the ventilator circuitry can be assessed through either mainstream (in-line) or sidestream analyzers. Probably the most important measurement is the **inspired** O_2 concentration (FiO_2) to ensure that the oxygen supply system is performing properly. Another common measurement is exhaled CO_2. The CO_2 at end expiration (end-tidal CO_2) correlates with arterial PCO_2 and can be used to trend ventilation effectiveness when tidal volume and expiratory time are held nearly constant.[6, 7] The mixed expired CO_2 can be used in the Bohr equation to calculate functional dead space. Finally, by comparing both O_2 and CO_2 concentrations in inspired and expired gas, oxygen consumption, and CO_2 production can be calculated.

In the future, ventilators also may have integral monitors for other gases. Examples might be inert gases (e.g., He or CH_4) for lung volume determinations and soluble gases (e.g., C_2H_2) for pulmonary blood flow determinations.

Calculations From Pressure/Flow/ Volume Monitors

A number of important calculated parameters can be monitored and displayed using pressure, flow, and volume measurements.[8, 9] These are defined subsequently and discussed in detail in Chapter 6.

Compliance

Static compliance reflects system distensibility and is expressed as a volume delivered per pressure applied. Total compliance of the respiratory system (C_{RS}) is $V_T/(P_{PLAT}-PEEP)$. Lung compliance (C_L) is determined from transalveolar pressure measurements and is $V_T(P_{PLAT}-P_{ES}-PEEP)$. A so-called "dynamic" compliance substitutes peak pressure for plateau pressure ($V_T/(P_{PEAK}-PEEP)$). Although a simpler measurement, the calculation of "dynamic" compliance includes flow-resistive pressures that are not reflective of system distensibility.

System distensibility can be described more carefully by constructing a static pressure–volume curve during both inflation and deflation (see Fig. 6–3). This is a complex procedure requiring multiple plateau pressure measurements over a range of increasing and then decreasing volumes. If done properly, however, it not only depicts compliance (slope of the pressure–volume relationship), but also may show inflection points suggesting alveolar recruitment and alveolar overdistension pressures.[10] Optimally, measured pressure should be referenced to P_{ES} to eliminate chest wall effects and thus depict only lung mechanical properties. Note that many ventilators display pressure–volume relationships during each breath. These "dynamic" pressure–volume relationships, however, include both flow-resistive and distending pressures and thus are not a substitute for the static curve in assessing lung parenchyma and chest wall mechanics. These concepts are discussed more in Chapter 6.

Resistance

Airway resistance (R_{AW}) is affected by both the length and (especially) the diameter of the airways (both natural and artificial). During inspiration, $R_{AW}=(P_{PEAK}-P_{PLAT})$/inspiratory flow. Resistance during expiration can be measured in several ways. A simple expression is P_{PLAT}/peak expiratory flow. Another approach is to calculate a time constant from the exponential expiratory flow pattern and insert the known C_{RS} to solve for a "mean" expiratory resistance. R_{AW} also can be assessed by plotting a flow–volume loop. These concepts are discussed in more detail in Chapter 6.

Breathing Loads

Breathing loads can be borne by either the ventilator (machine-controlled ventilation), the patient (patient-unassisted ventilation), or shared (patient–ventilator interactive ventilation).[11] Patient and ventilator loads can be quantified in one of two ways: a pressure–time product (PTP) or a work (W) calculation. PTP is the integral of pressure over time (see Fig. 6–11); W is the integral of pressure over volume (see Fig. 6–12). During machine-controlled ventilation (pas-

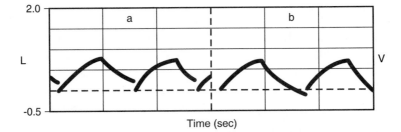

FIGURE 5–3

Ventilator circuit volume measurements over time. In the *a* breaths, delivered volume is greater than returned volume. This may reflect circuit leaks or bronchopleural fistulas. In the *b* breaths, delivered volume is less than returned volume. This may reflect gas flow introduced into the circuitry beyond the ventilator (e.g., nebulizer flow, tracheal gas insufflation).

sive patient), loads calculated using airway pressure reflect respiratory system loads on the ventilator, and loads calculated using esophageal pressure reflect chest wall loads on the ventilator. During patient-unassisted ventilation, loads calculated using esophageal pressure reflect lung loads on the patient. These measurement concepts are discussed in more detail in Chapter 6.

Timing

Ventilators can calculate, monitor, and display the various phases of the breath cycle (see Fig. 5–2). Commonly monitored parameters are inspiratory time (T_I), expiratory time (T_E), inspiratory time as a fraction of total cycle time (T_I/T_{TOT}), inspiratory:expiratory time ratio (I : E), and breathing frequency (f, or $1/T_{TOT}$).

Spontaneous Breathing Parameters

The breathing pattern during spontaneous breathing (with or without low-level continuous positive airway pressure [CPAP] or pressure support) can be described not only by frequency and tidal volume but also by f/V_T ratios, $f \cdot V_T$ product (minute ventilation), vital capacity, and maximal voluntary ventilation. During spontaneous trials, inspiratory pressure against a closed demand valve after 100 msec of effort ($P_{0.1}$), and with maximal effort (MIF) also can occur. Use of these assessments during the ventilator discontinuation process is discussed in Chapter 20.

Normal and Abnormal Pattern Recognition

Clinicians must recognize abnormal monitored values as well as abnormal graphic patterns.[12] Descriptions of several important patient–ventilator mechanical abnormalities that can be recognized by appropriate graphic monitoring follow.

Trigger Problems

Demand value sensitivity and responsiveness to patient effort during breath triggering are discussed elsewhere (see Chapter 9). The most important monitoring parameter for these valve properties are airway (circuit) pressure and the PTP of the breath triggering phase (see Fig. 9–2).[13] In the patient with severe airflow obstruction, the presence of air trapping (intrinsic or auto-PEEP) can act as a significant inspiratory threshold load. Under these conditions, ventilator triggering delay can be detected when comparing P_{ES} with P_{AW} (see Fig. 9–4).[14]

Flow Dys-Synchrony

When patient demand exceeds ventilator flow delivery during interactive breaths, considerable imposed loading can occur.[15] The best way to recognize this is to compare a controlled breath (passive passive) and a patient-triggered breath using P_{ES} and/or P_{AW} graphic displays (see Fig. 9–5). In the setting of inadequate ventilator flow during patient-triggered breaths, both these pressure tracings can be used to calculate the imposed load. Moreover, these tracings can be used to set the ventilator flow delivery pattern to ensure maximal synchrony. This is discussed in more detail in Chapter 9.

Cycle Dys-Synchrony

During interactive breaths, another source of patient ventilator dys-synchrony is with the cycling criteria. Breaths of excessive duration may elicit patient expiratory activity. Breaths that are of too short a duration may leave patients demanding more flow after the ventilator flow delivery has ceased. Flow and pressure tracings can depict this (see Fig. 9–11) and help guide setting the cycle criteria.

Alveolar Overdistension

Alveolar overdistension and volutrauma are thought to increase in incidence when regions in the lungs are distended beyond their normal maximal transpulmonary pressure. A simple way to assess this is the plateau pressure, which can be assessed graphically during an inspiratory hold or pause (see Fig. 5–2). Values greater than 35 cm H_2O may indicate excessive regional distension.[16] Another way to detect overdis-

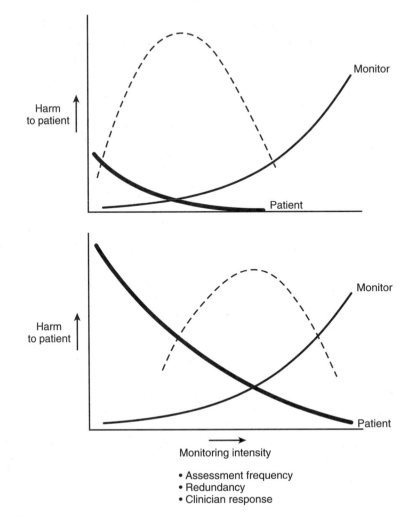

FIGURE 5–4
The cost-effectiveness of monitoring intensity is determined by patient risk and monitoring system properties. Harm can come from both patient disease events ("patient" line) and monitoring system events ("monitor" line). As monitoring intensity increases, patient harm should decrease. Increasing monitoring intensity, however, increases costs, the risk of monitor-induced injury, and the false-positive rate—all forms of potential patient harm. The dotted curve represents cost-effectiveness when these different factors are considered. The upper panel depicts a situation in which risk of harm due to patient disease is low, such that a lower level of monitoring intensity is cost-effective. The bottom panel depicts a situation in which patient harm due to patient disease is high, such that a higher level of monitoring intensity is cost-effective. (Reprinted with permission from MacIntyre NR: Levels of intensity of intensive care unit monitoring. In: Tobin M (ed): Principles and Practices of Intensive Care Monitoring, New York: McGraw-Hill, 1997.)

tension is with a static pressure–volume plot (optimally with P_{AW} referenced to P_{ES}) that reveals an upper inflection point (see Chapter 6).

Alveolar Under-Recruitment

Collapsed alveoli in parenchymal lung injury can be recruited with a positive pressure breath and then be prevented from derecruiting by the application of expiratory pressure (PEEP). Optimal PEEP conceptually is PEEP that maintains stability in "recruitable" alveoli but does not overdistend healthier and more compliant alveoli. The static pressure–volume plot has been proposed as an ideal way to assess these mechanical effects of PEEP.[17] Conceptually, the optimal PEEP should be determined by the lower inflection point on this plot. Moreover, this inflection point probably is determined more appropriately on the deflation limb of the pressure–volume plot after a full inspiration to total lung capacity has recruited the "recruitable" alveoli. See Chapter 6 for further discussion of these concepts.

Air Trapping/Intrinsic Positive End-Expiratory Pressure

As discussed in Chapters 6 and 19, the risk for air trapping and the development of intrinsic PEEP is directly proportional to the minute ventilation, the respiratory system's mechanical time constant, and the I:E ratio.[18] Intrinsic PEEP has a number of mechanical consequences that can be detected graphically. First, the expiratory flow signal does not reach zero before the next breath is given (see Fig. 6–14). Second, in volume-targeted ventilation, the combination of intrinsic PEEP and a constant tidal volume increases peak and plateau pressures (Chapter 6, see Fig. 6–14). Third, in pressure-targeted ventilation, the combination of intrinsic PEEP plus a set airway pressure limit reduces the tidal volume (see Fig. 6–14). The expiratory hold maneuver also can be assessed graphically to determine intrinsic PEEP in a passive patient (see Fig. 5–2).

Circuit Leaks/Extraneous Circuit Flows

Leaks in the circuit or the lungs reduce the exhaled tidal volume compared with the delivered tidal volume (Fig. 5–3). Additional flow in the circuit (e.g., nebulizer, tracheal gas insufflation) increases exhaled tidal volume compared with delivered tidal volume (see Fig. 5–3).

VENTILATOR ALARM SYSTEMS

The goal of a mechanical ventilator **alarm** is to warn of *events*. An event is any condition or occurrence that requires clinician awareness or action. Events can be divided conceptually into two broad categories—

mechanical/technical events and patient-generated events.

Mechanical/technical events involve the ventilator system itself. Because these systems replace or support the patient's life-sustaining ventilatory efforts, an alarm is required for every potential mechanical event that could impact on this function.[1, 19] Moreover, the alarm must occur in time for prompt correction. In contrast, a patient event involves a change in the patient's clinical status. This may be a consequence of a mechanical/technical malfunction but more often reflects changes in the patient's underlying disease process. Monitors and alarms are reasonable for such patient events but should not be a required integral component of a mechanical ventilator system. Rather, these alarms should be individualized for each patient as a supplement to clinical decision-making.

Levels of Events and Alarm Strategies

Alarm goals and strategies should be categorized by the events that they are designed to warn of rather than by any technical features they may have. The discussion of ventilator system alarm strategies that follows, therefore, considers four levels, or priorities, of alarmed mechanical and patient events: (1) ventilator events (malfunction) with immediate life-threatening consequences, (2) ventilator events (malfunction) not immediately life-threatening, (3) patient events affecting the ventilator–patient interface, and (4) patient events not affecting the ventilator–patient interface (Table 5–2).

Level 1 Events and Alarm Goals: Warn of Ventilator Events with Immediate Life-Threatening Consequences

Mechanical ventilators are life-support systems. Patients requiring mechanical ventilation may have little or no ability to breathe if the ventilator suddenly stops. The expectation for this type of alarm is that it will warn of every event in time for prompt

TABLE 5–2. Alarm Features for Different Event Priorities

EVENT PRIORITIES	ALARM FEATURES				
	Integral Part of Ventilator	Must Be Redundant	Alarm Sites	Automatic Response Needed	Clinical Focus
Level 1—ventilator malfunction, life-threatening	Yes	Yes	1, 2, 3*	Yes	Machine
Level 2—ventilator malfunction, not immediately life-threatening	Yes	No	1, 2*	No	Machine
Level 3—patient event affecting ventilator–patient interface	Yes	No	2, 3*	No	Machine and patient
Level 4—patient event not affecting ventilator–patient interface	No	No	3*	No	Patient

*Site 1, ventilator system; site 2, patient–ventilator interface; site 3, patient.
From Day S, MacIntyre NR: Ventilator alarm system. Prob Respir Care 4:118–126, 1991.

corrections (Table 5–3). Because of the essential nature of this type of warning, alarms with redundant or overlapping function should be present. For instance, a failure to deliver gas should cause a low-volume alarm, a low-pressure alarm and, if practical, even a gas exchange alarm (e.g., capnography). This type of event should not be considered to have a "mild" form; it is a serious failure every time it occurs. The alarms in this category are thus mandatory, redundant, and noncanceling. The goal is to provide virtually 100% reliability of the life-support functions of the ventilator. Although machine failure is unavoidable, appropriate alarms should alert users to technical breakdowns.

With a level 1 event, machines should not simply alarm and shut down; rather, they should default to a condition in which the patient is at the very least not "locked out" and is able to breathe from a fresh gas source. A more sophisticated default condition could be a backup minimum ventilation mode. Both responses are designed to alert users to immediately replace the ventilator with as little harm as possible done to the patient during mechanical failure. Ventilators also should have battery-backed alarms for level 1 events in case of power source failure.

Level 2 Events and Alarm Goals: Warn of Ventilator Events that Are Not Immediately Life-Threatening

The events in this category can range from mild irregularities in the mechanical function of the ventilator to dangerous situations that, under the proper circumstances, could threaten the patient's safety or life if left uncorrected for a period of time (Table 5–4). An example of a level 2 event would be a circuit leak. A small leak (<10 ml/breath)

TABLE 5–3. Level 1 Events and Alarms: Ventilator Events, Life-Threatening (Mandatory, Redundant, Noncanceling)

EVENT	ALARM SENSOR
No gas delivery to patient	Pressure/flow transducer, CO_2 monitor, timing device
Excessive gas delivery to patient	Pressure/flow transducer, timing device
Exhalation valve failure	Pressure/flow transducer, mandatory rate
Loss of electric power	Battery-powered alarm

From Day S, MacIntyre NR: Ventilator alarm systems. Prob Respir Care 4:118–126, 1991.

TABLE 5–4. Level 2 Events and Alarms: Ventilator Event Not Immediately Life-Threatening

EVENT	ALARM SENSOR
Blender failure	FiO$_2$ sensor
Loss of PEEP or excessive PEEP	Pressure transducer
Autocycling	Timer/flow transducer, CO$_2$ sensor
Circuit leak	Flow transducer, pressure transducer
Circuit partially occluded	Pressure, flow transducer
Inappropriate I:E ratio	Timer, flow transducer
Inappropriate heater/humidifier function	Temperature probe

FiO$_2$, inspired oxygen concentration; I:E, inspiratory:expiratory time; PEEP, positive end-expiratory pressure.
From Day S, MacIntyre NR: Ventilator alarm systems. Prob Respir Care 4:118–126, 1991.

would not harm most adult patients, whereas a large leak (several hundred millimeters/breath) may cause serious hypoventilation.

These alarms are important and are included in some form on all modern ventilators. There may not be redundant counterparts for each, however, and alarm-canceling capabilities often exist.

Level 3 Events and Alarm Goals: Warn of Patient Events Affecting the Ventilator–Patient Interface

Level 3 events can have significant impact on the level of support given and on the pressure and volume consequences of that support (Table 5–5). Examples include changes in patient compliance or resistance. Sensors for these events are generally in the ventilator circuitry (e.g., pressure/flow/volume sensors), although direct patient monitors also are used. Modern ventilators usually include alarms for level 3 events, although redundancy is not considered essential.

This group of events often triggers the same alarms as those in levels 1 and 2, and the clinician must be capable of quickly determining the nature of the alarmed event. Because patient status can change either abruptly or more insidiously, the alarms for these events must be adjusted carefully for each patient and changed often to correlate with patient conditions to remain accurate enough to warn of significant problems.

Level 4 Events and Alarm Goal: Warn of Patient Events Not Affecting the Ventilator–Patient Interface

Events in this group are not a function of ventilator system malfunction, nor do they impact ventilator behavior. Alarm sites are

TABLE 5–5. Level 3 Events and Alarms: Patient Events Affecting Ventilator–Patient Interface

EVENT	ALARM SENSOR
Change in ventilatory drive (CNS, peripheral nerves, or muscle function)	Timer, flow transducer, pressure transducer, CO$_2$ analyzer
Change in compliance/resistance (air trapping, barotrauma)	Pressure transducer, flow transducer
AutoPEEP	Pressure transducer, flow transducer

CNS, central nervous system; PEEP, positive end-expiratory pressure.
From Day S, MacIntyre NR: Ventilator alarm systems. Prob Respir Care 4:118–126, 1991.

thus only on the patient. Because of this, many modern ventilators may not contain any such alarm system as an integral part of the device. These events, however, can have significant clinical impact, but they often must be detected by other types of critical care monitors, such as free-standing oximeters, cardiac monitors, or blood gas analyzers (Table 5–6).

Alarm Cost-Effectiveness

Maximizing Sensitivity and Specificity. Ventilator setup involves selecting alarm parameters that maximize sensitivity (i.e., percentage of events alarmed) and specificity (i.e., percentage of non-events not alarmed). A high sensitivity, however, often leads to a loss of specificity and a high rate of false-positive alarms. This false-positive rate may be quite acceptable for a single alarm (e.g., 5%), but if a number of alarms are used together with similar specificity, the chances of a false-positive alarm can rise dramatically.[20] False-positive alarms produce two important problems. First, a high rate of false-positive alarms can lead to clinicians ignoring alarms. Indeed, in one study of mechanical ventilation hazards, 9% of ventilator alarms had been disabled by clinicians, ostensibly to reduce noise "pollution."[21] A second problem is the costs and patient risks of inappropriate therapy or unnecessary diagnostic tests in response to the false-positive alarm condition.

Balancing sensitivity and specificity is the

goal of setting appropriate alarm parameters (Fig. 5–4).[22] One approach would be to arbitrarily set alarm parameters as a "standard" percentage of the targeted values (Table 5–7).[23] Although this approach is reasonable, the clinician still may want to individualize certain alarm ranges. In doing this, the clinician must consider the likelihood of an otherwise undetected event, the potential harm from such an event, and the precision with which the alarm setting can distinguish a real event from simple physiologic variability or artifact. In general, the higher the likelihood of an undetected event causing serious harm, the more sensitive (at the expense of specific) an alarm setting should be.

Interpreting and Responding to Alarm Conditions. Even if an alarm is set properly, clinical skills are vital in determining the cause of the alarm and in responding appropriately. It is of no use to have alarms if a clinical response is not readily available. As noted earlier, automated responses such as backup modes are available on some ventilators. These, however, should not be considered a substitute for prompt clinical assessment.

Other Alarm Issues. Two other issues are related to alarm cost-effectiveness: costs and reliability. Alarms have direct costs associated with the actual hardware and software involved. Costs also are involved in equipment maintenance and staff training. These costs must be balanced against the potential patient harm (with its attendant costs) of unrecognized events.

TABLE 5–6. Level 4 Events and Alarms: Patient Events Not Affecting Ventilator–Patient Interface

EVENT	ALARM SENSOR
Change in gas exchange	
$\dot{V}/\dot{Q}$	Capnograph
V_D/V_T	Oximeter, metabolic calculations
VO_2 demands	Arterial blood gases
Change in respiratory system impedances	Mechanics measurements
Change in muscle function	Respiratory pressures, ventilatory capabilities
Change in cardiovascular function	Hemodynamic measurements

V_D/V_T, deadspace volume/tidal volume; VO_2, oxygen consumption; $\dot{V}/\dot{Q}$, ventilation perfusion.
From Day S, MacIntyre NR: Ventilator alarm systems. Prob Respir Care 4:118–126, 1991.

TABLE 5–7. Examples of Alarm Auto-Set Parameters

ALARM	AUTO-SETTING
Low exhaled mandatory tidal volume	-25% to a minimum of 30 ml
Low exhaled spontaneous tidal volume	-25% to a minimum of 30 ml
Low exhaled minute volume	-25% to a minimum of 0.3 L
High exhaled minute volume	$+25\%$ or 1000 ml, whichever is greater
Low breath rate	-5 bpm to a minimum of 3 bpm
High breath rate	$+5$ bpm
Low peak normal pressure	-5 cm H_2O or preset PEEP/CPAP, whichever is greater, to a minimum of 3 cm H_2O
Low mean airway pressure	-5 cm H_2O
Low PEEP/CPAP pressure	-5 cm H_2O or 20%, whichever is less, to a minimum margin of 2 cm H_2O

PEEP/CPAP, positive end-expiratory pressure/continuous positive airway pressure.
From Day S, MacIntyre NR: Ventilator alarm systems. Prob Respir Care 4:118–126, 1991.

Alarm systems are generally quite reliable. However, like any other component of the ventilatory support system, an alarm can malfunction. This has been reported to occur in as many as 3.7% of patients[24] and is one of the reasons for redundancy in level 1 event strategies (see section on level 1 events).

REFERENCES

1. American Association for Respiratory Care Consensus Group: Essentials of mechanical ventilation. Respir Care 37:1001–1009, 1992.
2. Tobin MJ: Monitoring of pressure, flow, and volume during mechanical ventilation. Respir Care 37:1081–1096, 1992.
3. American Society for Testing and Materials: F29: standard specification for ventilators intended for use in critical care F1100. In: Annual Book for ASTM Standards. Philadelphia: American Society for Testing and Materials, 1993.
4. Baydur A, Behrakis K, Zin A, et al: A simple method for assessing the validity of esophageal balloon technique. Am Rev Respir Dis 126:788–791, 1982.
5. Sullivan WJ, Peters GM, Enright PL: Pneumotachographs: theory and clinical application. Respir Care 29: 736–749, 1984.
6. Rebuck AS, Chapman KR: Measurement and monitoring of exhaled carbon dioxide. In: Nochomovitz ML, Cherniack NS (eds): Non-invasive Respiratory Monitoring. New York: Churchill Livingstone, 1986, pp 189–201.
7. McLellan PA, Goldstein RS, Ramcharan V, et al: Transcutaneous carbon dioxide monitoring. Am Rev Respir Dis 124:199–201, 1981.
8. Hubmayr RD, Gay PC, Tayyab M: Respiratory system mechanics in ventilated patients: techniques and indications. Mayo Clin Proc 62:358–368, 1987.
9. Tobin MJ: Respiratory monitoring in the intensive care unit. Am Rev Respir Dis 138:1625–1642, 1988.
10. Metamis D, LeMaire F, Harf A, et al: Total respiratory pressure-volume curves in the adult respiratory distress syndrome. Chest 86:58–66, 1984.
11. Marini JJ: Lung mechanics determinations at the bedside: instrumentation and clinical application, Respir Care 35:669–696, 1990.
12. MacIntyre NR: Graphical Analysis of Flow, Pressure and Volume During Mechanical Ventilation, Riverside, CA: Bear Medical Systems, 1991.
13. Sassoon CSH: Mechanical ventilator design and function: the trigger variable. Respir Care 37:1056–1069, 1992.
14. Gay PC, Rodarte JR, Hubmayr RD: The effects of positive expiratory pressure on isovolume flow and dynamic hyperinflation in patients receiving mechanical ventilation. Am Rev Respir Dis 139:621–626, 1989.
15. Marini JJ, Smith TC, Lamb VJ: External work output and force generation during synchronized intermittent mechanical ventilation. Am Rev Respir Dis 138:1169–1179, 1988.
16. American College of Chest Physicians Consensus Group: Mechanical ventilation. Chest 104:1833–1859, 1993.
17. Amato MB, Barbas CS, Medeiros DM, et al: Effect of a preventative ventilator strategy on mortality in ARDS. N Engl J Med 338:347–354, 1998.
18. Marini JJ, Crooke PS: A general mathematical model for respiratory dynamics relevant to the clinical setting. Am Rev Respir Dis 147:14–24, 1993.
19. Day S, MacIntyre NR: Ventilator alarm systems. Prob Respir Care 4:118–126, 1991.
20. Hess D: Noninvasive monitoring in respiratory care-present, past, and future: an overview. Respir Care 35:482–499, 1990.

21. Zwillich CW, Pierson DJ, Creagh CE, et al: Complications of assisted ventilation: a prospective study of 354 consecutive episodes. Am J Med 57:161–170, 1974.
22. MacIntyre NR: Levels of intensity of intensive care unit monitoring. In: Tobin M (ed): Principles and Practice of Intensive Care Monitoring. New York: McGraw-Hill, 1997.
23. The Bear® Ventilator Instruction Manual. Riverside, CA: Bear Intermed, 1990.
24. Watson H, MacIntyre NR: Mechanical ventilator failure. Prob Respir Care 4:127–135, 1991.

SECTION
II

Physiology of Positive Pressure Ventilation

Respiratory System Mechanics

Neil R. MacIntyre, MD

RESPIRATORY SYSTEM
MECHANICS
Measurements
Lung Inflation and
    Respiratory System
    Mechanics
Mechanical Loads
INTERACTION OF
VENTILATOR SETTINGS AND
LUNG MECHANICS

Pressure- Versus Flow/
    Volume-Targeted Breaths
Delivered Minute
    Ventilation and $f \times V_T$
    Settings
Ventilation Distribution
REFERENCES

KEY TERMS

compliance
intrinsic positive end-
    expiratory pressure

minute ventilation
pressure-time product
resistance

ventilation distribution
work

During normal spontaneous ventilation, fresh gas is exchanged with alveolar gas by a convective to-and-fro pumping action. This "bulk flow" gas transport is driven by pressure gradients created by the ventilatory muscles and respiratory system elastic recoil.[1] Conventional mechanical ventilation tends to mimic this pattern. Specifically, a positive pressure ventilator produces a periodic pressure gradient across the lungs to drive discrete volumes (tidal volumes) of gas into the lung while respiratory system elastic recoil pressure and expiratory muscle activity drive these volumes back out of the lungs.

This chapter is divided into two broad areas of discussion regarding this process: (1) a basic review of respiratory system mechanics and (2) a discussion of the interaction of ventilator settings with these mechanical properties.

RESPIRATORY SYSTEM MECHANICS

Measurements

Before proceeding in this discussion, a brief review of terminology and measurement techniques is in order. The key parameters that are commonly measured during mechanical ventilation are ventilator and res-

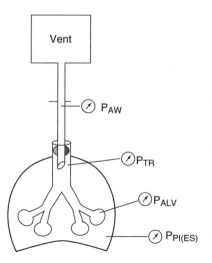

FIGURE 6–1
Sites of pressure measurements during mechanical ventilation.

piratory system pressures, gas flow in and out of the lung, and the consequent tidal volume delivered and returned.[2] Ventilator pressures are usually measured in the ventilator circuitry and often are expressed as airway pressures (P_{AW}). Pressure also can be measured in the esophagus (P_{ES}), which is often taken as a reflection of pleural pressure (P_{PL}). Pressure sometimes is measured at the distal end of the endotracheal tube as a reflection of tracheal pressure (P_{TR}). Under no-flow conditions (i.e., during an inspiratory or expiratory "hold" or "pause"), P_{AW} is termed a static, pause, or plateau pressure. Because there are no flow-resistive pressure gradients, this static P_{AW} measurement is equal to (P_{TR}) and is also equal to alveolar pressure (P_{ALV}). From these measurements, various pressure gradients (ΔP) can be calculated (Fig. 6–1): ΔP from P_{ALV} referenced to atmospheric pressure is transrespiratory system pressure, the pressure correlating with total respiratory system distension; ΔP from P_{ES} referenced to atmospheric pressure is trans-chest wall pressure, the pressure correlating with chest wall distension, and ΔP from $P_{ALV} - P_{ES}$ is transpulmonary pressure, the pressure correlating with alveolar stretch. During inspiratory gas flow, ΔP from $P_{AW} - P_{ALV}$ is trans-total airway pressure, the pressure correlating with total air flow resistance, and ΔP from $P_{AW} - P_{TR}$ is trans-upper airway

pressure during gas flow, the pressure correlating predominantly with artificial airway resistance.[3]

Gas flow usually is measured at the airway opening and can be separated into inspiratory and expiratory flow. Volume delivered (inspired) and volume returned (expired) are usually the integrals of the flow signal, although some ventilators have a volume spirometer to measure expired gas.[4]

Pressure, flow, and volume measurements can be plotted graphically over time or against each other (Fig. 6–2). The pressure volume relationship of the inspired gas is a particularly important plot in assessing alveolar recruitment and distension (discussed in Chapter 7). However, for this plot to be useful in this assessment, the measured pressure must be a reflection of P_{ALV} and thus a "static" pressure volume plot (i.e., a plot made using a range of lung vol-

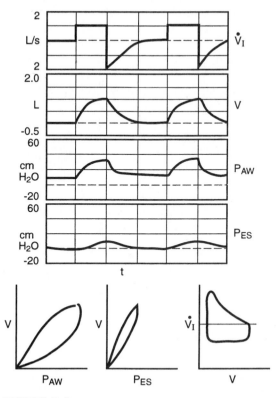

FIGURE 6–2
Pressure (airway: P_{AW}; esophageal: P_{ES}) flow (V_I), and volume (V) measurements can be plotted over time *(upper panels)* or vs. each other *(lower panels)*.

umes and measurements of P_{AW} under no-flow conditions) is required (Fig. 6–3).[5] Because this procedure is time consuming and often requires patient paralysis, alternative strategies have been proposed. One approach is to approximate P_{ALV} during a single slow (i.e., 10 L/min) inspiration by using either P_{TR} or P_{AW} and correcting for known airway resistance[6] (Fig. 6–4).

Lung Inflation and Respiratory System Mechanics

Lung inflation occurs when pressure and flow are applied at the airway opening during mechanical ventilation. These applied forces interact with respiratory system compliance (both lung and chest wall components), airway resistance, and, to a lesser extent, respiratory system inertness and lung tissue resistance. For simplicity, because inertness and tissue resistance are relatively small, they generally are ignored; thus, the interactions of pressure flow and volume with respiratory system mechanics can be expressed by the simplified equation of motion:

$$\text{Driving pressure} = (\text{flow} \times \text{resistance}) + \text{volume/system compliance}$$

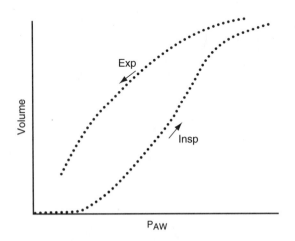

FIGURE 6–3
Static pressure volume plots. Airway pressure (P_{AW}) is measured during multiple inspiratory and expiratory pauses or holds as the lung is inflated and deflated during a mechanical breath. During the pause or hold, airflow is not occurring and thus, $P_{AW} = P_{ALV}$ (alveolar pressure).

In the mechanically ventilated patient, this relationship is expressed as:

$$P_{AW} = (V_I \times R) + (\dot{V}_T / CRS)$$

where P_{AW} is the pressure at the airway opening referenced to atmospheric pressure, V_I is the flow into the patient's lungs, R is the resistance of circuit, artificial airway, and natural airways, $\dot{V}_T$ is the tidal volume, and C_{RS} is the respiratory system compliance (Fig. 6–5). These mechanical components are discussed subsequently in more detail.

Compliance

Static compliance (and its inverse, elastance) describes the "willingness" of the components of the respiratory system to expand in response to delivery of alveolar pressure and volume.[1, 3] Static compliance of the respiratory system is expressed as the ratio of volume added to pressure applied in the alveoli ($C_{RS} = \Delta V / \Delta P_{ALV}$), elastance is the inverse of compliance and is expressed as the ratio of pressure applied to volume added ($E_{RS} = \Delta P_{ALV} / \Delta V$). A so-called dynamic compliance can be calculated using $\Delta V / \Delta P_{AW}$ while flow is occurring. Because the P_{AW} under these conditions reflects both compliance and airway resistance properties of the respiratory system (see Fig. 6–5), this measurement should not be used as a substitute for static compliance. Several features of C_{RS} must be considered in interpreting this value. Specifically, C_{RS} has *volume dependency*, C_{RS} has *hysteresis*, C_{RS} reflects two compliances in *series* (i.e., lung and chest wall), and the lung component of C_{RS} is actually a reflection of multiple *regional* compliances.

COMPLIANCE IS VOLUME DEPENDENT

In the human respiratory system, compliance is nonlinear and volume dependent.[3–7] This means that, because of surfactant behavior, the presence of regional collapse/atelectasis, and the nature of elastic tissue as it is stretched, the overall elastic properties of the respiratory system change as a function of lung volume, usually in a sigmoid

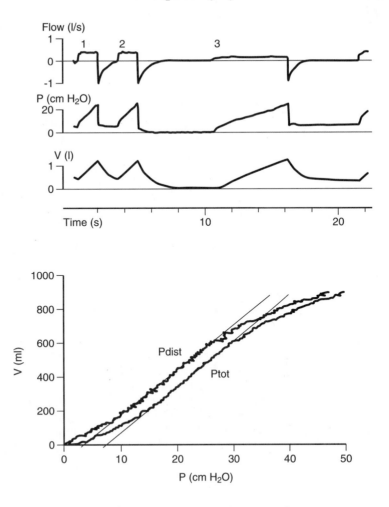

FIGURE 6–4

Approximating a static pressure-volume plot using a slow flow, single-breath technique. In the top panel, ventilator flow, pressure (P), and volume (V) are plotted during the maneuver. The measurement is done during breath 3. The low constant flow minimizes the effects of airway resistance on measured pressure. The bottom panel displays both the observed pressure-volume plot (P_{tot}) and a plot corrected for airway resistance effects (P_{dist}). (Reprinted with permission from Servillo G, Svantesson C, Beydon L, et al. Pressure volume curves in acute respiratory failure. Am J Respir Crit Care Med 155:1629–1636, 1997. © American Lung Association)

manner. (Note the nonlinearity of the pressure–volume plot of Fig. 6–3). For this reason, the volume at which C_{RS} is measured should be considered when assessing or comparing C_{RS} values.

COMPLIANCE HAS HYSTERESIS

Hysteresis refers to the phenomenon of a more steep (i.e., increased) compliance when measured during a deflation from near total lung capacity compared with measurement during inflation from near residual volume. (Note the difference in inflation and deflation in Fig. 6–3.) This is because the inflation maneuver may require a level of pressure to initially recruit collapsed alveoli and stabilize the surfactant layer. This "extra" pressure is not needed to prevent de-recruitment in alveoli during deflation. As a consequence of these effects, ventilation on the deflation limb is the most mechanically ad-

vantageous (i.e., requires the least pressure application).[7, 8] This is the rationale behind sigh breaths, "recruitment maneuvers," and providing positive end-expiratory pressure (PEEP) to prevent alveolar de-recruitment (see Chapter 7).[3, 9]

COMPLIANCE REFLECTS TWO COMPLIANCES IN SERIES

The lung sits within the thoracic cage, and each of these structures has its own compliance: lung compliance (C_L) and chest wall compliance (C_{CW}).[1, 10] The reciprocals of these two compliances are additive:

$$1/C_{RS} = 1/C_L + 1/C_{CW}.$$

These mechanical properties can be separated by comparing pleural (often represented by esophageal) pressure (P_{PL} and (P_{ES}) and airway pressures (P_{AW}) during pos-

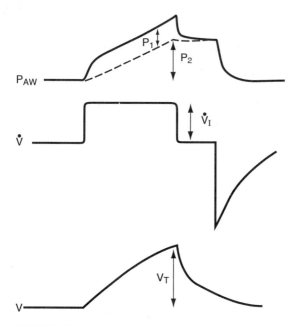

FIGURE 6–5
The equation of motion depicted graphically. P_{AW} is composed of both P_1 (pressure to overcome airflow resistance = $\dot{V}_IR$) and P_2 (pressure to distend respiratory system = V_T/C_{RS}). P_1 and P_2 can be separated by measuring P_{AW} during no-flow conditions (i.e., pause or hold). The end inspiratory P_{AW} (peak P_{AW}) is the sum of P_1 and P_2 and thus = $\dot{V}_IR + V_T/CRS$.

itive pressure ventilation (Fig. 6–6, *solid lines*). Specifically, during a passive, machine-controlled breath, static P_{AW} (i.e., during an inspiratory hold) can be taken as the distending pressures across the respiratory system, and thus, $\Delta V_T/\Delta P_{AW}$ = compliance of the respiratory system (C_{RS}). Under these same conditions, (P_{ES}) can be taken as pressure within the pleural space, and thus, $\Delta V_T/\Delta P_{ES}$ = compliance of the chest wall (C_{CW}). From the equation above, the reciprocal of C_L can be determined by subtracting the reciprocal of C_{RS} and C_{CW}. Calculations are different during a spontaneous breath. This is because the driving pressure gradient for gas flow is created in the pleural space by the inspiratory muscles instead of in the airway by the ventilator. Under these conditions (Fig. 6–6, *dashed line*), P_{AW} remains atmospheric and P_{ES} (referenced to passive recoil pressure) represents the driving transpulmonary pressures (i.e., it is no longer the passive chest wall distending

pressures). Thus, $V_T/\Delta P_{ES}$ during spontaneous breaths referenced to passive recoil pressure equals C_{RS} and referenced to atmospheric pressure (C_L).[1, 7, 10]

COMPLIANCE IS DETERMINED BY MANY DIFFERENT REGIONAL COMPLIANCES

In the normal upright human lungs, gravitational effects on lung water, lung stretch, and blood flow create lower compliance units in the base and higher compliance units in the apices.[1, 11] These differences account for the sequential filling and emptying of basilar and apical units in the normal lung.[11, 12] In lungs with parenchymal injury, there are often heavily injured regions with very poor compliance interspersed with healthier regions with more normal compliance.[13] Regional volume expansion from a positive pressure breath is heavily affected by these regional compliances. Specifically, severely injured lungs may have little ventilation delivered to stiffer regions and potential overdistension of healthier regions.[13, 14] This has given rise to the concept that parenchymal injury effectively creates "baby lungs," a description that emphasizes the

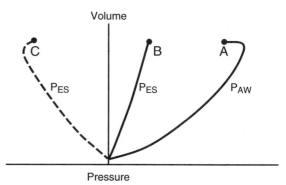

FIGURE 6–6
Determining C_{RS}, C_L, and C_{CW} during positive pressure breath and during spontaneous breath. Depicted are airway pressures (P_{AW}) and esophageal pressures (P_{ES}). With a positive pressure breath *(solid lines)*, P_{AW} at end inspiration under no-flow conditions (point A) reflects P_{ALV}. Thus, $C_{RS} = V_T/P_{AW}$ at point A and $C_{CW} = V_T/P_{ES}$ at point B. With spontaneous breath *(dashed lines)*, P_{ES} at point C referenced to atmosphere (point B) is used to calculate C_L; P_{ES} referenced to passive recoil pressure at point B is used to calculate C_{RS}.

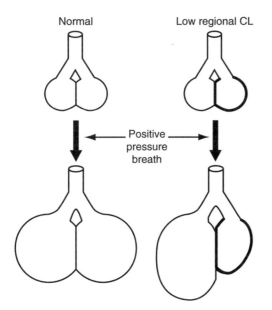

Normal   Low regional CL

Positive pressure breath

FIGURE 6–7
Regional compliance differences can create regions of poor inflation in diseased units while grossly overinflating healthier units during a positive pressure breath.

fact that only small portions of the lung may be available for ventilation (Fig. 6–7). Regional compliance differences, by producing regional differences in functional residual capacity, also may create the potential for shearing injury if one unit is filling proportionately faster or with markedly different volumes.

In practice, C_{RS} is often reported as a single value that usually is determined over the operational range of tidal ventilation (C_{RS} = V_T/static P_{AW} − PEEP), where V_T is the set tidal volume, static P_{AW} is the P_{AW} during the end inspiration hold, and PEEP is the total positive end-expiratory pressure in the alveoli (i.e., reflecting both set and intrinsic PEEP). Normal value for lung compliance is 200 ml/cm H_2O. Normal value for thoracic cage compliance is 200 ml/cm H_2O, and thus normal value for respiratory system compliance is 100 ml/cm H_2O. Severe lung injury is usually associated with values for C_{RS} less than 20 ml/cm H_2O. Usually, this reduction in C_{RS} is caused by lung disease (i.e., reductions in C_L), although chest wall injuries, surgical binders, and obesity can reduce C_{RS} through reduction in C_{CW}. The caveats of nonlinear behavior, hystere-

sis, and regional differences all should be considered when a single measurement of C_{RS} is interpreted.

Resistance

Resistance to airflow (R) is caused by both the natural and the artificial airways.[1, 3, 7] The determinants of resistance depend on whether flow is turbulent or laminar. In general, gas flow during positive pressure ventilation is treated as laminar flow such that $P_{AW} \approx R \times \dot{V}_I$.[3, 7] Under these conditions, airway (and circuit) diameter is the major determinant of resistance (i.e., R varies with the 4th power of the airway radius). Resistance also varies directly with airway (and circuit) length and gas density. Like compliance, R varies with lung *volume*, R differs during *inspiration and expiration*, R is a reflection of two resistances in *series* (i.e., artificial and natural airways), and R can have significant *regional* variation.

RESISTANCE VARIES WITH VOLUME

The effects of lung volume on airway resistance are depicted in Figure 6–8. As shown, as the lung is inflated, resistance falls as airways are pulled open by the increasing volume in the thorax.[1, 3]

RESISTANCE CHANGES WITH INSPIRATION AND EXPIRATION

During inspiration, the expanding lung tends to produce a larger airway diameter than during expiration, and thus, resistance generally is lower during inspiration.[15] Moreover, during expiration, smaller membranous airways can behave like starling resistors, creating so-called "flow-limited" segments.[16] Under these conditions, elastic recoil pressures are the driving force for gas flow because increases in pleural pressure greater than this only serve to compress these airways and increase resistance. In airway disease states, further narrowing of already pathologically narrowed airways during expiration can produce the phenomenon of air trapping and intrinsic positive end-expiratory pressure (**intrinsic PEEP**, or $PEEP_i$).[16, 17] The actual determinants of

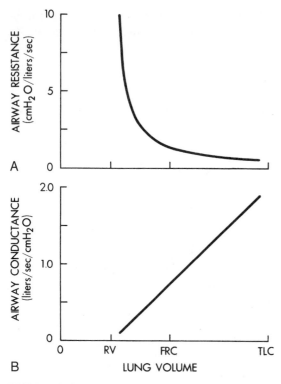

FIGURE 6–8
Schematic illustrations of the relationship between airway resistance (A) and airway conductance (B) and lung volume. The hyperbolic resistance-volume curve becomes a straight line when the same data are expressed as conductance-volume. (Reprinted with permission from Murray JF: Respiration. In: Smith LH, Thier S (eds): Pathophysiology. Philadelphia: WB Saunders, 1985, pp 753–854.)

PEEPi are the total minute ventilation, the inspiratory/expiratory ratio, and the mechanical factors involved in lung emptying (i.e., R and the elastic recoil driving pressure C_{RS}).[18] These lung-emptying mechanical factors are often expressed as a time constant, or tau (τ), which is the product of $C_{RS} \times R$. Short time constants favor rapid emptying and occur when C_{RS} and R are low (e.g., fibrosis); long-time constants favor slow emptying and occur when C_{RS} and R are high (e.g., emphysema).[18] These two relationships are depicted in Figure 6–9.

RESISTANCE REFLECTS THE ARTIFICIAL AND THE NATURAL AIRWAY'S RESISTANCE IN SERIES

In mechanically ventilated lungs, measured airflow resistance is influenced heavily by

the properties of the artificial airways.[19] Indeed, long narrow endotracheal tubes (ETs) can produce air flow resistance several times higher than normal airway resistance.[19] This ET resistance can have a number of important effects. First, ET resistance creates an inspiratory muscle load. Indeed, the resistance imposed by the ET may be of sufficient magnitude to fatigue a spontane-

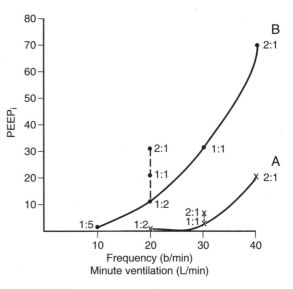

FIGURE 6–9
Examples of how intrinsic positive end-expiratory pressure (PEEPi) is a function of lung mechanics, minute ventilation, and I:E ratio. On the vertical axis is PEEPi predicted from a lung model and on the horizontal axis is frequency (f). In this model, tidal volume is set at 1 L and inspiratory time is 1 sec such that minute ventilation (MV) is determined by frequency and I:E increases as f and MV increase (representative I:E ratios are listed). Curve A illustrates the behavior of moderately restricted lung with only a slightly elevated resistance (CL = 30 ml/cm H_2O, insp R = 10 cm $H_2O/L/s$ and exp R = 10 cm $H_2O/L/s$). Note that significant PEEPi does not develop until f and MV exceed 30. Curve B illustrates the behavior of a severely obstructed lung (C = 70 ml/cm H_2O, insp R = 20 cm $H_2O/L/s$ and exp R = 40 cm $H_2O/L/s$). Note now that significant PEEPi develops at f and MV values of 20 (Model B) and 30 (Model A). Dotted lines depict the development of PEEPi as inspiratory flow is reduced and inspiratory line is lengthened with a constant minute ventilation. (Reprinted with permission from Marini JJ, Crooke PS: A general mathematical model for respiratory dynamics relevant to the clinical setting. Am Rev Respir Dis 147:14–24, 1993 © American Lung Association.)

ously breathing patient who otherwise might be able to tolerate extubation. This is the rationale for using small amounts of pressure support in intubated patients during spontaneous breathing trials.[20] Second, ET resistance creates a delay in achieving airway pressurization compared with circuit pressurization during ventilator gas delivery. In an actively breathing patient, this may cause discomfort.[21] To address this problem, a novel approach to pressure-targeted breaths is to move the ventilator-sensing site (and thus, pressure-targeting site) to the distal end of the ET (see Chapter 9).[22] Finally, ET resistance also produces expiratory resistance, which produces both an expiratory muscle load and an increased risk for air trapping.[18]

RESISTANCE HAS REGIONAL DIFFERENCES

In normal lungs, gravitational effects on lung water and required stretch make airway resistance slightly higher at the bases than at the apices.[11, 12] In disease states, airway resistance may have marked regional inhomogeneities. These can affect ventilation distribution and produce a shearing effect in adjacent regions with different filling patterns.

Clinically, airflow resistance can be measured during either inspiration or expiration. Inspiratory resistance generally is determined by using a constant flow breath (e.g., 1 L/sec) and then calculating the driving pressure as the difference between the P_{AW} during flow and without flow (e.g., peak P_{AW} − static P_{AW} at end inspiration).[4] Expressing this result with respect to volume (i.e., "specific resistance") takes into account the aforementioned effects of lung volume.[1, 4] Normal values are 4 to 6 cm H_2O/L/sec/L. Expiratory resistance is calculated in several ways.[23] A common approach is to use P_{ALV} − PEEP at end inspiration and divide peak expiratory flow by this value. Flow interrupters could be used to make similar calculations at different lung volumes during expiration. A more complex approach is to analyze the exponential decay characteristics of expiratory flow to calculate a time constant for a one-compartment

model (or two time constants for a two-compartment model). One then can use a known compliance value to solve for resistance.

Mechanical Loads

Mechanical loads describe the mechanical aspects of ventilation with a single number—an expression either of **work** (W) or of a **pressure–time product** (PTP). The concept of load is particularly useful in considering the inspiratory muscle energy requirement during spontaneous or interactive partial ventilatory support as mechanical loads correlate well with inspiratory muscle oxygen demands.[24] Moreover, when referenced to muscle strength and/or endurance properties, load tolerance is a useful guide to set levels of partial ventilatory support or predict the spontaneous breathing capabilities.[25, 26]

Work expresses load as the integral of pressure over volume (W = ∫PdV). Thus, compliance, resistance, and the size of the breath all contribute to the magnitude of the work per breath. As with compliance considerations (see Fig. 6–5), work calculations represent different loads during spontaneous breath or during controlled breaths. During spontaneous breaths, integrating P_{ES} over V_T (referenced to the passive recoil pressure) describes the work performed on the respiratory system by the inspiratory muscles. During a controlled breath, integrating P_{AW} over V_T describes the work performed on the respiratory system by the ventilator. During this same controlled breath, integrating P_{ES} over $\dot{V}_T$ describes the work performed on the chest wall by the ventilator.[3, 10] For a given, $\dot{V}_I$, $\dot{V}_T$, and set of respiratory system mechanics, total work should be identical regardless of whether measured during a spontaneous (patient work) or a controlled breath (ventilator work). Moreover, during interactive, partially supported breaths, where work is shared between patient and ventilator, the sum contributions of patient and ventilator work should be the same as during the controlled or spontaneous breath[27] (Fig. 6–10). Normal values for work are 4 to 6 joules/minute. Normal respiratory muscles gener-

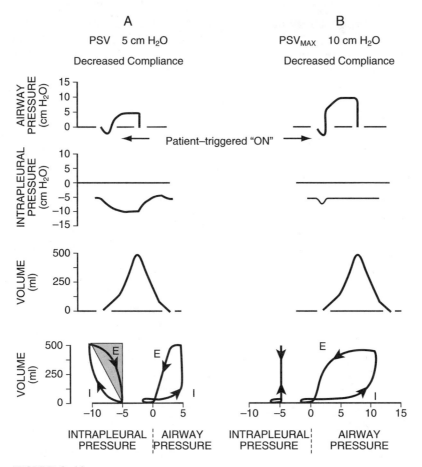

FIGURE 6–10

Work "shifting" using pressure support ventilation (PSV). In this example, chest wall compliance is ignored. (A) A PSV level of 5 cm H_2O is applied. Under this condition, work is performed in part by the patient and in part by the ventilator. Alternatively, all work may be provided by the ventilator by increasing the level of PSV to higher levels, e.g., 10 cm H_2O as in (B). (B) At this setting, the patient is relatively passive, intrapleural pressure does not change, and essentially no work is performed by the patient. (Reprinted from Banner MJ, Blanch PB, Kirby RR: Imposed work of breathing and methods of triggering a demand flow CPAP system. Crit Care Med 21:183–191, 1993.)

ally do not fatigue with work <20 to 25 joules/minute; abnormal respiratory muscles, however, may fatigue with even normal workloads.[24, 28]

The PTP expresses load as the integral of pressure over inspiratory time (PTP = ∫Pdt). Depending on whether the measured breath is spontaneous or ventilator controlled and whether pressure is P_{AW} or P_{ES}, the PTP (as in the aforementioned work discussion) can reflect properties of the lung, the chest wall, and the entire respiratory system and whether the load is borne by the patient or ventilator, or is shared (Fig. 6–11). Normal

values for the respiratory system are 4 to 6 cm H_2O × seconds per breath.[26]

As can be appreciated by their mathematical expressions, both work and PTP measurements of load are influenced by pressure requirements to ventilate. The work expression, however, incorporates the volume moved (muscle or ventilator "displacement") and ignores time while the PTP incorporates the duration of pressure generation but ignores the volume moved. Under heavy loading conditions (e.g., the patient with abnormal lung mechanics and thus high pressure requirements), duration of pressure (i.e., the PTP) correlates better with muscle energetics and fatigue potential than does volume moved with pressure (i.e., work).[24-26, 29] Indeed, during ventilation requiring high pressure, multiplying PTP by the T_I/T_{TOT} (inspiratory time as a fraction of total cycle time) and referencing this to the maximal pressure that the inspiratory muscles can generate (i.e., the maximum inspiratory force measurement), muscle fatigue can be expected if this value exceeds 0.15.[26] This concern with high pressure loads during partial ventilatory support is one of the rationales for providing ventilator pressure assistance with every spontaneous effort (i.e., pressure-assisted or supported breaths), as opposed to alternating fully supported breaths with unsupported breaths (i.e., intermittent mandatory ventilation).[30]

A simple way of calculating work or PTP for a given tidal volume and inspiratory time can use readily available airway pressure measurements during a ventilator-controlled breath. The simplest way is to use a constant flow, volume-controlled breath over

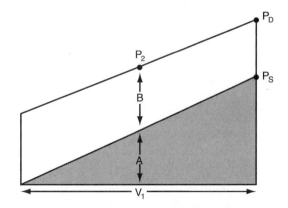

FIGURE 6–12
Pressure (P)–volume (VI) profile generated under the assumptions that airway resistance, flow, and thoracic compliance remain unchanged throughout inflation. The pressure of 1/2 VI, $P_2 = (A + B)$ is numerically equivalent to the mean inflation pressure and is composed of an element required to stretch the thorax to that volume ($A = 1/2\ P_s$), and an element needed to drive flow ($B = P_D - P_s$). (Reprinted with permission from Marini JJ, Rodriquez M, Lamb V: Bedside estimation of the inspiratory dynamics relevant to mechanical ventilation. Chest 89:56–62, 1986.)

1 second. An inspiratory pause measurement for static P_{AW} also is required. Mean inflation pressure can be calculated from simple geometric relationships (Fig. 6–12), and this pressure can be multiplied by either V_T (work/breath) or inspiratory time (PTP/breath).[31]

INTERACTION OF VENTILATOR SETTINGS AND LUNG MECHANICS

Pressure- Versus Flow/Volume-Targeted Breaths

As noted in Chapter 2, there are two basic approaches to delivering positive pressure breaths: pressure targeting and flow/volume targeting.[4] With pressure targeting, the clinician sets an inspiratory pressure target (with either time or flow as the cycling criterion) such that flow and volume are dependent variables (i.e., varying with lung mechanics and patient effort to maintain the pressure target). With flow/volume targeting, the clinician sets an inspiratory flow and cycling volume such that airway pres-

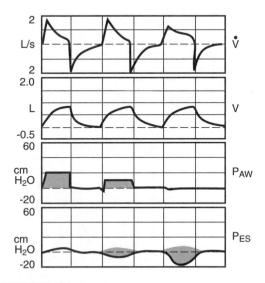

FIGURE 6–11
Load shifting as reflected in a Pressure Time (PTP). PTP is the integral of pressure over time *(shaded area)*. Load during the first breath is borne entirely by the ventilator; load during the third breath is borne entirely by the patient; load during the middle breath is shared. Note that the total PTP for this volume and inspiratory time is constant with all these breaths.

sure is the dependent variable (Fig 6–13). Changes of compliance or resistance cause a change of tidal volume (but not P_{AW}) with the pressure-targeted breath. In contrast, similar changes in compliance or resistance change P_{AW} (but not flow or volume) with a volume-targeted breath.

The concept of balancing lung stretch with volume guarantee is discussed more in Chapter 18. In general, if volume guarantee is more important than limiting stretch (e.g., central nervous system [CNS] injury with near normal lung mechanics), flow/volume targeting is appropriate. In contrast, if limiting stretch is more important than volume guarantee (e.g., a patient with adult respiratory distress syndrome [ARDS] who can tolerate some degree of hypercapnia), then pressure targeting is appropriate. The variable flow of the pressure-targeted breath also may synchronize with patient efforts during interactive breaths better than a fixed flow volume-targeted breath (see Chapter 9).

Pressure-targeted breaths and volume-targeted breath with decelerating flow patterns have lower peak pressures than constant or sine wave flow patterns. This is because flow decreases as the lung fills, thus decreasing the flow-resistive pressure at end inspiration. For a given tidal volume, however, this probably has little clinical sig-

nificance because it is the end inspiratory alveolar pressure that is important for lung distension and lung injury (see Chapter 11).

Delivered Minute Ventilation and the $f \times V_T$ Settings

Current generation ventilators can be shown to be capable of delivering more than 50 L/minute under a wide range of frequency (f) and V_T settings. As long as expiratory time is adequate for the lung to return to the "rest state" (i.e., functional residual capacity) determined by elastic recoil and applied PEEP, these machine capabilities can deliver this level of ventilation to the lungs. As noted above, however (see Fig. 6–9), under high minute ventilation delivery with short expiratory times and slow expiratory time constants (i.e., high compliance, high resistance conditions), intrinsic PEEP (air trapping) can develop. This may either be intentional (see long inspiratory time strategies in Chapter 18) or may be inadvertent (especially in patients with obstructive airway physiology). This intrinsic PEEP has different effects on pressure-targeted and volume-targeted ventilation. In pressure-targeted ventilation, intrinsic PEEP results in tidal volume loss, whereas in volume-targeted ventilation, it results in

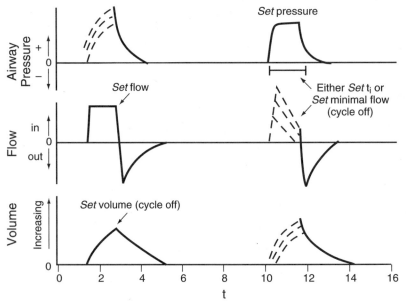

FIGURE 6–13
Flow-volume vs. pressure targeting. With flow/volume targeting *(left panels),* flow and volume are the independent (i.e., set) variables whereas pressure is the dependent variable. With pressure targeting *(right panels),* pressure is the independent (i.e., set) variable and flow and volume are dependent variables.

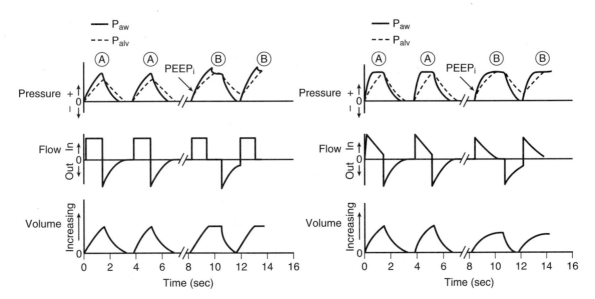

FIGURE 6–14

Effects of intrinsic PEEP (PEEPi) on volume-targeted *(left panel)* and pressure-targeted *(right panel)* ventilation. P_{ALV} = alveolar pressure, P_{AW} = airway opening pressure. In both panels, the first two breaths have adequate expiratory times and, thus, no trapping. In contrast, the second two breaths in both panels have inadequate expiratory times, and airway trapping (PEEPi) develops. With volume-targeted breaths, this increases airway opening pressures. With pressure-targeted breaths, this reduces tidal volume: (Reprinted with permission from Fulkerson WJ, MacIntyre NR: Problems in Respiratory Care Complications of Mechanical Ventilation. Philadelphia: JB Lippincott, 1991.)

airway pressure elevations (Fig. 6–14). Other signs of air trapping developing are the expiratory flow signal not returning to baseline (Fig. 6–14) and the expiratory hold maneuver in the passive patient (Fig. 6–15).

Intrinsic PEEP thus puts limits on the actual minute ventilation that can be delivered to patients under a given set of conditions (Fig. 6–16).[32] Intrinsic PEEP also can function as an inspiratory threshold load for

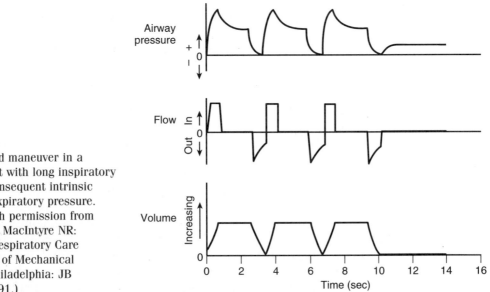

FIGURE 6–15

Expiratory hold maneuver in a passive patient with long inspiratory pauses and consequent intrinsic positive end-expiratory pressure. (Reprinted with permission from Fulkerson WJ, MacIntyre NR: Problems in Respiratory Care Complications of Mechanical Ventilation. Philadelphia: JB Lippincott, 1991.)

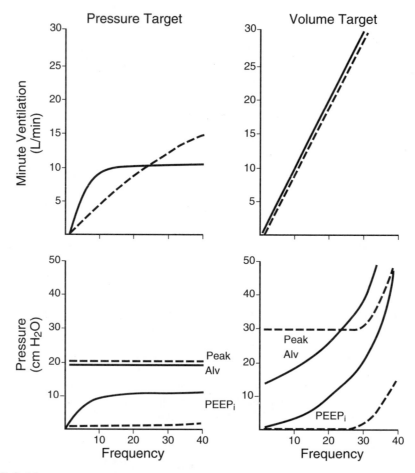

FIGURE 6–16

Examples of volume delivery *(top panel)* and pressure application *(bottom panels)* using pressure-targeted *(left panels)* and volume-targeted *(right panels)* breaths at different frequencies. Depicted pressures are peak alveolar (Peak Alv) and intrinsic positive end-expiratory pressure (PEEPi). Data are from a lung model similation restricted *(dashed lines)* and obstructed *(solid line)* physiology. Note that with pressure targeting, the development of PEEPi puts a limit on the minute ventilation capabilities. In contrast, volume targeting has rapidly rising peak alveolar pressures as PEEPi develops to guarantee the set volume. (Reprinted from Marini JJ, Crooke PS: A general mathematical model for respiratory dynamics relevant to the clinical setting. Am Rev Respir Dis 147:14–24, 1993. © American Lung Association.)

breath triggering during interactive ventilation (See Chapter 9).

Ventilation Distribution

A positive pressure tidal breath must distribute itself among the millions of alveolar units in the lung. Factors affecting this distribution include regional resistances, compliances, functional residual capacities, and the delivered flow pattern (including inspi-

ratory pause). In general, slower flows tend to distribute more evenly in obstructive inhomogeneities (although consequent shorter expiratory times may worsen air trapping) whereas faster flows (especially decelerating flows) tend to distribute more evenly in compliance inhomogeneities.[33] Inspiratory pauses also allow pendelluft action to fill slow-filling alveoli. It should be noted, however, that more uniform ventilation distribution does *not* necessarily mean better ventilation–perfusion matching (i.e., more even ventilation distribution actually may worsen ventilation–perfusion matching in a lung with perfusion inhomogeneities). Because of all these considerations, predicting which flow pattern and inspiratory:expiratory (I:E) ratio will optimize ventilation–perfusion matching is difficult and often an empirical trial-and-error exercise. How ventilation distribution affects ventilation–perfusion matching and gas exchange is discussed in more detail in Chapter 7.

SUMMARY

Respiratory system mechanics involve the interactions of resistance, compliance, patient effort, and positive pressure breath delivery strategy. In addition, regional mechanical behavior influences the distribution of ventilation and consequent ventilation–perfusion matching. The integration of these mechanical factors also allows for calculation of loads on the ventilatory muscles. Understanding these relationships is important in optimizing ventilatory support.[34]

REFERENCES

1. Murry JF: The Normal Lung, 2nd ed. Philadelphia: WB Saunders, 1986.
2. Truwit JD, Marini JJ: Evaluation of thoracic mechanics in the ventilated patient: part I, primary measurements. J Crit Care 3:133–150, 1988.
3. Truwit JD, Marini JJ: Evaluation of thoracic mechanics in the ventilated patient: part II, applied mechanics. J Crit Care 3:192–213, 1988.
4. American Association of Respiratory Care Consensus Group. Essentials of mechanical ventilation. Respir Care 37:999–1130, 1992.
5. Beydon L, Lemaire F, Jonson B: Lung mechanics in ARDS: compliance and pressure-volume curves. In: Zapol WM, Lemaire F (eds): Adult Respiratory Distress Syndrome. New York: Marcel Dekker, 1991, pp. 139–161.
6. Servillo G, Svantesson C, Beydon L, et al: Pressure volume curves in acute respiratory failure. Am J Respir Crit Care Med 155:1629–1636, 1997.
7. Salmon RB, Primiano FP, Saidel GM, Niewoehner DE: Human pressure-volume relationships: alveolar collapse and airway closure. J Appl Physiol 51:353–1162, 1981.
8. Sharp JT, Johnson FN, Goldberg NB, van Lith P: Hysteresis and stress adaption in the human respiratory system. J Appl Physiol 23:487–497, 1967.
9. Benito S, Lemaire F: Pulmonary pressure-volume relationship in acute respiratory distress syndrome in adults: role of positive and expiratory pressure. J Crit Care 5:27–34, 1990.
10. Agostoni E, Campbell EJM, Freedman S: Energetics. In: Campbell EJM, Agostoni E, Newsome-Davis J (eds): The Respiratory Muscles. Philadelphia: WB Saunders, 1970, pp 115–137.
11. Milic-Emili J, Henderson JAN, Dolovich MB, et al: Regional distribution of inhaled gas in the lung. J Appl Physiol 21:749–759, 1966.
12. Anthonisen NR, Robertson PC, Ross WRD: Gravity dependent sequential emptying of lung regions. J Appl Physiol 28:589–595, 1970.
13. Gattinoni L, Pesenti A, Torresin A, et al: Adult respiratory distress syndrome profiles by computed tomography. J Thorac Imaging 3:25–30, 1988.
14. Gattinoni L, Pesenti A, Baglioni S, et al: Inflammatory pulmonary edema and PEEP: correlation between imaging and physiologic studies. J Thorac Imaging 3:59–64, 1988.
15. Briscoe WA, Dubois AB: The relationship between airway resistance, airway conductance and lung volume in subjects of different age and body size. J Clin Invest 37:1279–1285, 1958.
16. Pride NB, Permutt S, Riley RL, Bromberger-Barnes B: Determinants of maximal expiratory flow from the lungs. J Appl Physiol 23:646–662, 1967.
17. Pepe PE, Marini JJ: Occult positive end-expiratory pressure in mechanically ventilated patients with airflow obstruction. Am Rev Respir Dis 126:166–170, 1982.
18. Tobin MJ, Ladato RF: PEEP, auto-PEEP, and waterfalls (editorial). Chest 96:449–451, 1989.
19. Wright PW, Marini JJ, Bernard GF: In vitro versus in vivo comparison of endotracheal tube airflow resistance. Am Rev Respir Dis 140:10–16, 1989.
20. Fiastro JF, Habib MP, Quan SF: Pressure support compensation for inspiratory work due to endotracheal tubes and demand continuous positive airway pressure. Chest 93:499–505, 1988.
21. Sasoon CSH: Mechanical ventilator design and function: the trigger variable. Respir Care 37:1056–1069, 1992.
22. Banner MJ, Blanch PB, Kirby RR: Imposed work of breathing and methods of triggering a demand flow CPAP system. Crit Care Med 21:183–191, 1993.
23. Marshall R: Objective tests of respiratory mechanics. In: Fenn WO, Rahn H (eds): Handbook of Physiology, Section 3, Respiration, vol. 2. Washington, DC: American Physiological Society, 1965, pp. 1404–1405.
24. MacIntyre NR, Leatherman NE: Mechanical loads on the ventilatory muscles. Am Rev Respir Dis 144:139–143, 1989.
25. Yang K, Tobin MJ: A prospective study of indexes predicting outcome of trials of weaning from mechanical ventilation. N Engl J Med 324: 1445–1450, 1991.

26. Field S, Sanci S, Grassino A: Respiratory muscle oxygen consumption estimated by the diaphragm pressure-time index. J Appl Physiol 57:44–51, 1984.
27. Banner MJ, Kirby RR, MacIntrye NR: Patient and ventilator work of breathing and ventilatory muscle loads at different levels of pressure support ventilation. Chest 100:531–533, 1991.
28. Bellemare F, Grassino A: Effect of pressure and timing or contraction on human diaphragm fatigue. J AppI Physiol 57:44–51, 1984.
29. Collett PW, Perry C, Engel LA: Pressure time product, flow, and oxygen cost resistive breathing in humans. J Appl Physiol 58:1263–1272, 1985.
30. MacIntyre NR: Weaning from mechanical ventilatory support: volume-assisting intermittent breaths versus pressure-assisting every breath. Respir Care 33:121–125, 1988.
31. Marini JJ, Rodriguez M, Lamb V: Bedside estimation of the inspiratory dynamics relevant to mechanical ventilation. Chest 89:56–62, 1986.
32. Marini JJ, Crooke PS: A general mathematical model for respiratory dynamics relevant to the clinical setting. Am Rev Respir Dis 147:14–24, 1993.
33. Macklen PT: Relationship between lung mechanics and ventilation distribution. Physiology 16:580–588, 1973.
34. Fulkerson WJ, MacIntyre NR: Problems in Respiratory Care: Complications of Mechanical Ventilation. Philadelphia: JB Lippincott, 1991.

Alveolar Capillary Gas Transport

Neil R. MacIntyre, MD

STEADY-STATE
ALVEOLAR–CAPILLARY
PRESSURE GRADIENTS FOR
CARBON DIOXIDE AND
OXYGEN
VENTILATION–PERFUSION
MATCHING
Concept
POSITIVE PRESSURE
VENTILATION EFFECTS ON
VENTILATION–PERFUSION
MATCHING
Positive End-Expiratory
Pressure

Inspiratory Flow Pattern
and Inspiratory–
Expiratory Time
Relationship Effects on
Ventilation–Perfusion
Intrathoracic Pressures
and Perfusion
ALVEOLAR-CAPILLARY GAS
TRANSPORT IN THE
CONTEXT OF OVERALL
OXYGEN DELIVERY
REFERENCES

KEY WORDS

inspiratory:expiratory ratios
oxygen delivery
positive end-expiratory
  pressure (PEEP)

pressure gradient
ventilation-perfusion
  relationship

Alveolar capillary gas transport is one of several steps that take place in the overall process of delivering oxygen to and removing carbon dioxide from the tissues (Fig. 7–1). Metabolic demands are quantified by tissue oxygen consumption (V_{O_2}) and tissue carbon dioxide production (V_{CO_2}).[1] In oxidative metabolism, depending on the caloric substrate, V_{CO_2} is generally 0.7 to 0.9 of V_{O_2} (the "R" value). The demands on the alveolar–capillary transport system thus are to provide for an influx of oxygen to equal metabolic V_{O_2} and to provide an efflux of carbon dioxide to equal metabolic V_{CO_2}. Calculated values for V_{O_2} and V_{CO_2} generally are referenced to body surface area. Representative normal values for V_{O_2} are 100 to 150 ml/min/m^2 and for V_{CO_2} are 80 to 120 ml/min/m^2.

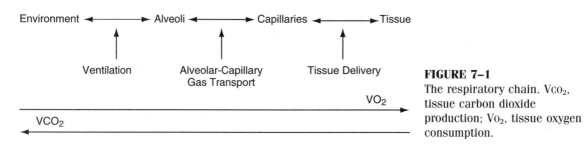

FIGURE 7–1
The respiratory chain. V_{CO_2}, tissue carbon dioxide production; V_{O_2}, tissue oxygen consumption.

STEADY-STATE ALVEOLAR–CAPILLARY PRESSURE GRADIENTS FOR CARBON DIOXIDE AND OXYGEN

The steady-state **pressure gradient** for capillary–alveolar CO_2 transport is the incoming mixed venous P_{CO_2} (P_{VCO_2}) with respect to the mean alveolar P_{CO_2} (P_{ACO_2}). Under normal conditions, P_{VCO_2} is 45 torr and P_{ACO_2} is 40 torr. The determinant of these two pressures is V_{CO_2}, with respect to the ventilation delivered to perfused alveoli (functional or alveolar ventilation [VA]). This relationship often is expressed in terms of alveolar P_{CO_2}.[1]

$$P_{ACO_2} \propto \frac{V_{CO_2}}{VA} \qquad (1)$$

This relationship is plotted in Figure 7–2 and, as can be seen, P_{ACO_2} is related linearly to V_{CO_2} and related inversely to VA. Thus, for example, doubling V_{CO_2} ($2 \times V_{CO_2}$ in Fig. 7–2) doubles the P_{ACO_2}, whereas doubling the VA halves the P_{ACO_2}.

Because of the high diffusibility of CO_2 and the near linear relationship of P_{CO_2} and CO_2 content in blood, CO_2 alveolar–capillary gas transport is affected only minimally by the **ventilation–perfusion relationship**[1-3] (see later discussion). Thus, in both normal and abnormal lungs, arterial P_{CO_2} (P_{aCO_2}) is virtually identical to P_{ACO_2}. Because of this, P_{aCO_2} can also be expressed as a function of V_{CO_2} and VA, as in equation 1 and in Figure 7–2.

The steady-state pressure gradient for alveolar–capillary O_2 transport is mean alveolar P_{O_2} (P_{AO_2}) and the incoming mixed venous P_{O_2} (P_{VO_2}). Under normal conditions, P_{VO_2} is 40 torr and P_{AO_2} is 100 torr. Like CO_2, P_{VO_2} is affected by tissue O_2 consumption (V_{O_2}), and P_{AO_2} is affected by ventila-

tion delivered to perfused alveoli (VA). P_{AO_2} also is affected by the inspired P_{O_2} (P_{IO_2}). The interaction of these factors is expressed as:

$$P_{AO_2} \propto P_{IO_2} - \frac{V_{O_2}}{VA} \qquad (2)$$

This relationship is plotted in Figure 7–3. Note that in contrast to CO_2, decreases in V_{O_2} and/or increases in VA increase P_{AO_2}, but P_{AO_2} will asymptote on P_{IO_2} (partial pressure of inspired O_2). This is why increasing alveolar ventilation has progressively less effect on P_{AO_2} and O_2 transport. Equation 2 also can be rearranged using R as the ratio of V_{CO_2}/V_{O_2} and VA as a function of P_{aCO_2} (equation 1), to give the simplified alveolar gas equation for P_{AO_2}:

$$P_{AO_2} = P_{IO_2} - \frac{P_{aCO_2}}{R} \qquad (3)$$

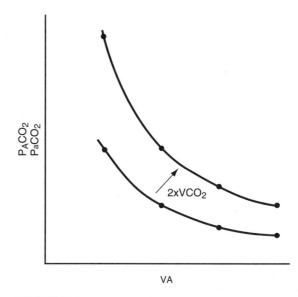

FIGURE 7–2
The relationship of alveolar (and arterial) partial pressure of carbon dioxide (P_{CO_2}) to V_{CO_2} and alveolar ventilation (VA).

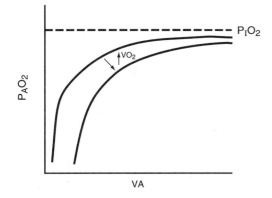

FIGURE 7-3

The relationship of alveolar partial pressure of oxygen (Po_2) to Vo_2, inspired Po_2 and VA.

Ventilation–perfusion matching has much more effect on alveolar–capillary O_2 transport than on CO_2 transport. As discussed subsequently in more detail, this is because the relationship between Po_2 and O_2 content is not linear (hemoglobin is saturated at Po_2 ≈ 100 torr) and the fact that O_2 is less diffusible than CO_2. Substantial differences in alveolar and arterial oxygen pressure thus can develop in the presence of ventilation–perfusion mismatch. Arterial Po_2 therefore, cannot be substituted into equation 2 or 3 for PAo_2. Instead, an "alveolar–arterial oxygen difference" (A–aDo_2) can be calculated to reflect this phenomenon:

$$A-aDO_2 = \left(PIO_2 - \frac{PaCO_2}{R} \right) - PaO_2 \quad (4)$$

A small A–aDo_2 gradient exists even in normal lungs (up to 25 torr with room air breathing), but it can increase many times in disease states.[3, 4] Thus, the A–aDo_2 gradient can be used to quantify the degree of lung injury.

VENTILATION–PERFUSION MATCHING

Concept

The concept of ventilation–perfusion ($\dot{V}/\dot{Q}$) matching is depicted in Figure 7–4.[2, 5-7] Ideal $\dot{V}/\dot{Q}$ is near 1 (i.e., ventilation and

perfusion are equal to each other). At the extremes are shunts ($\dot{V}/\dot{Q} = 0$) and dead space ($\dot{V}/\dot{Q} = \infty$). In normal upright human lungs, gravitational effects on lung water, perfusion, and ventilation create a vertical distribution of $\dot{V}/\dot{Q}$ relationships ranging from near 5 at the apex to near 0.5 at the bases.[2, 5-7] In diseased lungs, this distribution can be many times larger.[2, 5-7] A useful way to express this distribution is to use six gases of different solubilities and measure their lung and blood concentrations to construct a lung model with 50 $\dot{V}/\dot{Q}$ units.[5] The logarithmic standard deviation (sigma or σ) of this distribution then is used to quantify the degree of $\dot{V}/\dot{Q}$ inhomogeneities in the lung. Normal values for σ are less than 0.5, whereas values for σ of 2 or greater can be seen in severe disease.[2, 5-7]

The effects of $\dot{V}/\dot{Q}$ mismatching on Pco_2 and Po_2 are different. In general, as noted previously, CO_2 is more diffusible than oxygen, and its partial pressure in blood is roughly linearly related to its content. High $\dot{V}/\dot{Q}$ units thus can "compensate" for low $\dot{V}/\dot{Q}$ units such that even moderately abnormal $\dot{V}/\dot{Q}$ distributions have only small effects on $Paco_2$ (Fig. 7–5). Because of this behavior, CO_2 is the gas used to quantify functional or alveolar ventilation (VA). Specifically, as long as there is measurable ventilation and perfusion to a lung unit, CO_2 transport occurs, and that alveolar–

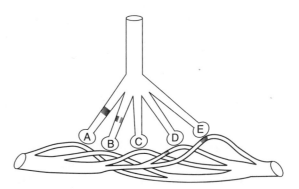

FIGURE 7-4

Conceptual depiction of ventilation-perfusion ($\dot{V}/\dot{Q}$) matching using a 5-unit lung model. Unit A is a $\dot{V}/\dot{Q}$ of 0 (a shunt), unit B is a low $\dot{V}/\dot{Q}$ unit (< 1), unit C is a normal $\dot{V}/\dot{Q}$ unit of 1, unit D is a high $\dot{V}/\dot{Q}$ unit (> 1), and unit E is a $\dot{V}/\dot{Q}$ of ∞ (dead space).

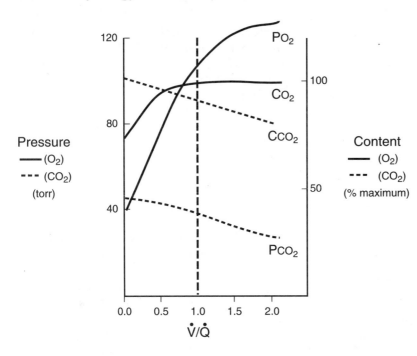

FIGURE 7–5

Effect of ventilation-perfusion ($\dot{V}/\dot{Q}$) ratios on arterial P_{O_2}, P_{CO_2}, O_2 content, and CO_2 content. Note that carbon dioxide pressure and content vary linearly with $\dot{V}/\dot{Q}$. High $\dot{V}/\dot{Q}$ units thus can "compensate" for low $\dot{V}/\dot{Q}$ units in overall CO_2 transport. In contrast, because hemoglobin is fully saturated with oxygen at $\dot{V}/\dot{Q}$ near 1, high $\dot{V}/\dot{Q}$ cannot "compensate" for low $\dot{V}/\dot{Q}$ in overall O_2 transport.

capillary unit can be considered functional. Extending this concept, physiologic dead space is defined as alveolar–capillary units in which no measurable CO_2 transport occurs. This is the basis for the Bohr equation that separates alveolar (functional) ventilation from wasted or dead-space ventilation (i.e., ventilation going to units with $\dot{V}/\dot{Q} = \infty$):[1]

$$\frac{VD}{VT} = \frac{Pa_{CO_2} - P_{E}{CO_2}}{Pa_{CO_2}} \quad (5)$$

where VD/VT is the dead space/tidal volume ratio and P_{ECO_2} is mixed expired P_{CO_2}. When the tidal volume and respiratory frequency (f) are known, alveolar ventilation can be expressed as the proportion of total delivered ventilation (VE) that is not "wasted" in dead-space ventilation:

$$VA = VE - f \times VD \quad (6)$$

In contrast to CO_2 behavior, oxygen is more sensitive to $\dot{V}/\dot{Q}$ abnormalities. The most important reason for this is the fact that hemoglobin, the major transport vehicle for O_2, is nearly fully saturated at $\dot{V}/\dot{Q}$ values near 1. P_{O_2} and oxygen content thus are not related linearly. This means that, unlike CO_2, high $\dot{V}/\dot{Q}$ units cannot compensate for low $\dot{V}/\dot{Q}$ units (Fig. 7–5) and a wid-

ened A–aDO_2 develops in disease states.[4, 6, 7] For this same reason, increasing the inspired oxygen concentration (FiO_2) has progressively less effect on Pa_{O_2} as $\dot{V}/\dot{Q}$ worsens (Fig. 7–6).[3] The physiology of oxygen supplementation also is discussed in further detail in Chapter 8.

As already noted, oxygen transport abnormalities can be quantified by the A–aDO_2 gradient. A simpler (although less precise) reflection of this same phenomenon is the Pa_{O_2}/FiO_2 ratio (P/F ratio). This ratio has been used by a number of consensus groups to define and quantify lung injury.[8] Specifically, acute lung injury can be defined by a P/F ratio of less than 300, whereas acute respiratory distress syndrome (ARDS) requires a P/F less than 200. Another technique to quantify alveolar–capillary oxygen transport abnormalities is to calculate an effective shunt. A relatively simple way to do this requires breathing 100% O_2. As long as arterial blood has near 100% hemoglobin saturation, the resultant Pa_{O_2} can be used in the simplified shunt equation:[1]

$$\frac{Q_S}{Q_T} = \frac{(A - aDO_2 \text{ gradient})(0.0031)}{A - aDO_2 \text{ gradient}) + (0.0031)} \quad (7)$$

where Q_S/Q_T is the fraction of total pulmonary blood flow that is "shunted" through $\dot{V}/\dot{Q}$ units near zero.

POSITIVE PRESSURE VENTILATION EFFECTS ON VENTILATION–PERFUSION MATCHING

Positive pressure ventilation can affect $\dot{V}/\dot{Q}$ relationships in a number of ways. Following are discussions on positive end-expiratory pressure (PEEP), the inspiratory–expiratory flow relationships, and the perfusion effects of intrathoracic pressure.

Positive End-Expiratory Pressure

Definition

Positive end-expiratory pressure is defined as an elevation of transpulmonary pressures at the end of expiration. PEEP is generally produced in one of two ways: applied or intrinsic.[9] Applied PEEP is produced in the ventilator circuitry generally through expiratory valves. Intrinsic PEEP is produced either when expiratory time is inadequate to return the lung to its "rest point" (functional residual capacity [FRC]) or when airway obstruction prevents alveoli from fully emptying.[9, 10] Expiratory muscle contraction can also raise intrathoracic pressures at end expiration, but this should not be considered PEEP because it is not a transpulmonary pressure (i.e., alveolar–pleural pressure).

Rationale

In infiltrative lung diseases, alveolar inflammation and edema coupled with dys-

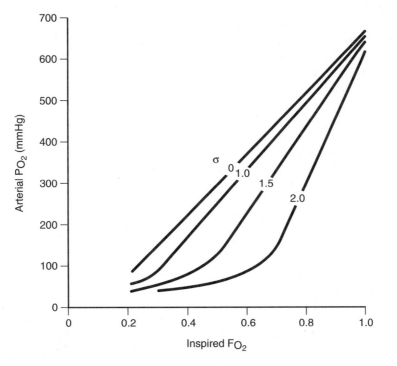

FIGURE 7–6

Graph showing the effects of changing inspired O_2 concentration (F_{O_2}) on arterial P_{O_2} in the presence of varying amounts of ventilation-perfusion inequality. When ventilation and perfusion are evenly matched (σ near 0), the relationship between inspired F_{O_2}, from 21 to 100%, is linear. As ventilation-perfusion inequalities worsen (σ = 1.0–2.0), the effect of breathing a given F_{O_2} is progressively less. Note that when the ventilation-perfusion abnormality is severe (σ = 2.0), breathing gas with an F_{O_2} as high as 0.7 has little effect on arterial P_{O_2}. (Reprinted with permission from West JB, Wagner PD: Pulmonary gas exchange. In: West JB, Wagner PD (eds): Bioengineering Aspects of the Lung. New York: Marcel Dekker, 1977, pp 361–457.)

functional surfactant produce poorly ventilated regions as well as regions that
actually collapse during all or part (i.e., end-
expiratory phase) of the ventilatory cycle.
Functionally, these units behave as low $\dot{V}/\dot{Q}$
units or shunts.[9, 11, 12] The rationale behind
applying expiratory pressure is that if such
units can be opened with a tidal breath (i.e.,
recruited), the PEEP will prevent subsequent re-collapse. In this sense, PEEP functions as a strategy to prevent de-recruitment (Fig. 7–7).

Recruited alveoli provide several benefits
to patient management.[9] First, recruited alveoli improve $\dot{V}/\dot{Q}$ matching and gas
exchange.[11, 12] Second, as discussed in more
detail in Chapter 11, patent alveoli throughout the ventilatory cycle appear to have less
risk of injury from the shear stress of repeated opening and closing.[13] Third, PEEP
prevents unstable surfactant monolayers in
alveoli that repeatedly open and shut and
thus improves lung compliance.[14]

PEEP can also be detrimental. Because
the tidal breath is delivered on top of the
baseline PEEP, end-inspiratory pressures
are raised by PEEP application. This must
be considered if the lung is at risk for
overstretch injury (Chapter 11). Moreover,
because alveolar injury is often quite heterogeneous, appropriate PEEP in one region
may be suboptimal in another and excessive
in yet another[15] (Fig. 7–8). Thus, optimizing
PEEP is a balance between recruiting the
recruitable alveoli in diseased regions without overdistending already recruited alveoli
in healthier regions.[16] Another potential
detrimental effect of PEEP is that it also
raises mean intrathoracic pressure. This
can compromise cardiac filling in susceptible patients (see Chapter 10).[17]

Strategies to Apply Positive End-Expiratory Pressure

There are a number of potential approaches
to optimizing PEEP that focus either on gas
exchange goals or mechanical goals.[9, 12, 18, 19]

Gas exchange goals are the traditional approach to setting PEEP.[9, 18] When using gas
exchange goals, the idea is to use FiO_2 requirements, PaO_2, or the calculated shunt
fraction as the target. An FiO_2–PaO_2 strategy, for instance, would be to apply whatever PEEP is necessary to attain a minimally acceptable PaO_2 at the lowest possible
FiO_2. A PEEP–FiO_2 nomogram (see Fig.
18–4, for example) could be used under
these circumstances.[20] A more aggressive
gas exchange goal would be to normalize
(or at least minimize) shunt fraction.[9] This
approach often requires very high levels of
PEEP (i.e., in excess of normal maximal
transpulmonary pressure). This approach
has lost popularity, however, because it has
become apparent that overdistending
healthier lung regions is probably an unacceptable trade-off for aggressive shunt
reduction.[8, 13] Moreover, some of the apparent shunt reduction that occurs with high

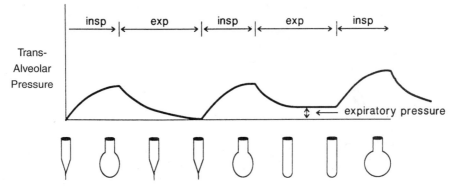

FIGURE 7–7
Conceptual action of positive end-expiratory pressure (PEEP) to prevent de-recruitment and
maintain alveolar patency throughout the ventilatory cycle. (Reprinted with permission from
MacIntyre NR: Oxygenation support. In: Dantzker D, MacIntyre NR, Bakow E (eds):
Comprehensive Respiratory Care. Philadelphia: WB Saunders, 1995.)

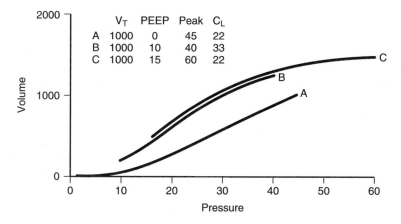

FIGURE 7–8

Mechanical changes in collapsed alveoli when ventilated with increasing levels of positive end-expiratory pressure (PEEP). Curve A represents alveoli that remain collapsed until 5–10 cm H_2O pressure is applied (opening pressure). Subsequent delivery of a 1000-ml tidal volume (V_T) produces a peak pressure of 45 cm H_2O and a calculated compliance (C_L) of 22 ml/cm H_2O PEEP improves C_L (curve B). Levels of PEEP above this opening pressure, however, serve only to overdistend the alveoli, thereby worsening C_L (curve C). (Reprinted with permission from MacIntyre NR: Oxygenation support. In Dantzker D, MacIntyre NR, Bakow E (eds): Comprehensive Respiratory Care. Philadelphia: WB Saunders, 1995.)

PEEP levels may be a consequence of reduced cardiac output from the high intrathoracic pressures[21] (see Chapter 10).

Mechanical goals for PEEP applications have the appeal of setting ventilator pressures in accordance with respiratory system mechanical behavior. This approach actually dates back several decades when "best compliance" was proposed as a reasonable way to set proper PEEP (note that curve B in Fig. 7–8 has the highest compliance).[12] Currently, the goal is similar but more specifically focused on inflection points in the static pressure volume curve[19] (see Chapter 6). The concept behind this is to use the lower inflection point as the marker for an optimal pressure that prevents de-recruitment. Because this measurement generally is taken on the inflation limit of the curve, it may overestimate this pressure requirement as measured on the deflation limit. A corollary to this is that it may be beneficial to first perform a "volume recruitment" maneuver (i.e., A 1 minute period of 25 to 40 cm H_2O PEEP) before returning to the desired PEEP level. This combined approach of volume recruitment followed by PEEP settings above the lower inflection point has been tied to an "open lung" ventilatory strategy that in preliminary work seems to improve outcome over traditional gas exchange–based conventional strategies.[19]

Because static pressure volume curves are time consuming and often require heavy sedation and/or paralysis, simpler ways of determining the de-recruitment pressure requirement are being investigated. Potential approaches include a very slow (e.g., 10 L/min) constant flow breath and record a single dynamic pressure–volume (PV) curve (see Chapter 6). Because flow is so slow, flow-resistive pressure is minimized and the curve approximates a static curve. Corrections for endotracheal tube–resistive pressure can be subtracted mathematically, or pressures can be recorded from the distal end of the endotracheal tube. Studies on mechanically targeted PEEP suggest that the operational PEEP in infiltrative lung disease is 8 to 25 cm H_2O with average first-day requirements in the 10- to 20-cm H_2O range.[19]

Inspiratory Flow Pattern and Inspiratory–Expiratory Time Relationship Effects on Ventilation–Perfusion

Inspiration from a positive pressure breath consists of a flow magnitude, a flow profile, and, if desired, a pause (inspiratory hold). Each of these can affect $\dot{V}/\dot{Q}$ matching to a certain extent. In general, rapid initial flows (a consequence of set decelerating flow profiles or pressure-targeted breaths) pressurize the lung most rapidly and thus produce the highest *mean* inspiratory alveolar pressure for a given end-inflation pressure. Although theoretically this may affect $\dot{V}/\dot{Q}$, studies showing improved gas exchange with this rapid filling strategy are few.[22]

Prolonging inspiratory time, generally by adding a pause and often used in conjunction with a rapid decelerating flow (i.e., pressure targeted) breath, also increase

mean inflation pressure and lengthen gas-mixing time in the lung. Moreover, if the resultant expiratory time is inadequate for the lung to return to its relaxed volume (i.e., FRC), intrinsic PEEP (air trapping) develops. These effects are depicted in Figures 7–9 and 7–10.

There are several physiologic effects of prolonging inspiratory time. First, the aforementioned increased gas-mixing time may improve $\dot{V}/\dot{Q}$ matching in infiltrative lung disease.[23] Second, intrinsic PEEP has similar effects to applied PEEP and, indeed, much of the improvement in gas exchange associated with long inspiratory time strate-

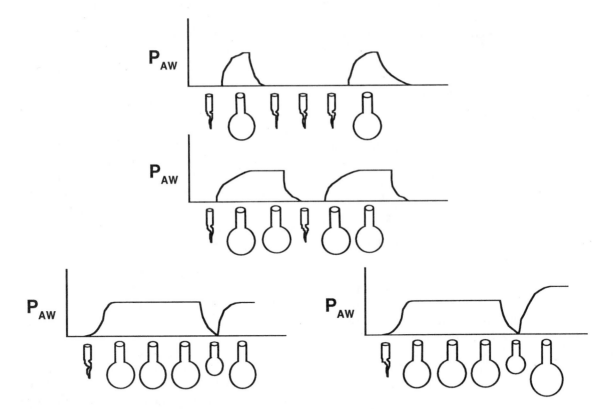

FIGURE 7–9

Airway pressure effects of longer inspiratory times. Plotted are airway pressure (P_{AW}) tracings over time with corresponding depictions of alveolar volume. In the top panel, the inspiratory and expiratory ratios are such that alveoli are at baseline volume for three fourths of the time. In the middle panel, inspiratory time has been extended so that alveoli are at inspiratory volume for a longer fraction of time, yet expiratory time is adequate for return to baseline volume. Under these circumstances, mean alveolar pressure is increased, but peak and baseline alveolar pressures are not affected. In the bottom panels, inspiratory time has been extended to the point that expiratory time is inadequate for a return to baseline volume. Under these circumstances, mean alveolar pressure has increased further. However, baseline alveolar pressure also has increased (i.e., "intrinsic" PEEP), which either reduces tidal volume (pressure-targeted breath in left panel) or increases end inspiratory alveolar pressures (volume-targeted breath in right panel).

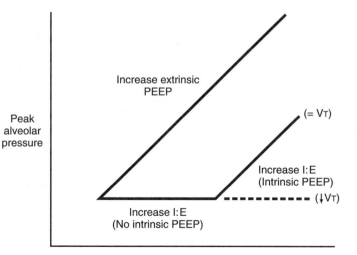

FIGURE 7–10

Relationship of peak alveolar pressure to mean alveolar pressure using various strategies to increase mean alveolar pressure. With increases in extrinsic or applied positive end-expiratory pressure (PEEP), the relationship is linear. With increases in inspiratory time that do not produce air trapping (intrinsic PEEP), mean airway pressure is increased without increases in peak alveolar pressure. However, when air trapping and intrinsic PEEP develop, either a higher peak alveolar pressure is needed for a constant V_T *(solid line)* or V_T diminishes for a constant peak alveolar pressure *(dotted line)*. (Reprinted with permission from MacIntyre NR: Oxygenation support. In Dantzker D, MacIntyre NR, Bakow E (eds): Comprehensive Respiratory Care. Philadelphia: WB Saunders, 1995.)

gies may be merely a PEEP phenomenon[24] (Fig. 7–11). Third, because these long inspiratory times significantly increase total intrathoracic pressures, cardiac filling and cardiac output also may be reduced. Finally, **inspiratory:expiratory ratios** that exceed 1:1 (so-called inverse ratio ventilation [IRV]) are uncomfortable, and patient sedation/paralysis often is required.[23, 24]

Intrathoracic Pressures and Perfusion

In addition to affecting ventilation and ventilation distribution, intrathoracic pressure applications from positive pressure ventilation can also affect both total perfusion and perfusion distribution. In general, as mean intrathoracic pressure is increased, cardiac filling is decreased and cardiac output/pulmonary perfusion decreases.[17] Reduced perfusion can make $\dot{V}/\dot{Q}$ matching appear better even though total oxygen delivery may fall (i.e., reduced blood flow may reduce

shunt flow).[21] These concepts are discussed in more detail in Chapter 10.

Intrathoracic pressures also can influence distribution of perfusion. The relationship of alveolar pressures to perfusion pressures in a four-zone lung model help explain this[25] (Fig. 7–12). Specifically, the supine human lung is generally in a West zone 3 (distension) state. As intrathoracic pressures increase, however, zone 2 and zone 1 regions can appear, creating high $\dot{V}/\dot{Q}$ units. Indeed, increases in dead space (i.e., zone 1 lung) can be a consequence of ventilatory strategies employing high ventilatory pressures. Thus, although high ventilatory pressure strategies such as IRV may *decrease* dead space by better gas mixing, they also can *increase* dead space by creating zone 1, high $\dot{V}/\dot{Q}$ units.

ALVEOLAR–CAPILLARY GAS TRANSPORT IN THE CONTEXT OF OVERALL OXYGEN DELIVERY

Thus far, the discussion has focused on the alveolar–capillary gas transport—the "mid-

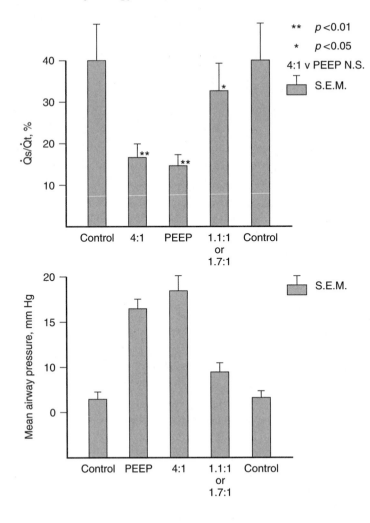

FIGURE 7–11

Comparison of shunt reduction *(upper panels)* and mean airway pressures *(lower panels)* in patients receiving four ventilatory strategies. "Control" ventilation had no intrinsic PEEP. "PEEP" ventilation was control plus applied PEEP. "4:1" was control plus sufficient inspiratory time to create a 4:1 I:E ratio and intrinsic PEEP. Note the similar reduction in shunt and elevation in mean airway pressure using either applied or intrinsic PEEP. Note also that the fourth strategy ("1.1:1"), a strategy that lengthened inspiratory time but did not produce intrinsic PEEP, also improved shunt and raised mean pressures but to a much lesser extent than either PEEP strategy. (Reprinted with permission from Cole AGH, Weller SF, Sykes MD: Inverse ratio ventilation compared with PEEP in adult respiratory failure. Intensive Care Med 10:227–232, 1984.)

dle link" in the respiration chain of Figure 7-1. This discussion would be incomplete, however, without a brief discussion of oxygen transport from the alveolar capillaries to the ultimate utilization site for oxygen, the tissues.[26]

Tissue delivery is the product of content times blood flow. **Oxygen delivery** (Do_2) is thus the product of arterial hemoglobin saturation (Sao_2) times hemoglobin concentration (Hb) times Hb–O_2 affinity (1.34 ml O_2/dl Hb) times cardiac output (CO). Thus:

$$Do_2 = Sao_2 \times Hb \times 1.34 \times CO \quad (8)$$

Normal values generally are referenced to body surface area and are 300 to 400 ml/min/m². Do_2 can be increased several-fold through increases in cardiac output or oxygen content. However, cardiac output manipulations have the greatest effect on O_2

delivery. Indeed, this is the reason that aggressively pushing the Pao_2 above 60 torr (a level that avoids pulmonary vasoconstriction and tissue hypoxia) usually offers little clinical Do_2 benefit.

Oxygen delivery often is assessed in reference to oxygen consumption. Generally, oxygen consumption is 25% of oxygen delivery. This is the so-called extraction ratio that also can be expressed as the arterial–venous oxygen difference (A–Vo_2). The normal A–Vo_2 is 5 ml/dl of blood. Normal tissues can increase the extraction ratio to 50% when oxygen demands are high or oxygen delivery is low. In conditions such as the systemic inflammatory response syndrome (SIRS), however, this capability to increase extraction is lost.[27] Thus, tissue hypoxia may exist even in the setting of high oxygen delivery. This is the reason that the A–Vo_2 difference, although useful in managing patients with

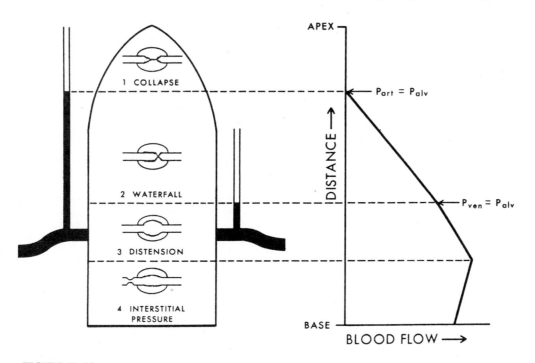

FIGURE 7–12

Schematic representation of the four zones of the lung in which different hemodynamic conditions govern blood flow. Alveolar pressure (P_{alv}) is assumed to be 0; the heights of the black columns on the left and right of the lung represent the magnitude of pulmonary arterial (P_{art}) and pulmonary venous (P_{ven}) pressures, respectively. (Reprinted with permission of Elsevier Science from Hughes JM, West J, Wagner P, et al: Effect of lung volume on the distribution of pulmonary blood flow in man. Respir Physiol 4:58–72, 1968.)

primary cardiovascular compromise, becomes potentially misleading in SIRS. For example, a narrow A–VO_2 difference (i.e., < 5 ml O_2/dl) in a patient with cardiogenic shock suggests good function, whereas this same A–VO_2 difference in a septic patient may reflect poor extraction capabilities from the systemic disease.

Cardiorespiratory support strategies using DO_2 can be useful. This may depend, however, on the patient population being treated. Specifically, strategies aimed at "supranormal" DO_2 have shown benefit in young surgical or trauma patients.[28] In contrast, medical patients may have untoward complication from excessive cardiac stimulation and thus may be managed better using a more normal DO_2 target.[29]

Finally, in disease states with severe reduction in DO_2, a concomitant reduction in VO_2 has been reported ("supply dependency").[30] Whether this represents a tissue metabolic response or a measurement arti-fact (mathematical "coupling" because DO_2 and VO_2 share several common measurements) is not clear. Thus, managing patients using DO_2/VO_2 relationships probably is not justified at the present time.

REFERENCES

1. Roughton FJW: Transport of oxygen and carbon dioxide. In: Fenn WO, Rahn H (eds): Handbook of Physiology, Section 3. Respiration. Vol I. Washington, DC: American Physiological Society, 1964, pp 767–825.
2. West JB: Ventilation-perfusion relationships. Am Rev Respir Dis 116:919–943, 1977.
3. West JB, Wagner PD: Pulmonary gas exchange. In: West JB, Wagner PD (eds): Bioengineering Aspects of the Lung. New York: Marcel Dekker, 1977, pp 361–457.
4. Mellemgaard K: The alveolar-arterial oxygen difference: its size and components in normal man. Acta Physiol Scand 67:10–20, 1966.
5. Wagner PD, Laravuso RB, Uhl RR, West JB: Continuous distributions of ventilation-perfusion ra-

tios in normal subjects breathing air and 100% O_2. J Clin Invest 54:54–68, 1974.

6. West JB: Ventilation-perfusion inequality and overall gas exchange in computer models of the lung. Respir Physiol 7:88–110, 1969.

7. Wagner PD: Ventilation-perfusion relationships. Annu Rev Physiol 42:235–247, 1980.

8. Slutsky AS: ACCP concensus conference: mechanical ventilation. Chest 104:1833–1859, 1993.

9. Kacmarek RM, Pierson DJ (eds): AARC conference on positive end expiratory pressure. Respir Care 33:419–527, 1988.

10. Pepe PE, Marini JJ: Occult positive end expiratory pressure in mechanically ventilated patients with airflow obstruction, the auto-PEEP effect. Am Rev Respir Dis 126:166–170, 1982.

11. Gattinoni L, Pelosi P, Crotti S, et al: Effects of positive end expiratory pressure on regional distribution of tidal volume and recruitment in adult respiratory distress syndrome. Am J Respir Crit Care Med 151:1807–1814, 1995.

12. Suter PM, Fairley HB, Isenberg MD: Optimum end-expiratory pressure in patients with acute pulmonary failure. N Engl J Med 292:284–289, 1975.

13. Webb HH, Tierney DF: Experimental pulmonary edema due to intermittent positive pressure ventilation with high inflation pressures: protection by positive end-expiratory pressure. Am Rev Respir Dis 110:556–565, 1974.

14. Wyszogodski I, Kyei-Aboagye K, Taeusch HW Jr, Avery ME: Surfactant inactivation by hyperventilation: conservation by end-expiratory pressure. J Appl Physiol 38:461–466, 1975.

15. Gattinoni L, Presenti A, Torresin A, et al: Adult respiratory distress syndrome profiles by computed tomography. J Thorac Imaging 3:25–30, 1988.

16. Gattinoni L, Presenti A, Baglioni S, et al: Inflammatory pulmonary edema and PEEP: correlation between imaging and physiologic studies. J Thorac Imaging 3:59–64, 1988.

17. Pinsky MR, Guimond JG: The effects of positive end-expiratory pressure on heart-lung interactions. J Crit Care 6:1–15, 1991.

18. MacIntyre NR: Oxygenation support. In: Dantzker D, MacIntyre N, Bakow E (ed): Comprehensive Respiratory Care. Philadelphia: WB Saunders, 1995.

19. Amto MS, Barbas CSV, Medeivos DM, et al: Effect of a protective-ventilation strategy on morality in the acute respiratory distress syndrome. N Engl J Med 338:347–354, 1998.

20. NIH ARDS Network: Respiratory Management Protocol. Baltimore: 1996.

21. Lynch JP, Mhyre JG, Dantzker DR: Influence of cardiac output on intrapulmonary shunt. J Appl Physiol 46:315–321, 1979.

22. Abraham E, Yoshihara G: Cardiorespiratory effects of pressure controlled ventilation in severe respiratory failure. Chest 98:1445–1449, 1990.

23. Armstrong BW, MacIntyre NR: Pressure controlled inverse ratio ventilation that avoids air trapping in ARDS. Crit Care Med 23:279–285, 1995.

24. Cole AGH, Weller SF, Sykes MD: Inverse ratio ventilation compared with PEEP in adult respiratory failure. Intensive Care Med 10:227–232, 1984.

25. Hughes JM, West J, Wagner P, et al: Effect of lung volume on the distribution of pulmonary blood flow in man. Respir Physiol 4:58–72, 1968.

26. Vincent JL: The relationship between oxygen demand, oxygen uptake and oxygen supply. Intensive Care Med 16:s145–s148, 1990.

27. Astiz ME, Rackow EC, Falk JL, et al: Oxygen delivery and consumption in patients with hyperdynamic septic shock. Crit Care Med 15:26–28, 1987.

28. Shoemaker WC, Appel PL, Kram HB, et al: Prospective trial of supranormal values of survivors as therapeutic goals in high risk surgical patients. Chest 94:1176–1186, 1988.

29. Hayes MA, Timmins AC, Yau EHS, et al: Elevation of systemic oxygen delivery in the treatment of critically ill patients. N Engl J Med 330:1717–1722, 1994.

30. Danek SJ, Lynch JP, Weg JG, et al: The dependence of oxygen uptake on oxygen delivery in the adult respiratory distress syndrome. Am Rev Respir Dis 122:387–395, 1980.

CHAPTER 8

Supplemental Oxygen

Yuh-Chin T. Huang, MD

THE OXYGEN PATHWAY
Oxygen Uptake
Oxygen Transport
Oxygen Consumption
RATIONALE FOR OXYGEN THERAPY
Physiologic Mechanisms of Hypoxemia
Causes of Tissue Hypoxia
TECHNIQUES FOR OXYGEN ADMINISTRATION
Delivery of Supplemental Oxygen
Monitoring During Oxygen Therapy

ADVERSE EFFECTS OF OXYGEN THERAPY
Blunting of Hypoxic Drive
Pulmonary Oxygen Toxicity
SPECIAL APPLICATIONS OF OXYGEN THERAPY
High Altitude
Carbon Monoxide Poisoning
Helium–Oxygen
Nitric Oxide Inhalation Therapy
REFERENCES

KEY WORDS

oxidant injury
oxygen
oxygen toxicity

shunting
ventilation–perfusion relationships

Oxygen (O_2) is the most essential chemical element for human life. It comprises 49.2% of the earth's crust by weight and 20.9% by volume in the atmosphere. The discovery of oxygen is usually credited to Joseph Priestley, who in 1774 extracted "air" that had a remarkably vigorous flame.[1] He termed this new gas "dephlogisticated air" because it required five times as much nitric oxide to saturate it as ordinary air. Before Priestley, however, a Swedish pharmacist, Carl Wilhelm Scheele, actually had discovered what he termed "fire air." He noted that "fire air" supported respiration as well as combustion. Lavoisier in 1777 recognized the chemical significance of oxygen and changed its name to "principe acidifiant" or "principe oxygine" in the mistaken belief that all acids contained oxygen. The word *oxygen* (oxys = acid, gene = to produce) became standard even before it had been proved that all acids do not contain oxygen.

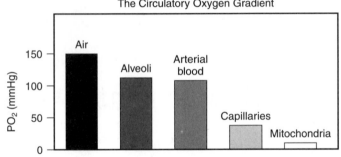

FIGURE 8–1

The O_2 gradient from the alveolar space to the mitochondria. Note that there is a stepwise decrement in PO_2 from 100 mm Hg in the alveolar space to values of a few mmHg at the mitochondria, where most of the O_2 is consumed. (Reprinted with permission from Piantadosi A, Huang YC: Respiratory functions of the lung. In: Baum GL, Crapo JD, Celli BR, Karlinsky JB (eds): Textbook of Pulmonary Diseases, 6th ed. Philadelphia, Lippincott-Raven, 1998.)

Priestley first wrote about the therapeutic use of oxygen in 1775: "From the greater strength and vivacity of the flame of a candle, in this pure air (oxygen) it might be conjectured, that it might be particularly salutary to the lungs in certain morbid cases, when common air would not be sufficient to carry off the phlogistic putrid effluvium quickly enough . . . perhaps, we may also infer from these experiments that . . . pure dephlogisticated air (oxygen) might be very useful as a medicine." The most enthusiastic early proponent of oxygen therapy was Beddoes, who produced the first textbook of oxygen therapy entitled *Considerations on the Medicinal Use and Production of Factitious Airs* in 1796. This enthusiasm, however, was tempered by its misuse and the toxic effects noted by Lavoisier in 1785, and, by the end of the 18th century, therapeutic use of oxygen was in decline. Since then, interest in oxygen therapy has waxed and waned, but research has continued to add to our understanding of how oxygen works in the human body. In this chapter, the physiologic basis of supplemental oxygen therapy and its complications are discussed. Oxygen therapy in several special conditions also is reviewed.

THE OXYGEN PATHWAY

The use of oxygen by the body occurs by a relatively simple physical pathway. This oxygen pathway begins in the atmosphere, where the partial pressure of oxygen (PO_2) is approximately 160 mm Hg, and ends at the mitochondria, where PO_2 is only a few millimeters of mercury (Fig. 8–1). Inspired PO_2 decreases as soon as the ambient gas reaches conducting airways because of its saturation with water vapor. Once the inspirate reaches the terminal respiratory units, gas exchange takes place. The blood in the pulmonary capillaries leaving the alveoli contains approximately the same PO_2 as the gas phase of the terminal units. The PO_2 in arterial blood is slightly lower because local matching of ventilation and perfusion in normal lungs is imperfect and unoxygenated blood is added to pulmonary capillary blood from postpulmonary shunt. Oxygen then is delivered to the systemic capillaries and diffuses into the cells to support aerobic metabolism. The bulk of molecular oxygen is consumed in the mitochondria (about 90%).

Oxygen Uptake

Oxygen is taken up via respiration by the lung's approximately 300 million alveoli, each of which is about 300 μm in diameter. The huge surface area (approximately 75 m²) and the thinness of the septa (< 0.5 μm thick) of the alveoli provide an extremely efficient mechanism for the human body to take up oxygen from the ambient air. With each inspiration, approximately 500 ml of air enters the lungs (tidal volume). If anatomic dead space is 150 ml and the respiratory rate is 12 breaths per minute, then alveolar ventilation would be (500 ml–150 ml) times 12, or 4.2 L per minute.

Oxygen in the alveolar space continuously diffuses into the pulmonary capillaries, where it binds the hemoglobin in the erythrocytes and enters the systemic circulation. Each erythrocyte traverses the pulmonary microcirculation in approximately three quarters of a second. Within the first third of this brief transit time, the hemoglobin becomes virtually completely oxygenated. At the same time, carbon dioxide (CO_2), formed constantly in the body tissues, is removed continuously from the pulmonary capillaries by ventilation. Slightly more O_2 is removed from the alveolar space than CO_2 is added (normal respiratory exchange ratio = 0.8). The efficiency of O_2–CO_2 exchange is determined primarily by the **ventilation–perfusion** ($\dot{V}A/\dot{Q}$) **relationship** of the lung units. Low $\dot{V}A/\dot{Q}$ units and right-to-left shunt ($\dot{V}A/\dot{Q}$ = 0) are associated with impaired oxygen uptake from the alveolar space, whereas high $\dot{V}A/\dot{Q}$ units and dead space ($\dot{V}A/\dot{Q}$ = infinity) result in inefficient elimination of CO_2 from the pulmonary arterial blood.

Oxygen Transport

Once oxygen diffuses into the blood, it binds rapidly to hemoglobin. The affinity of hemoglobin for oxygen increases with increasing oxygen saturation, and the hemoglobin–oxygen equilibrium curve has a sigmoid shape (Fig. 8–2). The amount of oxygen transported in the blood to the peripheral tissues (oxygen delivery [$\dot{D}O_2$]) is determined primarily by hemoglobin concentration, its oxygen saturation, and cardiac output (CO):

$$\dot{D}O_2 = 1.39 \times CO \times [Hb] \times \%sat + 0.003 \times PaO_2$$

The amount of oxygen carried by hemoglobin is 1.39 ml/g. Given the normal concentration of hemoglobin of 15 g/100 ml and 100% saturation with oxygen (PO_2 of 100 mm Hg), 100 ml blood can transport approx-

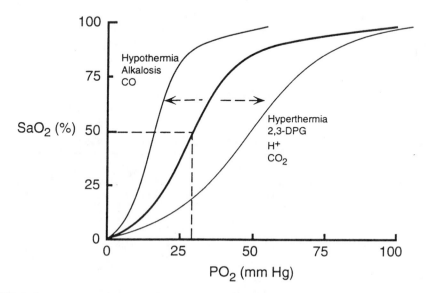

FIGURE 8–2

OEC of hemoglobin. The normal P_{50} value is indicated by the *dashed lines*. The changes in position of the OEC associated with various effector molecules are indicated by the *dashed arrows*. (Reprinted with permission from Piantadosi A, Huang YC: Respiratory functions of the lung. In: Baum GL, Crapo JD, Celli BR, Karlinsky JB (eds): Textbook of Pulmonary Disease, 6th ed. Philadelphia, Lippincott-Raven, 1998.)

imately 20 ml of oxygen in combination with hemoglobin (oxygen content). This is in contrast to the very low amount of oxygen physically dissolved in the plasma (0.003 × 100 or 0.3 ml per 100 ml). Thus, without hemoglobin, one would need a cardiac output of at least 80 L/min to support the normal resting oxygen consumption of 250 ml/min. The sigmoid shape of the hemoglobin-oxygen dissociation curve also suggests that when hemoglobin saturation is more than 90% (i.e., at the plateau of the curve), additional oxygen does not enhance oxygen delivery significantly because the percent saturation of hemoglobin cannot exceed 100%. It simply increases the amount of oxygen dissolved in the plasma.

A number of conditions can displace the oxygen–hemoglobin equilibrium curve to the right or the left of its normal position ($P50$, or PaO_2 at 50% saturation, of 27 mm Hg) (Fig. 8–2). Increased 2,3-diglycerophosphate (2,3-DPG), acidosis, and hyperthermia shift the curve to the right and facilitate the unloading of oxygen in the peripheral tissues. In contrast, decreased 2,3-DPG, alkalosis, and hypothermia shift the curve to the left and help maintain oxygen saturation in the arterial blood.

Oxygen Consumption

The mitochondria consume approximately 90% of the oxygen used by the cell. Other subcellular organelles (lysosomes, nucleus, cell membrane) use the other 10%. In the mitochondria, molecular oxygen receives electrons from the respiratory chain and is reduced to water. This reduction of oxygen is the primary function of cytochrome c oxidase, the last enzyme in the electron transport chain. High-energy phosphate compounds—for example, adenosine triphosphate (ATP)—are generated by electron transport in the process of oxidative phosphorylation. ATP provides most of the energy for biologic function.

At the tissue level, the relationship between the transport and the consumption of oxygen was described first by Fick in 1870. According to the Fick principle, oxygen consumption ($\dot{V}O_2$) of the tissues can be calculated as follows:

$$\dot{V}O_2 = CO \times (CaO_2 - CvO_2)$$

where CO is cardiac output, CaO_2 is arterial oxygen content, and CvO_2 is venous oxygen content. Increased extraction of oxygen from the blood leads to a lower CvO_2 and frequently a lower PvO_2 (normal PvO_2 is 35–40 mm Hg, with an oxygen saturation of approximately 75%). Resting blood and oxygen supply of various organs is shown in Table 8–1. As can be seen, brain tissue and cardiac muscle extract much more oxygen from the blood than do other organs. These two organs are most susceptible to ischemia and hypoxia.

TABLE 8–1. Oxygen Supply and Consumption of Various Organs

ORGAN	BLOOD FLOW (ml/min) (% CARDIAC OUTPUT)	BLOOD FLOW (ml/100 g)	A–V DIFFERENCE (VOLUME %)
Heart	210 (4)	70	11.4
Brain	760 (15)	50	6.3
Kidney	1220 (24)	400	1.3
Liver	510 (10)	29	4.1
Gastrointestinal tract	715 (14)	35	4.1
Skeletal muscle	760 (15)	2.5	6.4
Skin	215 (4)	9.5	1.0
Other organs (fat, etc.)	715 (14)	—	—
Total cardiac output	5100 ml		

A–V, arterial–venous.
Adapted from Jain KK, Fischer B: Oxygen in Physiology and Medicine. Springfield, IL: Charles C Thomas, 1989.

RATIONALE FOR OXYGEN THERAPY

Supplemental oxygen usually is given to correct alveolar hypoxia and arterial hypoxemia. The human body has only a negligible reserve of oxygen, which amounts to approximately 1.5 L. This would last for only 6 minutes in case of circulatory arrest (assuming a body oxygen consumption is 250 ml/min). Hemoglobin contains about half of the oxygen reserve (800 ml), whereas alveoli account for about half of the remainder. In a gas volume of 3.5 L in the alveoli, there is approximately 400 ml of oxygen. During a breath-hold, this would last for about 1½ minutes. If 100% oxygen has been breathed before the breath-hold, this can be extended to 10½ minutes. Other smaller reserves of oxygen are those bound to myoglobulin (250 ml) and those dissolved in tissues (50 ml).

There are few clinical controlled trials documenting the effectiveness of supplemental oxygen in acute hypoxia. The rationale for starting supplemental oxygen under acute hypoxic conditions is based on extensive clinical experience, which shows that untreated hypoxemia leads to tissue hypoxia and irreversible changes in vital organ function. As a general rule, supplemental oxygen is indicated when arterial PO_2 falls below 60 mm Hg or hemoglobin saturation is less than 90%. Exceptions occur in individuals adapted to high altitude who do not need oxygen even if arterial oxygen pressure (PaO_2) is less than 60 mm Hg. The decision for using supplemental oxygen can be facilitated greatly by understanding the physiologic mechanisms of hypoxemia and the mechanisms of tissue hypoxia of the underlying conditions.

Physiologic Mechanisms of Hypoxemia

In general, arterial hypoxemia is defined as PO_2 values less than 80 mm Hg in adult breathing room air at sea level. Hypoxemia usually indicates a defect in the gas exchange function of the lung, although a normal PO_2 does not exclude the presence of lung diseases. A more sensitive index to detect the presence of lung diseases is the alveolar–arterial O_2 gradient ($A–aDO_2$). $A–aDO_2$ can be calculated from the alveolar gas equation:

$$PAO_2 = (PB - PH_2O) \times FiO_2 - PACO_2/R$$
$$A–aDO_2 = PAO_2 - PaO_2$$

where PAO_2 is alveolar PO_2; PB is barometric pressure (760 mm Hg at sea level); PH_2O is water vapor pressure (47 mm Hg at 37°C); FiO_2 is oxygen fraction in the breathing air (21% in room air); $PACO_2$ is alveolar PCO_2 (frequently replaced by $PaCO_2$); and R is the respiratory exchange ratio (0.8). Normal $A–aDO_2$ is age dependent and is equal to the smaller of either 0.5 × age or 25.[2]

There are five physiologic mechanisms of hypoxemia. They are hypoventilation, ventilation–perfusion mismatch, right-to-left shunt, diffusion impairment, and decreased mixed venous oxygen content.

Hypoventilation

Hypoventilation decreases the arterial PO_2 and increases the arterial PCO_2. If $\dot{V}A/\dot{Q}$ distribution remains uniform, no alveolar–arterial difference develops for either O_2 or CO_2. The common causes of hypoventilation-associated hypoxemia are depression of the central nervous system from anesthesia or narcotics and neuromuscular diseases that affect respiratory muscle function. Although hypoxemia caused by hypoventilation can be corrected by supplemental oxygen, the primary treatment should be directed to supporting alveolar ventilation.

Ventilation–Perfusion Mismatch

Ventilation–perfusion mismatch (low $\dot{V}A/\dot{Q}$ regions) is the most common cause of hypoxemia in lung disease. Figure 8–3 illustrates the effects of $\dot{V}A/\dot{Q}$ mismatch on hypoxemia using a two-compartment lung model. In this example, the total ventilation is 4 L/min but unit A receives four times as much the ventilation as unit B (3.2 L/min vs. 0.8 L/min). If the distribution of perfusion is uniform (2.5 L/min for each unit), the $\dot{V}A/\dot{Q}$ ratio for unit A becomes 1.3 and that for unit B is 0.3. Oxygen tension and

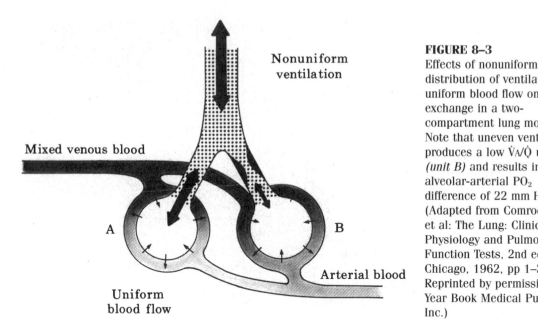

FIGURE 8–3
Effects of nonuniform distribution of ventilation with uniform blood flow on gas exchange in a two-compartment lung model. Note that uneven ventilation produces a low $\dot{V}_A/\dot{Q}$ unit *(unit B)* and results in an alveolar-arterial PO_2 difference of 22 mm Hg. (Adapted from Comroe JH Jr et al: The Lung: Clinical Physiology and Pulmonary Function Tests, 2nd ed. Chicago, 1962, pp 1–390. Reprinted by permission from Year Book Medical Publishers, Inc.)

saturation must decrease in blood, leaving unit B with low $\dot{V}_A/\dot{Q}$; oxygen saturation must rise in blood, leaving unit A with high $\dot{V}_A/\dot{Q}$. Because of the sigmoid shape of the hemoglobin dissociation curve, high PO_2 in the blood leaving high $\dot{V}_A/\dot{Q}$ in unit A is not sufficient to compensate for the low PO_2 contributed by low $\dot{V}_A/\dot{Q}$ in unit B. The final PO_2 in the pulmonary venous blood, which is derived from blood flow-weighted average of oxygen content, decreases. The arterial blood then would have a PO_2 of 84 mm Hg instead of 100 mm Hg, as in the ideal lung. Hypoxemia caused by $\dot{V}_A/\dot{Q}$ mismatch usually responds to supplemental oxygen well because a higher alveolar PO_2 increases PO_2 in the blood, leaving low $\dot{V}_A/\dot{Q}$ units.

Right-to-Left Shunt

A shunt is defined as a region where there is blood flow from the right heart to the left heart but no ventilation ($\dot{V}_A/\dot{Q} = 0$). The effects of a right-to-left shunt on gas exchange are shown schematically in Figure 8–4. In this example, 33% of the total blood flow (2.0 L/min) is shunt. Although gas exchange in units A and B is unimpaired, the net result from mixing of blood from these two units and the shunt pathway is a reduction of arterial PO_2 and the creation of the alveolar–arterial O_2 gradient. This effect on

PO_2 is similar to that caused by $\dot{V}_A/\dot{Q}$ mismatch. Because of the absence of ventilation in the shunt pathway, however, hypoxemia resulting from right-to-left shunt cannot be corrected by breathing 100% O_2. Thus, breathing 100% O_2 allows $\dot{V}_A/\dot{Q}$ mismatch to be differentiated from shunt as the cause of hypoxemia.

When a healthy person breathes 100% O_2, an alveolar–arterial PO_2 difference of approximately 50 mm Hg usually can be detected. This results from the presence of a physiologic shunt of approximately 2% to 3% of the cardiac output. Most of the physiologic shunt in normal subjects occurs distal to the gas exchange units, that is, a "postpulmonary shunt." The main sources of the normal postpulmonary shunt are bronchial and mediastinal veins that empty into pulmonary veins and the thebesian vessels of the left ventricle, which empty directly into the left ventricular cavity. When **shunting** occurs in patients with lung disease, it usually is accounted for by the perfusion of nonventilated lung regions through relatively normal vascular channels (intrapulmonary shunt). Sometimes shunt flow may occur through intracardiac communications, for example, a patent foramen ovale, when the pressure in the right atrium is increased because of pulmonary hypertension with right ventricular failure (intracardiac shunt).

Diffusion Impairment

In normal subjects at rest, O_2 equilibrates quickly between the blood and gas phases in the alveolar region of the lung, and there is no diffusion limitation. This is true for healthy persons at sea level and at low altitude. During exercise at higher altitudes ($> 10,000$ ft), the alveolar–arterial PO_2 difference can increase in normal individuals because of diffusion dysequilibrium as a result of low ambient O_2 and shortened capillary transit time.[3] Exercise-induced diffusion abnormalities in patients with lung diseases more commonly result from a decrease in pulmonary blood volume in combination with an increase in the rate of blood flow, thus shortening the capillary transit time for the erythrocytes. Similar to $\dot{V}A/\dot{Q}$ mismatch, hypoxemia caused by diffusion impairment can be corrected by having the individual breathe 100% oxygen.

Decreased Mixed Venous Oxygen Content

The O_2 content of pulmonary artery (mixed venous) blood usually has little effect on arterial PO_2 in persons with healthy lungs. In the presence of a substantial amount of either $\dot{V}A/\dot{Q}$ mismatch or a large right-to-left shunt, or both, the oxygen content in the mixed venous blood has a considerable effect on arterial PO_2. For a given amount of $\dot{V}A/\dot{Q}$ mismatch, the lower the mixed venous oxygen content, the lower the arterial PO_2. This mechanism of hypoxemia is particularly important in critically ill patients with serious cardiopulmonary diseases. The response to supplemental oxygen clearly depends on the relative contribution of $\dot{V}A/\dot{Q}$ mismatch and right-to-left shunt to hypoxemia.

Causes of Tissue Hypoxia

A complex disturbance of cellular function can be produced by hypoxia, primarily as a result of inadequate production of high-energy phosphate compounds (e.g., ATP). When oxygen is insufficient, glucose can only be metabolized anaerobically to pyruvate and lactate. Organs that use large amounts of oxygen, such as the brain and the heart, are more susceptible to hypoxia (Table 8–2). When blood oxygen tension is reduced acutely, symptoms and signs of cerebral hypoxia (impaired judgment, motor incoordination, altered mental status) and cardiac hypoxia (myocardial ischemia, arrhythmias) tend to manifest themselves

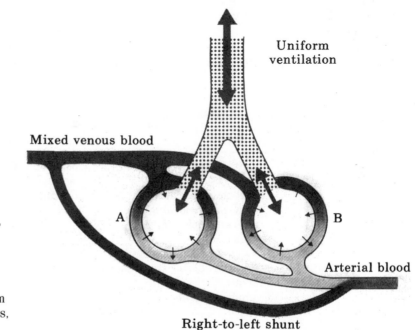

FIGURE 8–4
Effects of right-to-left shunt on gas exchange in a two-compartment lung model. (Adapted from Comroe JH Jr et al: The Lung: Clinical Physiology and Pulmonary Function Tests, 2nd ed. Chicago, 1962, pp 1–390. Reprinted by permission from Year Book Medical Publishers, Inc.).

TABLE 8–2. Arterial Oxygen Pressure (PO_2) and Oxygen (O_2) Content for Venous Blood of Different Organ Systems

ORGAN SYSTEM	PvO_2 (mm Hg)	% SATURATION	CvO_2	$(CaO_2–CvO_2)$ (ml/dl)
Brain	37	69	13.9	6.3
Heart	30	56	8.8	11.4
Intestine	45	80	16.1	4.1
Kidney	74	94	18.9	1.3
Skeletal muscle	32	60	12.2	8.0
Skin	75	95	19.2	1.0

CaO_2, arterial oxygen content; CvO_2, venous oxygen content; PvO_2, mixed venous oxygen tension.
Assuming PaO_2 = 100 mm Hg; hemoglobin = 15 g/dl; cardiac output = 6 L/min; and CaO_2 = 20.2 ml/dl.

first. When hypoxia becomes more severe and prolonged, the respiratory centers of the brainstem are affected, and death usually occurs as a result of respiratory failure. The goal of supplemental oxygen therapy thus is to prevent these detrimental consequences of tissue hypoxia.

Although tissue hypoxia may be associated with a variety of clinical conditions, there generally are four classic mechanisms that cause it (Table 8–3).

Hypoxic hypoxia results from an inadequate amount of oxygen in the blood (i.e., reduced PaO_2) caused by either lung disease or decreased oxygen in the inspired air (e.g., at high altitude). Supplemental oxygen may correct tissue hypoxia by raising the oxygen tension in the blood in most cases (except in right-to-left shunt).

Anemic hypoxia results from a reduction in the oxygen-carrying capacity of hemoglo-

bin, which may be caused by severe anemia, or the presence of dyshemoglobin states (carboxyhemoglobin, methemoglobin), which decreases the affinity of oxygen for the hemoglobin molecule. In anemia, PO_2 remains normal, but the absolute amount of oxygen transported per unit volume of blood is diminished. Because the hemoglobin is well saturated with oxygen, supplemental oxygen provides little benefit in augmenting oxygen delivery to the tissues unless the PO_2 in the arterial blood is raised to very high levels. Carbon monoxide poisoning not only decreases the oxygen-binding capacity of hemoglobin but also shifts the hemoglobin dissociation curve to the left, impairing the unloading of oxygen at the peripheral tissues. Oxygen is useful in carbon monoxide poisoning because it displaces carbon monoxide from hemoglobin and decreases the half-life of carboxyhemoglobin.

TABLE 8–3. Mechanisms of Tissue Hypoxia

CAUSES OF HYPOXIA	EXAMPLES	RESPONSE TO OXYGEN
Hypoxic	Lung diseases, high altitude	Good in most cases (except in right-to-left shunt)
Anemic	Severe anemia, carbon monoxide poisoning, methemoglobinemia	Generally useful depending on the arterial PO_2
Stagnant	Cardiac failure, hypovolemia, peripheral vascular diseases, cardiac arrest	Poor
Histotoxic	Cyanide poisoning	Poor

PO_2, partial pressure of oxygen.

Stagnant hypoxia is a result of poor tissue perfusion, as may be seen in severe cardiac failure, hypovolemic shock, cardiac arrest, or peripheral vascular diseases. Tissue edema associated with poor perfusion increases the distance through which oxygen has to travel before it reaches the cells and contributes to localized hypoxia. Supplemental oxygen is usually not helpful unless tissue perfusion can be restored.

Histotoxic hypoxia is an inability to use oxygen at the cellular level, as in cyanide or sulfide poisoning. These chemical poisons produce cellular hypoxia by inhibiting electron-transfer function by cytochrome oxidase so that it cannot pass electrons to oxygen. The oxygen that is delivered to the tissues by the blood is not extracted, and as a consequence, the venous blood tends to have a high oxygen tension. Obviously, supplemental oxygen has little benefit in this case unless the underlying toxic process can be reversed.

TECHNIQUES FOR OXYGEN ADMINISTRATION

Delivery of Supplemental Oxygen

Nasal Cannulae

Nasal cannulae are capable of delivering low-flow oxygen and provide FiO_2 in the range of 0.23 to 0.35. In general, 1 L/min of nasal cannula oxygen flow is approximately equivalent to an FiO_2 of 24% with each additional liter of flow, increasing the FiO_2 by approximately 3%. Flow rates exceeding 4 L/min, however, are not tolerated well because of drying of the nasal mucosa. An advantage of a nasal cannula is that the patient can eat and drink while receiving oxygen. Actual FiO_2 for a given oxygen flow, however, may fluctuate depending on whether the patient breathes by mouth or by nose. Although nasal cannulae usually are considered safe, complications, such as mucosal perforation leading to submucosal emphysema with airway obstruction, have been reported.

Simple Masks

A simple oxygen mask can provide flow rates greater than nasal cannula. It can deliver an oxygen concentration of up to 50%. The flow rate needs to be at least 5 to 6 L/min to avoid accumulation of CO_2 in the mask. The disadvantage of the simple mask is that it interferes with eating, drinking, talking, and expectoration.

Venturi Masks

Venturi masks can provide accurate FiO_2 by varying the size of the downstream orifice and creating specific air–oxygen entrainment ratios. Usual FiO_2 values delivered with these masks are shown in Table 8–4. The disadvantage of the Venturi mask is similar to that of a simple mask. Occasionally, the fixed flow rate of Venturi masks may not meet the flow demand of a tachypneic patient.

Partial Rebreathing and Nonrebreathing Masks

Partial rebreathing and nonrebreathing masks are capable of delivering high concentrations of oxygen. Both types of mask are equipped with a reservoir bag that serves as a source of 100% oxygen from which the patient can breathe. For nonbreathing masks, there is a one-way valve on each side of the mask between the reservoir bag and the mask. The one-way valves close during inspiration, thus allowing the patient to draw from the reservoir bag only. FiO_2 values as high as 0.90 can be achieved with nonrebreathing masks. For partial rebreathing masks, there is no one-way valve on each side of the mask. The mixing of exhaled gas with the source gas lowers the FiO_2 to 0.60 to 0.80.

Continuous Positive Airway Pressure

Continuous positive airway pressure (CPAP) commonly is delivered by a tight-fitting mask with a continuous gas-flow rate (usually 15–30 L/min at a specified FiO_2), a reservoir bag, a one-way valve, a humidifier,

TABLE 8–4. Inspired Oxygen Concentration (FiO$_2$) Provided by Venturi Masks

FiO$_2$	AIR–OXYGEN ENTRAINMENT RATIO	FLOW RATE (L/min)	
		Oxygen	Total
0.24	20:1	4	84
0.28	10:1	4	44
0.31	6:1	8	56
0.35	5:1	8	48
0.40	3:1	8	32
0.50	1.7:1	12	32

Adapted from Malloy R, Pierce M: Oxygen therapy. In Dantzker DR, MacIntyre NR, Bakow ED (eds): Comprehensive Respiratory Care. Philadelphia, WB Saunders, 1995.

and an expiratory pressure valve. Many patients, however, cannot tolerate a CPAP mask because of claustrophobia, aerophagia, or hemodynamic instability. In these patients, endotracheal intubation should be considered.

Monitoring During Oxygen Therapy

Patient's Clinical Status

Monitoring patients receiving oxygen therapy should begin with a routine history and physical examination. Special attention should be paid to symptoms and signs of hypoxia (dyspnea, diaphoresis, restlessness, cyanosis, heart rate, respiratory rates, breathing pattern, and mental status, and so on). Subjective relief of dyspnea may indicate successful intervention. Conversely, paradoxical movement of abdominal muscles and excessive use of accessory muscles are warning signs of impending respiratory arrest.

Arterial Oxygenation

Because one of the major goals of supplemental oxygen is to correct hypoxemia, arterial oxygenation should be measured periodically. This can be achieved by measuring arterial PO$_2$ by arterial blood gas analysis or by monitoring arterial oxygen saturation by pulse oximetry. Arterial blood gas analysis is invasive but provides additional information such as pH, PCO$_2$, and abnormal hemoglobin states (carboxyhemoglobin, methemoglobin). Pulse oximetry is noninva-

sive. Correlation between arterial oxygen saturation (SaO$_2$) measured by pulse oximetry and that measured by co-oximetry is good in general, however, pulse oximetry is reliable only if SaO$_2$ values are between 65% and 90%. Otherwise, it is inaccurate and overestimates the SaO$_2$ at lower values.[4] Brown, red, and other colored nail polishes may reduce the reading. Elevated bilirubin levels also may interfere with the reading. Pulse oximetry does not detect the presence of carboxyhemoglobin or methemoglobin. Thus, oxygen saturation measured by pulse oximetry in carbon monoxide poisoning or methemoglobinemia overestimates the true oxygen content of the arterial blood. Arterial oxygenation should be maintained at an arterial PO$_2$ of at least 60 mm Hg or an oxygen saturation of at least 90% using the lowest FiO$_2$. Arterial oxygenation status obtained by either arterial blood gas analysis or pulse oximetry always should be interpreted in the context of the patient's overall clinical status.

Tissue Oxygenation

BIOCHEMICAL MARKERS

The adequacy of tissue oxygenation may be tested indirectly by monitoring the biochemical sequelae of tissue hypoxia. For example, lactate accumulation may reflect an increase in anaerobic metabolism induced by hypoxia. The accumulation of lactate in the plasma, however, may not always indicate tissue hypoxia. The plasma lactate level is known to increase in liver failure, where the hepatic uptake of lactate is impaired, or in sepsis, where hypermetabolism produces a large quantity of lactate.

MIXED VENOUS OXYGEN TENSION (PvO_2) OR SATURATION (SvO_2)

PvO_2 or SvO_2 does not always reflect tissue oxygenation status. As can be seen by rearranging the Fick equation, PvO_2 and SvO_2 tend to decrease when SaO_2 falls or decreased Hb concentration is undercompensated by cardiac output. PvO_2 and SvO_2 may be normal or high despite inadequate tissue oxygenation in diseases such as sepsis and cirrhosis, in which shunting of arterial blood is believed to occur in the peripheral tissues. Nonetheless, a low PvO_2 or SvO_2 should prompt proper reassessment of the patient's condition, especially if it is part of a rapidly deteriorating trend. The reliability of PvO_2 and SvO_2 as hemodynamic or prognostic indices tends to vary with the type of disease process. In cardiogenic shock and with response to cardiopulmonary resuscitation, SvO_2 correlates with prognosis.[5, 6]

TISSUE OXYGEN MEASUREMENT

Because the ultimate goal of supplemental oxygen is to prevent or correct tissue hypoxia, measuring tissue PO_2 would be a more direct assessment of tissue oxygenation. Various methods of measuring tissue PO_2 have been developed and are summarized in Table 8–5. These methods have been used to assess and monitor tissue PO_2 in various organs, such as skeletal muscles, the brain, and the heart. Measurement of local tissue PO_2 on the surface of various organs gives direct information on the function of the capillary exchange area. These techniques, however, are often cumbersome and sometimes labor intensive when used routinely in clinical monitoring.

ADVERSE EFFECTS OF OXYGEN THERAPY

Adverse effects of oxygen therapy are listed in Table 8–6. The effects of oxygen therapy on blunting of hypoxic drive and pulmonary

TABLE 8–5. Methods of Measuring Tissue Partial Pressures of Oxygen

METHODS	IN VIVO APPLICATIONS
Polarographic techniques	
Invasive: needle electrodes and catheters	Muscles
Noninvasive: surface electrodes	Wounds
Optical techniques:	
Near infrared (NIR) spectroscopy	Brain, muscles
Mass spectrometry	Liver, muscles
Magnetic resonance imaging	Brain, kidney
Oxygen sensitive microchips (lanthanum oxide)	Giant neurons of aplasia

oxygen toxicity are discussed in the following section.

Blunting of Hypoxic Drive

Supplemental oxygen should be used with caution in any patient with known or suspected chronic hypercapnea, for example, chronic obstructive pulmonary diseases and neuromuscular diseases. In these patients, high PaO_2 may result in respiratory depression by blunting the hypoxic respiratory

TABLE 8–6. Adverse Effects of Oxygen

Accidental fires and burns of upper respiratory tract

Drying of mucous membranes of upper respiratory tract

Respiratory depression due to blunting of hypoxic drive in CO_2 retainers

Pulmonary oxygen toxicity

Retrolental fibroplasia and bronchopulmonary dysplasia in premature infants

Oxygen paradox; sudden transient loss of consciousness on breathing pure oxygen in acute hypoxic states drive.[7] Respiratory depression worsens CO_2 retention and respiratory acidosis. The PaO_2 of these patients should be maintained at 50 to 55 mm Hg with low-flow oxygen. The risk of tissue hypoxia in these patients is relatively low at these levels of PaO_2 because the hemoglobin dissociation curve usually is shifted to the right, which may facilitate unloading of oxygen molecules in the systemic capillaries.

Pulmonary Oxygen Toxicity

Joseph Priestley, who discovered oxygen, first predicted the adverse effects of oxygen: ". . . for, as a candle burns out much faster in dephlogisticated than in common air, so we might, as might be said, live out too fast, and the animal powers be too soon exhausted in this pure kind of air. . . ." In 1878, Paul Bert first documented the central nervous system toxicity produced by hyperbaric oxygen. Pulmonary oxygen toxicity was not discovered until 1899 by Lorraine Smith and retrolental fibroplasia of prematurity until 1942 by Terry.[8]

The development of pulmonary oxygen toxicity has been attributed in part to the increased production of reactive oxygen species (ROS), which overcomes the body antioxidant defenses. Reactive oxygen species (superoxide $[O_2^-]$, hydrogen peroxide $[H_2O_2]$, hydroxyl radical $[OH]$) are derived from incomplete reduction of molecular oxygen. ROS may react with many biologic target molecules, including lipids, proteins, nucleic acids, and may result in oxidative damages to cell membrane and structural proteins, inactivation of enzymes, and altered cellular metabolism. Some important biological sources of ROS are listed in Table 8–7.

The pathologic response to prolonged exposure to oxygen occurs throughout the respiratory system. The temporal sequence of progressive histologic injury has been studied well in rodents and nonhuman primates.[9] The initial production of ROS damages many biologic structures and causes a secondary cellular inflammatory response. Pathologic descriptions of human oxygen toxicity, however, have been limited because

TABLE 8–7. Biologic Sources of Reactive Oxygen Species (ROS)

SITES	EXAMPLES OF SOURCES OF ROS
Intracellular	Mitochondrial electron transport chain
	Cytochrome P_{450}, lipoxygenase, cyclooxygenase, xanthine oxidase, indoleamine dioxygenase, monoamine oxidase
	Auto-oxidations (hydroquinones, catecholamines, thiols, etc.)
Plasma membrane-associated	NADPH/NADH oxidase
Extracellular	Inflammatory cells-associated (myeloperoxidase)

NADH, reduced form of nicotinamide-adenine dinucleotide; NADPH, reduced form of nicotinamide-adenine dinucleotide phosphate.

of the presence of coexisting pulmonary diseases as well as variability in the concentration–time profile of oxygen exposure. One of the earliest findings after hyperoxic exposure appears to be an increase in proteins in bronchoalveolar lavage fluid, which was noted after an average of 17 hours of exposure. The increased proteins in the lavage fluid are no longer present after a 2-week recovery period.[10] Pathologic changes at a later stage of oxygen exposure resemble those found in subhuman primates, including alveolar epithelial injury, endothelial cell injury, alveolar septal inflammation, and interstitial and alveolar edema. Clinically, the earliest manifestations of pulmonary oxygen toxicity in healthy humans are cough and mild chest discomfort exacerbated by inspiration suggestive of the development of tracheobronchitis.[11] With prolonged oxygen exposure, functional abnormalities develop, including decreases in lung volumes, compliance, and DLCO (diffusing capacity of the lung for carbon monoxide), as well as impaired gas exchange.[12, 13]

Defining a "safe level" of oxygen exposure has been problematic in part because of the limited data in lower primates and normal humans. Baboons exposed to 60% O_2 for 2 weeks show evidence of pulmonary fibrosis 8 weeks later.[14] In nonsmoking human volunteers, inhaling 50% oxygen for a mean time of 44 hours has been shown to produce evidence of pulmonary oxidant stress, as demonstrated by increase in lipid peroxidation in the bronchoalveolar lavage fluid.[15] In another study, mechanically ventilated patients randomly assigned to receive 50% oxygen showed significantly lower oxygenation after extubation than did patients who were given the lowest possible FiO_2.[16] Thus, it seems that an FiO_2 of 0.50 or greater should be considered "toxic."

Oxygen toxicity may be enhanced by many factors, including drugs (bleomycin, paraquat), some pathophysiologic states (hyperthermia, hyperthyroidism), prematurity of the newborn, vitamin E deficiency, and protein deficiency. In the presence of these conditions, pulmonary oxygen toxicity may develop even after exposure to a "nontoxic" range of oxygen levels.

Although progress has been made in developing new treatments for pulmonary oxygen toxicity,[17–21] the efficacy of these therapies has not been tested in clinical trials. Thus, the best strategy for treating pulmonary oxygen toxicity is to prevent it from developing by avoiding undue exposure to high concentrations of oxygen for prolonged periods. The concentration of supplemental oxygen should be maintained as low as possible to maintain an optimal PO_2.

SPECIAL APPLICATIONS OF OXYGEN THERAPY

High Altitude

A decrease in the PO_2 in the breathing air is the main cause of hypoxia at high altitude, where barometric pressure is lower. For example, at 5500 m (18,000 ft), the barometric pressure decreases by approximately 50% (379 mm Hg) and the PO_2 in the inspired air decreases from 160 mm Hg at sea level to 70 mm Hg. At this altitude, the arterial oxygen saturation would drop from 97% at sea level to approximately 75%. This altitude also happens to be the highest level of continuous human habitation.

Acute ascent from sea level to elevations higher than 2500 m can produce headache, nausea, vomiting, and insomnia, which are referred to as acute mountain sickness. The most severe forms of acute mountain sickness may lead to high-altitude pulmonary edema (HAPE) and high-altitude cerebral edema (HACE). Hypoxia, which may result in inhomogeneous vasoconstriction and hyperperfusion of unconstricted vessels, is believed to play an important role in the pathogenesis of HAPE.[22, 23] Conversely, local vasodilatation of cerebral vessels caused by hypoxia may increase fluid leak from the capillaries into the brain tissue, contributing to cerebral edema.[24, 25] The definitive treatment of HAPE and HACE is descent. Supplemental oxygen may be a life-saving temporizing measure.

Carbon Monoxide Poisoning

Carbon monoxide is the leading cause of death from accidental poisoning. Carbon monoxide is absorbed and excreted primarily by the lungs. On entry into the blood stream, it combines with hemoglobin to form carboxyhemoglobin (COHb). The affinity of carbon monoxide for hemoglobin is approximately 240 times greater than that of oxygen, thus it interferes with O_2 transport. This causes a number of biochemical effects of carbon monoxide, which are summarized in Table 8–8.

The formation of COHb not only decreases the binding sites available for O_2 but also induces allosteric changes of the hemoglobin molecules. The allosteric modification of the heme group results in left shift of the oxygen hemoglobin equilibrium curve. The combined effects on tissue oxygenation are greater than would result from loss of oxygen-carrying capacity alone. In addition, carbon monoxide also binds during hypoxia to the reduced form of cytochrome c oxidase, the terminal enzyme of the mitochondrial electron transport chain, thus

TABLE 8–8. Biochemical Effects of Carbon Monoxide

EFFECTS ON BLOOD

Increase of COHb levels
Shift of oxygen dissociation curve to the left

ACTIONS AT CELLULAR LEVEL

Cellular hypoxia
Inhibition of cytochrome c oxidase
Inhibition of cytochrome P_{450}
Formation of carboxymyoglobin

COHb, carboxyhemoglobin.

blocking cellular respiration during reoxygenation.[26]

The symptoms and signs of carbon monoxide poisoning range from dyspnea, headache, emotional changes, clumsiness to respiratory depression, myocardial ischemia, arrhythmia, confusion, and coma. Although the severity of clinical manifestations of carbon monoxide poisoning in general vary with COHb levels, the correlation is not perfect. The emphasis should be placed more on history and clinical features than on COHb values when evaluating patients with carbon monoxide poisoning.

Immediate administration of supplemental oxygen is essential in the initial management of carbon monoxide poisoning. Oxygen helps dissociate carbon monoxide from hemoglobin and counteracts hypoxemia. The half-life of COHb in patients breathing room air is approximately 6 hours. With 100% oxygen, the half-life is decreased to about 1.5 hours. With the application of hyperbaric oxygen (2 ATA), the half-life is reduced further to 20 minutes. In mild carbon monoxide poisoning, treatment with normobaric oxygen is frequently sufficient. Care should be taken that the exhaled air (containing carbon monoxide) is not rebreathed if oxygen is administered by a mask. For severe carbon monoxide poisoning (COHb > 25% or carbon monoxide < 25% but with neurologic signs or symptoms), hyperbaric oxygen should be the treatment of choice.

Helium–Oxygen

Helium can be mixed with oxygen to form a low-density breathing gas mixture. Helium–oxygen (Heliox) that contains 80% helium and 20% oxygen has a density of approximately one third that of air with only slight increase in viscosity. Because the airway resistance to turbulent flow is related to gas density for a given driving pressure, helium–oxygen mixtures may reduce airway resistance and decrease work of breathing. Thus, helium–oxygen mixtures may be used as a temporizing measure while awaiting the resolution of the primary diseases or definitive treatment of conditions associated with upper airway obstruction, such as postextubation stridor,[27] tracheal stenosis or extrinsic compression,[28] and angioedema.[29] Helium–oxygen mixtures have little effect on lower airway obstruction, in which flow is less density dependent.

There are limitations on the use of helium–oxygen gas mixtures. To effectively reduce gas density, the helium concentration in the helium–oxygen mixture must be at least 60%, which limits oxygen concentration in the gas mixtures to a maximum of 40%. Helium–oxygen gas mixtures cannot be delivered by nasal cannula. Flowmeters that are calibrated for oxygen may underestimate helium–oxygen flow because of the low density of the gas.[30] In addition, the helium–oxygen mixtures are expensive and are not widely available. Prolonged use of helium–oxygen mixtures (> 24 hours) may result in hypothermia unless the gas is actively warmed to body temperature because of the high thermal conductivity of helium.[31]

Nitric Oxide Inhalation Therapy

Nitric oxide (NO) is a reactive molecule produced endogenously in the body by NO synthase from L-arginine. Since the first description of NO as the endothelium-derived relaxing factor (EDRF) mediating vasodilatation,[32–34] NO has been shown to be involved in a variety of biologic effects ranging from immunoregulation, neurotransmission, modulation of platelet function, and leukocyte adhesion to intracellular and transcellular signaling.

In the environment, NO gas can be formed from incomplete combustion, where it quickly is oxidized to nitrogen dioxide

(NO$_2$). NO is lipophilic and has strong affinity for heme groups. The affinity of NO for the heme group of hemoglobin is 1500-fold higher than that of carbon monoxide, or 40,000-fold higher than that of oxygen for the heme group. Such an avid reaction of NO with hemoglobin in the blood, which leads to rapid "inactivation" of NO, forms the physiologic basis for use of NO inhalation as a "selective pulmonary vasodilator."[35-37]

The first clinical applications of NO inhalation therapy in patients with acute respiratory distress syndrome (ARDS) was reported in 1993.[38] The results of this preliminary study showed that inhaled NO is equivalent to intravenous prostacyclin in reducing the pulmonary vascular resistance, but unlike prostacyclin infusion, it does not produce any change in systemic hemodynamics. Arterial oxygenation improved significantly, indicating a better ventilation–perfusion matching. Although no severe side effects were noted in this small study, concerns have been raised about the potential toxicity of NO inhalation to the lungs, particularly in patients with ARDS who frequently require high FiO$_2$. The enthusiasm for NO inhalation therapy in ARDS also is tempered by recent studies showing that oxygenation improvement with inhaled NO is short-lived (1–2 days).[39-41]

It is known that NO is oxidized to NO$_2$ by contact with O$_2$ in a dose- and time-dependent manner. NO$_2$ is a toxic gas that causes bronchiolitis. Acute exposure to high concentrations of NO$_2$ may cause pulmonary edema and death. Long-term exposure to very low concentrations of NO$_2$ (0.3–1.0 ppm for 6 months) has also been demonstrated to cause significant morphologic effects and biochemical changes in the mouse lung.[42] Although human data are more limited, exposure to 2.3 ppm of NO$_2$ for 5 hours in healthy nonsmokers decreases the blood antioxidant activity (glutathione peroxidase).[43]

NO, being a free radical, also may react with other oxygen-derived free radicals, such as superoxide (O$_2^-$).[44] The reaction between NO and O$_2^-$ is extremely rapid (nearly diffusion-limited). The reaction product, peroxynitrite (OONO$^-$), is a stronger oxidant than NO or O$_2^-$ and has

been shown to produce oxidation and nitration of biological molecules, such as proteins, DNA, and membrane lipids. Although the toxicity of peroxynitrite in vivo has not been proven directly, concerns over the potential adverse effects of peroxynitrite are justified based on experimental evidence. More research is needed to define how NO inhalation therapy interacts with supplemental oxygen.

REFERENCES

1. Jain K, Fischer B: History of oxygen. In: Jain K, Fischer B (eds): Oxygen in Physiology and Medicine. Springfield, IL: Charles C Thomas, 1989, pp 3–11.
2. Mellemgaard K: The alveolar-arterial oxygen difference: its size and components in normal man. Acta Physiol Scand 67:10–20, 1966.
3. Torres-Bueno J, Wagner P, Saltzman H, et al: Diffusion limitation in normal humans during exercise at sea level and simulated altitude. J Appl Physiol 58:989–995, 1985.
4. Sidi A, Rush W, Gravenstein N: Pulse oximetry fails to accurately detect low levels of arterial hemoglobin oxygen saturation in dogs. J Clin Monit 2:257, 1987.
5. Kandel G, Aberman A: Mixed venous oxygen saturation: its role in the assessment of the critically ill patient. Arch Intern Med 143:1400, 1983.
6. Kasmitz P, Druger G, Yorra F: Mixed venous oxygen tension and hyperlactatemia survival in severe cardiopulmonary disease. JAMA 236:570, 1976.
7. Dunn W, Nelson S, Hubmayr R: Oxygen-induced hypercarbia in obstructive pulmonary disease. Am Rev Respir Dis 144:526–530, 1991.
8. Terry T: Extreme prematurity and fibroblastic overgrowth of persistent vascular sheath behind each crystalline lens: I, preliminary reports. Am J Ophthalmol 25:203, 1942.
9. Fracica P, Knapp M, Crapo J: Patterns of progression and markers of lung injury in rodents and subhuman primates exposed to hyperoxia. Exp Lung Res 14:869–885, 1988.
10. Davis W, Rennard S, Bitterman P, Crystal R: Pulmonary oxygen toxicity: early reversible changes in human alveolar structures induced by hyperoxia. N Engl J Med 309:878–883, 1983.
11. Clark J, Lambertsen C: Pulmonary oxygen toxicity: a review. Pharmacol Rev 23:37–133, 1971.
12. Caldwell P, Lee W, Schildkraut H, Archibald E: Changes in lung volume, diffusing capacity, and blood gases in men breathing oxygen. J Appl Physiol 21:1477–1483, 1966.
13. Barber R, Lee J, Hamilton W: Oxygen toxicity in man: a prospective study in patients with irreversible brain damage. N Engl J Med 283:1478–1484, 1970.

14. Crapo J, Hayatdavoudi G, Knapp M, et al: Progressive alveolar septal injury in primates exposed to 60% oxygen for 14 days. Am J Physiol 267:L797–L806, 1994.

15. Griffith D, Garcia J, James H, et al: Hyperoxic exposure in humans: effects of 50 percent oxygen on alveolar macrophage leukotriene B4 synthesis. Chest 101:392–397, 1992.

16. Register S, Downs J, Stock M, Kirby R: Is 50% oxygen harmful? Crit Care Med 15:598–601, 1987.

17. Huang Y-C, Sane A, Simonson S, et al: Artificial surfactant attenuates hyperoxic lung injury in primates: I, physiology and biochemistry. J Appl Physiol 78:1816–1822, 1995.

18. Piantadosi C, Fracica P, Duhaylongsod F, et al: Artificial surfactant attenuates hyperoxic lung injury in primates: II, morphometric analyses. J Appl Physiol 78:1823–1831, 1995.

19. Robbins C, Horowitz S, Merritt T, et al: Recombinant human superoxide dismutase reduces lung injury caused by inhaled nitric oxide and hyperoxia. Am J Physiol 272:L903–L907, 1997.

20. Simonson S, Huang Y, Welty-Wolf K, et al: Aerosolized manganese superoxide dismutase decreases hyperoxic pulmonary injury in primates: I, physiology and biochemistry. J Appl Physiol 83:550–558, 1997.

21. Welty-Wolf K, Simonson S, Huang Y, et al: Aerosolized manganese superoxide dismutase decreases hyperoxic pulmonary injury in primates: II, morphometric analysis. J Appl Physiol 83:559–568, 1997.

22. Hultgren H: High altitude pulmonary edema. In: Hegnauer A (ed): Biochemical Problems of High Terrestrial Altitudes. Springfield, VA: Federal Scientific and Technical Information, 1967, pp 131–141.

23. Staub N: Overperfusion edema. N Engl J Med 302:1085–1086, 1980.

24. Severinghaus J, Chiodi H, Eger E II, et al: Cerebral blood flow in man at high altitude. Circ Res 19:274–282, 1966.

25. Sutton J, Lassen N: Pathophysiology of acute mountain sickness and high altitude pulmonary edema. Bull Eur Physiopathol Respir 15:1045–1052, 1979.

26. Brown S, Piantadosi C: Recovery of energy metabolism in rat brain after carbon monoxide hypoxia. J Clin Invest 89:666–672, 1992.

27. Kemper K, Ritz R, Benson M, Bishop M: Helium-oxygen mixture in the treatment of postextubation stridor in pediatric trauma patients. Crit Care Med 19:356, 1991.

28. Curtis J, Mahlmeister M, Fink J, et al: Helium-oxygen gas therapy: use and availability for the treatment of inoperable airway obstruction. Chest 90:455, 1986.

29. Boorstein J, Boorstein S, Humphries G, Johnston C: Using helium-oxygen mixtures in the emergency management of acute upper airway obstruction. Ann Emerg Med 18:688, 1989.

30. Curtis J, Orr J: Helium-oxygen gas mixtures in the management of patients with airway obstruction. Ear Nose Throat J 67:866, 1988.

31. Fleming J, Weigelt J, Brewer V, McIntire D: Effect of helium and oxygen on airflow in a narrowed airway. Arch Surg 127:956, 1992.

32. Furchgott R, Zawadzki J: The obligatory role of endothelial cells in the relaxation of arterial smooth muscle by acetylcholine. Nature 288:373–376, 1980.

33. Ignarro L, Buga G, Wood K, et al: Endothelium-derived relaxing factor produced and released from artery and vein is nitric oxide. Proc Natl Acad Sci USA 84:9265–9269, 1987.

34. Palmer R, Ferrige A, Moncada S: Nitric oxide release accounts for the biological activity of endothelium-derived relaxing factor. Nature 327:524–526, 1987.

35. Pepke-Zaba J, Higenbottam T, Dinh-Xuan A, et al: Inhaled nitric oxide as a cause of selective pulmonary vasodilation in pulmonary hypertension. Lancet 338:1173–1174, 1991.

36. Frostell C, Fratacci M, Wain J, et al: Inhaled nitric oxide: a selective pulmonary vasodilator reversing hypoxic pulmonary vasoconstriction. Circulation 83:2038–2047, 1991.

37. Pison U, Lopez F, Heidelmeyer C, et al: Inhaled nitric oxide selectively reverse hypoxic pulmonary vasoconstriction without impairing pulmonary gas exchange. J Appl Physiol 74:7287–7292, 1993.

38. Rossaint R, Falke K, Lopez F, et al: Inhaled nitric oxide in adult respiratory distress syndrome. N Engl J Med 328:399–405, 1993.

39. Dellinger R, Zimmerman J, Taylor R, et al: Effects of inhaled nitric oxide in patients with acute respiratory distress syndrome: results of a randomized phase II trial. Inhaled Nitric Oxide in ARDS Study Group. Crit Care Med 26:15–23, 1998.

40. Michael J, Barton R, Saffle J, et al: Inhaled nitric oxide versus conventional therapy: effect on oxygenation in ARDS. Am J Resp Crit Care Med 157:1372–1380, 1998.

41. Troncy E, Collet J, Shapiro S, et al: Inhaled nitric oxide in acute respiratory distress syndrome: a pilot randomized controlled study. Am J Resp Crit Care Med 157:1483–1488, 1998.

42. Nakajima T, Hajame O, Kusumoto S, Nagomi H: Biological effects of nitrogen dioxide and nitric oxide. In Lee SD (ed): Nitrogen Oxides and Their Effects on Health. Ann Arbor, MI: Ann Arbor Science, 1980, pp 121–141.

43 Rasmussen T, Kjaergaard S, Tarp U, Pedersen C: Delayed effects of NO_2 exposure on alveolar permeability and glutathione peroxidase in healthy humans. Am Rev Respir Dis 146:654–659, 1992.

44 Crow J, Beckman J: Reactions between nitric oxide, superoxide, and peroxynitrite: footprints of peroxynitrite in vivo. Adv Pharmacol 34:17–43, 1995.

CHAPTER 9

Patient–Ventilator Interactions

Neil R. MacIntyre, MD

DETERMINANTS AND CHARACTERISTICS OF THE SPONTANEOUS VENTILATORY PATTERN

VENTILATOR TRACKING OF SPONTANEOUS EFFORT

INTERACTIVE VENTILATOR DESIGN FEATURES

Ventilator Breath Triggering

Ventilator-Delivered Flow Pattern

Ventilator Flow Termination

Imposed Expiratory Loads

Backup Ventilator Breaths

FUTURE APPROACHES TO IMPROVING PATIENT–VENTILATOR SYNCHRONY

REFERENCES

KEY WORDS

cycle synchrony
flow synchrony
responsiveness

sensitivity
spontaneous ventilatory drive
triggering

In the acute phases of respiratory failure, near total mechanical ventilator support is required to provide adequate gas exchange and unload fatigued ventilatory muscles.[1] This often requires depressing or ablating the patient's spontaneous ventilatory activity with heavy sedation and/or neuromuscular blockade. As gas exchange abnormalities stabilize and the neuromuscular system recovers its ability to provide some level of activity, however, ventilatory support modes that permit some degree of spontaneous ventilatory activity can be used as an alternative to controlled, total support.[2] These modes often are termed "interactive" modes

because patients can affect various aspects of the mechanical ventilator's functions.

Patient–ventilator interactions can range from simple triggering of mechanical breaths to more complex processes affecting delivered flow patterns and breath timing. Advantages to interactive modes of support versus controlled modes of support are twofold: first, lower ventilator pressures generally are required with interactive modes; and second, interactive modes generally require less sedation. This latter benefit, coupled with avoidance of neuromuscular blockers, may reduce long-term mental status abnormalities and muscle dysfunction.[2, 3]

189

Interactive modes can be either synchronous or dys-synchronous with patient efforts.[2, 3] Synchronous interactions mean that the ventilator is *sensitive (sensitivity)* to the initiation and termination of a patient's ventilatory effort and is *responsive (responsiveness)* to the flow characteristics of the patient's ventilatory demand.[1-3]

Dys-synchronous interactions occur when ventilator gas delivery and patient efforts are not coordinated or are out of phase. Synchronizing patient–ventilator interactions is important to avoid "imposed" muscle loading that can occur when ventilator gas delivery and patient efforts are not matched.[3, 4] Synchronous interactions prevent unnecessary ventilatory muscle oxygen consumption and often improve patient comfort because patients are not "fighting" the ventilator.[3, 5]

The remainder of this chapter addresses patient–ventilator interactions by considering the determinants of the spontaneous ventilatory drive, by considering ventilator sensors, and by reviewing the design characteristics of currently available interactive ventilatory support modes.

DETERMINANTS AND CHARACTERISTICS OF THE SPONTANEOUS VENTILATORY PATTERN

The ventilatory control system is located in the brainstem and receives input from several sources.[6, 7] Among these are gas exchange sensors (e.g., pH, PaO_2), stretch receptors in the lung and thoracic cage, irritant and J receptors within the lung, cortical influences, and other factors (e.g., hormonal influences, cardiac output, and so on). The output of the ventilatory control system can be characterized by the timing and intensity of the phrenic nerve signal.[6-9] Timing often is described by the inspiratory and expiratory time partitioning (T_i and T_e, respectively) and the inverse of $T_i + T_e$, the respiratory frequency.[6-9] The intensity of the tidal breath signal is reflected in the electromyogram (EMG) signal, the airway occlusion pressure at 100 msec ($P_{0.1}$), the dP/dt of the inspiratory muscles, and the actual magnitude of the tidal volume.[6-9]

The overall goal of the ventilatory control system is to generate a breathing pattern that provides the best gas exchange for the least amount of ventilatory muscle energy utilization (the "minimal work" concept).[10] This simple construct, however, can be altered by the other aforementioned factors. Specifically, as muscles become overloaded or as irritant receptors become more active (dyspnea), the frequency may increase beyond the "minimal work" constraint.[7, 10-14] In addition, poor cardiac function can lead to bradypnea or apnea, and hyperinflation may result in a lengthening of T_e to improve lung emptying.

The ventilatory control system also responds to the effects of mechanical ventilation. For instance, as respiratory muscles become unloaded with appropriate mechanical ventilation, the abnormal mechanical input to the ventilatory control center may be lessened and an abnormal ventilatory pattern (e.g., tachypnea) may revert to a more normal one.[15] This is the physiologic basis for setting levels of mechanical ventilation according to ventilatory pattern endpoints (e.g., "set pressure support level to keep spontaneous ventilatory rate < 30 or 35"). Similarly, the ventilatory control system also may respond to loads imposed by dys-synchronous mechanical ventilator settings. This response is often similar to the response to other causes of excess muscle loading (e.g., tachypnea, dyspnea, and abdominal paradox).

Positive end-expiratory pressure (PEEP) also can influence the ventilatory control system. Atelectasis from suboptimal applied PEEP (or continuous positive airway pressure [CPAP]) can increase inspiratory work and impair gas exchange, thereby affecting patient comfort (dyspnea) and drive.[16] Conversely, excessive PEEP (either applied or intrinsic) can overdistend significant amounts of lung, putting muscles at suboptimal "resting" lengths and worsening the sense of patient discomfort.[16]

VENTILATOR TRACKING OF SPONTANEOUS EFFORT

For proper patient–ventilator synchrony, the mechanical ventilator needs the capa-

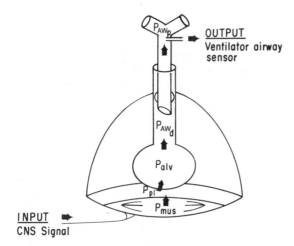

FIGURE 9–1
"Barriers" between the actual patient input signal into the muscles and the sensing site for patient activity by the ventilator. (From MacIntyre NR: Synchronous and dys-synchronous patient-ventilator interactions. In: Vincent JL (ed): Yearbook of Intensive Care and Emergency Medicine. New York, Springer, 1992.)

bility to monitor or track the pattern of the patient's **spontaneous ventilatory drive**.[17] This usually is done through measurements of flow or pressure at the patient's airway opening. Synchrony then is aimed at optimizing interactions with these parameters. As shown in Figure 9–1, however, there are important "barriers" between the patient's ventilatory control center signal and this sensing site. These barriers can

"dampen" the magnitude of patient effort and ventilator responsiveness, thereby introducing lags between patient demand and gas delivery even under the best of circumstances. Future interactive features may be improved by sensors placed in the patient's airway, the pleural space, or perhaps on the phrenic nerve itself.[18] Until such reliable sensors are developed, however, patient–ventilator synchrony with current systems must rely on synchronization of the mechanical ventilator to proximal airway signals.

INTERACTIVE VENTILATOR DESIGN FEATURES

Five aspects of patient–ventilator interactions are considered. The first three deal with mechanical breath parameters (Table 9–1): ventilator breath triggering (trigger criteria), ventilator-delivered flow pattern (target criteria), and ventilator flow termination (cycling criteria). Two additional considerations also are discussed: imposed expiratory loads and "backup" ventilator breaths.

Ventilator Breath Triggering

Interactive mechanical ventilation needs to sense a spontaneous effort to initiate gas

TABLE 9–1. Ventilator Breath Parameters

COMMON NAME	TRIGGER	TARGET	CYCLE
Volume control	Set ventilator timer	Set ventilator flow	Set ventilator volume
Volume assist	Patient effort	Set ventilator flow	Set ventilator volume
Pressure control	Set ventilator timer	Set ventilator pressure	Set ventilator timer
Pressure assist	Patient effort	Set ventilator pressure	Set ventilator timer
Pressure support	Patient effort	Set ventilator pressure	Flow decrease (cessation of patient effort)
Unassisted/ unsupported	Patient effort	Baseline patient airway pressure	Flow decrease (cessation of patient effort)

flow (triggering).[19] This often is accomplished by detecting the decrease in airway pressure that occurs with the beginning of a spontaneous effort (pressure triggering). An alternative approach is to detect the development of inspiratory flow by the patient drawing gas from the ventilator circuit (flow triggering). Note that there is a certain inherent dys-synchrony in the triggering process, regardless of technique (Fig. 9–2). This is due to several factors. First, a certain level of insensitivity must be put in the sensor to avoid allowing artifacts to trigger the ventilator (i.e., "auto-cycling"). Second, as

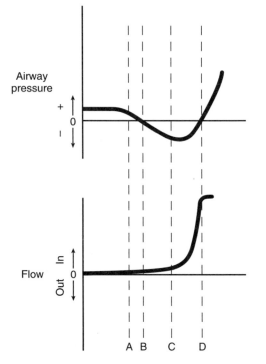

FIGURE 9–2
Trigger sensitivity and responsiveness. Depicted are airway pressure and flow during a patient-triggered breath. At point A, patient effort begins. Airway pressure drops until point B, where the set pressure trigger sensitivity (solid horizontal line) is achieved and the ventilator flow system is activated. The pressure time product between points A and B describes the muscle loads due to sensitivity of the system. The duration between points B and C reflects delays in the valving system between activation and actual valve opening to deliver flow. The duration between points C and D reflects delays in the valving system achieving the set flow. The pressure-time product between points B and D describes the muscle load due to responsiveness of the system.

noted in Figure 9–1, the patient's pleural pressure change is dampened as it is transmitted across lung parenchyma to the ventilator circuitry. Third, even when the patient effort has been sensed, demand valve systems have a certain inherent delay (up to 100 or more msec) before they physically open and achieve target flow into the airway (valve responsiveness). All these factors can result in significant "isometric-like" pressure loads on the ventilatory muscles during the triggering process[20] (Fig. 9–3). In addition, in the setting of air trapping and PEEP (intrinsic PEEP), the elevated alveolar pressure at end expiration can serve as a significant triggering threshold load on the ventilatory muscles (Fig. 9–4).[21]

Several strategies can be used to minimize the magnitude of the dys-synchrony induced during breath triggering. First, using ventilators with microprocessor flow controls can result in significantly better valve characteristics than those obtained on older-generation ventilators.[22] Second, continuous flow systems superimposed on the demand systems can improve demand system responsiveness in patients with high ventilatory drives (although such flows can *reduce* sensitivity in patients with very weak ventilatory drives).[20] Third, flow-based triggers have been shown to produce a more sensitive and responsive breath-triggering process in mechanical lung models.[19] Fourth, a small amount of applied inspiratory pressure support usually increases the ventilator's initial flow delivery and thereby can improve response characteristics of the demand valve system.[19] Fifth, in the setting of intrinsic PEEP creating an inspiratory threshold load, applied PEEP below the intrinsic PEEP level can help equilibrate the end-expiratory alveolar and circuit pressures and improve triggering (Fig. 9–4, right panel).[21] Finally, as noted previously, sensors in the airways, in the pleural space, or on the phrenic nerve may improve trigger sensitivity on future systems.[18]

Ventilator-Delivered Flow Pattern

Using the schema of Table 9–1, interactive breaths can be termed "assisted" (patient triggered, ventilator targeted, ventilator cy-

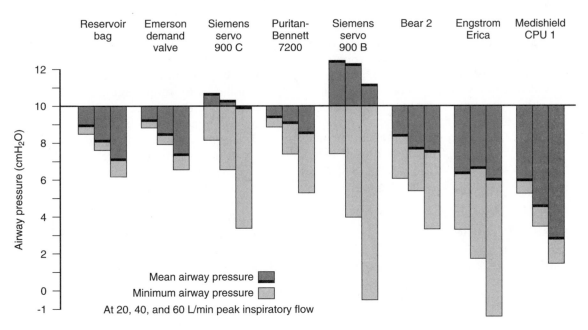

FIGURE 9–3
Airway pressure changes required to trigger various continuous positive airway pressure (CPAP) systems set at 10 cm H$_2$O using different stimulated inspiratory flow demands. (Reprinted with permission from Katz J, Kraemer R, Gjerde GE: Inspiratory work and airway pressure with continuous positive airway pressure delivery systems. Chest 88:519–526, 1985.)

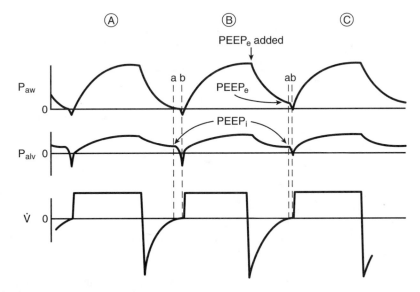

FIGURE 9–4
Impact of intrinsic positive end-expiratory pressure (PEEP$_i$) on triggering. Plotted are airway pressure (P$_{AW}$), alveolar pressure (P$_{ALV}$) and flow (V̇) in a patient with significant PEEP$_i$. To trigger a machine breath, alveolar pressure (P$_{ALV}$) must fall by the amount of PEEP$_i$ plus the set trigger sensitivity. The large drop in P$_{ALV}$ between a and b on breath B reflects this effort. The addition of extrinsic PEEP (PEEP$_e$) downstream from dynamically compressed airways reduces the P$_{ALV}$-P$_{AW}$ gradient and attenuates the triggering effort between a and b on breath C, without a significant increase in end-inspiratory P$_{ALV}$.

cled), "supported" (patient triggered, ventilator targeted, patient cycled), or "unassisted/unsupported" (patient triggered, patient targeted, patient cycled).[17]

Ventilator flow during these breath delivery strategies can be provided to meet one of three goals: (1) fully unload ventilatory muscles, (2) partially unload ventilatory muscles, or (3) not affect ventilatory muscle loads. Synchronous flow interactions can be defined according to one of these three goals.

Breaths Designed to Fully Unload Ventilatory Muscles

For an interactive breath to *fully* unload ventilator muscles, the patient should be required to trigger only the ventilator and then have the ventilator supply all the work of the breath. In considering breaths designed to fully unload ventilatory muscles, remember that diaphragmatic contraction does not cease with the onset of a patient-triggered, ventilator-delivered breath.[23] The goal of synchrony during a fully unloading breath thus is to deliver adequate flow over the entire inspiratory effort to totally unload the contracting muscles. Achieving this goal can be assessed by comparing the pressure pattern of the patient-triggered breath with a machine-triggered breath (i.e., a breath occurring without patient activity). Synchronous flow delivery should produce

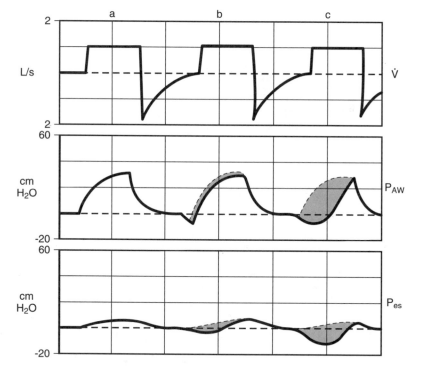

FIGURE 9–5

Manifestations of flow dys-synchrony of a ventilator breath. Plotted are flow *(upper panel)* and pleural pressure as reflected by esophageal pressure *(lower panel)* over a single ventilatory cycle. Breath a represents a control breath (no patient activity). Breath b represents a patient-triggered breath during which ventilator flow is adequate to almost totally unload fully the contracting ventilatory muscles. The dotted curve mimics passive breath a. As can be seen in both the airway and esophageal pressure tracings, the only appreciable difference between curves a and b is the triggering effort at the beginning of the breath. Breath c represents a patient-triggered breath during which ventilator flow is inadequate to unload fully the contracting ventilatory muscles. The dotted line again mimics the passive breath a. In contrast to the synchronous breath b, there is marked disparity in both airway and esophageal pressure tracings between breaths c and a. These differences can be quantified as a pressure time product (shaded area) reflecting the imposed muscle load from flow dys-synchrony.

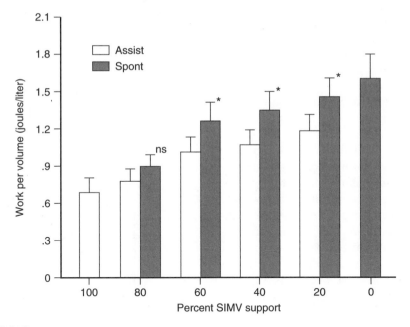

FIGURE 9–6
Patient work per liter of ventilation (mean inflation pressure) during the unassisted/unsupported breaths (hatched bars) and the ventilator-assisted breaths (open bars) at various levels of synchronized intermittent mandatory ventilation (SIMV) in a group of dyspneic patients. One hundred percent SIMV support reflects volume assist control ventilation. There is significant imposed work from flow dys-synchrony during all assisted breaths in these patients, and it increases as the level of ventilator assistance (%SIMV support) is reduced. (Reprinted with permission from Marini JJ, Smith TC, Lamb VJ: External work output and force generation during synchronized intermittent mechanical ventilation. Am Rev Respir Dis 138:1169–1179, 1988. © American Lung Association.)

nearly identical pressure waveforms (Fig. 9–5).

Patient-triggered breaths can be unloaded fully with either assisted or supported breaths that are either flow or pressure targeted. The interactive flow-targeted, volume-cycled breath supplies a clinician-set flow and volume in response to the patient's effort (the volume assist breath). To fully unload ventilatory muscles, these breaths must be given with every patient effort (often with a backup ventilator control rate), and the ventilator mode is termed *volume assist-control ventilation* (VACV). In contrast, pressure-targeted breaths supply a clinician-set airway pressure in response to the patient's effort and are either flow-cycled (pressure support [PS]) or time-cycled (pressure assist [PA]) (see cycling section). To fully unload ventilatory muscles with a pressure-targeted breath, the level of

pressure must be sufficient to supply all the work of a breath. Note that both the PS and the PA breath also can have backup control breaths in modes such as PS + intermittent mandatory ventilation or pressure assist-control ventilation (PACV).

Synchrony of a flow-targeted breath (**flow synchrony**) requires careful clinician selection of the flow magnitude and pattern. Arbitrary settings (e.g., constant flow of 40–60 L/min) are not always adequate. Indeed, in dyspneic patients on VACV, Marini and associates[23] calculated loads of 5 to 15 joules per minute (2 to 3 times normal) from flow dys-synchrony (Fig. 9–6, 100% SIMV). Synchrony of flow-targeted breaths can be improved by careful adjustments of the set flow using both patient observations (e.g., perceived effort, tachypnea) and airway pressure/flow graphics (see Fig. 9–5). In addition, use of a decelerating flow pattern also may be helpful because a patient's inspiratory effort tends to peak soon after breath initiation.

Pressure-targeted breaths may be easier to synchronize than flow-targeted breaths for two reasons.[15] First, because the ventilator has a pressure target, there is a rapid pressurization of the airway as gas is delivered with high initial flows. This tends to match the pressure changes occurring in the pleura more rapidly than that which takes place with currently available set flow patterns. Second, because pressure is the independent variable, flow is adjusted continuously by the ventilator to maintain a constant airway pressure. This serves to provide a more constant pressure application to the pleural space during a patient effort and thus a more continuous, or steady, pressure boost to the contracting muscles.

Although a conceptual step forward in patient–ventilator synchrony, pressure targeting has potential problems. First, a ventilator maximum initial flow may not be optimal in all patients.[24] Specifically, it appears that although patients with very active ventilatory drives require rapid initial flows for synchrony, patients with less active drives actually may be more synchronous if lower initial flows are applied.[24] The capability to adjust initial flows (and thus the rate of rise to the pressure target) may be of benefit in addressing this (Fig. 9–7). Second, the pressure target for the ventilator is the proximal airway while the patient's muscle effort actually is generated in the pleural space. This separation by a series of resistive elements (i.e., endotracheal tube and airways, see Fig. 9–1) introduces an inherent under-responsiveness of ventilator flow to patient effort. This would be a theoretical reason for targeting ventilator pressure to the distal endotracheal tube or the pleural space instead of the ventilator circuitry. Indeed, experimental systems using carinal or pleural pressure sites for pressure targeting appear to significantly reduce imposed loading and improve synchrony.[18, 25] Third, because pressure-targeted breaths consist only of an applied inspiratory pressure, fluctuations in patient

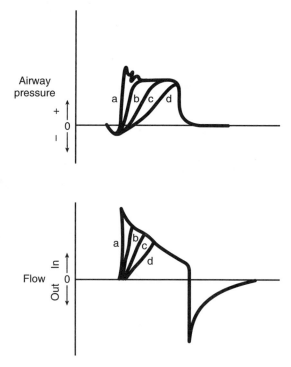

FIGURE 9–7
Airway pressure *(upper panel)* and flow *(lower panel)* illustrating effects of changing the pressure rise time during a pressure-supported (PS) breath. Curve a has the fastest rise time whereas curve d has the slowest. Note that the faster rise time also has the fastest initial flow. Because PS breaths generally terminate based on a percentage of peak initial flow, rise time adjustment also can affect breath duration. In general, patient ventilator synchrony is optimal when the pressure wave form has a smooth square configuration (curve b in this example).

effort and ventilatory system impedances can affect the delivered minute ventilation.

There are several clinical studies that have attempted to compare the synchrony effects of volume-targeted versus pressure-targeted breaths.[26–28] In general, careful selection of flow and pressure settings can provide good patient–ventilator synchrony with either breath type. In the patient with a vigorous ventilatory demand, however, many of these same studies suggest that a pressure-targeted breath may be more synchronous (Fig. 9–8).

Breaths to Partially Unload Muscles

Partial unloading of ventilatory muscles can be provided in one of three general ways:

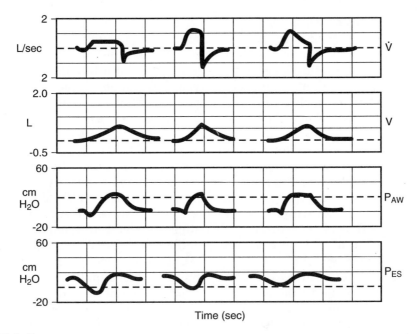

FIGURE 9–8
Ventilator flow ($\dot{V}$), tidal volume (V), airway pressure (P_{AW}), and esophageal pressure (P_{ES}) tracings in a ventilated patient. The patient is receiving ventilator flow set at 30 L/min to induce flow dys-synchrony *(left panels)*. This dys-synchrony is demonstrated by a markedly negative esophageal pressure tracing during inspiration. The airway pressure tracing also appears "pulled" down. The set ventilator flow has been increased to 75 L/min, and the esophageal pressure tracing can be seen to improve *(middle panels)*. A pressure-limiting feature of 22 cm H_2O above set positive end-expiratory pressure has been given *(right panels)*. With this approach, the dys-synchronous esophageal pressure can be seen to improve even further. (From MacIntyre NR, McConnell R, Cheng KG, Sane A: Patient-ventilator flow dys-synchrony: flow limited versus pressure limited breaths. Crit Care Med 25:1671–1677, 1997.)

first, an intermittent mandatory ventilation (IMV) approach (either flow-/volume-targeted or pressure-targeted fully unloaded breaths alternating with unassisted breaths); second, a stand-alone pressure-targeted approach (partial support/assist of every breath using PS or PA breaths); or third, a mixed approach of PS + IMV.

The IMV approach partially unloads by intermittently shifting all the work for a given effort between patient and ventilator. Synchronization of the assisted breaths during IMV has similar considerations to synchronization during VACV or PACV. However, the intermittence of breaths during IMV can add additional difficulty.[24, 29] This is because mechanical input to the ventilatory control center changes from breath to breath (i.e., unassisted breaths are alternating with assisted breaths). An "optimal"

ventilatory pattern is thus impossible for the ventilatory control center to establish. This, coupled with the increased ventilatory drive intensity often associated with unassisted breaths, can result in further dys-synchrony during the assisted breaths. In Marini's patients, there was a doubling of patient muscle work during the assisted breaths as the IMV assisted breath rate was reduced to 20% of the VACV rate[24] (Fig. 9–6). An interesting variant of IMV is airway pressure release ventilation (APRV), which holds the lung at a moderate level of inflation and provides intermittent mandatory ventilation through periodic brief deflations. Unassisted/unsupported breaths can occur during both inflation and deflation phases. APRV has been termed "upside down" IMV, and synchrony issues may be similar during APRV and IMV.

The pressure-targeted approach to partial unloading requires the patient to trigger the ventilator and then "share" the work of every breath with the ventilator. This is accomplished by giving a level of inspiratory pressure lower than that which totally unloads the muscles. Lower levels of inspiratory pressure thus are *designed* to have the patient's ventilatory muscles perform some level of work during each assisted/supported breath. Indeed, this is how muscles are "reloaded" during a pressure-targeted weaning protocol (see Chapter 20). Synchrony under these circumstances thus is *not* a process of total muscle unloading as it is during full assist/support. Rather, synchrony under these circumstances is defined as the process of ventilator flow continuously adjusting to keep a constant pressure "bias" on the contracting ventilatory muscles.

The combined PS + IMV approach conceptually improves patient–ventilator synchrony during IMV by providing pressure support to the spontaneous efforts that alternate with pressure- or volume-targeted assist/control breaths. However, many of the aforementioned concerns about IMV dyssynchrony remain, and this combination mode is inherently more complex for clinicians to adjust (especially during weaning). One advantage to the PS + IMV combination is that a low IMV rate can function as a "backup" if the patient's respiratory drive is unreliable.

Breaths That Do Not Affect Muscle Loads

For an interactive breath to not affect ventilatory muscle loads (i.e., the patient breathes entirely on his or her own), the ventilator should only provide sufficient gas flow during an inspiratory effort to maintain a constant level of airway pressure throughout the ventilatory cycle (CPAP). This interactive breath can be used during the spontaneous breaths of IMV (see previous discussion) or in patients not requiring ventilatory support but who need a constantly elevated airway pressure to maintain alveolar stability.

The goal of synchrony with unassisted/unsupported breaths is for the ventilator not to provide assist or support but rather

to ensure that adequate flow is delivered to minimize (or eliminate) any imposed loading. Indeed, the ideal CPAP system is one with large bore tubing and a high continuous flow. Under these circumstances, any patient effort merely draws off the continuous flow. Because there is no sensor or valve, synchrony is less of an issue. However, with this type of system, high patient demands can exceed the continuous flow capability (induce flow dys-synchrony), and monitoring can be difficult.

Demand valve systems (with or without a superimposed continuous flow) are a viable option for CPAP. Triggering of the valve is required, however, and the ventilator must be capable of rapidly responding to patient effort to maintain CPAP. With any CPAP system, significant flow dys-synchrony can be detected by observing decreases in inspiratory airway pressure tracings (i.e., perfect synchrony should result in a truly constant airway pressure).

With either a continuous flow or a demand valve system, recognize that a constant airway pressure measured in the ventilator circuit during the ventilatory cycle (apparent flow synchrony) is usually *not* a constant airway pressure if measured at the trachea (Fig. 9–9).[18] This is because the endotracheal tube can have significant resistive properties and thus produce an imposed load. Reducing (or eliminating) this load is the rationale for adding a small amount of inspiratory PS to CPAP breaths—it creates tracheal CPAP (see Fig. 9–9, breath b and breath c). The appropriate amount of PS can be estimated from endotracheal tube size and spontaneous flow rates (Fig. 9–10).[30] A more direct approach, however, is to target the ventilator pressure to tracheal pressure[18] (see Fig. 9–9, breath c). As noted previously in the triggering discussion, an additional advantage to using a small amount of PS to produce tracheal CPAP is that the ventilator demand valve responsiveness is generally better when the inspiratory pressure target is above the baseline.

Ventilator Flow Termination

The process of terminating gas delivery is termed *cycling*. Synchronous cycling should

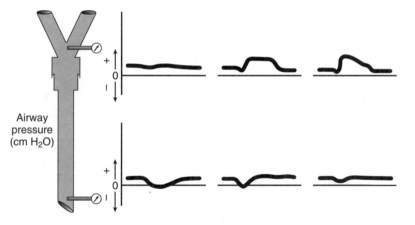

FIGURE 9–9

Schematic depiction of airway pressure tracings at the proximal and distal end of an endotracheal tube in which the clinical goal is to produce a continuous positive airway pressure (CPAP) of 5 cm H_2O. In the first breath, producing a CPAP of 5 cm H_2O at the proximal end of the tube results in a decrease in airway pressure at the distal end during patient inspiration to overcome tube resistance. Setting a pressure support (PS) level of 5 cm H_2O in the proximal airway during inspiration reduces some of the work to overcome tube resistance (second breath) and begins to produce true tracheal CPAP. Setting CPAP targeted to the distal airway, however, using a distal tube pressure sensor (third breath) actually produces a decelerating PS pattern in the proximal airway and results in true tracheal CPAP.

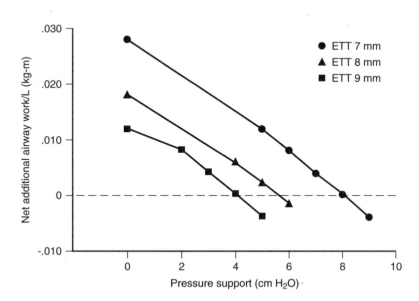

FIGURE 9–10

Imposed work caused by endotracheal tube resistance *(vertical axis)* plotted against level of pressure support using different endotracheal tube (ETT) sizes. Data are for a respiratory rate of 20 breaths per minute and a tidal volume of 500 ml. The appropriate pressure support to minimize imposed ETT work in this study ranged from 4–8 cm H_2O. (From Fiastro JF, Habib MP, Quan SF: Pressure support compensation for inspiratory work due to endotracheal tubes and demand continuous positive airway pressure. Chest 93:499–505, 1988.)

be done in accordance both with patient demand and with adequacy of tidal volume. Premature termination may result in an inadequate tidal volume and/or a patient continuing to demand inspiratory flow but not getting it (an inspiratory imposed load) (Fig. 9–11, left breath). Delayed breath termination may result in excessive tidal volumes, inadequate expiratory time (and consequent air trapping), patients fighting the ventilator to "turn it off" (an expiratory imposed load), or patients actually initiating their next inspiratory effort just as the previous machine breath has terminated (see Fig. 9–11, right breath).

With conventional flow-targeted, volume-cycled breaths, breath termination occurs when the set volume is reached. Synchrony is attained by setting an appropriate volume. With pressure-targeted breaths,

breath termination can occur in several ways. The standard PS breath generally terminates at some low level of inspiratory flow (e.g., 5 L/min or 25–30% of peak flow). Duration and magnitude of patient effort thus can affect the T_i of a PS breath. However, other factors that affect the peak flow (e.g., the pressure support level and the rate of pressure rise, see Fig. 9–7) also can affect T_i. Therefore, the response of T_i to clinician manipulations of the PS breath sometimes can be difficult to predict.[31] Usually an adjustment in the inspiratory pressure or in the pressure rise time that results in more synchronous interactions produces a slowing of the ventilatory rate, an increase in the tidal volume, and maintenance or lengthening of the T_i.[24] Conversely, excessive inspiratory pressure levels may produce a premature termination of patient in-

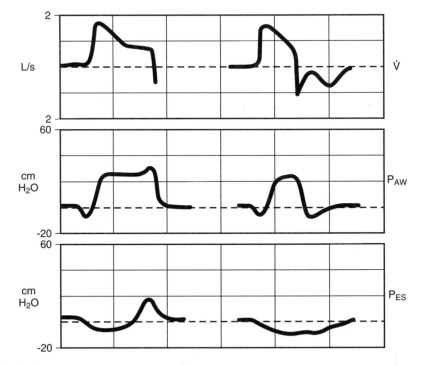

FIGURE 9–11

Two examples of cycling dys-synchrony. Depicted are airflow ($\dot{V}$, *upper panel*), airway pressure (P_{AW}, *middle panel*), and pleural pressure as estimated by esophageal pressure (P_{ES}, *lower panel*). In the left panel, breath cycling is delayed inappropriately for patient effort. As a consequence, patient expiratory effort is evident during the latter phases of ventilator gas delivery, elevating both P_{AW} and P_{ES}. In the right panel, breath cycling is inappropriately premature for patient effort. As a consequence, P_{AW} and P_{ES} are lowered during the ventilator expiratory phase, resulting in reduced expiratory flow (or even additional inspiratory flow). A subsequent premature triggering of a ventilator breath also could occur ("double pumping").

spiratory effort or even induce an expiratory effort.[24] An excessive rate of rise and peak flow also can cause premature termination because the cycling flow (25–30% of peak flow) is accordingly too high.

Two other ways also exist to affect termination of an interactive pressure-targeted breath. First, one can use the PA breaths (PACV with the mandatory rate set below the spontaneous rate). This allows the clinician to directly set the T_i. Both total and partial muscle unloading can be provided with the PA breath. This breath may be particularly useful in a patient in whom partial muscle unloading is appropriate but in whom cycling dys-synchrony occurs when standard pressure support is used. Second, one can provide a backup flow and volume guarantee during a pressure-targeted breath to ensure a minimal tidal volume.[27] This approach has been termed *volume-assured pressure support* (VAPS) or *pressure augmentation* and may be useful in adding pressure-targeted flow features to a patient in need of full unloading with volume-guaranteed breaths. It also may have utility in maintaining a minimal tidal volume in patients being weaned, using pressure-targeted breaths. A similar effect can be produced through feedback control of the inspiratory pressure level to ensure a desired tidal volume ("volume support" or "pressure-regulated volume control").

Imposed Expiratory Loads

Expiratory flow typically is generated from elastic recoil properties of the lung after termination of the inspiratory muscle activity. Expiratory muscles, however, also can contribute to expiratory alveolar pressure generation.

The only work associated with expiration should be that required to overcome airway resistance. In the ventilated patient, however, the endotracheal tube and exhalation valve assembly can produce a significant imposed load during expiration and interact with the patient's ventilatory drive accordingly.[31] Specifically, these expiratory loads can stimulate expiratory muscle contraction and affect the patient's ventilatory timing

mechanism—usually prolonging T_e with respect to T_i and increasing dyspnea and expiratory muscle energy expenditures. Wide-bore endotracheal tubes and threshold PEEP valves (instead of flow-resistive PEEP valves) commonly are used to reduce the potential dys-synchrony. Another approach is that of PEEP referenced to distal endotracheal tube pressures. Note that this approach may require the generation of a *negative* expiratory pressure in the circuit if tube resistance and/or expiratory flows are high.

Backup Ventilator Breaths

The purpose of a "backup" mandatory breath rate is to provide a minimal breath number guarantee during interactive modes. Several modes that have a clinician set breath rate already have been discussed. For instance, during volume or pressure-assist control, a minimal number of mandatory breaths are guaranteed if the patient's spontaneous rate falls below the set minimum ventilator rate. IMV (and APRV) also provides a set number of machine breaths. "Synchronized" IMV (SIMV) allows these breaths to be patient triggered if patient efforts are present. In SIMV, if the patient triggers the minimal number of assisted breaths, no mandatory controlled breaths are supplied.

A more sophisticated "backup" rate strategy activates mandatory breaths only if a certain minute ventilation is not achieved (e.g., mandatory minute ventilation, augmented minute ventilation, apnea ventilation). These strategies provide a guaranteed certain minimum minute ventilation that can increase to near total support if patient effort deteriorates. Ventilator breath synchrony of the ventilator delivered breaths depends on all the aforementioned factors.

FUTURE APPROACHES TO IMPROVING PATIENT–VENTILATOR SYNCHRONY

Future approaches to improving patient ventilator synchrony will be aimed at making interactive ventilatory support more sensitive and responsive to patient effort. One approach to this would be to improve the ability of the ventilator to sense patient effort. As noted previously, distal endotracheal tube sensors would seem to be a step forward, and pleural pressure signals would seem to be ideal.[18, 25] Clinically reliable sensors for such purposes, however, do not exist. Although theoretically attractive, phrenic nerve output as a driving signal for the ventilator pattern currently is not practical.

Improving valve sensitivity and responsiveness is also a goal for the future. Improved valve designs with better capabilities to separate noise from patient signal coupled with low resistance and low compliance circuitry are goals for the future.

Finally, an interesting alternate approach to flow- or pressure-targeted breaths has been the development of a flow-assist technique known as *proportional assist ventilation*.[32] This technique uses continuous feedback of inspiratory flow and then proportionally adjusts ventilator-delivered flow according to the desired level of muscle unloading. Provided that this feedback loop is sufficiently sensitive and responsive, this approach can offer a high level of patient–ventilator synchrony. Such systems, however, are only experimental at the present time.

REFERENCES

1. American College of Chest Physicians Consensus Group: Consensus conference on mechanical ventilation. Intensive Care Med 20:150–162, 1994.
2. MacIntyre NR: Synchronous and dys-synchronous patient ventilator interactions. In: Vincent JL (ed): Yearbook of Intensive Care and Emergency Medicine. Berlin: Springer-Verlag, 1992.
3. Marini JJ: Strategies to minimize breathing effort during mechanical ventilation. Crit Care Clin 6:635–661, 1990.
4. Banner MJ, Jaeger MJ, Kirby RR: Components of the work of breathing and implications for monitoring ventilator-dependent patients. Crit Care Med 22:515–523, 1994.
5. Ward ME, Corbert C, Gibbons W, et al: Optimization of respiratory muscle relaxation during mechanical ventilation. Anesthesiology 69:29–35, 1988.
6. Berger AJ, Mitchell RA, Severinghaus JW: Regulation of respiration. N Engl J Med 297:92–101, 1977.
7. Mead J: Control of respiratory frequency. J Appl Physiol 15:325–336, 1960.
8. Milic-Emili J: Recent advances in clinical assessment of control of breathing. Lung 160:1–17, 1982.
9. Bellemare F, Grassino A: Effect of pressure and timing of contraction on human diaphragm failure. J Appl Physiol 53:1190–1195, 1982.
10. Luijendijk SC, Milic-Emili J: Breathing patterns in anesthetized cats and the concept of minimum respiratory effort. J Appl Physiol 64:31–41, 1988.
11. Cohen CA, Zagelbaum G, Gross D, et al: Clinical manifestation of inspiratory muscle fatigue. Am J Med 73:308–316, 1982.
12. Tobin MJ, Perez W, Guenther SH, et al: The pattern of breathing during successful and unsuccessful trials of weaning from mechanical ventilation. Am Rev Respir Dis 134:1111–1118, 1986.
13. Gallagher CG, Hof VI, Younes M: Effect of inspiratory muscle fatigue on breathing pattern. J Appl Physiol 59:1152–1158, 1986.
14. Aubier M, Murciano D, Fournier M, et al: Central respiratory drive in acute respiratory failure of patients with chronic obstructive pulmonary disease. Am Rev Respir Dis 122:191–199, 1980.
15. MacIntyre NR, Leatherman NE: Ventilatory muscle loads and the frequency-tidal volume pattern during inspiratory pressure-supported ventilation. Am Rev Respir Dis 141:327–331, 1990.
16. American Association for Respiratory Care. Positive end expiratory pressure: state of the art after 20 years. Respir Care 33:417–500, 1988.
17. American Association for Respiratory Care: Consensus statement on essentials of mechanical ventilators. Respir Care 37:1000–1008, 1992.
18. Banner MJ, Blanch PB, Kirby RR: Imposed work of breathing and methods of triggering a demand flow CPAP system. Crit Care Med 21:183–191, 1993.
19. Sassoon C SH: Mechanical ventilator design and function: the trigger variable. Respir Care 37:1056–1069, 1992.
20. Katz J, Kraemer R, Gjerde GE: Inspiratory work and airway pressure with continuous positive airway pressure delivery systems. Chest 88:519–526, 1985.
21. Gay PG, Rodarte JR, Hubmayr RD: The effects of positive expiratory pressure on isovolumic flow and dynamic hyperinflation in patients receiving mechanical ventilation. Am Rev Respir Dis 139:621–626, 1989.
22. Hirsch C, Kacmarek RM, Stanek K: Work of breathing during CPAP and PSV imposed by the new generation mechanical ventilators: a lung model study. Respir Care 36:815–828, 1991.
23. Marini JJ, Smith TC, Lamb VJ: External work output and force generation during synchronized intermittent mechanical ventilation. Am Rev Respir Dis 138:1169–1179, 1988.
24. Ho L, MacIntyre NR: Effects of initial flow rate and breath termination criteria on pressure support ventilation. Chest 99:134–138, 1991.
25. MacIntyre NR, Nishimura M, Usada Y, et al: The

Nagoya conference on system design and patient–ventilator interactions during pressure support ventilation. Chest 97:1463–1466, 1990.

26. Tokioka H, Saito S, Kosaka F: Comparison of pressure support ventilation and assist control ventilation in patients with acute respiratory failure. Intensive Care Med 15:364–367, 1989.

27. Haas CF, Branson RD, Folk LM, et al: Patient determined inspiratory flow during assisted mechanical ventilation. Respir Care 40:716–721, 1995.

28. MacIntyre NR, McConnell R, Cheng KG, Sane A: Patient-ventilator flow dys-synchrony: flow limited versus pressure limited breaths. Crit Care Med 25:1671–1677, 1997.

29. Imsand C, Feihl F, Perret C, Fitting JW: Regulation of inspiratory neuromuscular output during synchronized intermittent mechanical ventilation. Anesthesiology 80:13–22, 1994.

30. Fiastro JF, Habib MP, Quan SF: Pressure support compensation for inspiratory work due to endotracheal tubes and demand continuous positive airway pressure. Chest 93:499–505, 1988.

31. Marini JJ, Kirk W, Culver BH: Flow resistance of the exhalation valves and PEEP devices used in mechanical ventilation. Am Rev Respir Dis 131:850–854, 1985.

32. Younes M: Proportional assist ventilation, a new approach to ventilatory support. Am Rev Respir Dis 145:114–120, 1992.

CHAPTER 10

The Effects of Respiratory Support on the Cardiovascular System

Jon N. Meliones, MD, MS, FCCM

GOALS OF THE CARDIORESPIRATORY SYSTEM

RESPIRATORY INTERVENTIONS

CARDIORESPIRATORY INTERACTIONS

Effect of Ventilatory Manipulations on Right Ventricular Preload

Effect of Ventilatory Manipulations on Right Ventricular Afterload

Effect of Ventilatory Manipulations on Left Ventricular Preload and Afterload

THERAPY FOR SPECIFIC PATHOPHYSIOLOGIC CONDITIONS

Right Ventricular Dysfunction and Pulmonary Artery Hypertension

Left Ventricular Dysfunction

RESPIRATORY FAILURE

REFERENCES

KEY WORDS

cardiopulmonary interactions
high-frequency jet ventilation
pulmonary artery

hypertension
right ventricular dysfunction

It is not uncommon for clinicians who care for patients with heart disease to underappreciate how alterations in respiratory physiology significantly have an impact on several important outcome variables in patients, including length of ventilation, length of stay, morbidity, and mortality.[1] Although the respiratory system is affected most by positive-pressure ventilation (PPV), the cardiovascular system also is affected. Cardiorespiratory interactions occur because pulmonary and systemic circulation are in series and the lungs and chest wall physically surround the heart and great vessels, exposing them to intrathoracic pressure. As a result of this intimate relationship, the cardiovascular and respiratory systems cannot be thought of independently and should be considered to function as a single unit. For a variety of reasons, the effects of **cardiopulmonary interactions** are exaggerated in patients with heart disease.[2] Therefore, providing effective respiratory support requires an understanding of the physiology of the respiratory system under normal and pathologic conditions and also the cardiorespiratory consequences of these processes. This chapter provides the basis for determining respiratory support by using the principles of cardiorespiratory interactions to develop a pathophysiology-based approach for respiratory support.

GOALS OF THE CARDIORESPIRATORY SYSTEM

The primary goals of the cardiorespiratory system are to provide adequate oxygen delivery to meet the metabolic demands and to eliminate the carbon dioxide that is generated.[3] Achieving these goals requires a variety of interactions between the cardiovascular and respiratory systems. If the cardiorespiratory system fails to supply adequate oxygen to meet the metabolic demands, anaerobic metabolism occurs, which results in acidosis and, ultimately, organ dysfunction.[3, 4] Therefore, a crucial balance develops between oxygen supply versus oxygen demands; the goal of cardiorespiratory management is to optimize this relationship. Abnormalities in the oxygen supply:demand ratio are the primary cause of abnormal convalescence.[2]

RESPIRATORY INTERVENTIONS

Respiratory interventions can increase oxygen delivery by increasing both oxygen content and cardiac output. A variety of respiratory manipulations increase oxygen content by increasing arterial oxygen percent saturation (SaO_2) and arterial oxygen pressure (PaO_2). These interventions are described in detail elsewhere; this chapter focuses on how respiratory manipulations alter cardiac output.[5]

The respiratory interventions used in patients can be categorized into three groups: different modes of conventional PPV, nonconventional ventilation, and inhaled medical gases.[6] Currently, there are multiple different modes of conventional PPV available in the intensive care environment. Because infants and children are sensitive to alterations in airway pressure, several nonconventional approaches have been used extensively in this patient population. A full discussion of these approaches is beyond the scope of this chapter, but several review articles present a more elaborate evaluation of these approaches.[5, 7] The two most common nonconventional modes of ventilation include **high-frequency jet ventilation** (HFJV) and high-frequency oscillatory ventilation (HFOV). By employing rapid respiratory rates and a lower peak inspiratory pressure (PIP), HFJV provides alveolar ventilation similar to conventional ventilation but allows a lower mean airway pressure.[7–9] The lowering of mean airway pressure, as described subsequently, may be beneficial in patients with ventricular dysfunction.[8, 9] In contrast, HFOV employs a higher mean airway pressure than conventional ventilation and should be used cautiously in patients with ventricular dysfunction.

CARDIORESPIRATORY INTERACTIONS

The importance of cardiorespiratory interactions in the management of critically ill patients with respiratory and cardiovascular disease is being realized only currently. Alterations in intrathoracic processes are transmitted to cardiac structures and can dramatically alter cardiovascular performance. Alterations in cardiovascular performance may be more dramatic in neonates and children than in adults for a number of reasons. First, ventricular dysfunction can be particularly severe in infants and children after cardiac surgery. In infants, the myocardium is immature and intrinsically noncompliant, and surgical interventions may require transmyocardial incisions and intracardiac repair. Congenital cardiac surgery also requires the placement of prosthetic material into the heart, which can disrupt normal myocardial architecture and function, resulting in myocardial injury, myocardial edema, and abnormal ventricular function.[2] These factors cause the neonatal myocardium to be sensitive to minor alterations in preload and afterload after cardiac surgery.

A second factor is the myocardial wall tension generated. The myocardium of neonates and young children generates a low pressure. Therefore, small changes in intrathoracic pressure can lead to large changes in transmural pressure gradients ($P_{transmural}$ = $P_{intracardiac}$ − $P_{pleural}$). In contrast, the adult myocardium generates a higher intraventricular pressure, resulting in only minimal changes in the transmural pressure gradients for a given change in intrathoracic pressure. Transmural pressure gradients affect cardiovascular performance because they contribute to myocardial wall tension. Because small changes in intrathoracic pressure result in a more dramatic change in myocardial wall tension, PPV has a more dramatic effect on ventricular function in infants and children than on adult patients.

Finally, the pulmonary and systemic circulations of neonates and children have a high smooth muscle content and are highly reactive to alterations in intrathoracic processes. Minor changes in intrathoracic pressure and lung volume can alter the afterload imparted on the right and left ventricle, which results in altered ventricular wall stress and performance.

Respiratory interventions primarily affect cardiac output by altering ventricular preload and afterload. Although minor alterations in heart rate and intrinsic contractility may be appreciated, they play a minimal role in modulating cardiac output.

Effect of Ventilatory Manipulations on Right Ventricular Preload

The initiation of PPV modifies cardiovascular performance by increasing intrathoracic pressure or altering lung volume. Important differences exist between the physiologic response of the right ventricle (RV) and left ventricle (LV) to alterations in intrathoracic pressures and lung volumes. The RV is extremely sensitive to alterations in intrathoracic pressure for a variety of reasons. Venous return to the right side of the heart is passive and occurs as a result of pressure gradients between the systemic venous system and the right atrium. When the right atrial pressure is 0 mm Hg, there is no resistance to flow from the systemic veins to the right atrium, and systemic venous return is maximum (Fig. 10–1). As right atrial pressure increases, there is an increase in resistance to blood flow to the right atrium, which results in a reduction of venous return and RV preload. During spontaneous breathing, right atrial pressure is low, impedance to blood flow to the

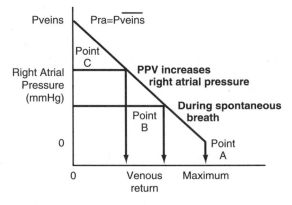

FIGURE 10–1

Venous return to the right heart occurs passively and is dependent on a pressure gradient from the systemic veins to the right atrium. When right atrial pressure (P_{ra}) is 0, there is no impedance to flow back to the right heart and venous return is maximum (point A). As right atrial pressure is increased and mean systemic venous pressure (P_{veins}) is held constant, there is a progressive reduction in venous return. When right atrial pressure exceeds mean systemic venous pressure, venous return ceases. During spontaneous breathing, right atrial pressure is low and systemic venous return is high (point B). During positive-pressure ventilation (PPV), intrathoracic pressure and right atrial pressure increase, resulting in a reduction of venous return (point C). P_{veins}, mean venous pressure. (Modified from Robotham JL, Lixfeld W, Holland L: The effects of PEEP on right and left ventricular performance. Am Rev Respir Dis 121:677, 1980. © American Lung Association.)

right heart is low, and venous return is high. PPV alters RV preload by increasing intrathoracic pressure. During PPV and/or positive end-expiratory pressure (PEEP), the increase in intrathoracic pressure is transmitted to the right heart, resulting in an increase in right atrial pressure. The increase in right atrial pressure causes an increase in resistance to flow into the right heart, and RV preload decreases. Therefore, PPV and PEEP may reduce RV performance by decreasing preload. Because there is no extrathoracic ventricular chamber that can compensate for changes in intrathoracic pressures, even small changes in intrathoracic pressure may result in significant alterations in RV filling.[8–10] In contrast to PPV, negative pressure ventilation has been shown to significantly increase right ventricular filling in conditions in which filling is decreased.[11] In a series of patients after surgery for tetralogy of Fallot, a significant increase in right ventricular filling and cardiac output was noted after conversion to negative pressure ventilation. This was the result of a reduction in right atrial and right ventricular end-diastolic pressure, which improves the venous return to the right heart.

Effect of Ventilatory Manipulations on Right Ventricular Afterload

The RV has been shown to be exquisitely sensitive to changes in intrathoracic processes that alter pulmonary vascular resistance. RV afterload is influenced by a variety of intrathoracic processes. One modulator of RV afterload is lung volume (Fig. 10–2). At low lung volumes, the lung is atelectatic, and pulmonary vascular resistance is high because of increased vascular resistance from hypoxic pulmonary vasoconstriction and the tortuous course of large- to medium-sized blood vessels that supply the lung.[10, 12, 13] As lung volume increases, the large vessels become linear, their capacitance increases, hypoxia subsides, and vascular resistance decreases. As lung volumes continue to increase, hyperexpansion of the alveoli and compression of the pulmonary capillaries occur, and vascular resistance in-

creases. The total pulmonary vascular resistance is the sum of these two forces. Pulmonary vascular resistance is high when the lung is atelectatic or overexpanded. PPV and/or PEEP can promote a reduction of RV afterload in patients with low lung volumes by expanding collapsed lung units and reducing vascular resistance. However, when tidal volume is excessive, PPV and/or PEEP can result in an increase in RV afterload because of alveolar expansion and compression of the capillaries. In patients with RV dysfunction and/or pulmonary artery hypertension, this response is exaggerated.[14]

RV afterload can be altered by increasing arterial pH. Both a metabolic alkalosis and a respiratory alkalosis cause a reduction in pulmonary artery pressure and RV afterload.[15] This implicates the hydrogen ion and not the $PaCO_2$ in modulating pulmonary vascular tone during alkalosis. Creating a metabolic alkalosis may be a preferred strategy because it allows a reduction in RV afterload without negatively affecting RV preload. In contrast, a respiratory alkalosis while reducing RV afterload may reduce RV preload by increasing intrathoracic pressure.

Another dramatic approach to altering RV afterload is the use of nitric oxide. The use of nitric oxide in a variety of clinical conditions is explained elsewhere. For the purpose of this chapter, however, it should be noted that in selected physiologic conditions, nitric oxide has been shown to lower pulmonary artery pressure and right ventricular afterload.[16–19]

Effect of Ventilatory Manipulations on Left Ventricular Preload and Afterload

The changes that occur in left ventricular preload in response to PPV are not well understood. Three physiologic principles have been proposed to explain why left ventricular preload is decreased in certain instances during PPV and PEEP. First, the LV can only eject the quantity of blood that it receives from the RV (ventricular interdependence).[20–22] Because RV cardiac output may be decreased during PPV, the LV re-

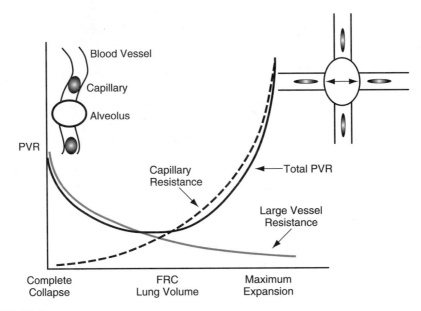

FIGURE 10–2

Pulmonary vascular resistance is dependent on lung volume and the sum of the resistance contributed by the large- to medium-sized pulmonary vessels and pulmonary capillaries. At lung volumes less than functional residual capacity, the lungs become atelectatic and pulmonary vascular resistance is high because of hypoxic pulmonary vasoconstriction and the increased resistance contributed by the tortuous large and medium-sized vessels. As lung volume increases, the alveoli become overexpanded and pulmonary vascular resistance falls. High lung volumes are associated with an increase in pulmonary vascular resistance because of increased resistance contributed by compression of the pulmonary capillaries. FRC, functional residual capacity; PVR, pulmonary vascular resistance. (Modified from West JB, Dollery CT: Distribution of pulmonary arterial flow variation during respiration. J Appl Physiol 19:713, 1964, with permission.)

ceives a decreased quantity of blood, and left ventricular preload falls. Second, RV afterload and RV systolic pressure increase during PPV. The increase in RV pressure results in conformational changes in the intraventricular septum and a decrease in left ventricular compliance and left ventricular preload. Finally, direct compression of the LV from the increase in intrathoracic pressure may further reduce preload. All these factors may contribute to a reduction of left ventricular preload during PPV and PEEP. This may be an advantageous strategy in patients with congestive LV failure.

One ventilatory strategy designed to improve left ventricular preload employs thoracic pump augmentation of left ventricular filling.[20–22] Thoracic pump augmentation of left ventricular filling is a phasic increase in thoracic pressure similar to what has been proposed as a mechanism for increasing cardiac output during chest compressions with cardiopulmonary resuscitation.[20–22] Unlike the RV, the LV derives its preload from intrathoracic sources. Therefore, a phasic increase in intrathoracic pressure is transmitted to the pulmonary circuit, resulting in an increase in pulmonary vascular pressures. Because the pulmonary vascular pressures are increased above left-sided filling pressures, an augmentation of left ventricular preload has been demonstrated.[20–22] Whether these transient changes in left ventricular filling result in tangible increases in cardiac output has not been resolved.

LV afterload can be altered by respiratory interventions through complex interactions. LV afterload is dependent on left ventricular myocardial wall tension.[20–22] LV wall tension is dependent on the pressure generated by the ventricle during systole and can be approximated by examining the difference between the left ventricular systolic pressure and intrathoracic pressure (left ventricular wall tension = $P_{LV} - P_{intrathoracic}$). LV wall tension can be reduced by either decreasing aortic pressure and, therefore, left ventricular pressure, or by increasing intrathoracic pressure. The effect of PPV on left ventricular wall tension is complex because the systemic arterial system consists of both intrathoracic and extrathoracic components. During PPV, the increase in intrathoracic pressure is transmitted rapidly to the intrathoracic arterial system. LV wall tension remains the same, however, because both the left ventricular pressure generated and the intrathoracic pressure generated are equal. For example, if LV wall tension = P_{LV} (100 mm Hg) $- P_{intrathoracic}$ (10 mm Hg) = 90 mm Hg, an increase in intrathoracic pressure by 30 mm Hg causes no net change in LV wall tension = P_{LV} (130 mm Hg) $- P_{intrathoracic}$ (40 mm Hg) = 90 mm Hg. However, the extrathoracic arterial system also develops an increase in arterial pressure because of propagation of the increased arterial pressure into the periphery. When the increase in intrathoracic pressure results in a significant increase in arterial pressure, aortic pressure is autoregulated because of baroreceptor stimulation. This results in a reflexive decrease in aortic pressure and a compensatory reduction of left ventricular pressure occurs. When aortic pressure returns to baseline as a result of this reflexive action, the left ventricular systolic pressure falls and the transmyocardial pressure gradient falls. Using the previous example, if LV wall tension = P_{LV} (100 mm Hg) $- P_{intrathoracic}$ (10 mm Hg) = 90 mm Hg, with an increase in intrathoracic pressure by 30 mm Hg and a return of aortic pressure to 100 mm Hg, LV wall tension = P_{LV} (100 mm Hg) $- P_{intrathoracic}$ (40 mm Hg) = 60 mm Hg. Therefore, the end result of a persistent increase in intrathoracic pressure is a decrease in left ventricular wall tension (decreased afterload), as a consequence of aortic pressure autoregulation. Under usual clinical conditions, intrathoracic pressure is low compared with left ventricular pressure, and inspiration occurs over only one to two cardiac cycles. This results in only minor phasic changes in left ventricular afterload because autoregulation may not occur. How-

ever, if intrathoracic pressure is high and the increased intrathoracic pressure occurs over multiple cardiac cycles (as occurs with PEEP), left ventricular afterload can be reduced. Clinicians should be aware of these interactions, especially in patients with congestive heart failure with ventricular dysfunction and concomitant respiratory dysfunction. Clinical signs that suggest that a patient may be experiencing these important cardiorespiratory interactions include wide fluctuations in arterial tracing during inspiration. If this is observed, and improvements in left ventricular performance are the goal, the clinician should consider respiratory strategies that optimize intrathoracic pressure to augment left ventricular performance.

THERAPY FOR SPECIFIC PATHOPHYSIOLOGIC CONDITIONS

Right Ventricular Dysfunction and Pulmonary Artery Hypertension

Patients with **RV dysfunction** and **pulmonary artery hypertension** benefit from manipulations of cardiorespiratory interactions designed to optimize RV preload and minimize RV afterload. Patients with RV dysfunction are particularly sensitive to changes in intrathoracic pressure because cardiac output is preload dependent. These patients may benefit from ventilation strategies that reduce intrathoracic pressure and increase preload, such as reducing the mean airway pressure and limiting PEEP. This can be accomplished by minimizing PIP, decreasing inspiratory time, and adjusting to the lowest PEEP that maintains functional residual capacity. The RV response to ventilatory manipulations is more dramatic in patients with concomitant hypovolemia because RV preload is already marginal. Therefore, strict attention to intravascular volume status is required in patients with RV dysfunction and elevated intrathoracic pressures. Pulmonary artery pressures and RV afterload may be reduced by hyperoxygenation and alkalinization. If a respiratory alkalosis requires an increase in airway pressure, a metabolic alkalosis should be created and alveolar partial pressure of carbon dioxide ($PaCO_2$) maintained in the low-to-normal range ($PaCO_2 = 30$–35 torr). Exogenous nitric oxide has become an important respiratory intervention in patients with pulmonary artery hypertension. In selected patients, nitric oxide has been shown to reduce pulmonary artery pressures and increase oxygen delivery.[16–19]

Because of the detrimental effects of PPV on RV dynamics, alternate modes of ventilation have been used in patients with pulmonary hypertension and RV dysfunction. Because HFJV reduces mean airway pressure and pulmonary vascular resistance while maintaining a similar or lower $PaCO_2$, it should be suited ideally for patients with RV dysfunction and/or pulmonary artery hypertension. In selected patients, HFJV has been shown to decrease mean airway pressure, decrease pulmonary vascular resistance, and increase oxygen delivery and should be considered when mean airway pressure is elevated.[8, 9] Negative pressure ventilation, as described previously, may have a dramatic benefit in selected patients with RV dysfunction.[11] Negative pressure ventilation appears to be the preferred mode of ventilation in patients with RV dysfunction.

Left Ventricular Dysfunction

In patients with left ventricular dysfunction, cardiorespiratory interactions should be directed at optimizing left ventricular function through a variety of approaches. The ventilatory strategy for patients with left ventricular dysfunction and decreased preload consists of using thoracic augmentation of left ventricular filling to augment filling. Reducing mean airway pressure as low as possible to permit appropriate filling of the ventricles also may prove beneficial in clinical conditions in which LV preload is low. In patients with congestive heart failure, however, increasing PEEP to limit LV preload may prove beneficial.

RESPIRATORY FAILURE

Respiratory failure occurs in patients with ventricular dysfunction. When respiratory failure does occur, a devastating combination of cardiorespiratory failure can ensue.[1] In these instances, it is essential to maintain lung volumes by titration of PEEP. However, this should be done cautiously because increases in PEEP may compromise cardiac output and necessitate administration of intravenous fluid to optimize oxygen delivery. These patients are best managed with Swan-Ganz catheterization directed at optimizing oxygen delivery. Nonconventional modes, including both HFJV and HFOV, may be considered when mean airway pressure is elevated significantly.

Respiratory support for patients requires a thorough understanding of cardiorespiratory performance. The primary goal of the cardiorespiratory system is to optimize the oxygen supply/demand relationship. If abnormal convalescence occurs, the presence of coexisting cardiovascular abnormalities must be considered. Using the principles of cardiac function, respiratory physiology, and cardiorespiratory interactions, a management strategy then can be developed that is matched to the pathophysiology that has caused the oxygen supply/demand abnormality. Using these principles, clinicians can maximize patient care and improve outcome variables.

REFERENCES

1. Kocis KC, Meliones JN, Dekeon MK, Bove EL: High-frequency jet ventilation for respiratory failure following congenital heart surgery. Circulation 84(suppl 4):II-142, 1991.
2. Meliones JN, Nichols D, Wetzel RC, Greeley WJ: Perioperative management of patients with congenital heart disease: a multidisciplinary approach In: Nichols D, Cameron DE, Greeley WJ, et al (eds): Critical Heart Disease in Infants and Children. St. Louis: Mosby–Year Book, 1998, pp 553–580.
3. Shoemaker WC, et al: Hemodynamic and oxygen transport monitoring to titrate therapy in septic shock. New Horizons 1:145–159, 1993.
4. Robotham JL, Lixfeld W, Holland L, et al: The effects of positive end-respiratory pressure on right and left ventricular performance. Am Rev Respir Dis 121:677, 1980.
5. Meliones JN, Martin LD, Barnes SD, et al: Respiratory support. In: Nichols D, Cameron DE, Greeley WJ, et al (eds): Critical Heart Disease in Infants and Children. St. Louis: Mosby–Year Book, 1998, pp 335–367.

6. Abrahams E, Yoshihara G: Cardiorespiratory effects of pressure controlled ventilation in severe respiratory failure. Chest 98:1445–1449, 1990.
7. Meliones JN, Leonard RA: High frequency ventilation in critical care. Trauma Q 14:24–28, 1994.
8. Meliones JN, et al: High-frequency jet ventilation improves cardiac function after the Fontan procedure. Circulation 84(suppl III):III-364–III-368, 1991.
9. Hayes JK, Smith KW, Port JD, et al: Comparison of tidal ventilation and high-frequency jet ventilation before and after cardiopulmonary bypass in dogs using two-dimensional transesophageal echocardiography. J Cardiothorac Vasc Anesth 51:320–326, 1991.
10. West JB, Dollery CT: Distribution of blood flow in isolated lung: relation to vascular and alveolar pressures. J Appl Physiol 19:713, 1964.
11. Shekerdemian LS, Shore DF, Lincoln C, et al: Negative-pressure ventilation improves cardiac output after right heart surgery. Circulation 94:II-49–II-55, 1996.
12. West JB: Respiratory Physiology—The Essentials. Baltimore: Williams & Wilkins, 1979.
13. Pinsky MR: Determinants of pulmonary arterial flow variation during respiration. J Appl Physiol 56:1237, 1984.
14. Tyler DC: Positive end respiratory pressure: a review. Crit Care Med 11:300–308, 1983.
15. Malik AB, Kidd SL: Independent effects of changes in H^+ and CO_2 concentrations on hypoxic pulmonary vasoconstriction. J Appl Physiol 34:318–323, 1973.
16. Wessel DL, Adatia I, Giglia TM, et al: Use of inhaled nitric oxide and acetylcholine in the evaluation of pulmonary hypertension and endothelial function after cardiopulmonary bypass. Circulation 88(5 part 1):2128–2138, 1993.
17. Roberts JD, Chen TK, Kawai N, et al: Inhaled nitric oxide in congenital heart disease. Circulation 87:447–553, 1993.
18. Wessel DL, Adaita I, Thompson JE, Hickey PR: Delivery and monitoring of inhaled nitric oxide in patients with pulmonary hypertension Crit Care Med 22:930–938, 1994.
19. Puybassett L, Stewart T, Rouby JJ, et al: Inhaled nitric oxide reverses the increase in pulmonary vascular resistance induced by permissive hypercapnia in patients with acute respiratory distress syndrome. Anesthesiology 80:1254–1257, 1994.
20. Pinsky MR, Summer WR: Cardiac augmentation by phasic high intrathoracic pressure support in man. Chest 84:370–375, 1983.
21. Pinsky MR, Summer WR, Wise RA: Cardiac augmentation by elevation of intrathoracic pressure. J Appl Physiol 54:950–955, 1983.
22. Meliones JN, Snider AR, Dekeon MK, et al: Effects of ventilation on diastolic filling after cardiac surgery. J Am Coll Cardiol 19:52A, 1992.

Lung Injury from Mechanical Ventilation

Nancy W. Knudsen, MD
William J. Fulkerson, MD

PNEUMOTHORAX,
PNEUMOMEDIASTINUM,
AND PULMONARY
INTERSTITIAL EMPHYSEMA
"STRETCH-INDUCED"
ACUTE LUNG INJURY

Experimental Studies
Clinical Studies
REFERENCES

KEY WORDS

barotrauma/volutrauma	overdistension	pressure-volume plots
lung protective strategy	permissive hypercapnia	recruitment

Mechanical ventilation has been a mainstay of intensive care support of patients with respiratory failure for decades. However, mechanical ventilation may be associated with serious lung injury. Modern case series of patients with acute respiratory distress syndrome (ARDS) reveal a mortality rate of approximately 40%, and some have questioned the contribution of current treatment modalities to the morbidity and mortality of respiratory failure. For years, ventilator-associated lung injury was synonymous with "**barotrauma**" manifested as pneumothoraces or pneumomediastinum. The potential for ventilator-induced endothelial and epithelial cell injury, which results in lung damage morphologically indistinguishable from other causes of ARDS, also has been recognized.

PNEUMOTHORAX, PNEUMOMEDIASTINUM, AND PULMONARY INTERSTITIAL EMPHYSEMA

Injuries secondary to mechanical ventilation can range from the emergent to the subtle. Pneumothorax, pneumomediastinum, and pulmonary interstitial emphysema are recognizable clinical and radiographic manifestations of alveolar **overdistention** and its sequelae.

Macklin and Macklin performed necropsies in a number of patients dying of respiratory failure with clinically recognized pneumomediastinum.[1] They found dissection of air along vascular sheaths passing to the mediastinum, subcutaneous tissue, and retroperitoneum. In other experiments, they were able to determine that the site of air escape was the alveolar base where it contacted the vascular sheaths. A gradient between the alveolus and vascular sheath was postulated to produce alveolar rupture and interstitial emphysema. Studies by Polak and Adams demonstrated that high airway pressure alone was insufficient to cause alveolar rupture.[2] Using a canine model, lungs were inflated with large volumes of air, but expansion of the lungs was limited by thoracic binding. The marked elevation of alveolar pressure was matched by elevation in the supporting pressure on the outside of the chest, thus avoiding a severe gradient between the intra-alveolar and extra-alveolar pressures. Under these conditions, the alveoli did not rupture.

Caldwell and associates likewise showed that the frequency of lesions induced by large alveolar volumes was decreased in animals with restricted chest movement.[3] They concluded that airway pressure itself was not the primary cause of perivascular interstitial emphysema and that excessive alveolar volume was the likely factor leading to alveolar rupture and air dissection.

One of the most common clinical manifestations of extra-alveolar air is pneumothorax. Zwillich and colleagues identified 15 episodes of pneumothorax in 354 patients mechanically ventilated for more than 24 hours.[4] Four of the 15 pneumothoraces occurred in patients with right mainstem bronchus intubation, emphasizing the importance of alveolar overdistension in the pathogenesis. In this series, pneumothorax did not correlate with decreased survival. There was a significant association between the patients' age and the incidence of pneumothorax, with more frequent complication in patients younger than age 30.

Fleming and associates reported a 15% incidence of pneumothorax in mechanically ventilated patients in the 24th Evacuation Hospital in Viet Nam.[5] In its most serious form, a pneumothorax can develop very high intrathoracic pressures that can seriously impair both ventilation and cardiac filling (tension pneumothorax) and can cause death if not treated rapidly. Pontoppidan noted that tension pneumothorax occurred more frequently in patients with underlying chronic obstructive lung disease who were on mechanical ventilation.[6]

Abnormal air collections must be recognized on the chest radiograph, especially if the patient is mechanically ventilated. As noted previously, spontaneous or iatrogenic pneumothoraces may enlarge rapidly with positive pressure ventilation, creating a tension pneumothorax. In a patient without pleural adhesions, air in a pneumothorax rises to the highest part of the pleural space. When the patient is erect, pleural air accumulates at the apex of the thorax. If the patient is supine when the radiograph is obtained, however, the highest part of the pleural space is over the anterior surface of the lung, and a small pneumothorax may be difficult to detect. A pneumothorax may appear only as a hazy lucency over the lung in this circumstance, but there are associated signs of increased volume in the affected hemithorax as the air collection enlarges. A characteristic finding, the *deep sulcus sign*, may be the only manifestation of an enlarging tension pneumothorax (Fig. 11–1). This results from air collecting and expanding over the anterior part of the lower lung field, causing depression of the ipsilateral diaphragm from expanding air

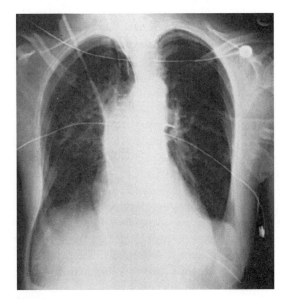

FIGURE 11–1

Supine chest radiograph illustrating the "deep sulcus" sign of a pneumothorax.

under pressure. A high degree of suspicion is necessary, and erect or decubitus views of the lung may be helpful, to investigate further the possibility of pneumothorax.

Subcutaneous emphysema is seen commonly in pulmonary barotrauma. It may be present with or without pneumothorax. Subcutaneous emphysema is usually most prominent in the head and neck. Palpable subcutaneous emphysema also can be found at very distal sites, however, such as the feet and abdomen. Although this usually is not a life-threatening complication, its presence should be interpreted by the clinician to mean that more serious and potentially life-threatening complications are likely unless the course of events is reversed or ventilator management is altered.

Pneumoperitoneum generally follows pneumomediastinum and results from air dissecting into the retroperitoneal space initially.[7] The periotoneum itself may rupture, leading to free intraperitoneal air. Occasionally, this may be painful and almost always presents a diagnostic dilemma that must be differentiated from a rupture of an intra-abdominal viscus. Severe pneumoperitoneum also may interfere with effective mechanical ventilation. Evacuation of a pneumoperitoneum occasionally is attempted, but it is usually unsuccessful. Pulmonary interstitial emphysema reflects the dissection of air along vascular sheaths after alveolar rupture. It frequently is difficult to recognize on the chest radiograph and may be mistaken for air bronchograms. A "salt-and-pepper" appearance of the radiograph is characteristic.

Less commonly, systemic air embolism can occur with disastrous results. Marini and Culver described two critically ill patients in whom recurrent episodes of cerebral infarction, myocardial infarction, and livedo reticularis developed while they were supported by mechanical ventilation.[8] In both patients, pre-existing extra-alveolar air collections had enlarged before the catastrophic clinical events took place. The pathophysiology of this event appears to be an extension of processes leading to interstitial emphysema and pneumothorax.

"STRETCH-INDUCED" ACUTE LUNG INJURY

Experimental Studies

Numerous investigators have shown pulmonary edema formation in animals after artificial ventilation employing high peak inspiratory pressure and tidal volumes.[9-17] Webb and Tierney were the first to convincingly demonstrate this phenomenon.[9] Rats were ventilated mechanically with peak inspiratory pressure (PIP) of 14, 30, and 45 cm H_2O. In those animals ventilated with 30 and 45 cm H_2O pressure, pulmonary edema developed rapidly. Parker and colleagues demonstrated increased microvascular permeability to fluid and protein after high peak inspiratory pressure (PIP) ventilation in dogs.[11] Various other animal models had no change in lung compliance when ventilated with PIP less than 25 cm H_2O for periods of up to 48 hours.[9-13] However, when PIP was greater than 25 cm H_2O, pulmonary edema and worsening lung compliance occurred.[9, 12, 15] Dreyfuss and associates investigated varying levels of inspiratory pressure and edema formation.[16] Thirty-two rats were divided into four groups and were ventilated for a total of 30 minutes at different levels of inspiratory pressure. High inspiratory pressures were achieved by increasing tidal volume and decreasing the respiratory rate as needed to prevent alkalosis. At the same time, labeled albumin and sodium were injected to monitor edema formation. Group I animals were ventilated for 30 minutes at PIP of 7 cm H_2O and a respiratory rate of 40 breaths/min; group II was ventilated for 25 minutes at PIP of 7 cm H_2O and 5 minutes at PIP of 45 cm H_2O; group III was ventilated for 20 minutes at PIP of 7 cm H_2O and 10 minutes at PIP of 45 cm H_2O; group IV was ventilated for 10 minutes at PIP of 7 cm H_2O and 20 minutes at PIP of 45 cm H_2O. The gross appearance of lungs was normal in all groups except for group IV, which showed marked congestion. There was also edema fluid present in the trachea in six of eight group IV animals. There was no difference in pulmonary edema between groups II and III. The albumin and sodium labeling demonstrated an association between increased pulmonary edema formation and duration of high PIP ventilation. Group IV animals were the only ones to demonstrate alveolar edema. The authors concluded that direct parenchymal injury and altered microvascular permeability is associated with high PIP and may result in pulmonary edema.

Kolobow and associates[12] observed the effects of PIP of 50 cm H_2O on sheep ventilated for 48 hours. Study end points were 48 hours of ventilation, death, development of pneumothorax, severe changes on chest radiography, a decrease in partial pressure of oxygen (PO_2) to less than 60 mm Hg, or a decrease in functional residual capacity (FRC) of 50%. The lungs were graded for atelectasis and pneumothorax by autopsy and chest radiography. Twenty-five sheep were divided into three groups. Group A consisted of nine sheep ventilated with tidal volumes of 8 to 15 ml/kg, respiratory rate of 15 breaths/min, inspired oxygen concentration (FiO_2) of 40%, positive end-expiratory pressure (PEEP) 6 to 8 cm H_2O, and PIP less than 20 cm H_2O; group B consisted of seven sheep with PIP of 50 cm H_2O and a respiratory rate of 1.5 to 3 breaths/min; group C consisted of nine sheep with PIP of 50 cm H_2O with addition of 3.8% carbon dioxide (CO_2). Three animals were given a respiratory rate of 3 breaths/min and six had a respiratory rate of 12 breaths/min. One animal in group A died, all in group B died within 2 to 35 hours of initiation of mechanical ventilation, and three of six animals in group C died. Chest radiographs in groups B and C showed evidence of atelectasis, which was more prominent at autopsy. The tidal volumes necessary to achieve the PIP in groups B and C were greater than 400% to 500% above baseline. These large tidal volumes (60–70 ml/kg) were believed to cause lung injury by overinflation of the airway structures.

Tsuno and colleagues[17] studied 27 sheep ventilated with moderate airway pressures. These animals were ventilated with FiO_2 of 40% for 48 hours or until PO_2 was less than 50 mm Hg, partial pressure of carbon dioxide was (PCO_2) greater than 50 mm Hg,

development of pneumothorax, or death. Group A consisted of 8 animals with PIP of 18 cm H_2O, tidal volume of 10 ml/kg, respiratory rate of 15 breaths/min, and PEEP of 3 to 5 cm H_2O; group B included 11 animals with PIP of 30 cm H_2O, respiratory rate of 4 breaths/min, and PEEP of 0; group C consisted of 8 animals with PIP of 30 cm H_2O, respiratory rate of 15 breaths/min, and PEEP of 0 cm H_2O. In group C, normocapnia was achieved by adding dead space to the circuit. Three animals in group B and two animals in group C died. Both groups B and C had a lower PO_2, more infiltrates, and a higher lung weight when compared with control group A. The same authors demonstrated a lower incidence of pneumothorax than a previous study using a PIP of 50 cm H_2O.[16] These authors also concluded that hyperinflation led to pulmonary parenchymal injury. The effect of PEEP in the control group was unknown, and the supposition was raised that low levels of PEEP may be protective against the formation of edema.

Webb and Tierney also investigated the possible role of PEEP in providing lung protection from stretch injury.[9] Rats ventilated with PIP of 45 cm H_2O and 0 cm H_2O PEEP were compared with those ventilated with 45 cm H_2O and 10 cm H_2O PEEP. Tidal volumes were lower in the 45/10 group to maintain a consistent PIP. All animals ventilated at 45/0 became cyanotic and moribund within 13 to 35 minutes. Histologically, the lungs exhibited marked perivascular edema and alveolar edema. Those animals ventilated at 45/10 showed less edema and cellular injury (Fig. 11–2).

Other investigators also have observed beneficial effects from PEEP in high-pressure lung injury models in which inspiratory pressures are constant and tidal volume is reduced.[18–20] This may be the result of improved **recruitment** at end-expiration or decreased tissue stress due to lower tidal volumes. If tidal volume is held constant, however, even small increases in PEEP above that required for optimal recruitment could be associated with worsening overdistension and additional lung injury.

Acute lung injury may be associated with

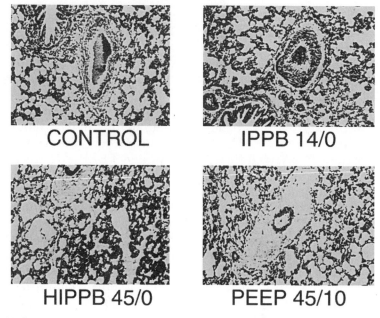

FIGURE 11–2

Lung tissue from rats ventilated with different strategies. Intermittent positive pressure breathing (IPPB) 14/0 delivered a peak pressure of 14 cm H_2O and a positive end-expiratory pressure (PEEP) of 0 cm H_2O; HIPPB delivered a peak pressure of 45 cm H_2O and a PEEP of 0 cm H_2O; and PEEP 45/10 delivered a peak pressure of 45 cm H_2O and a PEEP of 10 cm H_2O. Note that HIPPB has alveolar and perivascular edema, but PEEP 45/10 has only perivascular edema. (Reprinted with permission from Webb HH, Tierney DF: Experimental pulmonary edema due to intermittent positive pressure ventilation with high inflation pressures: protection by positive end-expiratory pressure. Am Rev Respir Dis 110:556–565, 1974. © American Lung Association.)

surfactant alteration and instability of terminal lung units due to edema, inflammation, and blood. This may be reflected in increased trapped gas volumes. In this situation, the slope of the inspiratory pressure–volume curve may change dramatically at low lung volumes during tidal volume ventilation, reflecting a threshold for opening collapsed lung units. Experimental studies with conventional ventilation of surfactant depleted lungs with various levels of PEEP suggest decreased lung injury when this threshold is exceeded by applied PEEP. This presumably results in decreased cyclic opening and closing of individual lung units—the "open lung" approach. Some have theorized that diminished cyclic reopening resulting from PEEP may decrease shear forces in terminal lung units and avoid further tissue injury.[21, 22]

Finally, there is convincing experimental data to support the theory that volume over-distension rather than airway pressure is the principal element responsible for tissue injury. Dreyfuss and associates subjected rats to large or low tidal volume ventilation with identical peak airway pressures.[23] The low tidal volume group had limited thoracoabdominal movement secondary to external restriction of thorax and abdominal movement. Pulmonary edema developed in rats subjected to high tidal volume/high pressure rats. It did not develop in rats subjected to low tidal volume/high pressure (Fig. 11–3).[24]

Rats ventilated at PIP of 45 cm H_2O and PEEP had less structural damage. In addition, lung injury developed in rats delivered high tidal volumes with a negative pressure ventilator. Therefore, excessive volume and alveolar overdistension seem most important in ventilator-associated lung injury, and the term **volutrauma** is appropriate to describe the sequelae. In the setting of acute

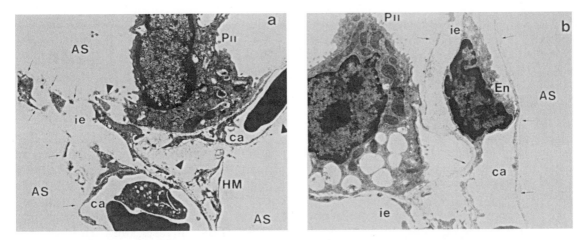

FIGURE 11-3
Ultrastructural aspects of the lungs of intact rats mechanically ventilated at 45 cm H_2O peak airway pressure with and without 10 cm H_2O positive end-expiratory pressure (PEEP). In the left panel, no PEEP was applied, and there is evidence of diffuse alveolar damage. In the right panel, 10 cm H_2O PEEP was applied, and the only abnormality is interstitial edema (ie). AS, alveolar space; ca, capillary; En, endothelial cell; HM, hyaline membranes; ie, interstitial edema. (Reprinted with permission from Dryfuss D, Soler P, Basset G, Saumon G: High inflation pressure pulmonary edema: respective effects of high airway pressure, high tidal volume, and positive end-expiratory pressure. Am Rev Respir Dis 137:1159–1164, 1988. © American Lung Association.)

lung injury, the distribution of ventilation may be uneven because of the heterogeneity of injury.[25] Tidal volumes are preferentially directed to more normal or recruitable lung units, and these areas may be more susceptible to overinflation, overdistension, and tissue injury.

Clinical Studies

The hypothesis that lung injury is caused by mechanical ventilation has been evaluated clinically by other investigators. Stocks and Godfrey found no differences in lung compliance between nonventilated infants and those infants ventilated with PIP less than 25 cm H_2O.[26] Gattinoni and colleagues studied 43 patients with ARDS treated with limitations on mechanical ventilation airway pressure and minute ventilation and extracorporeal CO_2 removal.[27] He reported decreased mortality in these patients compared with historic controls and predicted mortality based on Acute Physiology and Chronic Health Evaluation (APACHE) II estimates.[27] A subsequent controlled trial of extracorporeal CO_2 removal compared with conventional ventilatory strategies in patients with ARDS showed no survival advantage, however.[28] Hickling and colleagues retrospectively reviewed 50 patients with ARDS and an average lung injury score (LIS) greater than 2.5 who were treated with low volume, pressure-limited ventilation and **permissive hypercapnia**.[29] The reported mortality rate in this series was 16% compared with an expected mortality rate of 40% based on APACHE II estimates.

Hickling and associates[30] subsequently pursued a prospective study in 53 patients with severe ARDS and an LIS greater than 2.5. The tidal volume in these patients was 4 to 7 ml/kg, and PIP was limited to 30 to 40 cm H_2O. To achieve these goals, decreased alveolar minute ventilation and hypercapnia were tolerated. PEEP was used to try and maintain arterial oxygen percent saturation (SaO_2) greater than 90% with an FiO_2 less than 60%, but hemoglobin oxygen saturation levels in the mid 80s were tolerated in otherwise stable patients. Patients with severe head injury, intracranial hemorrhage, or spinal cord injury were excluded.

Of the 53 patients enrolled, the mortality rate was 26.4% (14/53), with an APACHE II-predicted mortality rate of 53.3% (p = 0.004). However, the survivors did have a significantly higher recorded mean pH (7.26), a higher mean lowest pH (7.18), and a lower mean base deficit (0.6). The highest PCO_2 was 63.6 mm Hg in survivors versus 74.3 mm Hg in nonsurvivors, which was not statistically significant. Nonsurvivors tended to have persistent metabolic acidosis.

Amato and colleagues reported on 28 patients with ARDS randomly assigned to a ventilatory strategy of limited airway pressure and tidal volume, as well as PEEP values determined by the lower inflection point on static pressure volume curves, to achieve the "open lung" approach compared with more conventional ventilatory management, including the least amount of PEEP necessary to improve oxygenation.[31] Thirteen patients received conventional ventilation and 15 patients were managed with the new approach. Conventional patients received volume assist ventilation (VAV) with tidal volumes of 12 ml/kg, respiratory rate 10 to 24 breaths/min, and initial PEEP of 5 cm H_2O with targets of PO_2 60 mm Hg to 100 mm Hg and PCO_2 25 mm Hg to 38 mm Hg. The experimental group received a pressure-limited mode of ventilation of either pressure support (PS), pressure control-inverse ratio ventilation (PC-IRV), or volume-assured pressure support ventilation (VAPSV). Peak inspiratory pressures were maintained at less than 40 cm H_2O, and tidal volume did not exceed 6 ml/kg. Respiratory rates were kept below 30 breaths/min, even in spontaneously breathing patients using sedation and paralyzing drugs. Static pressure volume curves were done to determine the lower inflection point, and PEEP was set at 2 cm H_2O above this point. The end points of the study were overall survival, ability to be weaned from mechanical ventilation, parameters of respiratory function, and deaths due to "progressive respiratory failure." There was no difference in overall survival between groups. Five of 15 subjects managed with the new approach, and 7 of 13 with conventional ventilation died (p = 0.45). Three of the

patients using the new approach died after successful extubation from unrelated complications, however. The authors did demonstrate faster rates of weaning, lower FiO_2 at death, improved lung compliance, and better $PaO_2:FiO_2$ ratios in those patients who received the lung protective strategy.

Four recent reports have explored the issue of "lung protection" methods further in patients with severe lung disease. Weg and colleagues analyzed data from 725 patients with ARDS who were subjects in a randomized trial of aerosolized surfactant for ARDS.[32] These investigators found no significant difference in ventilatory pressures or volumes between patients with evidence of pneumothorax or other barotrauma and those with no signs of barotrauma. In addition, there was no significant difference in mortality between patients with demonstrated air leaks and those without. Pressure measurements in this study were collected only for the first 5 days of mechanical ventilation.

Stewart and colleagues randomized 120 patients with ARDS to mechanical ventilation with a tidal volume of 8 ml/kg or less to maintain a PIP less than 30 cm H_2O or to tidal volumes of 10 to 15 ml/kg, allowing the PIP to rise as high as 50 cm H_2O.[33] No differences were noted in mortality, frequency of barotrauma, or the number of episodes of organ dysfunction. More patients in the protective strategy required paralyzing drugs. Both groups of patients had mean plateau pressures of less than 30 cm H_2O (28.5 cm H_2O control group and 22.3 cm H_2O limited ventilation group), however, which is below the concerning limits for pressure based on animal data. Therefore, **"lung protection strategies"** may not be necessary in patients with relatively low plateau pressures. Patients with high plateau pressures, however, may be at risk for overinflation and ventilator-related lung injury.

Amato and colleagues extended their earlier trial and analysis in another report.[34] Fifty-three patients were reported who were assigned randomly to a tidal volume of 6 ml/kg or less with airway pressures less than 20 cm H_2O above PEEP values compared with patients managed with a tidal volume of 12 ml/kg. In the experimental group, values for PEEP were determined as before with static **pressure-volume plot** curves on each patient. PEEP then was added equal to 2 cm above the lower inflection point on the static pressure-volume curve in the experimental group. The group receiving conventional treatment had PEEP added as needed to limit exposure to hyperoxia. The experimental group received more PEEP and had smaller tidal volumes, lower PIP, lower plateau pressures, lower minute ventilation, and higher PCO_2 values than the conventional group. The 28-day survival rate was 62% in the experimental group versus 29% in the conventionally treated patients (p = < 0.001). Survival to hospital discharge was not significantly affected, however. Concerns have been raised about the high mortality in the conventional group of this trial. In addition, the survival benefit appeared to be greatest in the first 3 days of mechanical ventilation, which would seem less likely attributable to ventilator-associated lung injury.

Finally, the National Institutes of Health (NIH) ARDS Network recently ended a trial of "high-stretch" versus "low-stretch" ventilation. As of this writing the results have yet to be published, but the initial data analysis from the 841 patients has shown a significant reduction in mortality in patients ventilated with a tidal volume of 6 ml/kg versus 12 ml/kg (mortality of 30% vs 39% respectively, P < .001).

Limiting tidal volume in patients with severe ARDS may lead to hypercapnia and respiratory acidosis. It is often difficult to maintain a minute ventilation that achieves normal PO_2 and avoids airtrapping in this patient population. Some have suggested that respiratory acidosis be corrected with sodium bicarbonate supplementation. Animal data suggest that intracellular acidosis is buffered rapidly and myocardial contractility is restored quickly after changes in PCO_2.[35, 36] Hypercapnia also may be beneficial because it shifts the oxygen–hemoglobin dissociation curve to the right and allows an increase in oxygen unloading to the tissues. Permissive hypercapnia appears to be a safe treatment modality in most patients with ARDS. It may be contraindicated in patients

at risk for high intracranial pressure and those with hemoglobinopathies associated with baseline rightward shifts of the oxyhemoglobin–dissociation curve.

The mechanisms of lung injury in the patient receiving mechanical ventilation may be multiple.[37–39] Animal studies have implicated large tidal volumes associated with PIP greater than 30 to 35 cm H_2O that results in alveolar overdistension. End-expiratory alveolar collapse with cyclic reopening during inspiration also may result in injury. Both processes appear to result in tissue damage and a morphologic pattern that is indistinguishable from ARDS. Other predisposing factors for lung injury include immaturity of lung and chest wall and surfactant deficiency or inactivation.

The human studies reported to date examining potential ventilator associated lung injury are stimulating, but there are no strong data to dictate the optimal way to avoid iatrogenic lung injury in patients receiving mechanical ventilation. Based on the clinical and experimental information available, we believe that it is prudent to avoid excessive plateau pressures in patients on mechanical ventilation (greater than 30–40 cm H_2O). We believe that this likely reflects high transalveolar pressures and hyperinflation of some lung units, which may contribute to alveolar–capillary damage. Lower alveolar minute ventilation and permissive hypercapnia should be tolerated to achieve this goal, except when contraindicated. Increased use of sedatives and possibly neuromuscular blockade may be necessary. Routine use of small tidal volumes and limited inspiratory pressures in patients with plateau pressures consistently less than 30 to 35 cm H_2O seems unwarranted and may have excess risks. The most appropriate use of PEEP is unclear. The report from Amato and associates argues for use of more liberal PEEP than is usual practice.[34] However, determination of static pressure–volume curves to determine potential levels of appropriate PEEP requires heavy sedation or paralysis, may not be reproducible, and must be done repeatedly. More studies are necessary to determine the most effective use of PEEP in patients with acute respiratory failure.

REFERENCES

1. Macklin M, Macklin C: Malignant interstitial emphysema of the lungs and mediastinum as an important occult complication in many respiratory diseases and other conditions. Medicine 23:281–358, 1994.
2. Polak B, Adams H: Traumatic air embolism in submarine escape training. U.S. Naval Med Bull 30:165, 1932.
3. Caldwell E, Powell R, Mullooly J: Interstitial emphysema: a study of physiologic factors involved in experimental induction of lesion. Am Rev Respir Dis 102:516–525, 1970.
4. Zwillich C, Pierson D, Creach C, et al: Complications of assisted ventilation. Am J Med 57:161–170, 1974.
5. Fleming W, Bowen J, Hatcher C: Early complications of long-term respiratory support. J Thorac Cardiovasc Surg 64:729–738, 1972.
6. Pontoppidan H: Treatment of respiratory failure in nonthoracic trauma. J Trauma 8:938–951, 1986.
7. Beilin B, Shulman D, Weiss A, et al: Pneumoperitoneum as the presenting sign of pulmonary barotrauma during artificial ventilation. Intensive Care Med 12:49–51, 1986.
8. Marini J, Culver B: Systemic gas embolism complicating mechanical ventilation in the adult respiratory distress syndrome. Ann Intern Med 110:699–703, 1989.
9. Webb HH, Tierney DF: Experimental pulmonary edema due to intermittent positive pressure ventilation with high inflation pressures: protection by positive end-expiratory pressure. Am Rev Respir Dis 110:556–565, 1974.
10. Staub N, Nagano H, Pearce M: Pulmonary edema in dogs, especially the sequence of fluid accumulation in the lungs. J Appl Physiol 22:227, 1967.
11. Parker JC, Hernandez LA, Longenecker GL, et al: Lung edema due to high peak airway pressures in dogs: role of increased microvascular filtration pressure and permeability. Am Rev Respir Dis 142:321–328, 1990.
12. Kolobow T, Moretti MP, Fumagalli R, et al: Severe impairment in lung function induced by high peak airway pressure during mechanical ventilation: an experimental study. Am Rev Respir Dis 135:312–315, 1987.
13. Thornton D, Ponhold H, Butler J, et al: Effects of pattern of ventilation on pulmonary metabolism and mechanics. Anesthesiology 42:4–10, 1975.
14. Coalson JJ, King RJ, Winter VT, et al: Oxygen and pneumonia-induced lung injury: I. Pathological and morphometric studies. J Appl Physiol 67:346–356, 1989.
15. Faridy EE, Permutt S, Riley RL: Effect of ventilation on surface forces in excised dogs' lungs. J Appl Physiol 21:1453–1462, 1966.
16. Dreyfuss D, Basset G, Soler P, Saumon G: Intermittent positive-pressure hyperventilation with high inflation pressures produces pulmonary microvascular injury in rats. Am Rev Respir Dis 132:880–884, 1985.
17. Tsuno K, Prato P, Kolobow T: Acute lung injury from mechanical ventilation at moderately high airway pressures. J Appl Physiol 69:956–961, 1990.
18. Sandhar BK, Niblett DJ, Argiras EP, et al: Effects of positive end-expiratory pressure on hyaline membrane formation in a rabbit model of the neonatal respiratory distress syndrome. Intensive Care Med 14:538–546, 1988.
19. Sohma A, Brampton W, Dunhill M, Sykes M: Effect of ventilation with positive end-expiratory pressure on hyaline membrane formation in a rabbit model of the neonatal respiratory distress syndrome. Intensive Care Med 14:538–546, 1988.
20. Argiras E, Blakeley C, Dunhill M, et al: High PEEP decreases hyaline membrane formation in surfactant deficient lungs. Br J Anaesth 59:1278–1285, 1987.
21. McCulloch PR, Forkert PG, Froese AB: Lung volume maintenance prevents lung injury during high frequency oscillation in surfactant-deficient rabbits. Am Rev Respir Dis 137:1185–1192, 1988.
22. Snyder JV, Froese A: The open lung approach: concept and application. In Snyder JV, Penski MR (eds): Oxygen Transport in the Critically Ill. Chicago: Year Book Medical Publishers, 1987, pp 374–395.
23. Dreyfuss D, Soler P, Basset G, Saumon G: High inflation pressure pulmonary edema: respective effects of high airway pressure, high tidal volume, and positive end-expiratory pressure. Am Rev Respir Dis 137:1159–1164, 1988.
24. Dreyfuss D, Saumon G: Ventilator-induced lung injury. Am J Respir Crit Care Med 157:294–323, 1998.
25. Gattinoni L, Pesenti A, Avalli L, et al: Pressure volume curve of the total respiratory system in acute respiratory failure: computed tomography study. Am Rev Respir Dis 136:730–736, 1987.
26. Stocks J, Godfrey S: The role of artificial ventilation, oxygen, and CPAP in the pathogenesis of lung damage in neonates: assessment by serial measurements of lung function. Pediatrics 57:352–362, 1976.
27. Gattinoni L, Pesenti A, Macheroni D, et al: Low frequency positive-pressure ventilation with extracorporeal carbon dioxide removal in severe acute respiratory failure. JAMA 256:881–886, 1986.
28. Morris AH, Wallace CJ, Clemmer T, et al: Extracorporeal CO_2 removal therapy for adult respiratory distress syndrome patients: a computerized protocol controlled trial. Reanimation Soins Intensits Medium d' Urgence 6:485–490, 1990.
29. Hickling KG, Henderson SJ, Jackson R: Low mortality associated with low volume pressure limited ventilation with permissive hypercapnia in severe adult respiratory distress syndrome. Intensive Care Med 16:372–377, 1990.
30. Hickling KG, Walsh J, Henderson S, Jackson R: Low mortality rate in adult respiratory distress syndrome using low-volume pressure-limited ventilation with permissive hypercapnia: a prospective study. Crit Care Med 22:1568–1578, 1994.

31. Amato MBP, Barbas CSV, Medelros DM, et al: Beneficial effects of the "open lung approach" with low distending pressures in acute respiratory distress syndrome. Am J Respir Crit Care Med 152:1835–1846, 1995.
32. Weg JG, Anzueto A, Balk RA, et al: The relation of pneumothorax and other air leaks to mortality in the acute respiratory distress syndrome. N Engl J Med 338:341–346, 1998.
33. Stewart TE, Meade MO, Cook DJ, et al: Evaluation of a ventilation strategy to prevent barotrauma in patients at high risk for acute respiratory distress syndrome. N Engl J Med 338:355–361, 1998.
34. Amato MBP, Barbas CSV, Medelros DM, et al: Effect of a protective-ventilation strategy on mortality in acute respiratory distress syndrome. N Engl J Med 338:347–354, 1998.
35. Foex P, Fordham RM: Intrinsic myocardial recovery from the negative inotropic effects of acute hypercapnia. Cardiovasc Res 6:257–262, 1972.
36. Tang W, Weil MH, Gazmuri RJ, et al: Reversible impairment of myocardial contractility due to hypercarbic acidosis in the isolated perfused rate heart. Crit Care Med 19:2:218–224, 1991.
37. Hernandez LA, Coker PJ, May S, et al: Mechanical ventilation increases microvascular permeability in oleic acid-injured lungs. J Appl Physiol 69:2057–2061, 1990.
38. Adkins KW, Hernandez LA, Coker PJ, et al: Age affects susceptibility to pulmonary barotrauma in rabbits. Crit Care Med 19:390–393, 1991.
39. Parker JC, Hernandez LA, Perry KJ: Mechanisms of ventilator-induced lung injury. Crit Care Med 21:131–143, 1993.

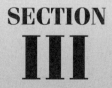

SECTION
III

Adjunctive Therapy During Mechanical Ventilation

CHAPTER 12

Nutrition in the Patient on Mechanical Ventilation

Stephen A. McClave, MD
Harvy L. Snider, MD
Larry G. Dukes, RPh
Leslie Campbell, BA

EFFECT OF UNDERFEEDING

EFFECT OF OVERFEEDING

NUTRITIONAL ASSESSMENT

NUTRITIONAL REQUIREMENTS

PERFORMANCE OF INDIRECT CALORIMETRY

DESIGN OF THE NUTRITION SUPPORT REGIMEN

MONITORING RESPONSE AND PATIENT TOLERANCE

REFERENCES

KEY WORDS

Acute Physiology and Chronic Health Evaluation (APACHE)

indirect calorimetry
respiratory quotient

resting energy expenditure

Patients on mechanical ventilation are under significant physiologic stress and are at risk for deterioration of nutritional status. The patient's nutritional state is vitally important to outcome because it is fundamentally associated with overall pulmonary status, immune competence, and the patient's ability to mount an overall stress response.[1] Caloric requirements and nutritional needs are not easily anticipated clinically or accurately predicted by conventional equations. Complications occur from both under- and overfeeding, and the clinical consequences of inappropriate feeding are not always readily discernible at the bedside by the health care practitioner.[2] **Indirect calorimetry**, therefore, becomes a useful tool for designing nutrition support regimens that precisely meet caloric requirements.

In this chapter, the effects of inappropriate feeding in the patient with respiratory failure requiring mechanical ventilation are enumerated. A clinically useful nutritional assessment with the means for determining nutritional requirements is discussed. Performance of indirect calorimetry, design of an appropriate nutritional support regimen, and monitoring the patient for response and tolerance to the nutritional support regimen are outlined.

EFFECT OF UNDERFEEDING

An important perspective is obtained by reviewing the effects of underfeeding as they relate to the underlying mechanisms of respiratory failure. A traditional way of viewing respiratory failure is to separate the disease process into hypercapnic and hypoxemic varieties. Both categories include patients who may require mechanical ventilatory support. In considering the effects of nutrition on patients, the mechanisms responsible for producing the respiratory failure should be kept in mind. Hypercapnic variety is caused by hypoventilation, which results from one or more of the following: (1) inadequate respiratory center drive; (2) inadequate transmission of the respiratory center drive to the myoneural junction; (3) interference with transmission of the signal across the myoneural junction; and (4) muscle weakness. Hypoxemic respiratory failure typically results from increased perfusion of unventilated lungs (i.e., pulmonary shunt). It is further pertinent to assess any effects of nutrition on lung anatomy and host defense mechanisms. We attempt to briefly summarize the findings as they relate to these underlying mechanisms.

We are unaware of studies directly evaluating respiratory center drive or conduction of the signal to the muscle (by diaphragmatic electromyogram [EMG] or phrenic nerve conduction studies) in the setting of underfeeding. Weissman and colleagues[3] looked at an indirect measure of this in subjects deprived of protein for 7 days. A 26% decrease in the ratio of tidal volume/inspiratory time (V_T/T_I or mean inspiratory flow rate) was found. Intravenous administration of an amino acid solution for 24 hours resulted in reversal. Because ventilatory response to chemical stimuli as measured by minute ventilation could be impaired by decreased respiratory drive or impaired muscle function, studies measuring only this parameter do not differentiate effects produced by one or another of these mechanisms. A study by Doekel and associates[4] involved this methodology and found that a semistarvation diet for 10 days resulted in a 58% reduction in hypoxemic ventilatory response. Refeeding with a normal diet reversed this effect.

A number of studies have addressed the effects of underfeeding on respiratory muscle function. In a group of patients dying after a chronic illness, those patients whose body weight was normal had minimal loss of diaphragmatic muscle mass compared with a control group of individuals who had experienced sudden death. A second group of patients dying after a chronic illness who had sustained loss of body weight (down to a mean 71% of ideal body weight) had a 43% reduction in diaphragmatic muscle mass compared with the control group experiencing sudden death.[5] In a study of healthy volunteers placed on modest caloric restriction for almost 6 months, Keys and associates[6] found a mean reduction in vital capacity of 8%. This improved to near baseline the following 12 weeks of refeeding.[6] In another group of patients who had sustained substantial weight loss, respiratory muscle strength appeared to be affected, as evidenced by maximal inspiratory pressures that were 35% and maximal expiratory pressures that were 59% of normal values. On the average, vital capacity was 63% and respiratory muscle strength was 37% of those values seen in healthy controls.[7] Similarly, Grant found that malnourished patients had reductions to 59% of predicted for maximum expiratory pressures and 43% predicted for maximal inspiratory pressures.[1] Two weeks of total parenteral nutrition (TPN) therapy produced significant but not complete normalization of these parameters. As a frame of reference, in normal lungs of patients who had proximal myopathies, reductions in vital capacity to less than 55% predicted or respiratory muscle strength to less than 30% of normal was associated with hypoventilation.[8] Further evidence that nutritional support may improve respiratory muscle strength was provided by Whitaker and colleagues,[9] who found increases in maximal inspiratory pressure and mean sustained inspiratory pressure in chronically ill malnourished patients with chronic obstructive pulmonary disease (COPD) given dietary supplements, compared with a control group not receiving the supplement.

Deterioration of nutritional status has been shown in other studies to result in physiologic and anatomic changes in the lung. Patients who were nutritionally depleted showed evidence of higher tracheal colonization and greater tracheal cell adherence by bacteria[10, 11] when compared with well-nourished controls. When nutritionally depleted patients undergoing elective gastrointestinal (GI) surgery were compared with well-nourished controls undergoing the same operation, these changes corresponded to a higher rate of pneumonia and longer hospital stays.[12] Morphologic changes and structural damage to the lung have been demonstrated in response to underfeeding. In an animal model in which rats were exposed to 3 weeks of semistarvation, decreases in alveolar wall surface tension, surfactant production, and overall elastic compliance were seen.[13] Adequate refeeding corrected the changes in surfactant, but the morphologic emphysematous changes in the lungs were not corrected.[13] Similar evidence has been shown in humans, world famines have resulted in emphysematous changes even in young adults.[1, 14]

These deleterious changes in the respiratory response to nutritional deterioration correlate to adverse effects on patient outcome. In patients with COPD with severe nutritional deficits, there were less frequent hospitalizations for those patients who successfully ingested a high-calorie diet compared with those patients who refused to eat.[15] Weaning capability in patients on mechanical ventilation improved with adequate nutritional support. Combining the results of two studies, successful weaning occurred in 88% of patients (22 of 25) who received adequate feeding but in only 32% (10 of 31) who failed to receive an adequate regimen.[16, 17]

EFFECT OF OVERFEEDING

A number of clinical problems arise from overfeeding patients in respiratory failure on mechanical ventilation. At the outset, overfeeding may promote fluid overload, hyperlipidemia, hyperglycemia, and azotemia.[2] Overfeeding actually may increase the overall stress response and raise energy expenditure for the critically ill patient on mechanical ventilation. The increased energy response is caused by increases in diet-induced thermogenesis related to overfeeding. The degree to which energy expenditure is increased is related to the degree to which the fixed rate of carbohydrate metabolism is exceeded.[18, 19] Once the fixed rate of carbohydrate metabolism is exceeded, the additional calories must be converted to either glycogen or fat. Lipogenesis to a greater extent than glycogenesis accounts for the dramatic increase in energy expenditure, with increases in diet-induced thermogenesis of up to 25% to 26%.[20] The hypermetabolic response is accompanied by increases in catecholamine secretion.[21, 22]

Overfeeding, which results in lipogenesis, promotes excessive carbon dioxide (CO_2) production, which may overwhelm respiratory function in individuals with reduced ventilatory capacity. In one study using parenteral nutrition, significant elevation in CO_2 production was seen as total caloric provision and was increased from 1.0 to 1.5 to 2.0 times the **resting energy expenditure** (REE).[23] In case series, high caloric loads provided through parenteral nutrition actually precipitated hypercapnia, respiratory acidosis, and respiratory failure, requiring placement on mechanical ventilation.[24-26] Increases in CO_2 production and minute ventilation were greater in patients who were adequately nourished before injury compared with those with evidence of depleted nutritional status.[25] Patients with mild to moderate injury showed greater increases in minute ventilation in response to overfeeding than patients with a greater severity of injury.[25] In studies with indirect calorimetry, the effects of overfeeding on substrate utilization are seen, as is the evidence of increased load to the pulmonary system. In a retrospective review of 78 patients on mechanical ventilation receiving TPN, those patients with a **respiratory quotient** (RQ) of greater than 1.0 (suggesting lipogenesis from overfeeding) showed that they received carbohydrate infusions that were 31.6% higher, had a minute ventilation that was 27.5% higher, and required intermittent minute ventilation

(IMV) settings that were 210% greater than patients whose measured RQ was less than 1.0.[27] Even in those patients on mechanical ventilation who received enteral tube feedings, a direct correlation was seen between overfeeding (percentage calories provided/required) and increasing RQ.[28] When the RQ increased in response to overfeeding, patients developed shallow, rapid respirations.[28] In general, these changes in response to overfeeding result in effects on minute ventilation, increase dead-space ventilation, promote respiratory failure, and delay weaning from mechanical ventilation.

NUTRITIONAL ASSESSMENT

Nutritional assessment in the patient on mechanical ventilation should focus on three main areas: (1) a determination of level of physiologic stress, as measured by the **Acute Physiology and Chronic Health Evaluation** (APACHE) scoring system; (2) a brief clinical examination of current nutritional status and respiratory muscle function; and (3) a thorough evaluation of the status of the GI tract in anticipation of use for enteral access. More traditional markers of nutritional assessment (i.e., anthropometry, immune markers, and visceral protein levels) have very little value in the stressed critically ill patient on mechanical ventilation.[29, 30] Anthropometric measures (such as mid arm circumference and tricep skin-fold thickness) and immune markers (i.e., total lymphocyte count and anergy panel) tend to be inaccurate and poorly reproducible, rarely reflect true nutritional status, and almost never affect the design of the nutrition support regimen.[30] Decreases in visceral protein levels (albumin, prealbumin, and transferrin) in the critically ill patient reflect the stress response and are related not only to decreased production of these proteins by the liver but also to extravasation of the proteins out of the vascular space.[31] Use of the visceral proteins as a marker of nutritional status in the critically ill patient is fallacious.[31] In theory, bioelectric impedance should be helpful in determining body composition and in differentiating lean body mass from

fat mass, but it has diminished usefulness in the critical care setting because of the significant error introduced by volume shifts and the presence of edema.

Level of stress is the single greatest factor affecting risk of nutritional deterioration and ultimate patient outcome. The more critically ill the patient, the more likely that even subtle aspects of nutritional support (such as route of nutrient administration[32] and control of hyperglycemia[33]) would have an impact on patient outcome.[33, 34] The APACHE scoring systems are the most carefully researched and commonly used marker for degree of critical illness and overall physiologic stress.[35-37] Whether the more convenient APACHE II system[36] or the more comprehensive (and possibly more reliable for serial use) APACHE III system is used,[37] these scores correlate to increased energy expenditure, overall stress response, development of nosocomial infection and multiple-organ failure, and ultimately, mortality.[35-38] These scoring systems indicate the degree of risk of nutritional deterioration and the urgency with which nutritional support should be instigated.

A brief clinical examination with attention to actual body weight (ABW) as a percentage of ideal body weight (IBW) and simple bedside tests for respiratory muscle function provide valuable clues as to the patient's current nutritional status. ABW as a percentage of IBW or usual body weight should be determined because weight loss correlates with acuity of respiratory failure and partial pressure of carbon dioxide (PCO_2) levels.[39] Patients with COPD with acute respiratory failure have been shown to have significantly lower percent IBW than stable patients with COPD.[40] In a large group of patients with acute respiratory failure, 56% were shown to have ABWs less than 80% of IBW.[29] Muscle atrophy tends to parallel weight loss. Patients who had profound nutritional depletion at a mean 71% of IBW were shown to have 43% less diaphragmatic muscle mass than healthy controls.[5] A simple bedside measure of respiratory muscle function is the maximal inspiratory and expiratory pressure. Absolute values reflect respiratory muscle strength, whereas sustaining pressures indicate endurance. In patients with COPD, respiratory endurance usually is affected more than the absolute inspiratory/expiratory pressures.[41] Serial inspiratory pressure measurements are one parameter reflecting response of muscle strength to nutritional support.

The need to obtain enteral access to maintain gut integrity and to contain the stress response with enteral feeding makes assessment of the GI tract imperative. The enteral route of nutrition support has been shown to reduce cost, nosocomial infection, multiple-organ failure, length of hospitalization, and mortality when compared with the parenteral route.[34] The term "ileus" and the axiom "If the gut works, use it" are outdated, misleading, and inaccurate, and should be avoided in the nutritional assessment of the patient on mechanical ventilation. The gut is always "working"; it never stops absorbing nutrients that are infused into its lumen. At times, it may not be safe for the gut to absorb luminal nutrients, particularly in the patient with systemic hypotension on pressor agents such as norepinephrine, dopamine, and dobutamine. Feeding through the enteral route in these circumstances may promote a shift of blood flow to the splanchnic circulation and may promote even further deterioration into clinical shock. It may be more appropriate to wait until these patients are no longer being given pressor agents or are at least being given renal perfusion doses of dopamine to initiate enteral feeding.

The more important factor to be addressed by nutritional assessment relates to which segments of the GI tract have adequate contractility. With an acute physiologic insult, the small bowel is the last segment of the GI tract to stop contracting and the first to return to contractility as the acute event abates. Residual volumes and nasogastric output from a saline sump tube are good clinical markers of gastric contractibility. Passage of stool and gas per rectum are good measures for colonic contractility. Although the presence of bowel sounds indicates small bowel contractility, bowel sounds are not required to initiate feeding into the jejunum. Assessment of contractility of the various segments of the GI tract

helps determine which feeding tube is required and at what level feedings need to be infused. Significant gastric atony often is accompanied by duodenal atony and often requires feeding into the jejunum with or without simultaneous aspiration and decompression of the stomach. Finally, some assessment of the degree of gut disuse and villous atrophy (estimated by the time period in which there are no luminal nutrients) should be made to determine the need for a specialized small peptide hydrolyzed formula (over a more standard formula).

NUTRITIONAL REQUIREMENTS

A number of factors in the critical care setting lead to hypermetabolism and increased energy expenditure in the respiratory failure patient on mechanical ventilation.[42] The disease process itself, with its concomitant stress response, may increase energy expenditure through stimulation of the sympathetic nervous system and the release of catecholamines. Other factors contributing to the increase in energy expenditure include fever, futile substrate cycling, medications (aspirin, pressor agents, catecholamines), release of counter-regulatory hormones (glucagon, cortisol, adrenocorticotropic hormone), inflammatory cytokines, shivering thermogenesis, and increased work of breathing.[42] The work of breathing, which may represent only 2% to 3% of energy expenditure in a healthy person, may increase up to 25% to 26% of energy expenditure in a patient in respiratory failure before placement on mechanical ventilation.[43, 44] Weight loss and nutritional deterioration of the patient with COPD may increase energy expenditure further compared with similar patients with COPD who remain well nourished at a stable weight.[45–47] COPD by itself may cause defects in diet-induced thermogenesis (DIT). Increased DIT was shown in patients with COPD compared with undernourished (non-COPD) controls,[48] indicating that greater energy expenditure was required to metabolize the same amount of nutrients (and thus less calories were available as fuel for muscles and lean body mass). Additionally, patients with COPD may have defects of certain adaptive mechanisms, lacking the ability to become hypometabolic during periods of fasting or caloric deprivation.[46] A misconception for some clinicians is that providing mechanical ventilation to a patient in respiratory failure markedly increases REE,[29] but it is really the underlying respiratory failure that causes the increase in energy expenditure. A patient on mechanical ventilation who is weaned successfully usually demonstrates an increase in energy expenditure as the patient assumes the work of breathing done previously by the machine.[43, 44]

Not all patients who are critically ill on mechanical ventilation manifest a hypermetabolic response. In multiple studies in the critical care setting, only 35% to 62% of patients were shown to be hypermetabolic (> 110% of the Harris-Benedict predicted REE).[43, 49–51] The rest were normometabolic (within 10%) or even hypometabolic (< 90% of the Harris-Benedict value). This seemingly inappropriate hypometabolic response may be explained by a number of factitious reasons,[42] such as pharmacologic treatment, choice of predictive formula, inaccurate weights, timing of the study, issues related to nutritional support, and even level of consciousness. However, progressive, inappropriate low metabolism may imply impending septic shock, and patients should be evaluated for underlying infection.[42, 52, 53]

More than 200 equations have been published in the literature, using a variety of clinical factors, to predict REE.[54] Surprisingly, none of these equations are more accurate than the time-honored Harris-Benedict equation,[54] despite modification of the equation for patient activity,[29] disease process,[55, 56] level of stress,[57] and even ventilatory status.[58] Use of the Harris-Benedict equation alone (which was developed in healthy volunteers) tends to underpredict measured REE,[50] but correcting the equation by a metabolic injury factor, such as those derived by Grant[55] or Elwyn and colleagues,[56] results in overprediction of measured REE.[50] Patients on mechanical ventilation have been shown in one study to have a mean measured REE greater than 105%

of predicted, the range being 70% to 140% of predicted.[43]

Use of predictive equations in the individual patient is inherently inaccurate because these equations are based on faulty clinical presumptions. Patients do not respond identically to a single disease process. Owen and associates have described the concept of a "metabolic signature" or "fingerprint," whereby patients inherit their own unique metabolic machinery, which causes them to respond differently to the same disease process or similar extent of injury.[59] In large studies of patients with the same disease process, the standard deviation for measured REE can range from 19% to 40% about a mean value, with variability from one patient to the next by up to 30% to 40%.[60–62] In an individual patient, energy expenditure is not constant, consistent, or easily predictable, with variation even in controls (without a disease process) of 12% to 25% when tested over several days to weeks.[63, 64] The metabolic response to an injury is not the same throughout the disease process.[43] Early in the course of the critically ill patient, daily energy expenditure may vary by up to 46% about a mean REE, whereas later in the patient's recovery process REE may vary up to only 12% about the mean.[43] Additional disease processes may complicate the "usual" metabolic response to respiratory failure. Organ failure, development of sepsis, or repeated surgical procedures may lead to increases in energy expenditure. Typically, recommendations based on predictive equations or tables for these various disease states tend to break down in the face of multiple concomitant disease processes.

PERFORMANCE OF INDIRECT CALORIMETRY

The best means to determine nutritional requirements is to measure energy expenditure by indirect calorimetry. Indirect calorimetry uses measurements of gas exchange parameters (O_2 consumption and CO_2 production) to indirectly, but accurately, predict energy expenditure. The physiologic principles that underlie conventional respiratory indirect calorimetry relate to the abbreviated Weir equation (REE = [$3.94 \times O_2$ consumption] + [$1.11 \times CO_2$ production]).[65] Indirect calorimetry has been shown to be as accurate as the large-chamber direct calorimeters, with the mean difference between the two methods for measuring REE at less than 3%.[66] Modern computerized portable instruments that are relatively inexpensive have facilitated the performance of indirect calorimetry in the critical care setting.

A slight modification of the principles of respiratory indirect calorimetry has led to the use and development of circulatory indirect calorimetry, in which the reverse Fick equation is used to derive O_2 consumption from cardiac output and arteriovenous O_2 difference using a Swan-Ganz catheter. A standard default RQ then is used with the O_2 consumption to calculate the REE. Multiple studies have shown that although measurements from both methods correlate significantly, the REE value obtained from the circulatory indirect calorimetry may underestimate the value obtained by respiratory indirect calorimetry by as much as 15%.[67-72] (The difference reflects the fact that the circulatory indirect calorimetry does not measure or account for the O_2 consumption by the pulmonary system.)

A number of routine steps should be taken to optimize test conditions at the time of an indirect calorimetric study.[73, 74] Patients should be tested in a quiet thermoneutral environment, and interruptions should be avoided. Patients receiving an oral diet should be fasted after midnight the night before, and patients not receiving continuous enteral or parenteral feedings should be switched to continuous infusion (which is maintained through the time of the testing). Standard physician orders are helpful and should alert staff and support personnel to the time of testing. Ventilator settings should not be changed for 90 minutes before the test, and any sedatives or analgesics should be administered 1 hour before the test. Patients with end-stage renal disease should not be tested on the day of hemodialysis. A multidisciplinary team that can be assembled to interpret results is a key factor in the success of an indirect calorimetry program.

The respiratory therapist must pay attention to a number of details when the patient on mechanical ventilation undergoes indirect calorimetry.[73, 74] The patient should be prepared by carefully suctioning the tracheostomy tube and ensuring a good seal on the trach cuff. The source of O_2 from the wall should be attached to an external O_2 blender to guarantee stable delivery of inspired oxygen concentration (FiO_2) throughout the testing period. The humidifier on the ventilator should be removed or bypassed. The gas sample line should be placed close to the patient or to the ventilator, depending on the specific manufacturer recommendations for the indirect calorimeter instrument. Indirect calorimeters should be calibrated carefully before testing with regard to the gas analyzers and volume transducers. Gas analyzers may be tested against reference tanks of known gas concentrations, and volume transducers usually are tested with a standard 3-L syringe. Further validation of instrument results may be done by using the indirect calorimeters to measure the RQ from a methanol-burning kit (which can be performed only on certain models) or placing the indirect calorimeter on an artificial lung machine (which simulates O_2 consumption and CO_2 production). Patients on mechanical ventilation should not be tested until the FiO_2 is 60% or less and the positive end-expiratory pressure or continuous positive airway pressure is less than 5 cm H_2O. Use of a pressure valve or baffles system to collect air samples may allow for patients to be tested at higher pressures.

Once indirect calorimetry is initiated, the end point of testing is achievement of steady state, defined by variation of the O_2 consumption and CO_2 production by less than 10%, and RQ by less than 5% over a consecutive 5-minute interval.[49, 50, 75] Extrapolating test results from this brief steady-state period out over 24 hours provides an adequate measure of caloric expenditure.[76] However, when the critically ill patient is tested, it may be more difficult to obtain or achieve steady state. The achievement of steady state ensures a greater degree of validity of measurements. In those patients who fail to achieve steady state, however, it may be more appropriate to take a mean value for REE over the entire testing period. This value obtained still provides a valuable reference point for clinicians in determining caloric requirements.

Recently, a commercial respiratory indirect calorimeter was developed that can provide continuous monitoring for up to 72 hours. The instrument connects directly into a mechanical ventilator produced by the same manufacturer, thus performing continuous monitoring of energy expenditure and allowing (by comparing to energy intake) the derivation of cumulative energy balance. The capability for continuous monitoring for up to 72 hours and the ability to download information into personal computer spreadsheets have made this instrument attractive for research. With the capability to monitor throughout a 24-hour period, strict control of test conditions is not necessary, and adjustments for fever and activity level or the achievement of steady state are not required.

A number of modifications may need to be made for proper interpretation of test results.[73, 74] Overall validity of the test should be evaluated by confirming that none of the values for RQ fall outside the physiologic range from 0.67 to 1.3.[77] Measured RQ values outside this range are nonphysiologic, represent significant error, and indicate an invalid test. In the presence of fever, the value obtained for measured REE should be reduced by 7% for each degree above 100° F.[55] The measured REE may be compared with the Harris-Benedict predicted value to provide the clinician with a sense of the metabolic response and the degree to which the patient is hypermetabolic or hypometabolic.[43, 49, 51] Total energy expenditure (TEE) is calculated by adding an activity factor to the measured REE—10% for bedridden patients and 15% for ambulatory patients.[78] Most importantly, the number of calories provided by the nutrition support regimen should be compared with the caloric requirements measured by the metabolic cart (TEE) to determine the appropriateness of current feeding.

DESIGN OF THE NUTRITION SUPPORT REGIMEN

An appropriate nutrition support regimen should meet basic requirements to fulfill the needs of the patient in respiratory failure on mechanical ventilation. The design of the nutrition support regimen and the speed with which it is initiated are determined by the level of stress and status of the gut. Measurement of caloric requirements is important to establish the goal of nutrition support with rapid advancement of the infusion rate to meet that goal. The nutrition support regimen should provide a mixed fuel regimen, should be infused through the enteral route, and must be adequate to enhance the weaning process. Finally, patients should be monitored throughout their infusion period for tolerance.

In designing the nutrition support regimen, the clinician must be aware that all three of the basic fuel substrates (carbohydrate, fat, and protein) individually can have deleterious effects on respiratory function. The individual effects of each substrate are probably much more pronounced when given by the parenteral route. With the enteral infusion of nutrients, formulas are more standardized, problems with absorption and assimilation may override theoretical problems with individual substrates, and the gut may act as its own governor, failing to absorb excesses of any one individual substrate.

The most pronounced effect on pulmonary function may come from excess carbohydrate infusion. The metabolism of carbohydrate is associated with a higher RQ than fat, which results from greater CO_2 production. High carbohydrate load given through the parenteral route has been shown to raise the RQ, CO_2 production, and minute ventilation to the point of actually precipitating hypercapnia, respiratory failure, and need for mechanical ventilation.[25] In one study, switching from 100% carbohydrate meal to a mixed fuel regimen (50:50 carbohydrate:fat ratio), CO_2 production was shown to decrease by 20% and minute ventilation by 26%.[79] Excess protein stimulates ventilatory drive and may increase the work of breathing because of its effect on increasing mean inspiratory flow, minute ventilation, and O_2 consumption.[80, 81] Use of branch chain amino acids may have an even greater effect on ventilatory drive than standard protein.[81] Theoretically, increasing protein provision may be used to stimulate ventilatory drive in weaning efforts, but pushing too hard with protein infusion in a patient with COPD (who already has an increased ventilatory drive) actually may precipitate fatigue and dyspnea.[29]

Excess infusion of fat—particularly over a short period of time—can also have a deleterious effect on respiratory function. High fat infusion actually may clog the reticuloendothelial system (RES) with deposition of fat in leukocytes and macrophages,[82–84] an effect that suppresses phagocytosis and bacterial killing. The rate of clearance of fat from the RES decreases as patient stress increases.[85, 86] There may be a cumulative dose response effect on the RES over several days of fat infusion.[29] Infusion of fat may lead to increased mean pulmonary artery pressure, increased shunting, increased pulmonary vascular resistance, increased vasoconstrictive response, and decreased arterial partial pressure of oxygen (PO_2).[87] Lipid-induced hyperlipemia actually can decrease pulmonary diffusion capacity.[88] Hyperlipemia may cause ventilation/perfusion inequalities, with decreases in the ratio of PaO_2:FiO_2, increases in the O_2 gradient, and pulmonary shunting.[89] A key concept in the infusion of lipids, particularly through the parenteral route, is to feed "low and slow." Many of these effects on the respiratory system can be avoided by using lower concentrations of fat infused over the entire 24-hour period.[90] Prolonged infusion of low concentrations of fat avoids lipemia, reduces clogging of the RES, and may enhance clearance and utilization.[29]

The basic principles by which to design the nutritional regimen partly depend on the type of pulmonary disease process that necessitated mechanical ventilation.[1] Patients maintained on mechanical ventilation because of respiratory muscle dysfunction or patients with hypoxemic respiratory failure may tolerate a fairly standard enteral formula or a parenteral regimen.[1] In these patients, a standard substrate profile is appropriate, with fat making up 20% to 30% of the calories, carbohydrates 40% to 50%, and protein the remainder. In patients with hypercapnic respiratory failure, however, the problems with excess carbohydrate infusion and consequent increases in CO_2 production must be avoided. In these patients, fat should make up a greater percentage of the nonprotein calories such that an overall profile with 40% fat, 40% carbohydrate, and 20% protein calories is more appropriate.[1]

The route of feeding is extremely important in the critical care setting. When compared with the parenteral route of feeding, early enteral feeding has been shown to decrease the overall stress response, hyperglycemia, and REE and actually increase visceral protein levels.[32, 34] Early enteral feeding decreases the cost of nutrition support and is associated with decreases in nosocomial infection, multiple-organ failure, length of hospitalization, and mortality when compared with the parenteral route.[32, 34, 91] Enteral feeding may provide the added benefit of stress ulcer prophylaxis in the patient on mechanical ventilation.[29] In an older retrospective study, Pingleton and Hadzima demonstrated significantly less evidence of GI bleeding in patients placed on enteral feeding when compared with patients placed on acid-reducing therapy or sucralfate (Carafate).[92] In a group of patients in the intensive care unit (ICU), the duodenal infusion of an enteral formula was shown to increase gastric pH with no change in serum gastrin levels when compared with the duodenal infusion of saline, an effect that was interpreted as providing some degree of stress prophylaxis.[93]

Standardization of enteral formulas avoids some of the problems seen with the infinite variations that occurred in the past with parenteral regimens. Specific pulmonary formulas are characterized by having increased protein and a lower carbohydrate:fat ratio (in which the ratio of carbohydrate:fat is decreased from 70:30 to 50:50). In one prospective randomized trial, patients treated with Pulmocare were shown to require an average of 62 fewer hours on mechanical ventilation and demonstrated a decrease of 16% in their $PaCO_2$ when compared with controls.[94] Use of pulmonary formulas has been criticized because of failure to show any impact on actual patient outcome. This criticism may not be warranted, because these formulas are inexpensive (costing less than 20% more than standard formulas) and have a substrate profile that makes physiologic sense for use in the patient on mechanical ventilation.

MONITORING RESPONSE AND PATIENT TOLERANCE

Fear of aspiration is often the greatest concern for clinicians when feeding patients through the enteral route in the critical care setting. The actual risk of aspiration, however, is overemphasized and should never limit the use of early enteral feeding in the ICU. Evidence of subclinical aspiration, in which gastric contents pass up into the esophagus or into the tracheal secretions, has been shown to occur in 36% to 44% of patients.[95, 96] However, the actual development of pneumonia with an infiltrate on chest radiograph, fever, and need for antibiotics occurs in only 1% to 4% of patients.[95, 96] The true risk of significant aspiration pneumonia is related more to misplacement of an enteral feeding tube into the lungs than it is to aspiration of gastric contents from a tube placed properly in the GI tract. Specific risk factors, which have been identified as increasing the risk of aspiration, include age older than 70 years, decreasing level of consciousness, location in the hospital (transfer from the ICU to a general ward), supine patient position, bolus style of infusion, increasing diameter of the feeding tube, and position of the feeding tube in the GI tract.[95, 96] Patients determined to be at high risk for aspiration on the basis of these factors should be managed by using the reverse Trendelenburg position, switching from bolus to continuous infusion of nutrients, placing the tube at or below the ligament of Treitz, adding metoclopramide monohydrochloride monohydrate (Reglan) or cisapride (Propulsid) to promote gastric emptying, and even switching to a combination tube that allows simultaneous aspiration and decompression of the stomach while feeding distally into the jejunum.

A number of clinical parameters should be followed in treating the patient on enteral feeding. Although it is important to monitor residual volumes, they are an important precise measure of gastric emptying. High residual volumes are often a single isolated event in patients otherwise tolerating their enteral feeding. Residual volumes have been shown to correlate poorly to physical examinations and abdominal radiographs.[97] The value of concern should be no less than 200 to 400 ml.[97] The management of patients who demonstrate high residual volumes should be to hold feedings, if concerned, only after the second residual volume above 200 ml. Feedings should be held for 2 hours before rechecking. If the patient demonstrates persistently high residual volumes over 8 to 12 hours, efforts should be made to place the tube at or below the ligament of Treitz. Above all, clinical judgment should be used in interpreting residual volumes. Low residual volumes do not always guarantee adequate tolerance and high residual volumes in the patient who is passing gas and stool with no nausea or vomiting may be of little concern.[97]

Diarrhea is a frequent problem in the ICU, but it is only rarely directly related to the tube feedings. Prospective studies evaluating the etiology of diarrhea in this setting reveal that the diarrhea is related to sorbitol in medications in 51% of cases, related to pseudomembranous colitis and *Clostridium difficile* in 17%, and only directly related to the feeding formula in 21% of cases.[98] Low-volume diarrhea in the ICU setting is often more a problem with incontinence, and rectal tubes or ostomy bags should be used readily. All patients should be evaluated to determine the etiology of the diarrhea. Stool studies should be obtained to rule out *C. difficile* infection, and medications should be reviewed to eliminate ingestion of sorbitol. Switching from standard formula to a small peptide formula may enhance assimilation and reduce the volume of stool output.

In general, the greatest problem to avoid is cessation of tube feedings.[99] "Down time" from enteral feeding may be reduced by avoiding placement of patients NPO after midnight for routine procedures and diagnostic testing. Feedings often can be continued up to within 4 hours of a procedure without a deleterious affect.[99] Tube displacement can be avoided by securing the tubes by bridling or placing a hemoclip on a string on the distal end of the feeding tube. Attention to hydration is warranted because adequate hydration promotes clearance of pulmonary secretions.[100] Indirect calorimetry can be used as a measure of respiratory tolerance of feeding, particularly in those patients intentionally being overfed to make up deficits. The patient whose RQ rises above 1.0 as feeding is initiated may be showing signs of pulmonary compromise and poor tolerance of the caloric load.[99]

CONCLUSIONS

Patients on mechanical ventilation allowed to experience compromise of nutritional status have fairly well-documented consequences, with respiratory muscle dysfunction, atrophy of respiratory muscle mass, and even structural changes of emphysema.[1] Providing adequate calories to meet requirements, especially through the enteric route, should be expected to help contain the stress response, promote weaning from the ventilator, and may help to reduce in-hospital complications, overall cost, and length of hospitalization.[32, 34] Indirect calorimetry is the most accurate means to determine the caloric goal, and careful attention to technique is important.[73] The efforts of the nutritionist in managing the patient with respiratory failure on mechanical ventilation should be to assess the level of stress and status of the gut, to achieve enteral access and maintain gut integrity, to determine caloric requirements by indirect calorimetry, to establish the goal of nutrition support, to monitor feedings closely, and to anticipate problems before they occur.

REFERENCES

1. Grant JP: Nutrition care of patients with acute and chronic respiratory failure. Nutr Clin Pract 9:11–17, 1994.
2. McClave SA: The consequences of overfeeding and underfeeding: indirect calorimetry plays a key role in designing nutrition regimens for mechanically ventilated patients. J Respir Care Pract Apr/May:57–64, 1997.
3. Weissman C, Askanazi J, Rosenbaum S, et al: Amino acids and respiration. Ann Intern Med 98:41–44, 1983.
4. Doekel RC Jr, Zwillich CW, Scoggin CH, et al: Clinical semi-starvation: depression of hypoxic ventilatory response. N Engl J Med 295:358–361, 1976.
5. Arora NS, Rochester DF: Effect of body weight and muscularity on human diaphragm muscle mass, thickness, and area. J Appl Physiol 52:64–70, 1982.
6. Keys A, Brozek J, Henschel A, et al: The Biology of Human Starvation. Minneapolis: University of Minnesota Press, 1950.
7. Arora NS, Rochester DF: Respiratory muscle strength and maximal voluntary ventilation in undernourished patients. Am Rev Respir Dis 126:5–8, 1982.
8. Braun NM, Arora NS, Rochester DF: Respiratory muscle and pulmonary function in polymyositis and other proximal myopathies. Thorax 38:616–623, 1983.
9. Whittaker JC, Ryan CF, Buckley PA, et al: The effects of refeeding on peripheral and respiratory muscle function in malnourished chronic obstructive pulmonary disease patients. Am Rev Respir Dis 142:283–288, 1990.
10. Niederman MS, Merrill WW, Ferranti RD, et al: Nutritional status and bacterial binding in the lower respiratory tract in patients with chronic tracheostomy. Ann Intern Med 100:795–800, 1984.
11. Niderman MS, Mantovani R, Schoch P, et al: Patterns and routes of tracheobronchial colonization in mechanically ventilated patients: the role of nutritional status in colonization of the lower airway by Pseudomonas species. Chest 95:155–161, 1989.
12. Windsor JA, Hill GL: Risk factors for postoperative pneumonia: the importance of protein depletion. Ann Surg 208:209–214, 1988.
13. Sahebjami H, Wirman JA: Emphysema-like changes in the lungs of starved rats. Am Rev Respir Dis 124:619–624, 1981.
14. Stein J, Fenigstein H: Anatomic pathologique de la maladie de famine. In: Apfelbaum E (ed): Maladie de famine. Rescherches cliniques sur la famine executees dans le ghetto de Varsovie en 1942. Warsaw: American Joint Distribution Committee, 1946, pp 21–77.
15. Braun SR, Dixon RM, Keim NL, et al: Predictive clinical value of nutritional assessment factors in COPD. Chest 85:353–357, 1984.
16. Bassili HR, Deitel M: Effect of nutritional support on weaning patients off mechanical ventilators. JPEN J Parenter Enteral Nutr 5:161–163, 1981.
17. Mattar JA, Velasco IT, Esgalb AS: Parenteral nutrition as a useful method of weaning patients from mechanical ventilation. JPEN J Parenter Enteral Nutr 2:50, 1978.
18. Elwyn DH, Kinney JM, Malayappa J, et al: Influence of increasing carbohydrate intake on glucose kinetics in injured patients. Ann Surg 190:117–127, 1979.

19. Burke JF, Wolfe RR, Mullany CJ, et al: Glucose requirements following burn injury: parameters of optimal glucose infusion and possible hepatic and respiratory abnormalities following excessive glucose intake. Ann Surg 190:274–285, 1969.

20. Heymsfield SB, Hill JO, Evert M, et al: Energy expenditure during continuous intragastric infusion of fuel. Am J Clin Nutr 45:526–533, 1987.

21. Askanazi J, Carpentier YA, Elwyn DH, et al: Influence of total parenteral nutrition on fuel utilization in injury and sepsis. Ann Surg 191:40–46, 1980.

22. Swinamer DL, Grace MG, Hamilton SM, et al: Predictive equation for assessing energy expenditure in mechanically ventilated critically ill patients. Crit Care Med 18:657–661, 1990.

23. Talpers SS, Romberger DJ, Bunce SB, et al: Nutritionally associated increased carbon dioxide production: excess total calories vs high proportion of carbohydrate calories. Chest 102:551–555, 1992.

24. Covelli HD, Black JW, Olsen MS, Beekman JF: Respiratory failure precipitated by high carbohydrate loads. Ann Intern Med 95:579–581, 1981.

25. Askanazi J, Rosenbaum SH, Hyman AI, et al: Respiratory changes induced by the large glucose loads of total parenteral nutrition. JAMA 243:1444–1447, 1980.

26. Amene P, Sladen R, Feeley T, Fisher R: Hypercapnia during total parenteral nutrition with hypertonic dextrose. Crit Care Med 15:171–172, 1987.

27. Liposkey JM, Nelson LD: Ventilatory response to high caloric loads in critically ill patients. Crit Care Med 22:796–802, 1994.

28. McClave SA, Lowen CC, Kleber MJ, et al: Is the respiratory quotient a useful indicator of over- or underfeeding? JPEN J Parenter Enteral Nutr 21:S113, 1997.

29. Mowatt-Larssen CA, Brown RO: Specialized nutritional support in respiratory disease. Clin Pharm 12:276–292, 1993.

30. Grant JP: Nutritional assessment in clinical practice. Nutr Clin Pract 1:3–11, 1986.

31. Fleck A: Acute phase response: implications for nutrition and recovery. Nutrition 4:109–117, 1988.

32. Kudsk KA, Croce MA, Fabian RC, et al: Enteral versus parenteral feeding—effects on septic morbidity after blunt and penetrating abdominal trauma. Ann Surg 215:503–511, 1992.

33. Baxter JK, Babineau TJ, Apovian CM, et al: Perioperative glucose control predicts increased nosocomial infection in diabetics. Crit Care Med 18:S207, 1990.

34. Zaloga GP, MacGregory DA: What to consider when choosing enteral or parenteral nutrition. J Crit Illness 5:1180–1200, 1990.

35. Knaus WA, Zimmerman JE, Wagner DP, et al: APACHE—Acute Physiology and Chronic Health Evaluation: a physiologically based classification system. Crit Care Med 9:591–597, 1981.

36. Knaus WA, Draper EA, Wagner DP, Zimmerman JE: APACHE II: a severity of disease classification system. Crit Care Med 13:818–829, 1985.

37. Knaus WA, Wagner DP, Draper EA, et al: The APACHE III prognostic system: risk prediction of hospital mortality for critically ill hospitalized adults. Chest 100:1619–1636, 1991.

38. Brown PE, McClave SA, Hoy NW, et al: The Acute Physiology and Chronic Health Evaluation II classification system is a valid marker for physiologic stress in the critically ill patient. Crit Care Med 21:363–367, 1993.

39. Fiaccadori E, Del Canale S, Coffrini E, et al: Hypercapnic-hypoxemic chronic obstructive pulmonary disease (COPD): influence of severity of COPD on nutritional status. Am J Clin Nutr 48:680–685, 1988.

40. Driver AG, McAlevy MT, Smith JL: Nutritional assessment of patients with chronic obstructive pulmonary disease and acute respiratory failure. Chest 82:568–571, 1982.

41. Morrison NJ, Richardson J, Dunn L, et al: Respiratory muscle performance in normal elderly subjects and patients with COPD. Chest 95:90–94, 1989.

42. McClave SA, Snider HL: Understanding the metabolic response to critical illness: factors that cause patients to deviate from the expected pattern of hypermetabolism. New Horiz 2:139–146, 1994.

43. Weissman C, Kemper M, Askanazi J, et al: Resting metabolic rate of the critically ill patient: measured versus predicted. J Anesthesiol 64:673–679, 1986.

44. Weissman C, Kemper M, Damask MC, et al: Effect of routine intensive care interactions on metabolic rate. Chest 86:815–818, 1984.

45. Schols AM, Fredrix E, Soeters PB, et al: Resting energy expenditure in patients with chronic obstructive pulmonary disease. Am J Clin Nutr 54:983–987, 1991.

46. Schols AM, Soeters PB, Mostert R, et al: Energy balance in chronic obstructive pulmonary disease. Am Rev Respir Dis 413:1246–1252, 1991.

47. Goldstein SA, Thomashow BM, Kvetan V, et al: Nitrogen and energy relationships in malnourished patients with emphysema. Am Rev Respir Dis 138:636–644, 1988.

48. Goldstein S, Askanazi J, Weissman C, et al: Energy expenditure in patients with chronic obstructive pulmonary disease. Chest 91:222–224, 1987.

49. Feurer ID, Crosby LO, Mullen JL: Measured and predicted resting energy expenditure in clinically stable patients. Clin Nutr 3:27–34, 1984.

50. Makk LJK, McClave SA, Creech PW, et al: Clinical application of the metabolic cart to the delivery of total parenteral nutrition. Crit Care Med 18:1320–1327, 1990.

51. Van Lanschot JJB, Feenstra BWA, Vermeij CG, et al: Calculation versus measurement of total energy expenditure. Crit Care Med 14:981–985, 1986.

52. Kreymann G, Grosser S, Buggisch P, et al: Oxygen consumption and resting metabolic rate in sepsis, sepsis syndrome, and septic shock. Crit Care Med 21:1012–1019, 1993.

53. Abraham E, Bland RD, Cobo JC, et al: Sequential cardiorespiratory patterns associated with outcome in septic shock. Chest 85:75–80, 1984.

54. Foster GD, Knox LS, Dempsey DT, et al: Caloric requirements in total parenteral nutrition. J Am Coll Nutr 6:231–253, 1987.

55. Grant JP: Handbook of Total Parenteral Nutrition. Philadelphia: WB Saunders, 1975, pp 12–26.

56. Elwyn DH, Kinney JM, Askanazi J: Energy expenditure in surgical patients. Surg Clin North Am 61:545–556, 1981.

57. Long CL, Schaffel N, Geiger JW, et al: Metabolic response to injury and illness: estimation of energy and protein needs from indirect calorimetry and nitrogen balance. JPEN J Parenter Enteral Nutr 3:452–456, 1979.

58. Ireton-Jones CS, Turner WW Jr, Liepa GU, et al: Equations for the estimation of energy expenditures in patients with burns with special reference to ventilatory status. J Burn Care Rehabil 13:330–333, 1992.

59. Owen OE, Colliver JA, Schrage JP: Adult human energy requirements. Front Clin Nutr 2:1–8, 1993.

60. Swinamer DL, Grace MG, Hamilton SM, et al: Predictive equation for assessing energy expenditure in mechanically ventilated critically ill patients. Crit Care Med 18:657–661, 1990.

61. Baker JP, Detsky AS, Stewart S, et al: Randomized trial of total parenteral nutrition in critically ill patients: metabolic effects of varying glucose-lipid ratios as the energy source. Gastroenterology 87:53, 1984.

62. Cunningham JJ: Factors contributing to increased energy expenditure in thermal injury: a review of studies employing indirect calorimetry. JPEN J Parenter Enteral Nutr 14:649–656, 1990.

63. Leff ML, Hill JO, Yates AA, et al: Resting metabolic rate: measurement reliability. JPEN J Parenter Enteral Nutr 11:354–359, 1987.

64. McClave SA, Kaiser SC, Olash BM, et al: Variation in resting energy expenditure for normals over a two year period of study. Gastroenterology 100:A536, 1991.

65. Weir JB: New methods for calculating metabolic rate with special reference to protein metabolism. J Physiol 109:1–9, 1949.

66. Daly JM, Heymsfield SB, Head CA, et al: Human energy requirements: overestimation by widely used prediction equation. Am J Clin Nutr 42:1170–1174, 1985.

67. Williams RR, Fuenning CR: Circulatory indirect calorimetry in the critically ill. JPEN J Parenter Enteral Nutr 15:509–512, 1991.

68. Smithies MN, Royston B, Makita K, et al: Comparison of oxygen consumption measurements: indirect calorimetry versus the reversed Fick method. Crit Care Med 19:1401–1406, 1991.

69. Takala J, Keinanen O, Vaisanen P, Kari A: Measurement of gas exchange in intensive care: laboratory and clinical validation of a new device. Crit Care Med 17:1041–1047, 1989.

70. Liggett SB, St. John RE, Lefrak SS: Determination of resting energy expenditure utilizing the thermodilution pulmonary artery catheter. Chest 91:562–566, 1987.

71. Walsh BJ, Murley TF: Comparison of three methods of determining oxygen consumption and resting energy expenditure. J Am Osteopath Assoc 89:43–46, 1989.

72. Levinson MR, Groeger JS, Miodownik S, et al: Indirect calorimetry in mechanically ventilated patients. Crit Care Med 154:144–147, 1987.

73. McClave SA, Snider HL: Use of indirect calorimetry in clinical nutrition. Nutr Clin Pract 7:207–221, 1992.

74. McClave SA, Snider HL, Greene L, et al: Effective utilization of indirect calorimetry during critical care. Intensive Care World 9:194–200, 1992.

75. Zavala DC: In: Nutritional Assessment in Critical Care: A Training Handbook. Iowa City: University of Iowa Press, 1989, pp 41–59.

76. Isbell TR, Klesges RC, Meyers AW, Klesges LM: Measurement reliability and reactivity using repeated measurements of resting energy expenditure with a face mask, mouthpiece, and ventilated canopy. JPEN J Parenter Enteral Nutr 15:165–168, 1991.

77. Branson RD: The measurement of energy expenditure: instrumentation, practical considerations, and clinical application. Respir Care 35:640–659, 1990.

78. Weissman C, Kemper M, Elwyn DH, et al: The energy expenditure of the mechanically ventilated critically ill patient—an analysis. Chest 89:254–259, 1989.

79. Askanazi J, Nordenstrom J, Rosenbaum SH, et al: Nutrition for the patient with respiratory failure: glucose vs. fat. Anesthesiology 54:373–377, 1981.

80. Askanazi J, Weissman C, LaSala PA, et al: Effect of protein intake on ventilatory drive. Anesthesiology 60:106–110, 1984.

81. Takala J, Askanazi J, Weissman C, et al: Changes in respiratory control induced by amino acid infusions. Crit Care Med 16:465–469, 1988.

82. Hamawy KJ, Moldawer LL, Georgieff M, et al: The effect of lipid emulsions on reticuloendothelial system function in the injured animal. JPEN J Parenter Enteral Nutr 9:559–565, 1985.

83. Seidner DL, Mascioli EA, Istfan NW, et al: Effects of long-chain triglyceride emulsions on reticuloendothelial system function in humans. JPEN J Parenter Enteral Nutr 13:614–619, 1989.

84. Salo M: Inhibition of immunoglobulin synthesis in vitro by intravenous lipid emulsion (Intralipid). JPEN J Parenter Enteral Nutr 14:459–462, 1990.

85. Cerra FB, Siegel JH, Border JR, et al: The hepatic failure of sepsis: cellular versus substrate. Surgery 86:409–422, 1979.

86. Lundholm M, Rossner S: Rate of elimination of the Intralipid fat emulsion from the circulation in ICU patients. Crit Care Med 10:740–746, 1982.

87. Venus B, Smith RA, Patel CB, et al: Hemodynamic and gas exchange alterations during Intralipid infusion in patients with adult respira-

tory distress syndrome. Chest 95:1278–1281, 1989.

88. Greene HL, Hazlett D, Demaree R: Relationship between Intralipid-induced hyperlipemia and pulmonary function. Am J Clin Nutr 29:127–135, 1976.

89. Hwang TL, Huang SL, Chen MF: Effects of intravenous fat emulsion on respiratory failure. Chest 97:934–938, 1990.

90. Ota DM, Jessup JM, Babcock GF, et al: Immune function during intravenous administration of a soybean oil emulsion. JPEN J Parenter Enteral Nutr 9:23–27, 1985.

91. Charash WE, Kearney PA, Annis KA, et al: Early enteral feeding is associated with an attenuation of the acute phase/cytokine response following multiple trauma [abstract]. J Trauma 37:1015, 1994.

92. Pingleton SK, Hadzima SK: Enteral alimentation and gastrointestinal bleeding in mechanically ventilated patients. Crit Care Med 11:13–16, 1983.

93. Layon AJ, Florete OG, Day AL, et al: The effect of duodenojejunal alimentation on gastric pH and hormones in intensive care unit patients. Chest 99:695–702, 1991.

94. Al-Saady N, Blackmore C, Bennett ED: High fat, low carbohydrate enteral feeding reduced $PaCO_2$ and the period of ventilation in ventilated patients. Intensive Care Med 15:290–295, 1989.

95. Metheny N: Minimizing respiratory complications of nasoenteric tube feedings: state of the science. Heart Lung 22:213–223, 1993.

96. Metheny N: Preventing pulmonary complications during enteral feeding in the critically ill. Program Manual, ASPEN 18th Clinical Congress, Jan 30–Feb 2, 1994, San Antonio, TX, pp 318–322.

97. McClave SA, Snider HL, Lowen CC, et al: Use of residual volume as a marker for enteral feeding intolerance: prospective blinded comparison with physical examination and radiographic findings. JPEN J Parenter Enteral Nutr 16:99–105, 1992.

98. Edes TE, Walk BE, Austin JL: Diarrhea in tube-fed patients: feeding formula not necessarily the cause. Am J Med 88:91–94, 1990.

99. McClave SA, Sexton LK, Adams JL, et al: Enteral tube feeding in the intensive care unit: factors impeding adequate delivery. Gastroenterology 112:A892, 1997.

100. Chapman KM, Winter L: COPD: using nutrition to prevent respiratory function decline. Geriatrics 51:37–42, 1996.

CHAPTER 13

Airway Management

Michael S. Gorback, MD

AIRWAY ANATOMY
Upper Airway
Lower Airway
BASIC AIRWAY
MANAGEMENT
Simple Maneuvers to
Relieve Airway
Obstruction
Orpharyngeal and
Nasopharyngeal Airways
TRACHEAL INTUBATION
Assessing the Patient for
Intubation

Selecting Intubation
Equipment
Performing Intubation
Postintubation Procedures
Cricothyroidotomy
Changing Endotracheal
Tubes
Changing Tracheostomy
Tubes

KEY WORDS

airway anatomy
oropharyngeal and
  nasopharyngeal airways

esophageal obturator airway
tracheal intubation

endobronchial intubation
laryngoscope

Control of the airway is a critical component of mechanical ventilation.[1,2] To provide this control in a safe and effective manner, the clinician must have a working knowledge of airway anatomy and know the application of basic and advanced management techniques. This chapter reviews three important components of airway management:

- Basic anatomy of the upper and lower airways as it relates to airway management
- Basic airway management techniques
- Tracheal intubation

AIRWAY ANATOMY (Fig. 13–1)

Upper Airway

Oral Cavity

The tongue is attached anteriorly to the mandible and the hyoid bone. In the unconscious patient, the tongue often falls posteriorly because of loss of muscle tone and obstructs the airway. Basic airway management maneuvers are aimed at relieving this obstruction.

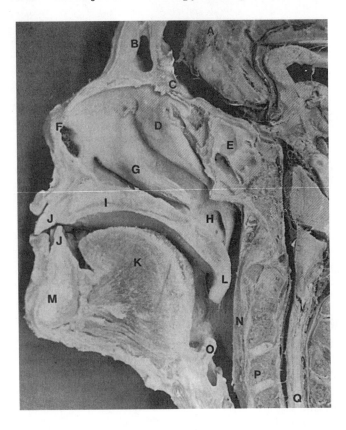

FIGURE 13–1

Anatomy of the upper airway depicted in a sagittal section of the head. *A,* brain; *B,* frontal sinus; *C,* cribriform plate; *D,* superior concha; *E,* sphenoid sinus; *F,* nostrils; *G,* inferior concha; *H,* eustachian tube; *I,* palate; *J,* teeth; *K,* tongue; *L,* uvula; *M,* mandible; *N,* posterior wall of pharynx; *O,* epiglottis; *P,* vertebral column; *Q,* spinal cord. (Reproduced with permission from Gorback MS: Emergency Airway Management. Philadelphia: BC Decker, 1990.)

The palate and the mandible provide the major bony framework of the oral cavity. The mandible serves as an anterior anchor for the tongue. The muscles of mastication insert on the ramus of the mandible.

Nose

The nasal cavity borders on the base of the skull. When there is basilar skull fracture, nasotracheal or nasogastric tubes may pass accidentally into the cranial cavity. The nasal mucosa is highly vascular and easily damaged. Topical vasoconstrictors and generous lubrication decrease the likelihood of epistaxis during manipulation of this portion of the airway. When the nasal route is being used for intubation, several anatomic relationships must be kept in mind. The distance from the nares to the carina is 27 cm in the average adult woman and 32 cm in the average adult man. Because the meatus of the paranasal sinuses and lacrimal ducts opens into the nasal cavity, prolonged intubation of the nose with nasogastric or nasotracheal tubes may cause sinus infections.

Nasogastric or nasotracheal tubes should be inserted perpendicular to the plane of the face because the floor of the nasal cavity runs parallel to the line of the teeth.

The relative patency of each side of the nose should be checked to determine the presence of obstruction, such as a deviated septum.

Pharynx

The oral cavity and nasopharynx are continuous with the oropharynx, which contains the uvula, tonsils, and proximal epiglottis. The major structures of the nasopharynx are the adenoids. The laryngopharynx begins at the tip of the epiglottis.

Larynx

The adult larynx is located at the level of C4 to C5; in infants it is higher, at C3 to C4. The larynx passes anteriorly, extending to the level of the cricoid cartilage. Posteriorly, the pharynx joins the esophagus at the same level.

As mentioned previously, the larynx ends

at the cricotracheal junction. The only circumferentially complete laryngeal cartilage is the cricoid cartilage, located at C6. Cricoid pressure, part of the Sellick maneuver, compresses the proximal esophagus between the cricoid cartilage and the anterior cervical spine. The narrowest part of the pediatric airway is the cricoid cartilage, whereas in the adult it is at the level of the vocal cords. The thyroid cartilage is a major anatomic landmark for both intubation and airway anesthesia. The superior laryngeal nerves can be blocked easily to provide supraglottic anesthesia. These nerves run past the superior horns of the thyroid cartilage as they enter the thyrohyoid membrane. The vocal cords are located inside the thyroid cartilage. The cricothyroid membrane is palpated easily between the thyroid and cricoid cartilages. This is the site of choice for emergency surgical access to the respiratory tract because of its relative avascularity and distance from the thyroid gland.

The epiglottis, a major landmark to look for during **laryngoscopy,** also impairs the view of the vocal cords. The upper part of the epiglottis is mobile, whereas the lower part attaches to the hyoid bone and the posterosuperior aspect of the thyroid cartilage.

Lower Airway

Trachea

The trachea is composed of 18 to 22 cartilaginous arches (approximately 2 rings per centimeter) joined by longitudinal elastic fibers, allowing it to stretch and contract as the lungs move during the respiratory cycle. The posterior or membranous wall is applied closely to the esophagus throughout its length. The trachea is 10 to 13 cm long in the adult.

Bronchi, Conducting Airways, and Alveoli

The right mainstem bronchus is approximately 2 cm long before it divides into the right upper lobe bronchus and the bronchus intermedius. The left mainstem bronchus is approximately 5 cm long before it divides into the left upper and lower lobe bronchi. Therefore, there is a greater likelihood of obstructing the upper lobe with right endobronchial intubation.

BASIC AIRWAY MANAGEMENT

Simple Maneuvers to Relieve Airway Obstruction

The first step to relieve airway obstruction is to establish a patent airway. Foreign material should be removed from the mouth and the oropharynx, either manually (finger sweep) or with suction.[1-3]

The presence of spontaneous respiration may dictate positioning. Apneic patients should be placed supine in anticipation of further airway support. An obtunded patient may be placed alternatively in the lateral decubitus position, with the head slightly down to prevent aspiration. Airway maneuvers such as the chin lift and jaw thrust are still possible in this position. A patient in respiratory distress frequently prefers the sitting position, with the neck extended and the head moved anterior to the plane of the torso. This position, which is similar to the sniffing position used for laryngoscopy, aligns the major axes of the airway. The sitting position removes the weight of the abdominal contents from the diaphragm. Forcing an awake dyspneic patient to lie flat may produce panic and struggling and may complicate management.

One of the simplest and most effective maneuvers to establish a patent airway is the chin lift. This maneuver is performed by placing the fingers under the chin and lifting upward to raise the chin while depressing the forehead with the other hand. The thumb may be used to depress the lower lip or mandible, thus opening the mouth. The jaw thrust is another effective technique for opening the airway. The fingers are placed behind the angle of the mandible, lifting upward to displace it forward. The thumbs may be used to hold the mouth open, to seal a mask on the face, or both. The chin lift and jaw thrust may be used together, with the thumbs employed to depress the mandible and open the mouth ("triple maneuver").

Oropharyngeal and Nasopharyngeal Airways

Simple Oropharyngeal Airways

The primary function of the simple oropharyngeal airway is to establish upper airway patency.[1,2] An airway that reaches from the corner of the mouth to the tragus of the ear when it is held next to the patient's face is most likely the proper size to use. There are two ways to insert a simple oropharyngeal airway. With the use of a tongue blade or a finger to depress the tongue, the airway may be slipped posteriorly. Alternatively, the airway may be inserted upside down (with the curvature facing the roof of the mouth) and rotated around into place. This

may require more mandibular excursion and also may dislodge loose teeth.

In a patient with intact gag reflexes, simple oropharyngeal airway insertion is a very provocative stimulus. Prior topical application of local anesthetic may alleviate this response. Obstructions can be exacerbated with these airways. The airway must be seated posterior to the tongue. If the airway is too small, the tip will be midway down the tongue, pushing it posteriorly against the back of the pharynx. Catching the tongue with the tip of the oral airway during insertion pushes the tongue posteriorly against the pharyngeal wall, causing obstruction.

The simple oropharyngeal airway usually is used to facilitate mouth-to-mouth or mask-to-mouth ventilation.

Simple Nasopharyngeal Airways

Simple nasopharyngeal airways, which are better tolerated by the awake patient, can

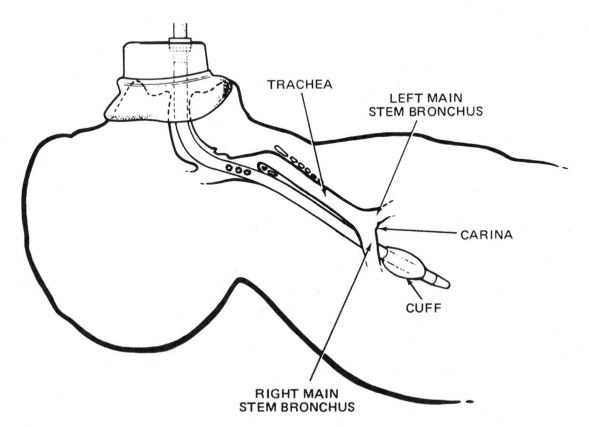

FIGURE 13-2
The esophageal obturator airway. (Reproduced with permission from Advanced Cardiac Life Support. Dallas: American Heart Association. Copyright American Heart Association, 1997.)

be inserted even if the patient is unable or unwilling to open his or her mouth.[1,2] Generous lubrication eases passage and prevents epistaxis. Topical vasoconstrictors may be used, but there is rarely time for their application. Topical anesthesia is not required, but coating the airway with lidocaine paste increases patient tolerance.

Esophageal Obturator Airways
(Fig. 13–2)

The esophageal obturator airway is a device consisting of a tight-fitting oronasal mask with a tube through it that is placed in the esophagus.[1,2] The distal end of this tube is designed to occlude the esophagus while ventilation is directed through a series of openings in the tube at the level of the larynx.

Proper placement must be ensured before the balloon cuff is inflated to occlude the esophagus. Problems associated with use of the device include esophageal injury, inadvertent tracheal intubation, tracheal compression from an overinflated cuff, and gagging/wretching. A tracheal tube can be inserted laryngoscopically with this device in place. The esophageal obturator airway should be considered a temporizing measure until a more secure tracheal tube can be placed.

Laryngeal Mask Airway (Fig. 13–3)

This device consists of a rigid curved tube that, when placed in the oropharynx, has its distal opening at the level of the larynx.[4] Around this distal opening is an inflatable "laryngeal mask" designed to surround the epiglottis and laryngeal structures. The tube is wide enough to allow subsequent passage of a standard tracheal tube. Alternatively, it can be used as a stand-alone airway to provide assisted ventilation.

Although shown to be an effective artificial airway, the laryngeal mask airway does not provide the same level of airway control and protection as does the standard cuffed tracheal tube. Other reported complications include posterior pharyngeal damage, gagging/vomiting, and ineffective ventilation from improper placement. Like the esopha-

geal obturator airway, this device should be considered a temporizing measure until a more secure tracheal tube can be placed.

TRACHEAL INTUBATION

Assessing the Patient for Intubation

A detailed evaluation often must be deferred in emergency situations (e.g., cardiac arrest). Unfortunately, management may be rushed needlessly when temporizing measures might have provided a few extra moments for thought and preparation. For example, a patient with impending respiratory failure may be assisted with a bag and mask while preparations are made for a more controlled, less stressful intubation. A small degree of preparation often tips the balance between an easy and a difficult procedure for both the clinician and the patient.

Patient History/Clinical Status

The clinician must determine whether the patient has any concurrent medical problems that could be exacerbated by the intubation procedure. The patient usually responds to intubation with hypertension and tachycardia. Occasionally, hypotension may ensue for several reasons: First, a patient with respiratory failure may have high circulating levels of catecholamines in response to hypoxia or hypercarbia. Relief of the blood gas derangements with assisted ventilation may cause a decrease in catecholamine levels and blood pressure. Second, hypotension from venodilation also may develop from the respiratory alkalosis produced by manual hyperventilation after intubation. Third, hypotension may result from decreased venous return caused by positive pressure ventilation. Finally, profound hypotension may occur after the administration of sedatives, hypnotics, or muscle relaxants.

The clinician must consider the impact of these responses on concurrent medical conditions. For example, patients with valvular disease, coronary artery disease, and

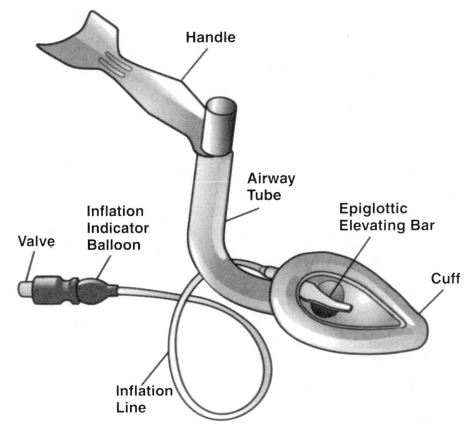

FIGURE 13–3
The laryngeal mask airway (Gensia Automedics, San Diego, CA).

congestive heart failure may respond poorly to increases in vasoconstriction or heart rate after intubation. Sudden elevations in arterial pressure may cause rupture of aneurysms. Patients with chronic hypertension often have a magnified pressor response to intubation. Conversely, beta-receptor antagonists, vasodilators, or diuretics taken for chronic hypertension may blunt compensatory responses. Patients with reactive airway disease (asthma, bronchitis, or allergy) often respond to intubation with bronchoconstriction, which can be severe. Tracheal stenosis may be mistaken for asthma, with the diagnosis often missed in an emergency situation. Signs of prior tracheal trauma, such as tracheostomy, may indicate this condition.

Intubation usually increases intracranial pressure. Precautions should be taken before intubation to blunt this response. Care should be taken to avoid giving sedatives or other drugs that might produce hyperten-

sion in the presence of cerebrovascular insufficiency. In patients with carotid disease, bradycardia, cerebral ischemia, or both can develop when the neck is extended for intubation.

Patients with myasthenia gravis have extreme sensitivity to nondepolarizing muscle relaxants.[5] Anticholinesterase drugs taken for myasthenia prolong the half-life of drugs metabolized by plasma cholinesterases, such as succinylcholine. Ester-type local anesthetics may produce toxic side effects at lower doses in the presence of anticholinesterases.

The disposition of drugs given during airway management is affected by renal or hepatic impairment. Diminished drug excretion caused by renal or hepatic impairment may significantly delay neurologic assessment after intubation. For example, pancuronium excretion is greatly impaired in the presence of renal failure. The action of drugs whose primary route of elimination is hepatic (e.g., narcotics, vecuronium, and lidocaine) may be prolonged by hepatic disease. Chronic ethanol or other drug abuse may cause increased tolerance to central nervous system depressants.

Coagulopathy (e.g., due to thrombocytopenia, anticoagulant administration, or a clotting factor deficiency) may cause uncontrollable hemorrhage after airway instrumentation (especially with nasal intubation) or the performance of nerve blocks.

Most airway management maneuvers cause or require neck motion. Musculoskeletal disorders of the cervical spine have a profound impact on airway management. Patients with cervical spine instability (e.g., caused by spinal trauma or rheumatoid arthritis) may suffer neurologic damage during airway manipulation. Patients with ankylosing spondylitis may suffer neck fractures during neck manipulation.

Limited mobility of the head, neck, larynx, and temporomandibular joint may be caused by arthritis, ankylosing spondylitis, previous fusion, or placement in a halo.[6] Infections such as epiglottitis or Ludwig's angina may precipitate airway compromise. Infections may complicate management if the infection is present at the site where a nerve block or tracheostomy is to be performed.

Aspiration risk factors include recent ingestion of food, gastric stasis (e.g., due to stress, anxiety, pain, gastric emptying disorders, or narcotic administration), gastroesophageal reflux, pregnancy, gastrointestinal obstruction, diminished level of consciousness (from any cause), and impaired protective reflexes (e.g., due to stroke).

Pregnancy produces changes in almost every major organ system.[7] Mucosal capillary engorgement narrows air passages and increases the tendency for bleeding during manipulation. Precautions include the use of gentle technique during suctioning or intubation and the use of a smaller tube. As the pregnancy progresses, functional residual capacity diminishes, physiologic anemia worsens, and cardiac output increases, all of which contribute to rapid arterial oxygen desaturation during apnea. Preeclampsia further complicates management because of the cardiovascular, renal, and central nervous system derangements superimposed on the physiologic changes of pregnancy. Severe airway edema, intracranial pathology, and coagulopathy are common.

A great deal can be learned from records of previous intubations. Intubation procedure notes or anesthesia records often record the degree of difficulty encountered. In consideration of possible future intubations, the clinician should document techniques and difficulties in the patient's record.

Physical Examination

Relative urgency often can be gauged with a brief determination of the patient's color, respiratory pattern, vital signs, level of distress, and level of consciousness. The autonomic stimulation of hypoxemia and hypercarbia produces hypertension, tachycardia, diaphoresis, and pallor. Hypotension and bradycardia are late signs. Drug overdose usually produces slow, deep, regular respiration. Metabolic acidosis accompanying diabetic ketoacidosis or renal failure (Kussmaul's breathing) also may produce this pattern.

Tachypnea is a nonspecific finding. Disorders of the conducting airways (asthma), parenchyma (pulmonary edema), vasculature (pulmonary embolism), respiratory muscles (fatigue), or extrapulmonary diseases (e.g., salicylate toxicity, shock, or hyperventilation syndromes) can produce tachypnea.

Asymmetrical thoracic movement may reflect pneumothorax, major unilateral bronchial obstruction (e.g., foreign body aspiration), splinting due to injury, or atelectasis. These disorders also may be noted on chest percussion. Discoordinate movement is abnormal and suggests airway obstruction or respiratory muscle fatigue. The chest and abdomen should rise and fall together. Cheyne-Stokes, Biot's, or apneustic respiration often points to central disorders.

A prolonged inspiratory time with inspiratory stridor is characteristic of variable extrathoracic obstruction, whereas expiratory stridor, prolonged expiratory time, or wheezing suggests variable intrathoracic obstruction or bronchoconstriction. Fixed obstruction may affect one or both respiratory phases. Stridor indicates severe narrowing of the airway. Voice changes may result from vocal cord edema or palsy, dislocation or injury of laryngeal cartilages, or foreign bodies.

Airway Examination

Examination of the mouth should include a search for loose or damaged teeth, dentures, and foreign bodies such as candy, chewing gum, tobacco, or food. According to one proposed scoring system,[8] if the soft palate, fauces, and uvula are visible when the patient opens the mouth wide, the glottis should be visible at laryngoscopy (Fig. 13–4). If only the soft palate and the uvular base are visible (or only the soft palate is visible), laryngoscopy may be difficult.

Temporomandibular joint mobility and mandibular morphology must be assessed.[9] In the healthy adult, mandibular excursion is approximately 50 mm (2 inches, or 3 fingerbreadths). When excursion is reduced to half of that, or approximately 25 mm, difficulty with laryngoscopy may be anticipated. The distance from the symphysis of the mandible to the hyoid bone also should be approximately 3 fingerbreadths. Two fingerbreadths or less usually indicates a retrognathic mandible. If nasal intubation is anticipated, the clinician should alternately compress each nostril as the patient breathes. This may provide a gross assessment of which passage is more patent. The patient may be able to indicate which nostril is the more patent.

Goiters, abscesses, tumors, cysts, hematomas, or other neck masses may deviate or compress the airway.[10] Neck mobility should be checked (provided that instability has been ruled out) because limited neck extension may hinder laryngoscopy. Patients with short, muscular ("bull") necks, morbid obesity, arthritis, radiation changes, or previous cervical fusion may have limited extension. Tracheostomy scars may indicate residual tracheal stenosis. Facial trauma

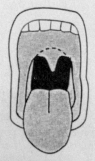

Class I: soft palate, uvula, fauces, pillars visible

No difficulty

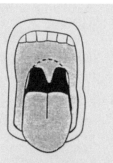

Class II: soft palate, uvula, fauces visible

No difficulty

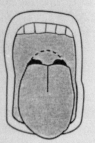

Class III: soft palate, base of uvula visible

Moderate difficulty

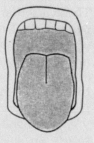

Class IV: hard palate only visible

Severe difficulty

FIGURE 13–4

Mallampati signs as indicators of difficult intubation. (Reproduced with permission from Mallampati SR, Gatt SP, Gugino LD, et al: A clinical sign to predict difficult tracheal intubation. Can Anaesth Soc J 32: 429–434, 1985.)

can cause airway obstruction, complicate airway management, and accompany other more serious injuries to the head and neck.

Chest radiography, arterial blood gas analysis, and pulmonary function tests are useful, time permitting. Electrocardiography, blood chemistry results, and hematologic profiles may be useful, but only tests used for evaluation for airway intervention are discussed here.

Arterial blood gas analysis findings must be interpreted in light of the clinical picture. Clearly, life-threatening hypoxemia and acidosis are reasons for emergent intubation. Conversely, an isolated oxygenation deficit may respond to oxygen (O_2) supplementation without intubation. Moreover, compensated hypercarbia is not necessarily an indication for intubation. Patients receiving narcotics may have moderate respiratory acidosis yet remain awake and stable.

Simple pulmonary function tests may be extremely useful,[11] especially when they indicate a trend. A vital capacity of less than 10 to 12 ml/kg may indicate impending respiratory failure in a progressive neurologic disorder. The peak expiratory flow rate is sensitive to upper airway obstruction. If the ratio of forced expiratory volume (FEV, in milliliters) to peak expiratory flow rate (in liters per minute) is greater than 10, upper airway obstruction should be suspected.

When upper airway compromise is suspected, soft tissue films of the head, neck, and chest may be useful in revealing pathology not apparent on physical examination. If airway obstruction is suspected, this should be noted on the requisition; routine anteroposterior and lateral neck radiographs usually are optimized for bone. Overpenetrated chest films help to delineate the tracheobronchial tree, whereas expiratory chest radiographs are useful for demonstrating postobstructive emphysema distal to a radiolucent foreign body. Computed tomography (CT) can be extremely useful in evaluating the upper airway, if time permits.

Selecting Intubation Equipment

Laryngoscopes

Most laryngoscopes are either curved (e.g., the MacIntosh laryngoscope) or straight (e.g., the Miller or Wisconsin laryngoscope).[12] The choice of blade is largely a personal one. The curved blade (Fig. 13–5) has a moderate curvature and a tapered flange along the left side. This blade elevates the epiglottis by stretching the hypoepiglottic ligament. Claimed advantages for the curved blade include

- Less dental trauma
- More room for passage of the tube
- Less chance of provocation of reflexes by pressing on the epiglottis

Straight blades (see Fig. 13–5), which come in a variety of configurations, are used in all age groups. The tip of a straight blade is use to lift the epiglottis directly to expose the vocal cords. Claimed advantages of this blade are greater exposure of the glottis and less need for a stylet.

Endotracheal Tubes

Contemporary high-volume, low-pressure, cuffed plastic endotracheal tubes have replaced low-compliance rubber tubes because the pressure required to obtain a good seal with the latter usually exceeds tracheal capillary pressure, thereby predisposing the patient to tracheal injury. By convention, size is determined by the inner diameter of the tube (in millimeters).

The endotracheal tube has evolved in many specialized forms. Pediatric endotracheal tubes with an internal diameter of less than 4 mm usually are uncuffed. Flexible armored tubes are available if kinking or compression of the tube is of concern. Pulling on the ring of a "trigger" tube with a finger (or thumb) flexes the tube, maneuvering the tube tip. Double-lumen tubes isolate the two sides of the tracheobronchial tree to:

- Prevent soiling of a healthy lung by pus or blood from the other
- Provide differential lung ventilation
- Perform lung lavage

Stylets and Guides

Stylets should be made of a malleable material (e.g., copper) and have a smooth sur-

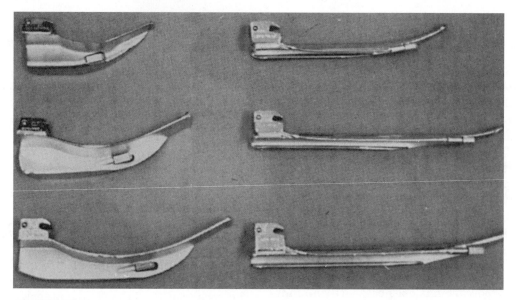

FIGURE 13–5
Laryngoscopic blades. Straight (Miller) blades are on the right, curved (MacIntosh) blades
are on the left. (Reproduced with permission from Gorback MS: Emergency Airway
Management. Philadelphia: BC Decker, 1990.)

face, either of polished metal or plastic coated.[12] After the lubricated stylet has been inserted into the tube, the tube is bent into the desired shape, usually a J or "hockey stick" configuration.

When the glottis cannot be seen, malleable plastic guides may be useful. The guide is shaped (usually into a J or hockey stick form, as with stylets) and slid under the epiglottis into the larynx. Flexible urethral sounds, nasogastric tubes, and suction catheters serve well. Dedicated bougies are also commercially available.

Fiberoptic Devices and Light Wands

The fiberoptic bronchoscope can be used for difficult or awake intubation.[13,14] Light wands are malleable stylets with a light source on the end to aid intubation by transillumination of the airway.[15,16] The Bullard laryngoscope, a rigid, curved fiberoptic device, is inserted like an oral airway, with the larynx being seen through its fiberoptic system. All three of these devices may be inserted orally in cases in which decreased mandibular excursion prevents conventional laryngoscopy. Flexible light wands are available for the nasal route.

Monitoring Devices

Pulse oximetry allows continuous noninvasive assessment of oxygenation during airway management. Capnography allows early detection of failed intubation by revealing the absence of carbon dioxide (CO_2) in exhaled gas. Semiquantitative chemical sensors attach inline to the end of the endotracheal tube and change color with pH, thereby detecting the presence of CO_2. These devices may be included in an emergency bag for convenient determination of the end-tidal CO_2 at any clinical location.

Performing Intubation

Once the decision to intubate has been made, the practitioner must decide the route of intubation and whether to intubate the patient awake or under anesthesia.

Choice of Route

The two major routes for intubation are oral and nasal. The advantages of oral intubation include faster execution, the use of a larger tube, and a minimal risk of bacterial infection. Oral intubation requires an open mouth (which dictates that the patient must be cooperative, paralyzed, or unconscious) and adequate mandibular excursion. Trauma to the teeth and lips is more likely to occur with oral intubation. The patient can occlude the tube by biting down, but this can be prevented with the insertion of an oral airway or another bite block after intubation. Although it is frequently taught that oral intubation produces more laryngeal damage, this is true only in the short term.

Nasal intubation is feasible even if the patient cannot or will not open his or her mouth. There are no hard data to support the truism that nasal intubation is more comfortable once the tube is in place. Although occlusion by the teeth is not possible, kinking in the nasopharynx has been known to occur. Because the tube position is more stable, short-term laryngeal damage is decreased. Mouth care is easier without the impediment of an orotracheal tube.

Nasal intubation usually takes longer to perform. A longer and narrower tube must be used, and the increased respiratory workload may impede subsequent weaning attempts. Fiberoptic bronchoscopes or even suction catheters may be too large to pass through a narrower or kinked tube. Nasal tubes also may be associated with a higher risk of sinusitis.[17]

Injury is probably more common during nasal intubation. As opposed to the occasional tooth or lip damage seen with oral intubation, nasal mucosal and turbinate damage are common with nasal intubation. Because the resultant epistaxis may be severe and difficult to control, coagulopathy is a contraindication to nasal intubation. Nasopharyngeal tumors, adenoids, and abscesses may be disrupted. Submucosal tunneling or other injury to the posterior pharyngeal wall may occur during nasal intubation. The tube may be passed into the cranial cavity in the presence of basilar skull fracture. Pressure necrosis of the nasal septum or alae may occur.[18]

Awake Versus Anesthetized

The advantages of awake intubation include maintenance of airway, spontaneous respi-

ration, and preservation of protective airway reflexes. If there is a question of central or peripheral nervous system derangement or damage, neurologic assessment is possible immediately after intubation. If sedation or local anesthesia is used, these advantages are compromised to various degrees.

Awake intubation requires patient cooperation, especially for oral intubation. Nasal intubation can be performed in an uncooperative patient if active restraint is used, but this is not recommended because autonomic stress responses (e.g., hypertension, tachycardia, and elevated intracranial pressure) are practically guaranteed unless sedation and regional anesthesia are used.

Intubation under anesthesia or heavy sedation (e.g., using barbiturates, etomidate, ketamine, benzodiazepines, propofol, or narcotics) eliminates the requirement for patient cooperation. The stress response is usually less than with awake intubation. The major disadvantage of heavy sedation or general anesthesia is the production of apnea or profound respiratory depression. Such techniques should be used only by experienced personnel because the patient's life depends on the respiratory support skills of the operator. Anesthesia (whether general, regional, or topical) also obtunds or abolishes protective airway reflexes; in addition, postintubation neurologic assessment is impossible until the central nervous system depressants wear off.

Preparation for Intubation

Pharmacologic preparation of the patient is beyond the scope of this chapter. Detailed descriptions may be found in other sources.

In all but the most urgent cases, all necessary equipment should be set up and checked. A basic setup includes:

- A laryngoscope and blade (or blades), with fresh batteries
- Endotracheal tubes of appropriate size, plus a few sizes larger or smaller
- A 5- or 10-ml cuff syringe
- An oxygen source capable of delivering 10 to 15 L/min, tubing, masks, and a bag–valve device
- Suction and suction catheter (Yankauer tip preferred)

- Stylets
- Intravenous access
- Emergency drugs
- A stethoscope

Oral Intubation

The occiput should be elevated approximately 5 cm. A folded blanket provides a firmer base than a pillow. The head is tilted back, aligning the axes of the larynx, pharynx, and mouth. Because this position mimics the posture of someone sniffing a flower, it often is called the sniffing position. With the middle finger of the right hand placed on the upper teeth and the thumb on the lower teeth, the two are spread apart ("scissors maneuver"). The laryngoscope blade is inserted on the right side of the mouth, aiming for the right tonsillar pillar. The tongue is kept to the left of the flange. A common mistake is to place the blade down the middle of the tongue, which is a frequent cause of difficult intubation. The blade is slid into the pharynx until the epiglottis can be seen.

Up to this point, laryngoscopy is the same with either type of blade. If a curved blade is used, the tip of the blade is inserted into the space between the base of the tongue and the epiglottis (vallecula) as far as it can go. The blade is then lifted at a 45-degree angle in the direction of the axis of the handle. Tension on the hypoepiglottic ligament lifts the epiglottis (Fig. 13–6).

When a straight blade is used, the tip of the blade is inserted under (posterior to) the epiglottis, with the blade used to lift the epiglottis directly (see Fig. 13–6). Again, the clinician lifts up on the handle: the laryngoscope should not be levered using the teeth as a fulcrum. With either type of blade, the tube is passed gently through the larynx until the cuff is seen to pass below the vocal cords.

Problems with Visualization

Poor technique is the most common cause of inadequate laryngoscopy.[19] The two most common errors are improper positioning and failure to keep the tongue to the left of the blade. Sometimes the novice inserts the blade too far, neglecting to look for the epi-

glottis on the way in. On withdrawal of the blade from the esophagus, the epiglottis falls into view. Displacing the glottis posteriorly toward the line of sight may be accomplished by pressure on the thyroid cartilage. The pressure should be applied such that the cartilage is not pinched, which closes the vocal cords. Suction should be used or the throat should be cleared manually of obstructing material. Magill forceps may be used to remove large pieces of solid material. Sometimes using a different blade makes the difference between a successful intubation and an unsuccessful one.

If the vocal cords still cannot be visualized but the epiglottis or the arytenoid cartilages can be seen, a malleable stylet is used to shape the tube into a J or hockey stick shape, and the practitioner tries to slide the tube along the underside of the epiglottis into the larynx. When the tube can be felt to pass through the vocal cords, the stylet is removed and the tube is advanced into the trachea.

The oral fiberoptic approach requires good topical anesthesia of the tongue. The use of a bite block or an intubating airway is highly recommended. The tongue should be displaced forward with an intubating airway, tongue traction, a jaw thrust maneuver, or a laryngoscope. An awake patient can be asked to protrude the tongue. Staying in the midline, the practitioner follows the tongue to the epiglottis.

Another approach in this situation is to intubate the larynx with a tube exchanger or another endotracheal guide and then to pass the endotracheal tube over it. Malleable urethral sounds, nasogastric tubes, and gum elastic bougies all have been used for this method.

The clinician should not persist in an intubation attempt for more than 15 to 30 seconds unless continuous oxygen saturation monitoring (pulse oximetry) indicates that oxygenation is adequate. Cyanosis, a late sign of desaturation, should not be used as an end point for an intubation attempt. Some practitioners have promulgated breath holding during intubation on the premise that when the intubator needs a breath, so does the patient. However, the following points should be considered:

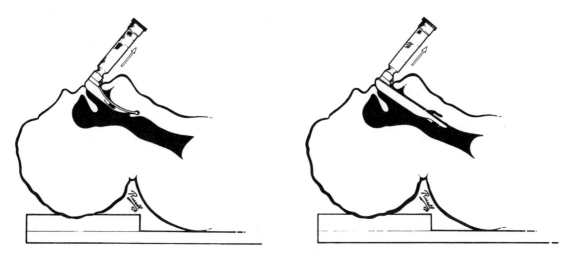

FIGURE 13-6
Proper positioning of the laryngoscope and the epiglottis using a curved blade *(left)* and a straight blade *(right)*. (Reproduced with permission from Advanced Cardiac Life Support. Dallas: American Heart Association. Copyright American Heart Association, 1997.)

- Breath holding impairs concentration.
- The intubator's tolerance for apnea is likely to differ from that of the patient.
- A dyspneic intubator is an impaired intubator.

Nasal Intubation

Anesthesia (either general or topical) and mucosal vasoconstriction are highly desirable. If nasal intubation is performed under general anesthesia, topical anesthesia is not as necessary, but it still helps to blunt the response to intubation, allowing a lower dose of general anesthetic. Topical vasoconstrictors are recommended, regardless of the choice of anesthetic.

The tube and the nasal passages should be lubricated generously. Insertion of a nasal airway lubricated with anesthetic paste (which also applies a final coat of lubrication and anesthetic) can help to determine patency as well. Through the insertion of successively larger nasal airways coated with anesthetic paste, the stimulus is gradually increased as more topical anesthesia is applied. Long cotton-tipped applicators also can be used to apply topical anesthesia and to explore the nasal passages. The tube is inserted with firm, steady pressure directed perpendicular to the face, not upward toward the forehead. Passage into the naso-

pharynx is usually accompanied by a sudden loss of resistance. The tube should not be forced if major resistance is encountered.

There are three general ways to perform nasal intubation:

- Blind
- Under direct vision
- With a fiberoptic scope

Blind nasal intubation requires no equipment other than the endotracheal tube itself. Contrary to popular belief, this technique often works in apneic patients, but success is more likely with spontaneous respiration. The practitioner advances the tube during inspiration while listening for breath sounds. If breath sounds are lost while the tube passes without resistance, esophageal placement is most likely. The tube should be withdrawn until breath sounds reappear. Extension of the neck directs the tip of the tube anteriorly. If the tube has gone laterally or anteriorly, the loss of sounds is accompanied by increased resistance. Rotating the tube guides it laterally, and flexion of the neck directs it posteriorly. A method of directing the tube anteriorly without neck manipulation is by inflation of the cuff. This technique may be used when the tube consistently passes posteriorly into the esophagus. The tube is withdrawn until breath sounds reappear, and then the cuff is inflated or overinflated. This displaces the tip of the tube away from the posterior wall of the pharynx. The tube is then advanced slightly. If it can be advanced past the point at which breath sounds were previously lost and if breath sounds continue to be present, the tip probably has entered the larynx. The cuff should be deflated and the tube advanced approximately 4 to 5 cm. This should place the tube below the vocal cords.

Nasal intubation may be performed under direct vision, but this requires laryngoscopy. Because this combines several disadvantages of both techniques, it is rarely a first choice for emergency intubation. It is useful for performing nasal intubation under controlled conditions, such as in changing an oral tube to a nasal one. Sometimes direct visualization is necessary when blind attempts fail but nasal intubation is the route of choice.

Nasal intubation with direct laryngoscopy is performed as for blind nasal intubation, except that the tube is advanced only into the pharynx. Laryngoscopy then is performed as described previously for oral intubation, advancing the tube under direct vision. The manipulations described previously for blind intubation may be used to guide the tube into the larynx. Alternatively, the tube is grasped above the cuff with Magill forceps and is guided into the larynx while an assistant advances the tube slowly. The cuff portion should not be grasped with the forceps because it may be torn.

Because the tongue is a major impediment to oral fiberoptic intubation, many prefer the nasal route. A disadvantage to the nasal route is that even slight amounts of blood impair visualization with the fiberoptic scope. Antisialagogues such as atropine or glycopyrrolate may be used to dry secretions in preparation for fiberoptic intubation. Elevation of the head helps to drain secretions and prevent posterior displacement of the tongue.

The dominant hand manipulates the controls while the nondominant hand controls the direction and depth of insertion. The scope must be rotated as a unit: it should be rotated by turning it with both hands.

As with other nasal intubations, anesthesia, vasoconstriction, and sedation are key elements to management. There are differences of opinion as to whether the tube or the scope should be passed first. If the scope is passed through the nose first, there often is less epistaxis to obstruct vision. The major problem with this technique is that one may successfully pass the scope into the trachea only to find that the tube will not fit through the nose. Conversely, if the tube is passed through the nose first, patency is ensured, but the operating field is more likely to be obscured by blood. If the tube is inserted first, it should be passed just far enough to feel the "give" as the tube bends into the nasopharynx. If the tube is inserted in this way, the larynx often is visible as the scope passes out of the end of the tube. If the tube is inserted too far initially, the first view from the end of the tube is the esophagus. Having the patient breathe through the nose moves the soft palate anteriorly, which aids in nasal intubation. After the larynx has been visualized, the patient should pant, which opens the larynx and decreases the cough and gag reflexes.

Tactile Orotracheal Intubation

The main danger with tactile orotracheal intubation is bitten fingers. This technique should be used only with paralyzed or deeply comatose patients or with the employment of a mouth prop or bite block. The tube is shaped into a J with a malleable stylet. Standing at the right side of the patient, the clinician inserts the left hand into the right side of the mouth and into the pharynx. The epiglottis (the only firm mobile structure in the pharynx) is palpated with the middle finger, and the endotracheal tube is passed down the left side of the mouth. The tube is guided into the glottis with the middle and index fingers. The stylet is withdrawn before the tube is introduced more than a few centimeters past the cords.

Endobronchial Intubation

Indications for endobronchial intubation[20] include:

- Preventing contamination of a healthy lung by a contaminated one
- Bronchopleural fistula
- Giant lung cyst
- Tracheobronchial disruption
- Operations on the lung or esophagus
- Pulmonary lavage
- Need for different tidal volumes or expiratory pressures in each lung

As described previously, the right upper lobe bronchus arises closer to the carina than the left upper lobe bronchus, so it is more likely to be occluded by the endobronchial cuff. Therefore, left-sided tubes are preferable.

Preparation for endobronchial intubation is similar to that for oral intubation with a single-lumen tube, with two major modifications:

1. Both cuffs (bronchial and tracheal) should be checked.

2. A stylet is inserted through the bronchial side of the catheter, giving it a slight curvature to the left toward the end of the tube.

With the airway adapters to the right, the distal part of the tube is inserted as if it were a single-lumen tube, and the stylet is withdrawn when the bronchial cuff passes through the vocal cords. The tube is rotated 90 degrees counterclockwise until the airway connectors are in the midline. This directs the endobronchial side to the left. The tube is advanced until it is seated in the bronchus, and the laryngoscope is removed. The point at which the two lumina join should be at the level of the teeth. Placement and function are confirmed by inflating the tracheal cuff first and checking breath sounds during manual ventilation. If only one lung is ventilated, the tracheal cuff is probably in one of the mainstem bronchi; the cuff is deflated and the tube withdrawn slightly. This is repeated until bilateral breath sounds are heard, and the bronchial cuff is inflated using no more than 3 ml of air. The pilot balloon is palpated during inflation to ensure that excessive pressure is not applied. Breath sounds still should be bilateral after inflation of the bronchial cuff. The tubing is clamped to the bronchial

side. Breath sounds should disappear on the left and be present on the right. The process is repeated on the other side: the findings should reverse. If bilateral breath sounds are heard with either side clamped, the tube is not positioned properly. If the tube seems to be well seated and bilateral sounds persist with one side clamped, the bronchial cuff may be distal to a secondary bronchus. This is more likely to occur with a right-sided tube because of the early takeoff of the right upper lobe bronchus. The tube is pulled back 1 or 2 cm at a time, with the intubator checking for proper function.

If both lumina are in one bronchus or if the tube is kinked, clamping one side abolishes breath sounds bilaterally. A remote possibility is occlusion of one of the ports. The intubator should try withdrawing the tube in 1- to 2-cm increments. If the tube has passed into the contralateral bronchus, ventilation will be absent on the right when the bronchial side is occluded. Positioning of the tube can be aided or confirmed by fiberoptic bronchoscopy. As viewed through the tracheal lumen, the right mainstem bronchus should be easily visible, whereas the endobronchial portion may be seen passing into the left mainstem bronchus. The tube may be withdrawn until the cuff is visible just distal to the carina, ensuring the proper position.

Light Wands

Lighted stylets (light wands)[15,16] are used to intubate by transillumination of the airway in a dim room. The light wand stylet is lubricated and passed through an endotracheal tube. The tube is shaped into a J. The jaw is pulled forward, and the light wand is advanced into the pharynx until a bright area of light is seen below the cricoid cartilage, indicating that the tube is in the trachea. The stylet is removed and the tube is advanced to the desired depth.

Postintubation Procedures

The clinician inflates the cuff while palpating the pilot balloon for excessive pressure. The cuff is deflated slowly until air can be heard escaping around it, and then just enough air is added to seal the leak. The following signs should be sought:

- Bilateral chest movement during ventilation
- Condensation of moisture in the tube during exhalation
- Loss of phonation in an awake patient

Both lungs are auscultated, and the practitioner listens over the epigastrium to rule out esophageal intubation. The latter produces coarse flatulent sounds over the stomach. Esophageal intubation often produces a belching sound during ventilation. The depth of the tube is checked: it should be approximately 22 ± 2 cm at the level of the incisors (oral intubation) and 27 ± 2 cm at the level of the nares (nasal intubation) in the typical adult.

Because there is usually no CO_2 in the stomach, the presence of end-tidal CO_2 is a good indicator that the tube is placed correctly. If a functioning capnograph fails to detect CO_2, it is almost certain that the tube is not in the trachea. One notable exception to this rule is in cardiac arrest: if there is no circulation, no CO_2 is delivered to the lungs, yielding a false-negative finding on capnography. Recent ingestion of carbonated beverages or antacids may yield transient false-positive results after esophageal intubation. The end-tidal CO_2 should disappear within a few breaths if this occurs. Hypoxemia (as indicated by pulse oximetry or cyanosis) due to esophageal or endobronchial intubation is a late sign. Tube placement also may be confirmed by bronchoscopy or laryngoscopy.

Persistent air leaks are usually the result of a leaky cuff or a malfunctioning pilot balloon valve. If an inordinate amount of air is required but the cuff is not leaking (i.e., the pilot balloon does not lose pressure), the tube may not be inserted far enough; the poor seal is the result of the cuffs being between or above the vocal cords.

Cricothyroidotomy

Cricothyroidotomy is performed when conventional intubation is impossible or contra-

indicated.[21-23] The cricothyroid membrane is palpable between the thyroid and cricoid cartilages. A common error is to mistake the thyrohyoid space for the cricothyroid space. The former is tucked up under the mandible, whereas the latter is usually in the mid to lower neck. A good way to identify the cricoid cartilage is to palpate in the suprasternal notch and walk the finger up until the cricoid cartilage is encountered. This structure is much larger and firmer than the tracheal rings. If time permits, the area is prepared and local anesthesia is administered. An incision is made through the skin and the cricothyroid membrane. This incision should not be too generous (perhaps 1.5–2 cm) because the carotid arteries lie laterally. Some prefer to make the skin incision vertically, allowing better palpation and identification of the cricothyroid membrane. The incision should be shallow so that the posterior larynx and the esophagus are not injured. The incision can be opened by twisting the scalpel handle in the incision, or a clamp may be used to spread the margins of the incision. Any hollow stent may be used to maintain patency; it does not have to be a tracheostomy tube, although this is preferable.

Complications of emergency cricothyroidotomy include incorrect placement (most commonly through the thyrohyoid membrane), false passage, hemorrhage, thyroid cartilage fracture, subcutaneous emphysema, and laryngeal and esophageal laceration.

Needle Cricothyroidotomy

Needle cricothyroidotomy is a temporizing measure to be used until more definitive airway control is achieved. A large-bore catheter attached to an oxygen source is inserted through the cricothyroid membrane (directed caudally). Intermittent occlusion of a Y connector or a side hole in the tubing allows insufflation of oxygen. Some setups have a springloaded valve that can be depressed intermittently. The clinician insufflates for 1 sec and releases for 4 sec.

The catheter can be connected to a conventional bag-valve setup. The connector from a small endotracheal tube (approximately 3 mm in diameter) fits into the hub of an intravenous catheter. Alternatively, a connector from a larger (7–8 mm in diameter) endotracheal tube fits the barrel of a 3-ml syringe. The syringe tip fits into the intravenous catheter. It is very difficult to apply enough pressure to provide adequate ventilation, but it is better than nothing.

Changing Endotracheal Tubes

The nature of the procedure of changing endotracheal tubes implies that airway control already has been established. This allows the luxury of using sedation and paralysis to obtain optimal conditions. If possible, the stomach is emptied with an orogastric or a nasogastric tube to prevent aspiration during the exchange. The administration of 100% oxygen for several minutes before the procedure should provide an oxygen reserve unless a severe oxygenation deficit is present. When the same route will be used, a simple exchange over a guide is possible.

Direct visualization with either a laryngoscope or a fiberoptic bronchoscope allows the same or a different route to be chosen for the new endotracheal tube. Heavy sedation, anesthesia, and paralysis are often necessary to ensure good operating conditions and patient comfort. The larynx should be well visualized before the old tube is removed. One disadvantage to using the fiberoptic scope is that secretions dragged along when the old tube is removed may obscure the area being observed. As a safety precaution, it is advisable to pass a tube exchanger down through the old tube first. Then, if airway control or visibility is lost before insertion of the new tube, a tube may be reinserted over the guide.

Tube exchanges can be performed by passing semirigid devices through an existing endotracheal tube. Some exchangers are hollow, allowing oxygen insufflation if difficulties arise in passing the new tube. An 18-F nasogastric tube with the suction ports cut off works very well. Some commercially available tube exchangers are very rigid and may cause tracheobronchial injury.

Changing Tracheostomy Tubes

A tracheostomy tube that has been in place less than 7 days should not be changed unless absolutely necessary. If a fresh tracheostomy tube needs to be changed, a surgeon (preferably the surgeon who performed the tracheostomy) and equipment for emergency intubation should be available.

Exchange may be performed over a guide, as with other endotracheal tubes. The practitioner should always be prepared for oral or nasal intubation in case control of the airway is lost during the exchange. In some cases, it may be preferable to intubate the patient from above before the exchange, placing the tube proximal to the tracheostomy but below the vocal cords. The endotracheal tube can then be advanced past the stoma to ensure ventilation if the exchange is unsuccessful. Inadvertent decannulation of a fresh tracheostomy may not leave a clear track for reinsertion, and attempts to recannulate the trachea may result in blind passage into deep tissue layers. The patient may require intubation by the oral or nasal route, emergency surgical exploration, or both. Some surgeons place silk sutures into the walls of the tracheal stoma. In an emergency, pulling on the sutures brings the tracheal stoma into approximation with the skin stoma.

Mature stomata do not require these special precautions.

CONCLUSIONS

To provide state-of-the-art respiratory care, practitioners must understand basic principles of airway management. This first requires a fundamental understanding of the relationships of the oral cavity, nose, pharynx, larynx, trachea, and lower airways. Skilled clinicians also should know how to assess the need for airway care and be able to supply a patent airway noninvasively using proper positioning and masks. Tracheal intubation is an important skill that can be both life saving and life supporting. A number of techniques and types of equipment are available that sometimes must be used in conjunction with pharmacologic therapy to sedate or paralyze the patient. Complications of tracheal intubation are important to recognize and treat promptly.

REFERENCES

1. Gorback MS: Emergency Airway Management. Philadelphia: BC Decker, 1990.
2. American Heart Association: Advanced Cardiac Life Support. Dallas: American Heart Association, 1995.
3. Guildner CW: Resuscitation-opening the airway: a comparative study of techniques for opening an airway obstructed by the tongue. J Am College Emergency Physicians 5:588–590, 1986.
4. Brimacombe JR, Berry A: The incidence of aspiration associated with the laryngeal mask airway: a meta-analysis of published literature. J Clin Anesth 7:297–305, 1993.
5. Viby-Mogensen J: Cholinesterase and succinylcholine. Dan Med Bull 30:129–150, 1983.
6. Brechner VL: Unusual problems in the management of airways: I. Flexion-extension mobility of the cervical vertebrae. Anesth Analg 47:362–373, 1968.
7. Cheek TG, Gutsche BB: Maternal physiologic alterations during pregnancy. In: Shnider SM, Levinson G (eds): Anesthesia for Obstetrics, 2nd ed. Baltimore: Williams & Wilkins, 1987, pp 3–13.
8. Mallampati SR, Gatt SP, Gugino LD, et al: A clinical sign to predict difficult tracheal intubation. Can Anaesth Soc J 32:429–434, 1985.
9. Block C, Brechner VL: Unusual problems in airway management: II. The influence of the temporomandibular joint, the mandible, and associated structures on endotracheal intubation. Anesth Analg 50:114–123, 1971.
10. Empey DW: Assessment of upper airways obstruction. Br Med J 3:503–505, 1972.
11. Miller RD, Hyatt RE: Evaluation of obstructing lesions of the trachea and larynx by flow-volume loops. Am Rev Respir Dis 108:475–481, 1973.
12. Ellis DG, Jakymec A, Kaplan RM, et al: Guided orotracheal intubation in the operating room using a lighted stylet: a comparison with direct laryngoscopic technique. Anesthesiology 64:823–826, 1986.
13. Murphy P: A fiberoptic endoscope used for nasal intubation. Anaesthesia 22:489, 1967.
14. Taylor PA, Toney RM: The broncho-fiberscope as an aid to endotracheal intubation. Anaesthesia 46:611, 1972.
15. Ducrow M: Throwing light on blind intubation. Anaesthesia 33:827–829, 1978.
16. Ellis DG, Jakymec A, Kaplan RM, et al: Guided orotracheal intubation in the operating room using a lighted stylet: a comparison with direct laryngoscopic technique. Anesthesiology 64:823–826, 1986.
17. Arens JF, Lejume FE, Webre DR: Maxillary sinusitis: a complication of nasal tracheal intubation. Anesthesiology 40:415–416, 1974.
18. Zwillich C, Peirson DJ: Nasal necrosis: a complication of nasotracheal intubation. Chest 64:376–377, 1973.
19. Latto IP, Rosen M (eds): Difficulties in Tracheal Intubation. London: Bailliere Tindall, 1984.
20. Benumof JL, Partridge BL, Salvatierra C, Keating J: Margin of safety in positioning modern double-lumen endotracheal tubes. Anesthesiology 67:729–738, 1987.
21. McGill J, Clinton JE, Ruiz E: Cricothyrotomy in the emergency department. Ann Emerg Med 11:361–364, 1982.
22. Weymuller EA, Pavlin EG, Paugh D, Cummings CW: Management of difficult airway problems with percutaneous transtracheal ventilation. Ann Otol Rhinol Laryngol 96:34–37, 1987.
23. Smith RB, Schaer WB, Pfaeffle H: Percutaneous transtracheal ventilation for anesthesia and resuscitation: a review and report of complications. Can Anaesth Soc J 22:607–612, 1975.

CHAPTER 14

Sedation and Paralysis in the Mechanically Ventilated Patient

Clyde I. Miyagawa, PharmD
Steven E. Pass, PharmD

SEDATION

BENZODIAZEPINES
Diazepam
Chlordiazepoxide
Midazolam
Lorazepam

ANESTHETIC AGENTS
Propofol

NARCOTICS
Morphine
Meperidine
4-Anilinopiperidines
  (Fentanyl, Sufentanil,
  Alfentanyl, Remifentanil)

NEUROLEPTICS

MONITORING ASPECTS OF
SEDATION

AGENT OF CHOICE FOR
SEDATION

PARALYZATION
Pancuronium
Vecuronium
Atracurium/Cisatracurium
Doxacurium
Rocuronium

ADVERSE EFFECTS

MONITORING OF
PARALYSIS

AGENT OF CHOICE

REFERENCES

KEY WORDS

lorazepam	pancuronium	sedation level score
midazolam	paralysis	train-of-four
myopathy	sedation	vecuronium

Critically ill patients require analgesia and sedation during their stay in an intensive care unit (ICU). They commonly experience agitation and anxiety secondary to a multitude of factors, such as sleep deprivation, sensory overload, inadequate pain management, invasive/noninvasive procedures (e.g., chest tube placement, hemodynamic monitoring, central line placement, dressing changes, bronchoscopy, and so forth), and especially mechanical ventilation. Reducing anxiety and agitation can help decrease oxygen consumption and improve gas exchange in patients requiring mechanical ventilation, as well as minimize those complications self-inflicted by the agitated patient.

A plethora of pharmacologic agents exists for the sedation and paralysis of mechanically ventilated patients. Unfortunately, such availability has resulted in the use of a vast array of sedative and paralytic combinations.[1-3] Issues that ultimately affect the selection of appropriate agents include the efficacy, safety profile, and cost of these various regimens. However, the selection of a particular agent has been historically based primarily on the personal experience of individual clinicians with little to no scientific literature to support or refute individual choices.[3] Additionally, accurate and reliable scientific methods do not exist to measure and assess the various drug regimens or the appropriate level of sedation and/or paralysis.[2-4] Consequently, in the current era of cost-containment and continuous quality improvement, many ICUs have attempted to develop protocols, guidelines, and policies to address and manage the issues of sedation and paralysis in mechanically ventilated patients.[5, 6]

SEDATION

The ideal sedative agent should have a rapid onset and short-acting effects. It should be easily titratable to patient response, with immediate reversibility or dissipation of effect. There should be no significant accumulation with minimal side effects, and it should not be associated with the development of tolerance, withdrawal symptoms, or addiction. Unfortunately, no such agent currently exists.

Sedatives are indicated in ICU settings for the management of agitation and anxiety, as adjuncts to narcotic analgesics, and to treat delirium. The sensory overload and stress associated with routine ICU care have to a large extent mandated some form of sedative therapy, either intermittent or continuous, to all patients in ICUs.[1, 7]

Benzodiazepines, opiates, barbiturates, neuroleptics, and general anesthetics all have been used in the management of agitation and anxiety in ICUs.[3] Opiate and benzodiazepine continuous infusions are the most popular agents used.[3] However, despite potent sedative effects that these agents possess, the pharmacodynamic effects of these agents are highly variable and unpredictable in this patient population, secondary to significant dynamic alterations in metabolism, volume of distribution, and clearance.[8, 9] Additionally, the development of tachyphylaxis is a commonly observed phenomenon with many of these agents. The end result is a highly variable dosing regimen requiring constant titration to achieve the desired end point.

BENZODIAZEPINES

Benzodiazepines traditionally have been the "workhorse" in the ICU.[1, 3] Despite their potent anxiolytic activity, benzodiazepines are devoid of analgesic effects and do provide anterograde amnesia, a most desirable effect in the critically ill patient. Although hypotension, respiratory depression, and tachycardia can be observed with this class of agents, the incidence is significantly lower than that observed with narcotic analgesics. Because all benzodiazepines sedate patients to a similar degree when equipotent doses are administered, the selection of the "ideal" benzodiazepine is dependent on pharmacokinetic, pharmacodynamic, and cost issues. The benzodiazepines available for intravenous use are listed in Table 14–1. The role of these agents in ICUs over the past two decades is an interesting chronicle of the pharmacokinetic development of this class of drugs, the pharmacodynamic effects observed in critically ill patients, and the effects of rising health care costs.

Diazepam

Marketed in the 1970s, diazepam is a long-acting lipophilic benzodiazepine that has

TABLE 14–1. Benzodiazepines

AGENT (HALF-LIFE IN Hr)	ACTIVE METABOLITE(S) (HALF-LIFE IN Hr)	DOSE	COST/DAY
Diazepam (20–50)	Desmethyldiazepam (200)	0.1–0.2 mg/kg	Low
	Oxazepam (8)	IVP q2–4hr	
	3-Hydroxydiazepam (5–20)		
Chlordiazepoxide (5–30)	Demoxepam (14–95)	**	Low
	Desmethylchlordiazepoxide (18)		
	Desmethyldiazepam (30–200)		
	Oxazepam (3–21)		
Midazolam (1–12.3)	1-Hydroxymethylmidazolam (1–1.5)	2–8 mg/hr	High
Lorazepam (10–20)	None	0.5–5 mg/hr	Low

IVP, intravenous push.
**Not recommended for use in the ICU setting

survived the test of time. Despite the development and release of subsequent benzodiazepines with superior pharmacokinetic profiles, diazepam has retained a major clinical role in the management of hospitalized patients. The sedative effects are seen within 2 to 3 minutes, with peak effects observed within 3 to 5 minutes. The clinical effects are rather short lived (0.5–1 hour) after the administration of single intravenous doses secondary to redistribution to peripheral tissues. When used in this manner, diazepam has been shown to be a cost-effective agent in critically ill patients.[10] However, with multiple doses or continuous infusions exceeding 2 days, saturation of peripheral compartments and central nervous system binding sites occur, resulting in a significantly prolonged sedative effect.[11] The extended half-lives of the two active metabolites contribute to a sustained sedative effect after discontinuation of the parent compound.[12] These pharmacokinetic and pharmacodynamic characteristics, along with diazepam's poor solubility profile, have deterred clinicians from routinely administering diazepam as prolonged continuous infusions in critically ill patients. Rather, its role has been limited to that of intermittent short-term administration.[10]

Chlordiazepoxide

Similar to diazepam, chlordiazepoxide is an effective long-acting benzodiazepine with an onset of action of 2 to 3 minutes. Metabolized to four active metabolites, each possessing long half-lives, chlordiazepoxide, as does diazepam, fails both pharmacokinetically and pharmacodynamically to meet the criteria of the ideal sedative for prolonged continuous infusions. The use of this agent in critically ill patients has largely been abandoned in most ICUs.

Midazolam

Before the release of **midazolam** in the mid 1980s, continuous infusions of benzodiazepines in critical care units were rare. Because of stability issues with diazepam, chlordiazepoxide, and lorazepam, most patients requiring sedation received intermittent intramuscular (IM) or intravenous push (IVP) doses of these agents.[13, 14] Unfortunately, this route of administration resulted in a "roller coaster" effect, and once sedation was terminated, patients often required prolonged periods of time to awaken.[15, 16]

The release of midazolam was greeted joyously by critical care clinicians, who proclaimed the drug to be the "ideal" benzodiazepine. Retaining an onset of activity similar to diazepam (2–3 min), a half-life significantly shorter than other existing benzodiazepines, initially thought to have no active metabolites, and demonstrating excellent water solubility characteristics, midazolam rapidly became the agent of choice in many ICUs for long-term sedation.[1, 8]

Over the next few years, however, the pharmacokinetic and pharmacodynamic advantages of midazolam that had been anticipated were not seen in intense clinical trials involving critically ill patients. Despite a relatively short half-life, peripheral drug redistribution sites are rapidly saturated with repeated bolus or continuous infusion therapy.[17] Additionally, the 1-hydroxymethyl metabolite was discovered to be an active metabolite with a half-life similar to that of the parent compound.[18] Clinical trials in critically ill patients demonstrated accumulation of both midazolam and its metabolite in patients with renal insufficiency, congestive heart failure, and decreased plasma albumin levels and in the elderly.[15, 16, 19–21] The end result was a significant prolongation of the sedative effect after discontinuation of the infusion, with awakening times ranging from 2 to 48 hours.[15, 16, 19, 21] Although not demonstrated in any specific clinical trial, it has been speculated that this prolonged sedative effect may increase the length of intubation and, consequently, the length of ICU stay, with a resultant increase in total health care costs.

The cost of midazolam is considerably higher than any other intravenous benzodiazepine currently available. However, the anticipated pharmacokinetic and pharmacodynamic advantages initially were believed to outweigh any cost issues associated with the drug. The recent discovery of prolonged sedation and awakening times coupled with an increased sensitivity by the medical community to rising costs has clouded the role of midazolam in ICUs. It has not been shown to be the "ideal" benzodiazepine that it had once been thought, as reflected by a recent survey demonstrating that midazolam was the benzodiazepine of choice in only 22% of the ICUs surveyed.[3] In fact, it no longer can be considered a "cost-effective" agent for continuous sedation of critically ill patients.

Lorazepam

Lorazepam is an intermediate-acting benzodiazepine available since the 1970s. Its role in continuous infusions in critically ill patients was limited, however, by an intermediate half-life and, most importantly, poor stability characteristics (lorazepam is formulated in a propylene glycol solvent). Therefore, its role in the early 1990s was confined predominantly to intermittent IVP administration. However, the pharmacodynamic properties of midazolam and rising costs of health care have forced clinicians to re-evaluate the role of older, less expensive benzodiazepines such as lorazepam.

Pharmacokinetically and pharmacodynamically, lorazepam has been shown to be superior to diazepam and midazolam.[20] Lorazepam is less lipophilic than diazepam or midazolam and penetrates the central nervous system more slowly, resulting in an increased time to peak effect.[22] However, the decreased lipophilic nature reduces its volume of distribution and consequently its potential for peripheral accumulation.[23] Additionally, lorazepam elimination is independent of renal or hepatic dysfunction, and it is metabolized through hepatic glucuronidation to inactive metabolites.[24]

Limited clinical trials in critically ill patients have demonstrated a more rapid awakening time with lorazepam than with midazolam.[20, 25, 26] Pohlman and colleagues observed a return to baseline mental status of 261 minutes with lorazepam and 1813 minutes with midazolam in patients requiring continuous sedation in a medical ICU.[20] In the current health care environment, lorazepam is rapidly becoming the most "cost-effective" and most widely used benzodiazepine for continuous infusion in critically ill patients.[3, 25, 26]

ANESTHETIC AGENTS

Anesthetic agents historically have played a minor role in the management of sedation in critically ill patients. Currently, propofol is the only agent that is used in this setting to any significant degree.

Propofol

Originally released as a short-acting intravenous general anesthetic for same-day surgical procedures, the pharmacokinetic (half-life 2–8 min) and pharmacodynamic properties of propofol are well suited for continuous sedation in the critically ill patient.[27, 28] It has a rapid onset of action (40 sec) and a short time to awakening and has been proved safe in patients with renal or hepatic dysfunction. Similar to benzodiazepines, propofol provides no analgesic effects. At doses between 10 and 80 μg/kg/min, it has been shown to be as effective as midazolam in sedating patients in medical, surgical, and cardiothoracic ICUs.[27, 29–32] Additionally, in comparison to midazolam, time to awakening and cost are significantly less with propofol.[27, 29–32]

However, propofol's role in ICUs can be limited by a number of factors. Hemodynamically, hypotension can be observed but is normally tolerable. Because of its lipophilicity, propofol requires a phospholipid emulsion vehicle, providing a source of calories (1.1 kcal/ml of propofol) above and beyond the nutrition patients already may be receiving. Depending on the rate of propofol infusion and the duration of infusion, modification of the rate and content of other nutrition sources must be considered. Additionally, the role of lipids and their effects on increased CO_2 production as well as a propofol-induced metabolic acidosis recently have been reported.[33–36]

NARCOTICS

Pharmacologically, narcotics are not classified as anxiolytics and should not be used in that manner. Anxiety is best managed with anxiolytics (benzodiazepines), and pain is best managed with analgesics (narcotics). However, a manifestation of analgesia is the provision of some degree of sedation. In the trauma/surgical arena, it is not uncommon to prescribe both an anxiolytic and an analgesic for the management of anxiety and pain, respectively.[3]

Ironically, critically ill patients often receive inadequate analgesia because of concerns about adverse effects (respiratory depression, decrease in GI motility, hypotension) and the development of dependence.[37] However, for postoperative patients

or those requiring painful invasive monitoring, the use of adequate analgesia is essential to minimize the clinical repercussions of pain-associated sympathetic discharge. In critically ill patients, the intravenous route of administration is preferred over the oral or intramuscular route secondary to variations in drug absorption. Additionally, these doses should be given on a scheduled basis, if not as continuous infusions. Table 14–2 lists the more commonly used narcotics for analgesia or sedation or both.

Morphine

Morphine is the most frequently used narcotic analgesic and the prototypical agent with which all others are compared.[3] It has enjoyed this enviable position because of its potency, efficacy, and cost-effectiveness. It has a low degree of lipid solubility, and therefore has a relatively slow onset of action (5–10 min). It is metabolized by the liver, and its metabolites are excreted renally. Caution must be exercised in patients with renal failure because of accumulation of the active metabolite morphine-6-glucuronide.[38] Adverse effects associated with morphine include histamine-mediated hypotension, vagally mediated bradycardia, and respiratory depression.

Meperidine

Other than a slightly more rapid onset of action (3–5 min) and a shorter duration of activity (2–4 hr), meperidine is comparable pharmacokinetically to morphine. Its side effects include sinus tachycardia, hypoten-

TABLE 14–2. Narcotics

AGENT	DOSE (INFUSION)	COST
Meperidine	**	Low
Morphine	0.03–0.15 mg/kg/hr	Low
Fentanyl	50–200 μg/hr	Low
Sufentanil	**	High
Remifentanil	0.025–0.2 μg/kg/hr	High
Alfentanyl	0.5–1 μg/kg/hr	High

**Not recommended for infusion

sion, and respiratory depression. The major potential adverse effect is the ability of the active metabolite normeperidine to produce central nervous system excitation (apprehension, tremors, and/or seizures), especially in elderly patients and those with renal insufficiency.[39] Therefore, the use of meperidine in the management of critically ill patients is highly discouraged.

4-Anilinopiperidines (Fentanyl, Sufentanil, Alfentanyl, Remifentanil)

The inherent hypotension associated with morphine-induced histamine release has forced many ICUs, especially those directed by anesthesiologists, to employ agents from the 4-anilinopiperidine class of narcotics. Fentanyl is the classic representative agent from this group and has largely become the 4-anilinopiperidine narcotic analgesic of choice. Associated with less histamine release than morphine and meperidine, fentanyl is a semisynthetic analgesic with a faster onset of action than morphine.[40] Because of its redistribution to muscle and fat, it has a short duration of action, making it an ideal agent for continuous infusion.

Pharmacokinetically, remifentanil, sufentanil, and alfentanyl are superior to fentanyl. However, with long-term use, these pharmacokinetic advantages are not realized pharmacodynamically. Cost issues prohibit the routine use of these agents for continuous sedation and/or pain control in ICUs, and fentanyl remains the agent of choice.

NEUROLEPTICS

Haloperidol, a butyrophenone used in the ICU specifically for the treatment of delirium and psychosis (including the condition of ICU psychosis), has little or no effect on respirations and few anticholinergic or hemodynamic side effects. Its sedative effect is significantly less than that observed with benzodiazepines and opiates. The onset of action is 2 to 5 minutes after doses of 1 to 20 mg IVP, depending on the level of agitation displayed by the patient. Adverse effects as-

sociated with haloperidol include central nervous system depression and hypotension, as well as the development of extrapyramidal side effects, manifested as muscle rigidity, drowsiness, and lethargy. Neuroleptic malignant syndrome, manifested as muscle rigidity, fever, and mental status changes, occurs rarely with haloperidol use but is associated with a high mortality rate.

The initial dose is 5 mg intravenously. If the patient continues to be agitated after 20 minutes, give double the previous dose. This may be repeated every 20 minutes until agitation subsides, a cumulative dose of 200 mg has been administered, or toxicity develops.[41]

MONITORING ASPECTS OF SEDATION

Sedation is a nonspecific term used to describe the action of an agent to move a patient toward a state in which the patient is calm and relaxed. However, interpretation of the term sedation is wide and variable. In the past, mechanically ventilated patients were often placed on a standard sedation regimen regardless of their weight, organ function, and mental status. Currently, the emphasis is on tailoring sedative requirements to meet patients' specific needs. In general, the goal is to titrate sedation to maintain the patient asleep but arousable or awake but not complaining. To ensure that the patient's individual needs are met, the depth and quality of sedation must be assessed regularly. This process has been addressed in many institutions in a multidisciplinary (physician, nurse, pharmacist, respiratory therapist) manner through the development of guidelines for sedation. The development and implementation of such guidelines can result in improvement in patient care as well as drug cost savings.[42]

No perfect method exists for objectively assessing the desired level of sedation. The Ramsay scale provides a subjective measure of the depth but not the quality of sedation.[43] It does not measure pain or cognitive dysfunction. However, in the absence of an ideal monitoring technique, many ICUs have adopted a modified Ramsay scale to assess their patients (Table 14–3). A level of 3 is the desired end point, and assessment is obtained at least thrice daily. The ideal level of sedation should result in a patient who is sleeping lightly but easily arousable. Doses of sedatives should be titrated to achieve the desired **sedation level score.**[41, 42]

AGENT OF CHOICE FOR SEDATION

Over the past few decades, sedatives such as midazolam with improved pharmacokinetic characteristics have been developed. Unfortunately, these advances have not resulted in the anticipated pharmacodynamic outcomes. Although narcotics are used frequently, benzodiazepines have been and continue to be the agents of choice for sedation.[3] In 1980, lorazepam was commonly used in ICUs simply because it was the only available agent. It was replaced in the mid 1980s by the pharmacokinetically superior agent midazolam. Ironically, the 1990s have seen a resurrection of lorazepam because of cost constraints and the lack of any pharmacodynamic advantage of midazolam. The Society of Critical Care Medicine has recommended the following: (1) midazolam or propofol for the short-term (<24 hours) treatment of anxiety in the critically ill patient, (2) lorazepam for the prolonged treatment of anxiety, (3) morphine for analgesia in hemodynamically stable patients, (4) fentanyl for analgesia in critically ill patients with hemodynamic instability, and (5) haloperidol for the management of delirium in the critically ill patient.[41] These recommendations are based on clinical trials as well as cost considerations and represent a multidisciplinary consensus regarding sedation of the critically ill patient.

TABLE 14–3. Modified Ramsay Scale

1. Agitated, anxious, restless
2. Calm, cooperative, oriented, tranquil
3. Responds to verbal commands
4. Brisk response to light touch
5. Unable to be assessed (paralyzed)

PARALYZATION

Through the past three decades, the role and utilization of neuromuscular blocking agents (NMBAs) in critically ill patients has been dictated enormously by the technologic development of mechanical ventilation. These agents have been used routinely in ICUs dating back to the 1960s when curare (d-tubocurarine) was used with diazepam and morphine in patients receiving controlled mechanical ventilation who could not breathe on their own secondary to ventilator design.[44] This inability to provide a mixture of spontaneous and mechanical ventilation commonly led to patient agitation, requiring sedation and in many instances **paralysis.** The late 1960s and early 1970s saw the development of intermittent mandatory ventilation and the beginning of the era of partial ventilatory support. This mode of ventilation resulted in a decreased need for neuromuscular blockade. The 1990s heralded the introduction of computerized ventilators and the techniques of pressure-control ventilation and pressure-control inverse-ratio ventilation. This era of "less ventilation" and new patterns of respiratory support may result in permissive hypercarbia with increased sedation and paralyzation requirements reminiscent of the 1960s.[44]

Composed of depolarizing and nondepolarizing agents, the NMBAs can be categorized into short-acting (10–20 min), intermediate-acting (40–60 min), and long-acting (90–180 min) agents based on their half-lives and duration of action (Table 14–4). Many of these have been evaluated for continuous neuromuscular blockade in critically ill patients and have been shown to be effective.[45, 46]

The selection of an NMBA for patients requiring mechanical ventilation depends on the following variables: (1) NMBA pharmacokinetic/pharmacodynamic profile, (2) NMBA cost, (3) NMBA adverse effect potential, and (4) patient organ function/dysfunction. Ideally, the agent of choice should have a rapid onset of action, short duration of activity, no cumulative drug effect, no dependence on renal/hepatic function, minimal adverse effect profile, and

TABLE 14–4. Neuromuscular Blocking Agents

AGENT	STRUCTURE	ACTIVE METABOLITES	DOSAGE REGIMEN	DURATION	COST/DAY
Pancuronium	Aminosteroid	3-OH and 17-OH pancuronium	LD 0.1 mg/kg MD 0.05–0.1 mg/kg/hr	Long	Low
Vecuronium	Aminosteroid	3-desacetyl-vecuronium	LD 0.1 mg/kg MD 0.05–0.1 mg/kg/hr	Intermediate	Moderate
Atracurium	Benzyliso-quinolone	No	LD 0.5 mg/kg MD 0.5–1 mg/kg/hr	Intermediate	High
Rocuronium	Aminosteroid	No	—	Intermediate	Moderate
Cisatracurium	Benzyliso-quinolone	No	LD 0.1 μg/kg MD 0.5–10 μg/kg/min	Intermediate	Moderate
Doxacurium	Benzyliso-quinolone	No	LD 0.03 mg/kg MD 0.01–0.03 mg/kg/hr	Long	Low

LD, loading dose; MD, maintenance dose.

minimal cost profile. Unfortunately, no such agent currently exists.

Pancuronium

Marketed in 1972, **pancuronium** was one of the first agents used for paralysis in critically ill patients. However, its use was associated with prolonged paralysis after discontinuation of the drug. This was attributed to the long half-life of the parent compound as well as the activity of the 3-hydroxy metabolite.[47] This effect was accentuated in patients with renal and hepatic failure in whom the elimination half-lives of both parent compound and metabolite were prolonged.[45–47] Additionally, pancuronium demonstrated significant hemodynamic alterations in a patient population least likely to tolerate any further changes. Vagolytic effects often resulted in tachycardia and increases in blood pressure, whereas mast cell degranulation and histamine release resulted in hypotension.[48] Despite these limitations, pancuronium continued to be used for paralyzation in ICUs mainly because of the lack of other, safer alternatives.

Vecuronium

The release of **vecuronium** in 1984 heralded an era in which neuromuscular block-

ers with dramatically improved pharmacokinetic (short half-life) and hemodynamic characteristics were introduced into clinical practice. Vecuronium provided an effective neuromuscular blocker without the cardiovascular manifestations of pancuronium. Additionally, because the active metabolite, 3-desacetylvecuronium, and the parent compound are eliminated extensively by the liver, vecuronium was believed to be safe in patients with renal insufficiency.[49] However, case reports have suggested prolonged effects in patients with renal insufficiency.[49, 50] Nonetheless, during the mid 1980s vecuronium rapidly became the agent of choice in many ICUs.

Atracurium/Cisatracurium

Atracurium and cisatracurium besylate are similar to vecuronium in duration of action and lack of cardiovascular side effects. However, unlike pancuronium and vecuronium, the metabolism and elimination of atracurium and cisatracurium is independent of renal and hepatic function. They are inactivated in the plasma by two nonoxidative pathways: (1) ester hydrolysis and (2) Hofmann elimination, a nonenzymatic chemical process that occurs at physiologic pH and temperature. These pharmacokinetic attributes have made atracurium and cisatracurium ideal NMBAs in patients with renal and hepatic insufficiency. Cisatracurium is one of 10 isomers of atracurium and, other than being available at a lower cost, does not differ clinically from atracurium when used as continuous infusions in critically ill patients.[51]

Doxacurium

Released in 1991, doxacurium is the most potent neuromuscular blocking agent currently available and has been shown to be effective in the ICU setting.[52, 53] It is a long-acting agent with a hemodynamic side effect profile similar to vecuronium. Because the drug is excreted renally, patients with renal failure may experience a prolongation of its normal pharmacologic effects.[52] The pharmacokinetics of doxacurium do not appear to be affected by hepatic failure. Doxacurium recently was compared with pancuronium in critically ill patients and was found to cause less tachycardia and a more rapid recovery of neuromuscular function than pancuronium.[52] Further studies are required to evaluate the cost-effectiveness of this agent in critically ill patients requiring continuous paralysis.

Rocuronium

Rocuronium is pharmacokinetically similar to vecuronium except for a more rapid onset of action (60 vs. 90 sec). It has not been studied in critically ill patients as continuous infusions but should produce results similar to those observed with vecuronium. Rocuronium provides no advantage pharmacokinetically or pharmacodynamically over vecuronium or cisatracurium.

ADVERSE EFFECTS

The adverse effects of all NMBAs are similar but vary in intensity among the individual agents. The two major adverse effects include hemodynamic manifestations and prolonged paralysis. Ganglionic blockade and histamine release can result in hypotension, whereas vagal stimulation can result in tachycardia.[48] These can be of major consequence in patients with underlying coronary artery disease. All available agents with the exception of pancuronium appear to be safe in this patient population.

A variety of neuromuscular disorders have been described in critically ill patients, including a sensorimotor axonal polyneuropathy (critical illness polyneuropathy), disuse atrophy, and steroid-induced **myopathy.** Since 1985, there have been numerous reports in the literature describing the development of a prolonged paralysis and/or muscle weakness for days to months after discontinuation of NMBAs.[54–59] This phenomenon has been characterized by two separate and probably unrelated events.[60, 61] The first event has been referred to as "short-term persistent paralysis" and is pharmacokinetically induced secondary to an overdose of the NMBA and/or accumulation of active metabolites that leads to persistent paralysis for hours to a few days. This problem is relatively easy to avoid with the development of dosing protocols and guidelines that use **train-of-four** monitoring (see under Monitoring of Paralysis). Protocols/guidelines of this nature have the ability to minimize the incidence of adverse effects while maximizing clinical effect with the least amount of NMBA.[5, 6]

The second event is more likely a "long-term persistent muscle weakness" or tetraparesis that can last for weeks or months. It is associated with marked increases in serum creatine kinase and diminished motor-evoked potentials.[62] Muscle biopsy examination has shown moderate-to-severe panfascicular necrotizing myopathy.[63] The cause of this prolonged muscle weakness is unknown but has been tentatively attributed to the structural classification of the neuromuscular agent and/or concomitant steroid use.[60, 64–66] Most case reports have involved patients receiving pancuronium or vecuronium (aminosteroids) and concomitant high-dose steroid therapy.[47, 55, 64–66] NMBAs and steroids alone have both been reported to cause myopathy. When co-administered, these agents appear to produce an even greater risk. Until the exact mechanism can be determined, caution must be exercised with all neuromuscular agents, especially with concomitant steroid use. The consequence of this myopathy can have a significant economic impact on the cost of patient care.[34] Rudis and colleagues reported an increase in ICU and hospital stay, continued mechanical ventilation, and disproportionate health care expenditures in excess of $60,000 per patient with NMBA-induced myopathy.[34]

The large number of reports documenting these adverse effects have tempered somewhat the cavalier paralyzation-prescribing habits of intensive care clinicians. The development of guidelines that incorporate a multidisciplinary approach to the management of these patients can no longer be considered a desirable but optional task. Rather, it should be viewed as a mandated necessity to ensure the safe and effective use of these agents.

MONITORING OF PARALYSIS

Patients receiving NMBAs require constant monitoring of their level of paralysis to avoid the development of prolonged paralysis and muscle weakness. Train-of-four stimulation with peripheral nerve stimulators has been used to quantify the degree of neuromuscular blockade in the operating room and ICUs.[3, 5, 6] During train-of-four, an electrical current activates a motor nerve and the mechanical response of the muscle innervated by that nerve is assessed. This practice can result in lower doses of NMBAs to maintain a desired depth of paralysis, a faster recovery of neuromuscular function and spontaneous ventilation, and overall lower patient costs.[34] Recently, the Society of Critical Care Medicine advocated the use of train-of-four monitoring in critically ill patients requiring paralysis.[67] However, correlation of train-of-four values with clinical assessment of paralysis (spontaneous respirations and muscle activity) does not occur consistently and often can result in overparalyzation of patients.[68, 69] Limitations of train-of-four monitoring include operator-dependent variables (consistency of individuals performing evaluation), patient-dependent variables (peripheral edema, skin integrity), and site of train-of-four monitoring (ulnar, facial nerves).[68, 69] It is recommended that in addition to routine train-of-four monitoring, neuromuscular blockade should be allowed to dissipate on a daily basis to provide an opportunity for clinical evaluation, to assess the adequacy of concomitant sedation and analgesia, and to determine whether continued paralysis is even necessary.[67, 69]

AGENT OF CHOICE

The ideal NMBA does not currently exist. On the basis of pharmacokinetic, pharmacodynamic, and hemodynamic issues, cisatracurium should be the agent of choice. However, cost of drugs is an important component in the provision of health care and must be included in the evaluation of pharmaceuticals. Pancuronium is the least expensive NMBA available. However, it is pharmacokinetically and hemodynamically inferior to agents such as vecuronium and cisatracurium. Ironically, the Society of Critical Care Medicine recently recommended pancuronium as the preferred NMBA for critically ill patients with no underlying cardiac disease.[67] This is largely because of the increased sensitization of clinicians to the adverse effect potential of NMBAs as a class and, equally as important, the development of usage guidelines and protocols that ensure the lowest dose necessary to achieve a maximal clinical benefit. These elements were not recognized or appreciated in the 1970s. In those patients with cardiac disease or hemodynamic instability in whom tachycardia may be deleterious, vecuronium is the preferred NMBA.[67] Similar to the scenario observed with the benzodiazepines, the 1990s has seen a resurgence of older, pharmacokinetically less desirable agents (pancuronium) in ICUs primarily because of cost restraints and improved monitoring techniques.

REFERENCES

1. Dasta JF, Fuhrman TM, McCandles C: Patterns of prescribing and administering drugs for agitation

and pain in patients in a surgical intensive care unit. Crit Care Med 22:974, 1994.

2. Hansen-Flaschen JH, Brazinsky S, Basile C, et al: Use of sedating drugs and neuromuscular blocking agents in patients requiring mechanical ventilation for respiratory failure: a national survey. JAMA 266:2870, 1994.

3. Watling SM, Dasta JF, Seidl EC: Sedatives, analgesics, and paralytics in the ICU. Ann Pharmacother 31:148, 1997.

4. Bion JF, Leddingham IM: Sedation in intensive care—a postal survey [letter]. Intensive Care Med 13:215, 1987.

5. Colosimo RJ, Fournier S: Established guidelines for the selection, use and monitoring of neuromuscular-blocking agents in intensive care unit patients [abstract P-7D]. In Programs and Abstracts of the 29th Annual American Society of Health-System Pharmacy Midyear Clinical Meeting, 1994, Miami, p 59.

6. Newman CH, Cohen IA, Lysaght L, et al: Development of hospital protocols for the use of continuous intravenous sedative and neuromuscular-blocking agents in intensive care unit patients [abstract P-6D]. In Programs and Abstracts of the 29th Annual American Society of Health-System Pharmacy Midyear Clinical Meeting, 1994, Miami, p 59.

7. Shelly MP, Sneyd R: Intensive care sedation: progress towards decreasing the mortality rate. Br J Intensive Care October:323, 1992.

8. Burns AM, Shelly MP, Park GR: The use of sedative agents in critically ill patients. Drugs 43:507, 1992.

9. Shapiro HM: Barbiturates in brain ischemia. Br J Anaesth 57:82, 1985.

10. Ariano RE, Kassum DA, Aronson KJ: Comparison of sedative recovery time after midazolam versus diazepam administration. Crit Care Med 22:1492, 1994.

11. Ritz R, Elsaser S, Schwander J: Controlled sedation in ventilated intensive care patients. Resuscitation 16(suppl):583, 1988.

12. Mandelli M, Tognoni G, Garattini S: Clinical pharmacokinetics of diazepam. Clin Pharmacokinet 3:72, 1978.

13. Hadbury AM, Hoyt JW: Promotion of cost-effective benzodiazepine sedation. Am J Hosp Pharm 50:660, 1993.

14. Hamcock BG, Black CD: Effect of a polyethylene-lined administration set on the availability of diazepam injection. Am J Hosp Pharm 42:335, 1985.

15. Oldenhof H, deJong M, Steenhoek A, et al: Clinical pharmacokinetics of midazolam in intensive care patients, a wide interpatient variability? Clin Pharmacol Ther 43:263, 1988.

16. Vree TB, Shimoda M, Driessen JJ, et al: Decreased plasma albumin concentration results in increased volume of distribution and decreased elimination of midazolam in intensive care patients. Clin Pharmacol Ther 46:537, 1989.

17. Malacrida R, Fritz ME, Suter PM, et al: Pharmacokinetics of midazolam administered by continuous infusion to intensive care patients. Crit Care Med 20:1123, 1991.

18. Driessen JJ, Vree TB, Guelen PJ: The effects of acute changes in renal function on the pharmacokinetics of midazolam during long-term infusion in ICU patients. Acta Anaesthesiol Belg 42:149, 1991.

19. Patel IH, Soni PP, Fukuda EK: The pharmacokinetics of midazolam in patients with congestive heart failure. Br J Clin Pharmacokinet 29:565, 1990.

20. Pohlman AS, Simpson KP, Hall JB: Continuous intravenous infusion of lorazepam versus midazolam for sedation during mechanical ventilatory support: a prospective randomized study. Crit Care Med 22:1241, 1994.

21. Shafer A, Doze VA, White PF: Pharmacokinetic variability of midazolam infusions in critically ill patients. Crit Care Med 18:1039, 1990.

22. Greenblatt DJ, Ehrenberg BL, Gunderman J: Kinetic and dynamic study of intravenous lorazepam: comparison with intravenous diazepam. J Pharmacol Exp Ther 250:134, 1989.

23. Simpson PJ, Eltringham RJ: Lorazepam in intensive care. Clin Ther 4:150, 1981.

24. Wilkinson GR: The effects of aging and liver disease on disposition of lorazepam. Clin Pharmacol Ther 24:411, 1978.

25. Cernaianu AC, Del Rossi AJ, Flum DR, et al: Lorazepam and midazolam in the intensive care unit: a randomized, prospective, multicenter study of hemodynamics, oxygen transport, efficacy, and cost. Crit Care Med 24:222, 1996.

26. Deppe SA, Sipperly ME, Sargent AI, et al: Intravenous lorazepam as an amnestic and anxiolytic agent in the intensive care unit: a prospective study. Crit Care Med 22:1248, 1994.

27. Aitkenhead AR, Pepperman ML, Willatts SM: Comparison of propofol and midazolam for sedation in critically ill patients. Lancet 2:704, 1989.

28. Ermakov S, Crippen D: Continuous propofol infusion for sedation in delirium tremens. Crit Care Med 20:S37, 1992.

29. Carrasco GC, Molina R, Costa J, et al: Propofol vs midazolam in short-, medium-, and long-term sedation of critically ill patients. Chest 103:557, 1993.

30. Chamorro C, de Latorre FJ, Montero A, et al: Comparative study of propofol versus midazolam in the sedation of critically ill patients: results of a prospective, randomized, multicenter trial. Crit Care Med 24:932, 1996.

31. Roman KP, Gallagher TJ, George B, et al: Comparison of propofol and midazolam for sedation in intensive care unit patients. Crit Care Med 23:286, 1995.

32. Vega RB, Soria MM, Garcia CM, et al: Prolonged sedation of critically ill patients with midazolam or propofol: impact on weaning and costs. Crit Care Med 25:33, 1997.

33. Parke TJ, Stevens JE, Rice ASC, et al: Metabolic acidosis and fatal myocardial failure after propofol in children: five case reports. BMJ 305:613, 1992.

34. Rudis MI, Guslits BJ, Peterson EL, et al: Economic impact of prolonged motor weakness complicating neuromuscular blockade in the intensive care unit. Crit Care Med 24:1749, 1996.

35. Strickland RA, Murray MJ: Fatal metabolic acidosis in a pediatric patient receiving an infusion of propofol in the intensive care unit: is there a relationship? Crit Care Med 23:405, 1995.

36. Venus B, Prager R, Palel CB: Cardiopulmonary effects of Intralipid infusion in critically ill patients. Crit Care Med 16:587, 1988.

37. Marks RM, Sachar EJ: Undertreatment of medical inpatients with narcotic analgesics. Ann Intern Med 78:173, 1973.

38. Chan GLC, Matzke GR: Effects of renal insufficiency on the pharmacokinetics and pharmacodynamics of opioid analgesics. Drug Intell Clin Pharm 21:773, 1987.

39. Shochet RB, Murray GB: Neuropsychiatric toxicity of meperidine. J Intensive Care Med 3:246, 1988.

40. Shafer A, White PF: Use of a fentanyl infusion in the intensive care unit: tolerance to its anesthetic effects. Anesthesiology 59:245, 1993.

41. Shapiro BA, Warren J, Egol AB, et al: Practice parameters for intravenous analgesia and sedation for adult patients in the intensive care unit: an executive summary. Crit Care Med 23:1596, 1995.

42. Devlin JW, Hollbrook AM, Fuller HD: The effect of ICU sedation guidelines and pharmacist interventions on clinical outcomes and drug cost. Ann Pharmacother 31:689, 1997.

43. Hansen-Flaschen JH, Cowen J, Polomano RC: Beyond the Ramsay scale: need for a validated measure of sedating drug efficacy in the intensive care unit. Crit Care Med 22:732, 1994.

44. Shapiro BA: A historical perspective on ventilator management. New Horiz 2:8, 1994.

45. Prielipp RC, Coursin DB: Applied pharmacology of common neuromuscular blocking agents in critical care. New Horiz 2:34, 1994.

46. Topulos GP: Neuromuscular blockade in adult intensive care. New Horiz 1:447, 1993.

47. Giostra E, Magistris MR, Pizzolato G, et al: Neuromuscular disorders in intensive care unit patients treated with pancuronium bromide. Chest 106:210, 1994.

48. Levy JH, Adelson DM, Walker BF: Wheal and flare responses to muscle relaxants in humans. Agents Actions 34:302, 1991.

49. Smith Cl, Humlin JM, Jones RS: Vecuronium infusion in patients with renal failure in an ICU. Anaesthesia 42:387, 1987.

50. Lynam D, Cronnelly R, Castognole K: The pharmacodynamics and pharmacokinetics of vecuronium in patients anesthetized with isoflurane with normal renal function or with renal failure. Anesthesiology 69:227, 1988.

51. Newman PJ, Quinn AC, Grounds RM, et al: A comparison of cisatracurium (51W89) and atracurium by infusion in critically ill patients. Crit Care Med 25:1139, 1997.

52. Murray MJ, Coursin DB, Scuderi PE, et al: Double-blind randomized multi-center study of doxacurium versus pancuronium in intensive care unit patients who require neuromuscular-blocking agents. Crit Care Med 23:450, 1995.

53. Prielipp RC, Robinson JC, Wilson JA, et al: Dose response, recovery and cost of doxacurium as a continuous infusion in neurosurgical intensive care unit patients. Crit Care Med 25:1236, 1997.

54. Gooch JL, Suchyta MR, Balbierz JM: Prolonged paralysis after treatment with neuromuscular junction blocking agents. Crit Care Med 19:1125, 1991.

55. Lagasse RS, Katz RI, Petersen M: Prolonged neuromuscular blockade following vecuronium infusion. J Clin Anesth 2:269, 1990.

56. Marik PE: Doxacurium-corticosteroid acute myopathy: another piece to the puzzle. Crit Care Med 24:1266, 1996.

57. Op de Coul AAW, Lambregts PCLA, Koeman J: Neuromuscular complications in patients given Pavulon (pancuronium bromide) during artificial ventilation. Clin Neurol Neurosurg 87:17, 1985.

58. Segredo V, Caldwell JE, Matthay MA: Persistent paralysis in critically ill patients after long-term administration of vecuronium. N Engl J Med 327:524, 1992.

59. Vandenbrom RHG, Wierda MKH: Pancuronium bromide in the intensive care unit: a case of overdosage. Anesthesiology 69:996, 1988.

60. Chingmuh L: Intensive care unit neuromuscular syndrome? Anesthesiology 83:237, 1995.

61. Hoyt JW: Persistent paralysis in critically ill patients after the use of neuromuscular blocking agents. New Horiz 2:48, 1994.

62. Ramsay DA, Zochodne DW, Robertson DM: A syndrome of acute severe muscle necrosis in intensive care unit patients. J Neuropathol Exp Neurol 52:387, 1993.

63. Wokke JAJ, Jennekens FGI, Van den Ooord CJM: Histological investigations of muscle atrophy and end plates in two critically ill patients with generalized weakness. J Neurol Sci 88:95, 1988.

64. Danon MJ, Carpenter S: Myopathy with thick filament (myosin) loss following prolonged paralysis with vecuronium during steroid treatment. Muscle Nerve 14:1131, 1991.

65. Fischer JR, Baer RK: Acute myopathy associated with combined use of corticosteroids and neuromuscular blocking agents. Ann Pharmacother 30:1437, 1996.

66. Kupfer Y, Namba T, Kaldawi E: Prolonged weakness after long-term infusion of vecuronium bromide. Ann Intern Med 117:484, 1992.

67. Shapiro BA, Warren J, Egol AB, et al: Practice parameters for sustained neuromuscular blockade in the adult critically ill patient: an executive summary. Crit Care Med 23:1601, 1995.

68. Tschida SJ, Hoey LL, Mather D, et al: Train-of-four: to use or not to use. Pharmacotherapy 15:546, 1995.

69. Tschida SJ, Hoey LL, Mather D, et al: Inconsistency with train-of-four monitoring in a critically ill paralyzed patient. Pharmacotherapy 15:540, 1995.

CHAPTER 15

Pharmacology of Respiratory Drugs Administered by Aerosol During Mechanical Ventilation

Karen L. Gunther, RN, BSN
Paul M. Dorinsky, MD
Theodore J. Witek, Jr., Dr PH

GENERAL THERAPEUTIC CONSIDERATIONS
BRONCHODILATORS
Sympathomimetics
Antimuscarinics
ANTI-INFLAMMATORY AGENTS
AGENTS WITH ANTI-INFECTIVE PROPERTIES
Aerosolized Antibiotics

Ribavirin
DEOXYRIBONUCLEASE (DNASE), SURFACTANT, AND OTHER AGENTS
Recombinant Human Deoxyribonuclease
Surfactant
Other Agents
REFERENCES

KEY WORDS

bronchodilator
surfactant

sympathomimetics

GENERAL THERAPEUTIC CONSIDERATIONS

This chapter reviews the pharmacology of the drugs that can be administered by aerosol during mechanical ventilation. Before individual drug classes are discussed, a brief discussion of general therapeutic considerations is provided.

Drug delivery by aerosol can be advantageous to patients with respiratory disorders because delivery to site of intended action can result in lower doses being administered, with the added benefit of reduction of systemic side effects. The patient requiring ventilatory support adds an important clinical dimension to administration of aerosol therapeutics because the interface between drug delivery device and the airway is altered significantly (Table 15–1). The technical aspects of aerosol delivery and mode of mechanical ventilation, which are discussed in detail in Chapter 4, underscore several important points to consider in the pharmacology of aerosol therapeutics. For example, the physical pathway of the ventilatory circuit can alter the amount of drug reaching the intended site of action, resulting in a therapeutic window that can be quite different from that which typically characterizes stable patients without artificial airways.

Two additional variables need to be considered in a discussion of aerosol pharmacology. First, aerosol drugs administered to a patient while in the supine position can affect aerosol distribution and ultimate response. Second, patients who require mechanical ventilatory support are, for the most part, at the extremes of disease severity. As a result of both respiratory (e.g., mu-

TABLE 15–1. Factors That Can Affect the Response to an Inhaled Agent During Mechanical Ventilation

PATIENT

Airway obstruction
  Degree of bronchospasm
  Degree of mucus plugging
Dynamic hyperinflation
Patient position

AGENT AND FORMULATION

Dose and dose frequency
Particle size distribution

PATIENT–AEROSOL GENERATOR INTERFACE

Placement of generator in circuit
Use of spacer/adapter
Size of artificial airway (e.g., endotracheal tube
  inner diameter)

VENTILATOR RELATED

Humidity of circuit gas
Ventilation settings (f, V_T, I:E)
Modes of operation (e.g., patient triggering)

f, breathing frequency; I:E, inspiratory:expiratory (time ratio); V_T, tidal volume.

cus plugging) and nonrespiratory (e.g., concomitant therapies) factors that may coexist in these patients, the efficacy of aerosolized agents may be altered.

Where do these added problems leave the practitioner? First, one must be a true practitioner and guide individual therapeutic regimens on the basis of clinical evaluation. Second, one must continue to appreciate the need for and contribute to clinical investigation into optimal dosing and evaluation of response in these patients.

BRONCHODILATORS

Sympathomimetics

Sympathomimetics are the most widely used bronchodilators in respiratory care. Although the antispasmatic properties of these drugs have been known for centuries, modern-day therapy has evolved primarily from alterations of the catecholamine structure of drugs such as epinephrine and isoproterenol. Currently, one has the choice between shorter-activity (i.e., 2–6 hours) beta-2-specific agonists and longer-acting (e.g., twice daily) agents.

The mechanism of action of **beta-2 agonists** is understood to involve interaction of the drug with a receptor that leads to exchange of guanosine triphosphate (GTP) for guanosine diphosphate (GDP). The GTP-activated G protein then activates adenylate cyclase, leading to the formation of cyclic adenosine monophosphate (cAMP). Among the initial events that result in a cellular response is the activation of protein kinase A, which phosphorylates various cellular proteins and regulates their activities. Details of this pharmacology can be found elsewhere.[1, 2]

Tissue responses after beta receptor stimulation include relaxation of bronchial smooth muscle, prevention of release of mediators from mast cells, increased mucus secretion from submucosal glands, and increased mucociliary transport. The acute bronchodilator properties of beta agonists are regarded as the most useful to the practitioner.

Clinical Utility

The goal of acute bronchodilation is best achieved through the inhalation of beta-2 agonists. Bronchodilator effects typically outweigh the known and suspected adverse effects of both short- and long-acting agents.[3, 4] Potential adverse effects from beta receptor stimulation include tachycardia, skeletal muscle tremors, and hypokalemia (Fig. 15–1). Patients with pre-existing cardiovascular disease—particularly the elderly—may be more prone to such reactions. Because these patients often represent a substantial portion of ventilated patients, one must monitor therapy, particularly with any dose titration regimens.

The provision of optimal pharmacotherapy is paramount in the goals of modern-day asthma therapy, and a stepwise approach currently is outlined in Clinical Practice Guidelines.[5] Short-acting clinical agents are indicated for relief of acute symptoms, whereas long-acting beta agonists added to **anti-inflammatory agents** are indicated for long-term symptom prevention (especially nocturnal symptoms). In chronic obstructive pulmonary disease (COPD), current pharmacologic care standards[6, 7] recognize the role of beta agonists for the relief of symptoms. Again, the potential for arrhythmias should be considered in using these agents in patients with cardiac disease, although serious complications with conventional dosages in the stable patient are regarded as rare.[6]

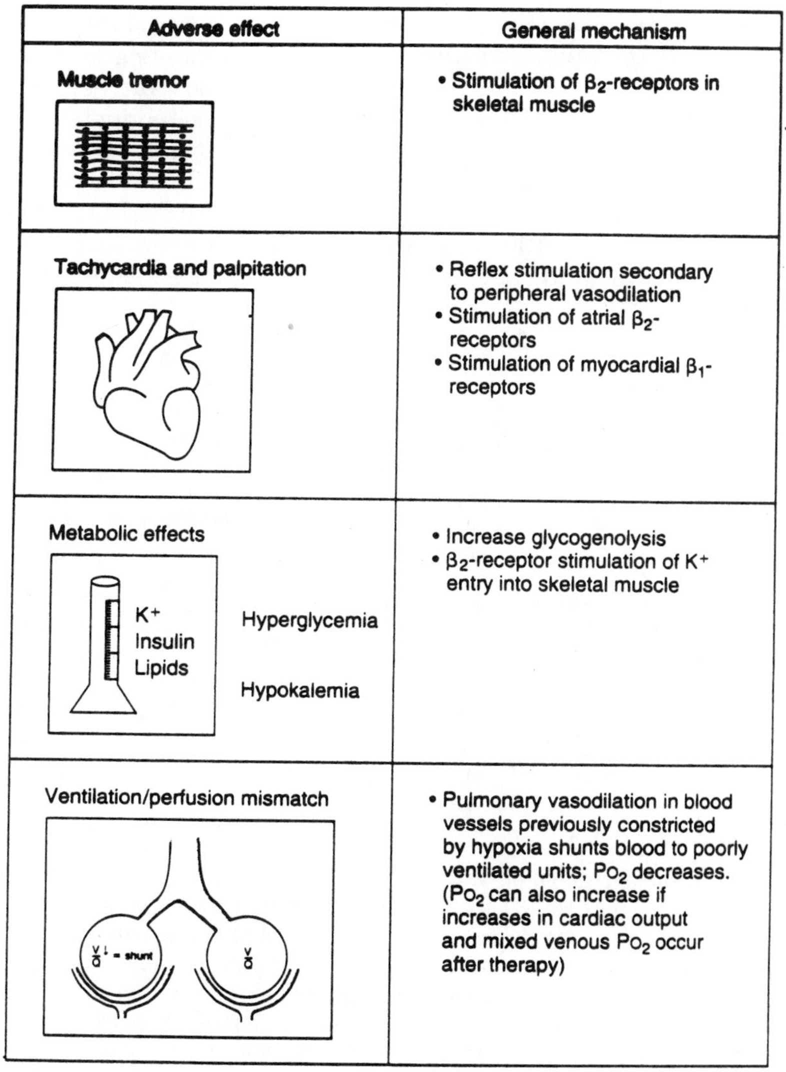

Adverse effect	General mechanism
Muscle tremor	• Stimulation of β_2-receptors in skeletal muscle
Tachycardia and palpitation	• Reflex stimulation secondary to peripheral vasodilation • Stimulation of atrial β_2-receptors • Stimulation of myocardial β_1-receptors
Metabolic effects K+ Insulin Lipids Hyperglycemia Hypokalemia	• Increase glycogenolysis • β_2-receptor stimulation of K^+ entry into skeletal muscle
Ventilation/perfusion mismatch	• Pulmonary vasodilation in blood vessels previously constricted by hypoxia shunts blood to poorly ventilated units; Po_2 decreases. (Po_2 can also increase if increases in cardiac output and mixed venous Po_2 occur after therapy)

FIGURE 15–1
Adverse effects and their general mechanisms that may be associated with sympathomimetic therapy. Po_2, partial pressure of oxygen; Q, blood flow; V, ventilation.

Aerosol Therapy During Mechanical Ventilation

Significant bronchodilation can be achieved with beta agonists when they are employed optimally in patients requiring mechanical ventilation.[8] Consensus statements presently support the use of either the nebulizer or the metered dose inhaler (MDI) as an acceptable method of delivery in mechanically ventilated patients.[9] Many, but not all, trials have demonstrated an improvement in airway pressure responses (e.g., airway resistance) after MDI administration of albuterol[10–14] or metaproterenol[15] in mechanically ventilated patients. In these trials, cohorts were generally small (N = 7–20) and included patients with COPD,[10, 12–14] acute respiratory distress syndrome (ARDS),[15] or mixed conditions.[11–13] The doses of beta agonists used in these studies varied (0.2–3.0 mg), as did the administrative and assessment techniques.

Dose response to MDI albuterol has been evaluated in patients who require mechanical ventilation. Manthous and associates[16] administered albuterol with cumulative exposure as high as 100 puffs (90 μg/puff) from an MDI and did not observe significant bronchodilator or toxic effects. In a subsequent trial with the use of a spacer,[13] they observed significantly reduced pressure responses after cumulative doses of 15 puffs (90 μg/puff) that were not improved further with 15 more puffs (total = 30 puffs). In a subsequent trial, Dhand and coworkers[14] observed significant differences in airway resistance in 12 patients with COPD after 4 puffs of albuterol (90 μg/puff) (Fig. 15–2) that were comparable to those seen after cumulative doses of both 12 and 28 puffs. Because heart rate was increased significantly after the cumulative dose of 28 puffs (mean of 89 beats/min after 28 puffs, 84 beats/min after 12 puffs, and 81 beats/min after 4 puffs; no increases greater than 110 beats/min) (Fig. 15–3), the investigators concluded that 4 puffs was the best dosage.

Taken together, the observations with albuterol administered to mechanically ventilated patients via MDI highlight several important aspects of therapeutics. First, the technique of delivery, the assessment of response, and the disease characteristics of the study population need to be considered in evaluating existing data. Second, one needs to assess carefully the individual therapeutic outcome by both monitoring the

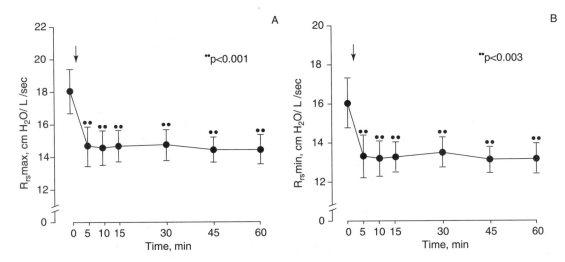

FIGURE 15–2

Effect of administration of four puffs on R_{rs}max (A) and R_{rs}min (B) in seven patients. A significant decrease in R_{rs}max and R_{rs}min occurred within 5 minutes of albuterol administration (p < 0.003 for both). The effect of albuterol persisted for 60 minutes (p < 0.003 for both R_{rs}max and R_{rs}min). R_{rs}, respiratory system resistance. (Reprinted with permission from Dhand R, Duarte AG, Jubran A, et al: Dose response to bronchodilator delivered by metered-dose inhaler in ventilator-supported patients. Am J Respir Crit Care Med 154:388–393, 1996. © American Lung Association.)

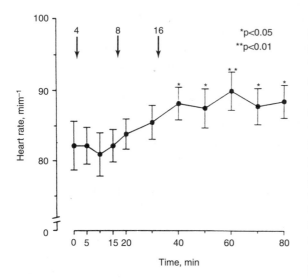

FIGURE 15–3

Effect of doubling doses of albuterol (4, 8, and 16 puffs) on heart rate. Heart rate did not change after administration of 4 puffs or a cumulative dose of 12 puffs ($p > 0.05$). After a cumulative dose of 28 puffs, heart rate increased significantly ($p < 0.01$) and was significantly higher at 80 minutes ($p < 0.05$) when compared with baseline values. Bars represent standard error* $p < 0.05$;** $p < 0.01$. (Reprinted with permission from Dhand R, Duarte AG, Jubran A, et al: Dose response to bronchodilator delivered by metered-dose inhaler in ventilator-supported patients. Am J Respir Crit Care Med 154:388–393, 1996. © American Lung Association.)

desired effect (e.g., decreased airway pressure) and the unwanted pharmacodynamic responses (e.g., tachycardia).

Antimuscarinics

Antimuscarinic bronchodilators were introduced into current practice with the development of ipratropium bromide. Like beta agonists, bronchodilatory properties of this class of drugs have been known for centuries. The prototype agent atropine, although occasionally administered via aerosol in the modern era, was hampered by its side effects. By contrast, the inability of ipratropium bromide to be absorbed across biologic membranes widens its therapeutic window; this has resulted in its widespread use for relief of the obstructed airway.[17]

Antimuscarinic pharmacology has been advanced over the past decade. Five muscarinic receptors have been cloned, four of which have been defined pharmacologically, and three of which have known functions.[18, 19] Mediation of cholinergic bronchoconstriction and glandular secretion occurs via the respiratory M_3 receptor. M_3 stimulation, via a G protein, activates phospholipase C (PLC) to release inositol 1,4,5-triphosphate (IP_3) and diacylglycerol (DAG). IP_3 results in release of intracellular calcium, whereas DAG activates protein kinase C (PKC), which leads to smooth muscle contraction. The bronchodilatory role of antimuscarinic drugs such as ipratropium bromide is based on inhibition of these postreceptor events.

Clinical Utility

As previously noted, antimuscarinic drugs have been used for centuries as bronchodilators,[20] but it was not until the introduction of ipratropium bromide in the 1980s that they became an integral part of the clinician's **bronchodilator** regimen. Ipratropium bromide has been used most extensively as a bronchodilator in the treatment of COPD,[21] for which both United States[6] and European[7] treatment guidelines highlight its role in maintenance treatment. Ipratropium bromide is not indicated for rapid relief of bronchospasm because its onset is somewhat slower than that of short-acting beta agonists. Because many patients with COPD are prescribed ipratropium bromide concurrently with a beta agonist, a single MDI with both agents has been developed and introduced.[22]

For asthma, current guidelines[5] recommend that ipratropium use be limited to that of a potential addition to acute therapy with short-acting agents such as albuterol. The benefits of antimuscarinics in patients with specific asthma symptoms such as nocturnal symptoms and cough are reviewed elsewhere.[23]

Aerosol Therapy During Mechanical Ventilation

The antimuscarinic drug ipratropium bromide is used extensively in maintenance care of the stable patients with COPD. There is one report[10] that describes significant improvements in pressure responses both 30 and 60 minutes after MDI administration of 0.04 mg of ipratropium bromide in COPD patients, most of whom had acute exacerbations of their underlying lung disease. Cardiovascular monitoring did not identify any significant changes, with the exception of a slight increase in systolic blood pressure that the authors speculated was related to sedation differences.

ANTI-INFLAMMATORY AGENTS

Oral and intravenous corticosteroid therapies remain effective and often life-saving forms of treatment for patients with a variety of acute and chronic pulmonary disorders. The long-term use of these agents, however, is limited by undesirable systemic effects. These include a large array of reactions, some potentially serious, such as adrenal insufficiency, fluid and electrolyte imbalances, glucose intolerance, gastric ulceration, osteoporosis, and growth impairment in children.[5, 24] The severe systemic side effects of chronic oral corticosteroid use prompted the development of inhaled preparations, with the goal of achieving a therapeutic effect in the lungs without the untoward systemic effects. Given the safety profile of inhaled therapy, increasingly widespread use of these agents has occurred over the past 2 decades.

Current guidelines for the treatment of obstructive lung disease indicate a primary role for inhaled corticosteroid therapy in asthma[5, 25] but a limited role in COPD.[6] The use of inhaled corticosteroids in the treatment of asthma is dictated by disease severity and is directed toward suppression of airway inflammation. The efficacy of these agents in the management of asthma is probably the result of their wide range of cellular anti-inflammatory effects.[24] Details of proposed cellular and molecular pathophysiologic mechanisms of airway inflammation and the therapeutic activity of corticosteroids can be found in several reviews.[24, 26–28]

Aerosolized corticosteroids, although effective as a maintenance therapy, have no role in the acute management of asthma exacerbations. As recommended in the Asthma Management Guidelines[5, 25] and observed in clinical practice, intravenous steroids are essential for the successful management of asthma patients with acute respiratory failure who require mechanical ventilation. After resolution of the acute episode, strategies for the transition to oral steroids and ultimately inhaled agents are based on the patient's clinical response to therapy.

For the most part, the use of inhaled corticosteroids in mechanically ventilated patients is not indicated. An exception to this practice would be in patients who require maintenance inhaled corticosteroid therapy and who are on mechanical ventilation for reasons other than acute respiratory failure. In these situations, inhaled corticosteroids could be administered via the endotracheal tube. However, to date, no clinical studies have been conducted that support the therapeutic value of inhaled corticosteroids in patients requiring ventilatory assistance.

AGENTS WITH ANTI-INFECTIVE PROPERTIES

Aerosolized Antibiotics

The conceptual basis for delivering antibiotics to the lower respiratory tract via aerosolization is compelling. Namely, aerosol administration of antibiotics to the lungs may enable very high concentrations of antibiotics to be delivered directly to the site of lung infection with minimal systemic absorption and, therefore, minimal systemic side effects. However, as discussed in subsequent sections, the hoped-for improvements in therapeutic efficacy generally have not been achieved with this form of therapy, mostly because of factors that affect the aerosol characteristics of antibiotics (e.g., surface tension, viscosity, and osmolality).[29]

Clinical Utility

Clinical trials with aerosolized antibiotics have yielded inconsistent results. As noted previously, these inconsistencies are due, in part, to physical and chemical factors that affect antibiotic aerosol delivery (Table 15–2) and that may limit the amount of antibiotic that reaches the lower respiratory tract.[29–31] Optimally, an antibiotic that is to be aerosolized should not be readily susceptible to oxidation and must not have an excessively high (will not form droplets) or low (causes foaming and diminishes aerosol production) surface tension. Likewise, as the concentration of antibiotic increases in the nebulized solution, there is a greater likelihood that osmolality and viscosity will also increase, leading to cough and a lower nebulization rate, respectively.[30] Finally, because the distribution and extent of lung consolidation may affect antibiotic distribution because the antibiotic will not be optimally delivered to lung units that are consolidated and/or poorly ventilated.[29]

Given these diverse factors affecting antibiotic aerosol delivery, it perhaps is not surprising that results of clinical trials have been inconsistent. Nonetheless, aerosolization of antibiotics has been shown to be clinically useful in the prevention of lung infection in stable patients with cystic fibrosis and may be useful as an adjunct to intravenous antibiotic therapy in cystic fibrosis patients with acute infection.[32] In this regard, Touw and colleagues[32] recently reviewed all

TABLE 15–2. Factors Affecting Antibiotic Aerosol Delivery

PHYSICAL PROPERTIES OF ANTIBIOTIC FORMULATION

- Antibiotic concentration
- Susceptibility to oxidation
- Surface tension
- pH
- Viscosity
- Osmolarity

METHOD OF AEROSOLIZATION

- Jet nebulizer
- Ultrasonic nebulizer

PATIENT FACTORS

- Respiratory rate and tidal volume
- Duration of breath-hold/inspiratory pause
- Underlying lung disease

studies published between 1965 and 1995 in which inhaled antibiotics were used to treat cystic fibrosis. Among the 12 studies in which inhaled antibiotics were used as maintenance therapy in stable outpatients, an improvement in lung function and/or a reduction in the number of hospital admissions was reported in four uncontrolled studies and in six of eight placebo-controlled studies.[32] By contrast, antibiotic aerosol therapy did not add to the clinical efficacy of intravenous antibiotics in cystic fibrosis patients hospitalized with acute infection.[32] Thus, despite the conceptual appeal of aerosol antibiotic therapy, its role in cystic fibrosis appears limited to preventive and maintenance therapy.

Aerosol Therapy During Mechanical Ventilation

Experimentally, conditions can be defined in which at least certain antibiotics achieve lung concentrations after aerosol delivery that exceed those which occur after intravenous infusion. Specifically, Hashimoto and associates[33] showed that aerosolized imipenem/cilastatin produced greater bronchoalveolar lavage (BAL) antibiotic concentrations in rats than did the intravenous infusions. More importantly, these investigators showed that aerosolizing antibiotics resulted in better bacterial killing and less lung injury than intravenous antibiotics in rats with *Pseudomonas aeruginosa* lung injury.[33] By contrast, aerosolized antibiotics used in mechanically ventilated intensive care unit (ICU) patients have not been effective and may, at times, be associated with deleterious consequences. Namely, although aerosolized antibiotics can reduce gram-negative colonization rates in intubated patients, their routine use in this patient population also can lead to the emergence of resistant bacteria and an increase in ICU mortality.[34, 35] As a result of these observations, aerosolized antibiotics are no longer used in ICU patients.

Conclusions

Currently, aerosolized antibiotics do not have an established role in the prevention or treatment of lower respiratory tract infections in mechanically ventilated patients. However, clinical studies are lacking in this patient population, in which newer antibiotic agents are employed and correlated to the amount of antibiotic that actually reaches the lower respiratory tract. Until this information is available, the clinical utility of aerosolized antibiotics in situations other than preventive therapy in stable patients with cystic fibrosis remains unclear.

Ribavirin

Respiratory syncytial virus (RSV) is a single-stranded RNA virus that replicates in the respiratory epithelium and causes a variety of respiratory illnesses. In adults and older children, RSV generally causes a cold-like illness or otitis media. However, in infants, RSV causes a more severe illness and generally results in bronchiolitis or pneumonia.

Ribavirin, a synthetic nucleoside analogue with antiviral activity against a broad spectrum of viruses including RSV, is the only agent indicated for the treatment of hospitalized infants and children with severe lower respiratory tract infection due to RSV.[36, 37] Because most healthy children with RSV infection recover without treatment or require only supportive care during hospitalization, the use of ribavirin generally is limited to infants with underlying conditions known to increase the risk of severe or fatal RSV infection (e.g., prematurity, immunosuppression, congenital heart disease, or underlying pulmonary disease).[38]

General Considerations

To ensure optimal penetration of an aerosolized drug designed to treat parenchymal disease, particles should exhibit a mass median aerodynamic diameter (MMAD) of 0.8 to 3.0 μm.[9, 39] However, ribavirin is administered using a Small Particle Aerosol Generator (ICN Pharmaceuticals, Costa Mesa, CA), which generates drug particles with an MMAD less than 1.5 μm.[9] Particles less than 0.8 μm generally are exhaled and pre-

sumably contribute little to the desired treatment effect. Additionally, aerosol delivery to the lower respiratory tract may also be reduced in the presence of an artificial airway, potentially leading to a diminished therapeutic effect. Despite these putative limitations, the recommended administration and dosing regimen is the same for infants who require mechanical ventilation as for those who do not. Ribavirin is reconstituted in sterile H_2O at a concentration of 20 mg/ml and administered as a continuous aerosol over 12 to 18 hours for a 3- to 7-day treatment period.[37] Because exposure to ribavirin has potential teratogenic and embryotoxic effects,[37] care must be taken to limit environmental exposure of the health care worker, especially women of childbearing potential.[9]

Aerosol Therapy During Mechanical Ventilation

Initially, ribavirin was not approved for use in infants and children with RSV infection who required assisted ventilation because of concerns related to drug crystal precipitation in the ventilator tubing and exhalation valve and a lack of clinical data in this patient population.[38] The technical problems have been circumvented through the use of one-way valves in inspiratory lines and a breathing circuit filter in the expiratory line.[38–40] However, establishment of clinical efficacy of ribavirin in mechanically ventilated infants and children with RSV infection was more difficult.

Smith and colleagues[41] conducted a small randomized, placebo-controlled trial consisting primarily of healthy term infants with RSV-associated respiratory failure. In this study, the use of ribavirin led to reductions in the duration of mechanical ventilation (4.9 vs. 9.9 days; p = 0.01), supplemental oxygen use (8.7 vs. 13.5 days; p = 0.01), and hospital length of stay (9.0 vs. 15.3 days; p = 0.005) compared with placebo. However, the validity of these results has been criticized, primarily because of the use of aerosolized water as a control and the concern that aerosolized water (i.e., a hypotonic solution) could produce bronchospasm.[42] In a later study, Meert and associates[43] conducted a similar trial but used an isotonic saline aerosol instead of sterile water as the placebo treatment. This trial failed to show a significant difference in the duration of mechanical ventilation, supplemental oxygen use, intensive care, or hospitalization between ribavirin- and placebo-treated groups. In contrast to the patients studied by Smith and colleagues,[41] who were largely immunocompetent (75%), most patients in the Meert study had significant underlying cardiopulmonary or neurologic disorders (59%) and/or were born prematurely (68%).

To definitively evaluate the use of aerosolized ribavirin in this clinical setting, a 38-center Pediatric Critical Care Study Group was formed and conducted a prospective multicenter cohort study to specifically examine the drug's effectiveness in reducing both the duration of mechanical ventilation and mortality rates in healthy infants.[44] A total of 223 immunocompetent infants were enrolled, and 91 (41%) received ribavirin therapy. Predicted Pediatric Risk of Mortality Scores (PRISMs) and actual mortality rates were not significantly different among the treated and untreated groups. Both the term and premature infant groups treated with ribavirin had a longer duration of hospitalization and ICU stay and prolonged time on mechanical ventilation. Thus, these data fail to support the clinical benefit of ribavirin therapy in well term or premature infants with RSV-associated respiratory failure.

Conclusions

Although ribavirin is approved for use in the treatment of hospitalized infants and children with severe lower respiratory tract infection due to respiratory syncytial virus, including patients requiring assisted ventilation, inconclusive evidence is available regarding the efficacy of this agent in mechanically ventilated patients. Perhaps future clinical studies and/or new delivery techniques will establish the efficacy of ribavirin therapy in RSV-infected patients who require mechanical ventilation.

DEOXYRIBONUCLEASE (DNASE), SURFACTANT, AND OTHER AGENTS

Recombinant Human Deoxyribonuclease

Recombinant human DNase I has been available for nearly a decade. It was cloned from human pancreatic cDNA using probes that were based on the amino acid sequence of bovine pancreatic DNase I.[45] The resultant product, when incubated with purulent sputum obtained from cystic fibrosis patients, dramatically improved sputum pourability (i.e., a qualitative sputum viscoelasticity assay) and sputum viscoelasticity (i.e., as measured quantitatively using a viscometer).[45, 46] Given these properties of human DNase I and the fact that it was developed for aerosol administration, this agent may have broad application to a variety of human diseases (e.g., cystic fibrosis, chronic bronchitis).

Clinical Utility

Altered clearance of purulent secretions contributes to the morbidity of a variety of airway inflammatory disorders, in particular, cystic fibrosis. DNA, which is released by neutrophils that accumulate in the airways during airway infection, is estimated to comprise nearly 10% of the dry weight of the respiratory secretions of cystic fibrosis patients, which corresponds to a DNA concentration of approximately 5.9 mg/mL.[47, 48] As noted previously, recombinant human DNase (dornase alfa) is highly effective in improving the viscoelastic properties of purulent sputum in vitro[45, 46] and thus has undergone clinical testing in several disease states.

Most of the clinical experience with aerosolized DNase is derived from patients with cystic fibrosis. In this regard, Ramsey and associates[49] administered three different doses of DNase (i.e., 0.6, 2.5, and 10.0 mg twice daily) or placebo via aerosol to 181 cystic fibrosis patients. In this phase II study, forced expiratory volume in 1 second (FEV$_1$) and forced vital capacity (FVC) improved by 10% to 15% and were greatest after the 2.5-mg and 10.0-mg doses. Subsequently, Fuchs and colleagues[47] studied 968 patients with cystic fibrosis in a double-blind, randomized, placebo-controlled study over a 24-week period during which DNase was administered via aerosol in either once- or twice-daily doses of 2.5 mg/dose. These patients were required to have an FVC of greater than 40% of predicted normal values at study entry. The data from this study indicated that, compared with controls, treated patients had a 28% to 37% decrease in the risk of developing an infectious exacerbation and a modest improvement in FEV_1 (i.e., 5–6%). Finally, McCoy and associates[50] studied aerosolized DNase (2.5 mg once daily) versus placebo in 320 cystic fibrosis patients whose FVC was required to be less than 40% of predicted normal values at study entry. In this study, treated patients had significant improvements in FEV_1 (9.4% vs. 2.1%) and FVC (12.4% vs. 7.3%) compared with controls. However, DNase did not result in a decreased incidence of infectious complications.

In summary, aerosolized DNase has been shown to be efficacious in patients with cystic fibrosis with moderate (FVC > 40% predicted) and advanced (FVC < 40% predicted) disease. Whether this aerosolized compound also may be effective in patients with other forms of inflammatory airway disorders and/or in patients who require mechanical ventilation remains, at present, unclear.

Aerosol Therapy During Mechanical Ventilation

As previously stated, patients in ICUs who require mechanical ventilation often have compromised pulmonary function and may have difficulty clearing secretions. However, difficulty in clearing secretions in this patient population generally suggests the presence of an underlying neuromuscular disorder and/or is the consequence of generalized weakness from a debilitating disease or a prolonged illness. As a result, therapy directed primarily at altering the viscoelastic properties of sputum either is not effective or is not sufficient to improve lung function. Nonetheless, disorders in which excessive secretions are the result of airway

pathology and that contribute to respiratory failure could, in theory, respond favorably to a therapeutic modality such as DNase.

Presently, little clinical information is available to support the use of DNase in ventilated patients, regardless of underlying disease. For example, chronic bronchitis is characterized by chronic mucopurulent sputum production. However, DNase has not been shown to clinically benefit these patients.[51] Likewise, although anecdotal reports of the benefits of DNase use in ventilated patients exist,[52] it has not been evaluated systematically as an adjunctive therapy in any group of ventilated patients. Finally, although DNase can be aerosolized to droplet sizes less than 6 μm, the optimal delivery system (jet vs. ultrasonic nebulizer) and particle size for DNase in ventilated patients has not been established.[53] Moreover, the deposition characteristics of DNase in the lower respiratory tract of patients during aerosolization through a ventilator circuit are unknown.

Conclusions

It is clear that aerosolized DNase is a potent recombinant product that dramatically improves the viscoelastic properties of purulent respiratory secretions. However, little data are available to support its use in patients other than nonintubated patients with cystic fibrosis. Recommendations for the use of DNase in ventilated or nonventilated patients with lung disorders other than cystic fibrosis must await appropriate, placebo-controlled clinical trials.

Surfactant

Surfactant is produced and secreted by type II pneumocytes and is composed of a mixture of lipids, proteins, and carbohydrates. Surfactant is primarily responsible for lowering alveolar surface tension, thereby permitting alveoli to empty evenly during deflation and lowering the distending pressures necessary to achieve any given lung volume.[54] Surfactant also has important immune effects, which include modulation of lymphocyte responsiveness and neutrophil chemotaxis and enhancement of macrophage antibacterial functions. Recently, it has become possible to replace surfactant via direct lung installation or aerosolization. As detailed in the remainder of this section, inadequate levels of surfactant are important in the pathophysiology of both the infant and the acute (adult) respiratory distress syndromes, and these conditions serve as the focal point for a discussion of surfactant replacement strategies.

Clinical Utility (Infants)

Infant or neonatal respiratory distress syndrome (RDS) is a disorder that occurs in premature infants as a result of inadequate production of surfactant. The result of inadequate surfactant production in these premature infants is alveolar collapse, decreased lung compliance, and the development of refractory hypoxemia (shunt physiology). This leads to respiratory failure and, in most cases, the need for mechanical ventilation. Although corticosteroids have been administered to mothers to augment prenatal surfactant production, the mainstay of therapy is administration of surfactant to infants with RDS.[55]

A detailed discussion of surfactant replacement in RDS is beyond the scope of this chapter and has been reviewed in detail elsewhere.[56-59] However, surfactant preparations differ considerably with respect to their source (natural vs. synthetic), composition (Table 15–3), and in vivo behavior.[56-59]

Nonetheless, the more than 40 randomized, controlled trials that have been reported in the past 15 years are generally consistent in showing that surfactant therapy improves gas exchange, reduces barotrauma, and improves survival in RDS.[56-59] Finally, although aerosol surfactant administration has not been evaluated fully in RDS, natural surfactants appear to outperform artificial surfactants in most trials.[57, 58]

Clinical Utility (Adults)

Acute (adult) respiratory distress syndrome (ARDS) occurs in the setting of diverse clinical disorders and is characterized by diffuse inflammatory lung injury, nonhydrostatic pulmonary edema, and refractory hypoxemia (paO_2 to FiO_2 ratio < 200). Recently, Gregory and colleagues[60] demonstrated that patients with ARDS have decreases in both total phospholipids and surfactant proteins (SP-A and SP-B) compared with controls. Subsequently, several large surfactant replacement trials have been completed in adults with ARDS. The largest trial was conducted by Anzueto and colleagues[61] and consisted of administering artificial surfactant (Exosurf) to 364 patients with ARDS via continuous aerosolization for up to 5 days. In this trial, aerosolized surfactant had no benefit as assessed by 30-day survival, physiologic parameters, or time on mechanical ventilation. Subsequently, Gregory and colleagues[62] administered natural surfactant (Survanta) in serial doses by en-

TABLE 15–3. Source and Composition of Commonly Used Surfactant Preparations

PREPARATION	SOURCE	COMPOSITION	ROUTE OF ADMINISTRATION	TRIALS IN RDS	TRIALS IN ARDS
Exosurf	Synthetic	DPPC	Aerosol instilled	Yes	Yes
Survanta	Bovine lung extract	Lung lipids, DPPC	Instilled	Yes	Yes
Infasurf	Calf lung lavage	Surfactant lipids, SP-B, SP-C	Instilled	Yes	No
Alveofact	Bovine lung lavage	Surfactant lipids, SP-B, SP-C	Instilled	Yes	Yes
Curosurf	Porcine lung extract	Lung lipids, SP-B, SP-C	Instilled	Yes	Yes

ARDS, adult (acute) respiratory distress syndrome; DPPC, dipalmitoylphosphatidylcholine; RDS, respiratory distress syndrome; SP-B, surfactant protein B; SP-C, surfactant protein C.

dotracheal instillation to 43 adult patients
with ARDS. Compared with controls, the
treated patients had a significant reduction
in 28-day mortality (18.8% vs. 43.8%; p =
0.075). Despite these encouraging results,
no phase III trial with Survanta currently
is planned.

With respect to the future of surfactant
replacement in ARDS, several important
factors need to be considered. First, surfactant preparations differ considerably in
their composition and in their ability to
modulate airway inflammatory responses.[63]
Second, the method of surfactant administration affects the amount of surfactant that
reaches the lower respiratory tract. For example, the percentage of aerosolized surfactant that reaches the lung has been found
to be a small percentage (<5%) of the initial
dose.[64] Finally, the distribution of surfactant
within the lungs, whether administered by
nebulization or direct instillation, may not
be uniform in ARDS, in which the extent
and severity of lung injury are not uniform.[56, 65]

Conclusions

Exogenous surfactant replacement has been
shown to be beneficial in the management of
preterm infants with RDS. However, despite
evidence for surfactant dysfunction in
ARDS, the efficacy of exogenous surfactant
replacement has not been established in
adults. Establishing a role for surfactant
therapy in ARDS ultimately may depend
on first identifying the optimal composition
(e.g., surfactant proteins with or without
phospholipids), route of administration
(aerosolized vs. direct installation vs. bronchoscopic instillation), dose, and underlying
disease (e.g., trauma, acid-aspiration, sepsis) for which it is beneficial.

Other Agents

A comprehensive discussion of all agents
that can be administered via aerosolization
and have potential for use in ventilated patients is beyond the scope of this chapter.
For example, aerosolized amiloride, a sodium channel blocker with the potential to

decrease mucus viscosity, currently is being
evaluated in patients with cystic fibrosis.
Likewise, the mucolytic agent N-acetylcys-
teine (Mucomyst) has not been shown to be
useful in the management of most respiratory disorders. Finally, other agents, which
include aerosolized manganese superoxide
dismutase for acute lung injury, aerosolized
amphoterecin for fungal lung infections and
aerosolized cyclosporine for lung transplantation, currently are being evaluated.
However, if these approaches are to be clinically useful, optimal delivery systems, drug
characteristics during aerosolization and
target patient populations will need to be
identified carefully.

SUMMARY

Several pharmacologic agents can be administered by aerosol to patients undergoing mechanical ventilation. These include
bronchodilators and agents that can alter
mucous viscosity or the composition of alveolar lining fluid.

Bronchodilators are the most commonly
used class of drugs administered to ventilated patients. Several reports have indicated improved airway pressure parameters
after their administration. However, because the patient–aerosol generator interface is altered significantly during mechanical ventilation because of the presence of an
artificial airway, the therapeutic window of
drugs established in stable patients can be
distinctly different. Hence, individual assessment of dose and dose frequency is required in this patient population and must
take into account both the efficacy and
safety of the dose titration scheme.

REFERENCES

1. Graham RM: Adrenergic receptors: structures and function. Cleve Clin J Med 57:481–491, 1990.
2. Rasmussen H, Kelley G, Douglas JS: Interaction between Ca²⁺ and cAMP messenger system in reg-ulation of airway smooth muscle contraction. Am J Physiol Lung Cell Mol Physiol 258:L279–L288, 1990.
3. Price AH, Clissold SP. Salbutamol in the 1980s: a re-appraisal of its clinical efficacy. Drugs 38:77–122, 1989.

4. AAAI Committee on Drugs: Position statement: safety and appropriate use of salmeterol in the treatment of asthma. J Allergy Clin Immunol 98:475–480, 1996.

5. National Heart, Lung and Blood Institute and World Health Organization: Global Initiative for Asthma. Bethesda, MD: National Institutes of Health, 1995, NIH Publication #95-3659.

6. American Thoracic Society: Standards for the diagnosis and care of patients with chronic obstructive pulmonary disease. Am J Respir Crit Care Med 152:S77–S120, 1995.

7. Siafakas NM, Vermeire P, Pride NB, et al: Optimal assessment and management of chronic obstructive pulmonary disease (COPD). Eur Respir J 8:1398–1420, 1995.

8. Dhand R, Tobin MJ: Bronchodilator delivery with metered dose inhalers in mechanically ventilated patients. Eur Respir J 9:585–595, 1996.

9. American Association for Respiratory Care: Aerosol consensus statement—1991. Respir Care 36:916–921, 1991.

10. Fernandez A, Lazaro A, Garcia A, et al: Bronchodilators in patients with chronic obstructive pulmonary disease on mechanical ventilation: utilization of metered-dose inhalers. Am Rev Respir Dis 141:164–168, 1990.

11. Mancebo J, Amaro P, Lorino H, et al: Effects of albuterol inhalation on the work of breathing during weaning from mechanical ventilation. Am Rev Respir Dis 144:95–100, 1991.

12. Dhand R, Jubran A, Tobin MJ: Bronchodilator delivery by metered-dose inhaler in ventilator-supported patients. Am J Respir Crit Care Med 151:1827–1833, 1995.

13. Manthous CA, Chatila W, Schmidt GA, et al: Treatment of bronchospasm by metered-dose inhaler albuterol in mechanically-ventilated patients. Chest 107:210–213, 1995.

14. Dhand R, Duarte AG, Jubran A, et al: Dose response to bronchodilator delivered by metered-dose inhaler in ventilator-supported patients. Am J Respir Crit Care Med 154:388–393, 1996.

15. Wright PE, Carmichael LC, Bernard GR: Effect of bronchodilators on lung mechanics in the acute respiratory distress syndrome (ARDS). Chest 106:1517–1523, 1994.

16. Manthous CA, Hall JB, Schmidt GA, et al: Metered-dose inhaler versus nebulized albuterol in mechanically-ventilated patients. Am Rev Respir Dis 148:1567–1570, 1993.

17. Gross NJ: Ipratropium bromide. N Engl J Med 319:486–494, 1988.

18. Baraniuk JN: Muscarinic receptors. In: Leff AR (ed): Pulmonary and Critical Care Pharmacology. New York: McGraw-Hill, 1996 pp 97–104.

19. Barnes PJ: New developments in anticholinergic drugs. Eur Respir Rev 6:290–294, 1996.

20. Gandevia B. Historical review of the use of parasympatholytic agents in the treatment of respiratory disorders. Postgrad Med J 51:13–20, 1975.

21. Ferguson GT, Cherniack RM: Management of chronic obstructive pulmonary disease. N Engl J Med 328:1017–1022, 1993.

22. Wilson JD, Serby CW, Menjoge SS, et al: The efficacy and safety of combination bronchodilator therapy. Eur Respir Rev 6:286–289, 1996.

23. Beakes DE: The use of anticholinergics in asthma. J Asthma 34:357–368, 1997.

24. Barnes PJ, Pederson S, Busse WW: Efficacy and safety of inhaled corticosteroids in asthma: new developments. Am J Respir Crit Care Med 157:S1–S53, 1998.

25. National Asthma Education and Prevention Program: Expert panel report II: guidelines for the diagnosis and management of asthma. February 1997.

26. Robinson DS, Geddes DM: Inhaled corticosteroids: benefits and risks. J Asthma 33:5–16, 1996.

27. Pederson S, O'Byrne P: A comparison of the efficacy and safety of inhaled corticosteroids in asthma. Allergy 529(suppl 39):1–34, 1997.

28. Pincus DJ, Beam WR, Martin RJ: Chronobiology and chronotherapy of asthma. Clin Chest Med 16:699–713, 1995.

29. Smith AL, Ramsey B: Aerosol administration of antibiotics. Respiration 62:19–24, 1995.

30. Weber A, Morlin G, Cohen M, et al: Effect of nebulizer type and antibiotic concentration on device performance. Pediatr Pulmonol 23:249–260, 1997.

31. Coates AL, MacNeish CF, Meisner D, et al: The choice of jet nebulizer, nebulizing flow and the addition of albuterol affects the output of tobramycin aerosols. Chest 111:1206–1212, 1997.

32. Touw DJ, Brimicombe RW, Hodson ME, et al: Inhalation of antibiotics in cystic fibrosis. Eur Respir J 8:1594–1604, 1995.

33. Hashimoto S, Wolfe E, Guglielmo B, et al. Aerosolization of imipenem/cilastatin prevents Pseudomonas-induced acute lung injury. J Antimicrob Chemother 38:809–818, 1996.

34. Greenfield S, Teres D, Bushnell LS, et al: Prevention of gram-negative bacillary pneumonia using aerosol polymyxin as prophylaxis: effect on colonization pattern of the upper respiratory tract of seriously ill patients. J Clin Invest 52:2935–2940, 1973.

35. Feeley TW, DuMoulin GC, Hedley-Whyte J, et al: Aerosol polymyxin and pneumonia in seriously ill patients. N Engl J Med 293:471–475, 1975.

36. Hall CB, McBride JT, Walsh EE, et al: Aerosolized Virazole treatment of infants with respiratory syncytial viral infection. N Engl J Med 308:1443–1447, 1983.

37. Virazole® Package Insert. Costa Mesa, CA: ICN Pharmaceuticals Inc., 1997.

38. American Academy of Pediatrics Committee on Infectious Diseases: Use of ribavirin in the treatment of respiratory syncytial virus infection. J Pediatr 92:501–504, 1993.

39. American Association for Respiratory Care. AARC clinical practice guideline: selection of a device for delivery of aerosol to the lung parenchyma. Respir Care 41:647–653, 1996.

40. Frankel LR, Wilson CW, Demers RR, et al: A technique for the administration of ribavirin to mechanically ventilated infants with severe respira-

tory syncytial virus infection. Crit Care Med 15:1051–1054, 1987.

41. Smith DW, Frankel LR, Mathers LH, et al: A controlled trial of aerosolized ribavirin in infants receiving mechanical ventilation for severe respiratory syncytial virus infection. N Engl J Med 325:24–29, 1991.

42. Moler FW, Bandy KP, Custer JR: Ribavirin therapy for acute bronchiolitis: need for appropriate controls. J Pediatr 119:509, 1991.

43. Meert KL, Sarnaik AP, Gelmini MJ: Aerosolized ribavirin in mechanically ventilated children with respiratory syncytial virus lower respiratory tract disease: a prospective, double-blind, randomized trial. Crit Care Med 22:566–572, 1994.

44. Moler FW, Steinhart CM, Ohmit SE, et al: Effectiveness of ribavirin in otherwise well infants with respiratory syncytial virus-associated respiratory failure. J Pediatr 128:422–428, 1996.

45. Shak S, Capon D, Hellmiss R, et al: Recombinant human DNase I reduces the viscosity of cystic fibrosis sputum. Proc Natl Acad Sci USA 87:9188–9192, 1990.

46. Shak S. Aerosolized recombinant human DNase I for the treatment of cystic fibrosis. Chest 107:655–705, 1995.

47. Fuchs HJ, Borowitz DS, Christiansen DH, et al: Effect of aerosolized recombinant human DNase on exacerbations of respiratory symptoms and/or pulmonary function in patients with cystic fibrosis. N Engl J Med 331:637–642, 1984.

48. Chernik WS, Barbero GJ: Composition of tracheobronchial secretions in cystic fibrosis of the pancreas and bronchiectasis. Pediatrics 24:739–745, 1959.

49. Ramsey BW, Astley SJ, Aitken ML, et al: Efficacy and safety of short-term administration of aerosolized recombinant human deoxyribonuclease in patients with cystic fibrosis. Am Rev Respir Dis 148:145–151, 1993.

50. McCoy K, Hamilton S, Johnson C: Effects of 12-week administration of dornase alfa in patients with advanced cystic fibrosis lung disease. Chest 110:889–895, 1996.

51. Hudson TJ. Dornase in the treatment of chronic bronchitis. Ann Pharmacother 30:674–675, 1996.

52. Kling S, Gie RP, Riphagen S: Dornase alfa in the management of a mechanically ventilated infant with cystic fibrosis [letter]. Pediatr Pulmonol 24:124–125, 1997.

53. Feil SB, Fuchs HJ, Johnson C, et al: Comparison of three jet nebulizer aerosol delivery systems used to administer recombinant human DNase I to patients with cystic fibrosis. Chest 108:153–156, 1995.

54. Lewis JF, Jobe AH: Surfactant and the adult respiratory distress syndrome. Am Rev Respir Dis 147:218–233, 1993.

55. Jobe AH: Pulmonary surfactant therapy. N Engl J Med 328:861–868, 1993.

56. Haas CF, Weg JG. Exogenous surfactant therapy: an update. Respir Care 41:397–415, 1996.

57. Halliday HL: Overview of clinical trials comparing natural and synthetic surfactants. Biol Neonate 67(Suppl 1):32–47, 1995.

58. Halliday HL: Controversies: synthetic or natural surfactant. The case for natural surfactant. J Perinat Med 24:417–426, 1996.

59. American Association for Respiratory Care: Perinatal–Pediatrics Guidelines Committee: surfactant replacement therapy. Respir Care 39:824–829, 1994.

60. Gregory TJ, Longmore WJ, Moxley MA, et al: Surfactant chemical composition and biophysical activity in acute respiratory distress syndrome. J Clin Invest 88:1976–1981, 1991.

61. Anzueto A, Baughman RP, Guntupalli KK, et al: Aerosolized surfactant in adults with sepsis-induced acute respiratory distress syndrome. N Engl J Med 334:1417–1421, 1996.

62. Gregory TJ, Steinberg KP, Spragg R, et al: Bovine surfactant therapy for patients with acute respiratory distress syndrome. Am J Respir Crit Care Med 155:1309–1315, 1997.

63. Tegtmeyer FK, Gortner L, Ludwig A, Brandt E. In vitro modulation of induced neutrophil activation by different surfactant preparations. Eur Respir J 9:752–757, 1996.

64. MacIntyre NR, Coleman RE, Schuller FS, et al: Efficiency of the delivery of aerosolized artificial surfactant to intubated patients with the adult respiratory distress syndrome. Am J Respir Crit Care Med 149:A125, 1994.

65. Lewis JF, Ikegami M, Jobe AH, Absolom D: Physiologic responses and distribution of aerosolized surfactant in a non-uniform pattern of lung injury. Am Rev Respir Dis 147:1364–1370, 1993.

CHAPTER 16

Positioning of the Patient

Joseph A. Govert, MD

EFFECTS OF POSTURE AND
POSITION ON HEALTHY
SUBJECTS
Lung Volumes
Regional Pleural Pressures
Regional Lung Inflation
Pulmonary Mechanics
Distribution of Ventilation
Distribution of Perfusion
Ventilation–Perfusion ($\dot{V}/\dot{Q}$)
    Relationships
EFFECTS OF POSTURE AND
POSITION ON PATIENTS
WITH RESPIRATORY
DISEASE
Neuromuscular Disease

Obstructive Airway Disease
Unilateral Lung Injury
Acute Respiratory Distress
    Syndrome—Physiologic
    Mechanism of Prone
    Positioning
Acute Respiratory Distress
    Syndrome—Clinical
    Effects of Prone
    Positioning
REFERENCES

KEY WORDS

abdominal pressure
pleural pressure

shunting

Frequent changes in body position and posture are universal in healthy animals and humans, even during sleep. Many practitioners believe that repositioning is also important during illness. They believe that frequent patient repositioning and early mobilization during illness and after surgical procedures help prevent complications such as pressure sores, musculoskeletal wasting, atelectasis, pneumonia, and thromboembolism. Despite these benefits, patients with respiratory failure requiring mechanical ventilation commonly remain in a supine horizontal position for days, weeks, or even months.

Both clinical experience and experimental evidence in animals and humans indicate that changes in position and posture alter the regional forces in the airways, alveoli, and pulmonary vasculature. Profound differences are noted in healthy patients mechanically ventilated for elective surgery and in patients with cardiopulmonary disease. Perhaps the most common clinical example of the effect of posture is the increased dyspnea and worsened oxygenation in patients with obstructive lung disease or heart failure when supine. Consequently, these patients often strongly prefer to remain upright or to sleep on a number of pillows. Mechanically ventilated patients often cannot express any sort of preference for certain body positions. As a consequence, they usually remain supine because it is almost always the most convenient for the caregiver.

Recently, there has been increased interest in the physiologic as well as clinical effects of body position in mechanically ventilated patients. It is likely that a combination of mechanisms are responsible for the changes in the distribution of ventilation and perfusion that occur in these patients when body position is altered. This chapter reviews several mechanisms, including improved regional lung inflation, alterations in lung compliance, regional variation in pleural pressure, redistribution of lung water, changes in functional residual capacity (FRC), and positional effects on diaphragmatic function. A number of clinical series demonstrating changes in oxygenation in mechanically ventilated patients who are placed in the lateral decubitus or prone positions also are described.

EFFECTS OF POSTURE AND POSITION ON HEALTHY SUBJECTS

Lung Volumes

In healthy subjects, moving from the sitting to the supine position reduces FRC by approximately 25%.[1] This is mainly due to the abdominal contents exerting greater pressure on the diaphragm. During mechanical ventilation and general anesthesia, decreased inspiratory muscle tone further reduces FRC. General anesthesia and mechanical ventilation also have an impact on diaphragmatic mechanics, which in turn affects FRC. Froese and Bryan[2] found that actively breathing, nonmechanically ventilated supine patients had more diaphrag-

matic movement in the posterior, or dependent, regions of the diaphragm. They suggest that the cause of this is the posterior diaphragm's decreased radius of curvature and the increased stretch of the muscle fibers in that region.[2] However, when patients in that series were mechanically ventilated during general anesthesia, the diaphragm moved passively with motion predominantly in the anterior, or nondependent, regions because of the decreased **abdominal pressure** in these regions.[2] This led to worsened ventilation–perfusion ($\dot{V}/\dot{Q}$) relationships and mild deterioration in oxygenation.[2]

In spontaneously breathing patients, moving from the horizontal supine position to the prone or lateral decubitus position increases FRC by 15% to 20%.[1, 3] This improvement is even more dramatic in mechanically ventilated patients. In a study of 17 healthy anesthetized and paralyzed patients undergoing elective surgery, Pelosi and associates found that FRC improved by approximately 50% when patients were shifted from the supine to the prone position.[4] At this time, the effects of body position on vital capacity and total lung capacity are studied less than the effects on FRC. However, both vital capacity and total lung capacity appear to decrease somewhat in recumbent, supine, spontaneously breathing individuals, probably because of the accumulation of intrathoracic blood.[3, 5] There are no data available on the effect of the prone position on vital capacity.

Regional Pleural Pressures

The **pleural pressure** (P_{pl}) surrounding the lung varies regionally mainly because of the effect of gravity on the lung and, to a lesser extent, on the structures of the mediastinum, chest wall, and abdomen.[6] The weight of the lung at any vertical height produces hydrostatic pressure, which significantly influences P_{pl} at that height. For example, in healthy upright individuals, P_{pl} increases linearly from the lung apex to the diaphragm. The P_{pl} gradient in healthy individuals is approximately 0.2 to 0.3 cm H_2O/cm, which is very close to normal lung density, suggesting that lung weight is the main determinant of the P_{pl} gradient.[6, 7] As a consequence of the P_{pl} gradient, lung alveoli are more distended in the apical, or nondependent, portions and less distended in the basilar, or dependent, portions of the normal upright lung. Although P_{pl} gradients have not been measured in humans in the prone, supine, or lateral decubitus positions, they have been measured experimentally in animals.[8, 9] In all instances, regardless of position, regional P_{pl} is less and alveolar distention is greater in the nondependent portions of the lung.

The position of the lung's surrounding structures also influences regional P_{pl}. For example, the heart rests primarily on the lungs during ventilation in the supine position, but it rests primarily on the sternum

in the prone position. As a result, the weight of the heart exerts less effect on P_{pl} in the region of the left lower lobe when patients are in the prone position. This partially explains the decreased pleural pressure gradients in both healthy and diseased animals in the prone position as compared to the supine position.[9, 10] Similarly, in the lateral decubitus position, the weight of the abdominal contents and mediastinum are distributed preferentially toward the dependent lung, causing decreased FRC and atelectasis in the dependent lung relative to the nondependent lung (Fig. 16–1).[11]

The effect of general anesthesia or mechanical ventilation on regional P_{pl} in humans is not well described, although it is known that muscle tone decreases during anesthesia, increasing chest wall resistance

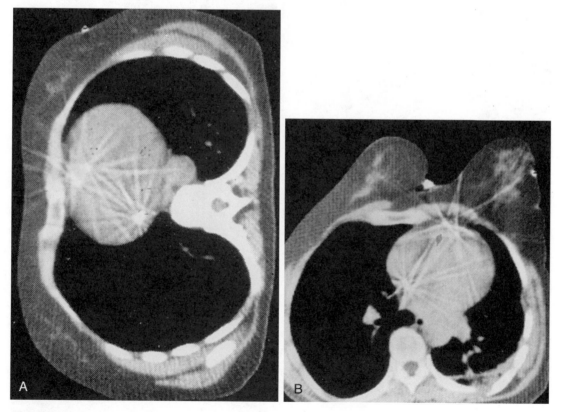

FIGURE 16–1
Computed tomographic images of the chest in supine and lateral decubitus positions. (A) Supine position before anesthesia. (B) Lateral decubitus position during anesthesia. Note the downward shift of mediastinal structures and loss of lung volume in the dependent lung in the lower panel. (From Klingstedt C, Hedenstierna G, Lundquist H, et al: The influence of body position and differential ventilation on lung dimensions and atelectasis formation in anaesthetized man. Acta Anaesthesiol Scand 34:315–322, 1990.)

and thus increasing P_{pl}.[4] This helps explain the diminished FRC and eventual development of atelectasis in the dependent regions of healthy subjects undergoing prolonged mechanical ventilation for elective surgery (Fig. 16–2).[4, 11]

Regional Lung Inflation

Regional lung inflation depends on the local transpulmonary pressure, which is the difference between the pressure in the alveoli and pressure at the pleural surface ($P_{transpulmonary} = P_{pl} - P_{alveolar}$). At FRC, alveolar pressure equals atmospheric pressure, so transpulmonary pressure is equal to P_{pl}, making any differences in regional transpulmonary pressures the result of differences in regional P_{pl}. Therefore, any gradient in regional P_{pl} results in a regional lung inflation gradient.

Over the past decade, Gattinoni and colleagues and Pelosi and associates have used computed tomography (CT) to measure regional lung inflation.[11–13] By quantitative analysis of CT density, they defined a gas/tissue ratio to describe regional lung density for a single CT section, usually at the base of the lung. This gas/tissue ratio also acts as an index of regional lung inflation. In healthy supine subjects, regional lung inflation decreases along the vertical gravitational axis with a constant exponential rate of change (13.9 $\pm$ 2.5 cm).[13] Consequently, the alveolar dimensions in the posterior or

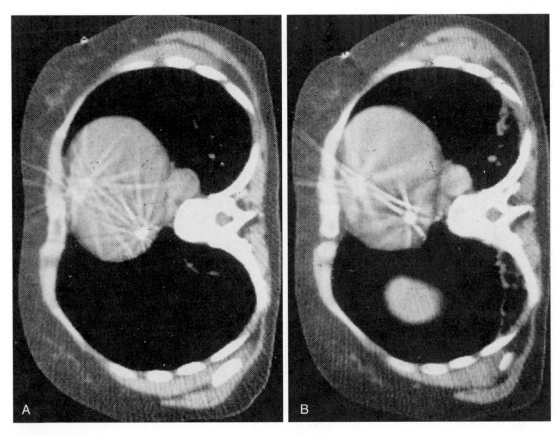

FIGURE 16–2
Computed tomographic image of the chest after anesthesia and mechanical ventilation. (A) Supine position before anesthesia. (B) Supine position after anesthesia. Note the development of atelectasis in the dependent, dorsal lung regions. (From Klingstedt C, Hedenstierna G, Lundquist H, et al: The influence of body position and differential ventilation on lung dimensions and atelectasis formation in anaesthetized man. Acta Anaesthesiol Scand 34:315–322, 1990.)

dorsal regions of the lung are only one third of those of the ventral surface.

When healthy subjects are turned into the prone position, regional inflation again decreases exponentially along the vertical axis, but more slowly (decay constant = 26.2 ± 2.2 cm) than when the subjects are supine.[13] These studies suggest that positional changes in FRC are related to regional lung inflation gradients, which in turn are the result of varying regional pleural pressures.[11-13]

Pulmonary Mechanics

Position and posture affect both lung and chest wall compliance as well as airway resistance.[14, 15] In healthy subjects, moving from a sitting to a supine position reduces lung compliance.[15] Although the mechanism remains unclear, some speculate that the pleural pressure and regional lung inflation gradients change when subjects are supine because of a combination of increased pulmonary blood volume, atelectasis, and small airway closure.[16] Moving from a supine to a lateral decubitus position improves lung compliance.[16] The effects of the prone position on lung compliance in healthy subjects is unknown, but a recent study suggests that in patients with acute lung injury, lung compliance does not change greatly when the position is altered. Unfortunately, this study was underpowered to detect small differences in lung compliance.[17]

The effect of position on chest wall compliance is more difficult to ascertain. In the supine position, the stiffening of the rib cage is offset by the softened resting tone of the abdominal muscles, making the abdomen/diaphragm compartment more compliant. Consequently, chest wall compliance in healthy upright subjects is similar to that in supine subjects.[18] This finding may vary greatly according to the individual's body habitus. Again, there are few data regarding the effects of prone positioning on chest wall compliance in healthy subjects, although a recent study suggests that chest wall compliance may decrease in prone patients with acute lung injury.[17]

Airflow resistance increases by 30% to 40% in healthy spontaneously breathing subjects in the supine as opposed to the upright position.[14, 16] Although the underlying cause of this change is not completely understood, diminished airway caliber related to decreased lung volumes is thought to play a significant role. Generally, changes in pulmonary mechanics are of little consequence to healthy individuals; however, increased airway resistance in the supine position contributes to the orthopnea seen in patients with flares of obstructive lung disease and may explain the prominence of nocturnal symptoms in asthmatics (gravitational effects). Currently, the effects of prone positioning on airway mechanics are not known.

Distribution of Ventilation

For healthy spontaneously breathing adults, regardless of position, ventilation is distributed predominantly to the dependent lung as a result of at least two factors.[6] First, regional lung inflation and alveolar inflation are greater in the nondependent portions of the lung, distending those alveoli and thereby placing them on the flatter, or less compliant, portion of the pressure–volume curve. This preferentially directs ventilation to the less distended, dependent alveoli.[18, 19] Second, Froese and Bryan[2] found that the greater displacement of the dependent hemidiaphragm shifted ventilation to the dependent lung, which is maintained in the upright, supine, prone, and lateral decubitus positions.[6, 20]

However, there are three conditions under which ventilation increases in the nondependent lung relative to the dependent lung. First, ventilation at low lung volumes shifts the pressure–volume relationships between the dependent and nondependent alveoli to favor alveoli in the nondependent lung.[19] Additionally, under these conditions, there is increased atelectasis in the dependent regions, driving ventilation preferentially toward the nondependent lung regions. Second, a high inspiratory flow rate or the use of accessory respiratory muscles preferentially distributes ventilation to the nondependent regions.[20] Third, in mechanically ventilated patients—especially those anesthetized or sedated—the abdominal contents restrict the dependent diaphragm, increasing the movement of the nondependent diaphragm and the nondependent portions of the lung.[2, 21] Unfortunately, the distribution of ventilation in mechanically ventilated prone patients is controversial, with markedly differing results among studies.[6, 21]

Distribution of Perfusion

The classic model of pulmonary perfusion in healthy lungs proposed by West in 1960 describes lung vasculature using three main compartments according to the relationships between pulmonary arterial (P_{art}), alveolar (P_{alv}), and pulmonary venous (P_{ven}) pressures (Fig. 16–3).[22, 23] In zone 1, vessels are held closed and there is no flow ($P_{alv} > P_{art}$). In zone 2 ($P_{art} > P_{alv} > P_{ven}$), the pressure gradient causing flow is arterial–alveolar, which increases linearly with grav-

ity; therefore, so does flow. In zone 3 ($P_{ven} > P_{alv}$), venous pressure exceeds alveolar pressure. Now the pressure gradient is arterial–venous, which is relatively constant, although there is some increase in blood flow according to a gravitational gradient caused by changes in transmural pressure.[23]

Many authors agree that zone 1 conditions do not exist in healthy subjects.[24–27] Zone 2 conditions occur in the upright and lateral positions; however, there remains significant debate regarding the presence of zone 2 conditions in supine or prone positions because of the lung's greatly reduced vertical lung dimension in these positions compared with upright or lateral positions.[24–27] These same investigators suggest that zone 3 conditions occur throughout the supine lung with relatively homogeneous perfusion, although small gravitational gradients do exist.[24–27] Little is known about the distribution of lung perfusion in prone humans. However, one dog model of acute lung injury identified no significant gravitational perfusion gradient.[28] That study posi-

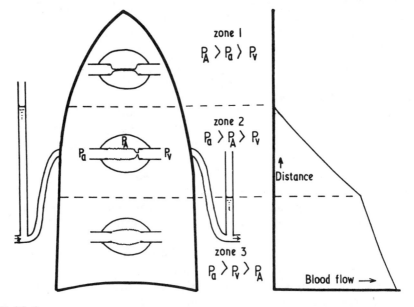

FIGURE 16–3

Classic three-zone model of pulmonary perfusion. The lung is divided into three zones according to the relative magnitudes of the pulmonary arterial (P_a), pulmonary venous (P_v), and pulmonary alveolar (P_A) pressures. In zone I, alveolar pressure exceeds arterial pressure. In zone 2, arterial pressure exceeds alveolar pressure, but alveolar pressure exceeds venous. In zone 3, venous pressure exceeds alveolar pressure. (Adapted with permission from West JB, Dollery CT, Naimark A: Distribution of blood flow in isolated lung: relation to vascular and alveolar pressures. J Appl Physiol 19:713–724, 1964.)

tively correlated regional blood flow in the supine and prone positions with blood flow preferentially distributed to the dorsal regions, rather than negatively as would be expected with a purely gravitational model.[28]

Ventilation–Perfusion ($\dot{V}/\dot{Q}$) Relationships

In healthy spontaneously breathing subjects, both ventilation and perfusion are highest in the dependent lung regions. Interestingly, $\dot{V}/\dot{Q}$ ratios tend to decrease along the vertical gradient in upright and prone positions but increase in the supine position.[24] During mechanical ventilation of healthy subjects, the distribution of perfusion remains unchanged; however, the overall $\dot{V}/\dot{Q}$ relationship is less favorable because of the tendency of ventilation to be distributed to the nondependent lung in these patients.[22, 29]

EFFECTS OF POSTURE AND POSITION ON PATIENTS WITH RESPIRATORY DISEASE

Neuromuscular Disease

Orthopnea is a common symptom in patients with diaphragmatic weakness or paralysis, with the degree of orthopnea correlating to the severity of disease.[30] When the patient is supine, the weight of the abdominal contents increases the inspiratory load on the already weakened diaphragm. With complete diaphragmatic paralysis, accessory inspiratory muscle contractions reduce pleural pressure, displacing the diaphragm paradoxically into the chest during inspiration. In the upright position, this displacement is opposed by the weight of the abdomen. However, in the supine position, it is enhanced by pressure from the abdominal contents.[30] As a result, the normal reduction in vital capacity associated with the supine position is accentuated markedly by diaphragmatic weakness, with vital capacity decreasing by more than 25% when a patient goes from upright to supine.[3] In contrast, patients who have quadriplegia but

intact diaphragmatic function may significantly increase vital capacity by shifting from upright to supine.[31] This is the result of the increased residual volume in the upright position created by outward bulging of the abdominal contents and consequent drop in the diaphragm.[31]

Atelectasis and secretion retention cause significant morbidity in patients with neuromuscular weakness. Multiple studies in both healthy and diseased subjects indicate that in the supine position, atelectasis tends to occur in the dorsal lung regions, where elevated pleural pressures cause decreased regional lung inflation. Prone positioning tends to expand the dorsal lung regions and may facilitate secretion drainage from dependent portions of the lungs.[32] In a study of patients with acute quadriplegia, a respiratory care program that included deep breathing, chest percussion, and prone positioning decreased the need for mechanical ventilation as well as the mortality rate when compared with historic controls.[32] Consequently, frequent position changes are recommended for patients with neuromuscular weakness.[32]

Obstructive Airway Disease

Position and posture may have important effects in patients with airway disease. In the upright position, there is a decrease in airway resistance. Conversely, in the supine position, the increase in airway resistance results in air trapping, which may explain why stable patients with chronic obstructive pulmonary disease (COPD) experience less of a decrease in FRC when supine compared with control patients.[1] In patients with severe COPD, hyperinflation flattens the diaphragm. Dyspnea sometimes is improved by leaning forward and contracting the abdominal muscles at expiration. Researchers hypothesize that the pressure from the abdominal contents generated by contracting the abdominal muscles causes a cephalad shift in the diaphragm, enhancing the length–tension relationship of the diaphragm.[33]

During acute crisis, patients with COPD and asthma tend to avoid lying flat.[33, 34] In one study of patients in acute asthmatic flare, no asthmatic with a peak expiratory flow of less than 150 L/min chose to be recumbent.[34] The many reasons for this include the increase in airway resistance while supine, as well as recruitment and optimization of accessory inspiratory and expiratory muscles in the upright position.[33]

In the absence of specific data for mechanically ventilated patients, practitioners extrapolate what is known in nonventilated patients with airflow obstruction to ventilated patients. As a result, it generally is recommended that actively weaning COPD patients be placed in the upright position. Unfortunately, there are no data describing the effects of the prone as opposed to the supine position in these patients.

Unilateral Lung Injury

As described previously, both perfusion and ventilation normally are distributed preferentially to the dependent portions of the lung. Extending this principle to patients with unilateral lung disease, a number of case series (Table 16–1) demonstrate that placing these patients in a "good lung down" lateral decubitus position significantly improves oxygenation in both spontaneously breathing and mechanically ventilated patients.[35–40] As shown in Table 16–1, there is a wide range of clinical responses to decubitus positioning.

Most, but not all, patients with unilateral lung disease benefit where the healthy lung is placed in the dependent position. Occa-sionally, critically ill patients require prompt return to the supine position because of arrhythmia, hypotension, or desaturation.[41] In patients with COPD and patients who are paralyzed, the benefit is suspect because ventilation is distributed preferentially to the nondependent lung. When these patients are positioned with the "good lung down," the greater perfusion in the dependent lung may create **shunting** in the dependent lung and increase dead space in the nondependent lung, effectively worsening $\dot{V}/\dot{Q}$ matching.[42] Another exception to the "good lung down" rule involves patients with unilateral pleural effusion, in whom lateral decubitus positioning does not appear to affect $\dot{V}/\dot{Q}$ matching or oxygenation.[43] Interestingly, in acute unilateral pulmonary embolism requiring mechanical ventilation, gas exchange improves when the affected lung is dependent.[44] Finally, "good lung down" positioning also is contraindicated in pulmonary hemorrhage and lung abscess because of the risk of spillage into the uninvolved lung.

Acute Respiratory Distress Syndrome—Physiologic Mechanism of Prone Positioning

In 1974, Bryan first proposed using prone positioning in the treatment of patients with acute respiratory distress syndrome (ARDS), speculating that the prone position improved diaphragmatic excursion in the dorsal aspect of the lung, improving FRC,

TABLE 16–1. Clinical Series Describing the Effect of "Good Side Down" Positioning in Unilateral Lung Disease

SERIES	NO. OF PATIENTS	NO. RESPONDING	pO$_2$ SUPINE (mm Hg)	pO$_2$—"GOOD SIDE DOWN" (mm Hg)	pO$_2$—"GOOD SIDE UP" (mm Hg)
Zack et al,[35] 1974	19	13	—	86	77
Dhainaut et al,[36] 1980	4	4	—	—	—
Remolina et al,[37] 1981	9	6	66 ± 3	106 ± 13	58 ± 3
Ibanez et al,[38] 1981	10	8	102 ± 23	144 ± 25	86 ± 15
Gillespie and Rehder,[39] 1987	4	4	—	101 ± 29	61 ± 10
Dreyfuss et al,[40] 1992	8	7	100 ± 14	156 ± 23	—

pO$_2$, partial pressure of oxygen.

$\dot{V}/\dot{Q}$ matching, and oxygenation.[45] In 1976, Piehl and Brown improved oxygenation in five patients with ARDS by shifting them from the supine to the prone position.[46] In their patients, the mean partial pressure of oxygen (pO_2) improved from 72 to 106, lasting for at least 4 hours. In 1977, Douglas and colleagues reported a similar series of six patients, in which five showed improved oxygenation, with a mean pO_2 increase of 69 mm Hg (range 2–178 mm Hg).[47] They speculated that the improved oxygenation might be due to a combination of causes, including better $\dot{V}/\dot{Q}$ matching, larger FRC, improved regional diaphragmatic movement, and enhanced secretion removal.[47]

Research on delineation of the mechanisms leading to improved oxygenation was not published until 1987, when Albert and associates found dramatic, reproducible improvement in oxygenation caused by prone positioning in a study of mongrel dogs with oleic acid–induced acute lung injury.[48] To explain the mechanism for the improved oxygenation, they studied regional diaphragm movement, $\dot{V}/\dot{Q}$ relationships, changes in FRC, and hemodynamics. As predicted by Bryan, diaphragmatic motion in the nondependent portions of the lung increased, regardless of whether the animals were supine or prone. However, turning initially prone animals to a supine position did not enhance oxygenation, as would be predicted if diaphragmatic motion was the sole mechanism causing improved oxygenation.[48] Using the multiple inert gas method, Albert and associates noted dramatic decreases in the shunt fraction of prone animals, suggesting that the improved oxygenation in the prone position was the result of improved $\dot{V}/\dot{Q}$ matching.[48] They found no significant change in FRC or hemodynamic variables.[48]

To study regional lung perfusion, Wiener and colleagues performed experiments in oleic acid–induced acute lung injury in dogs using radiolabeled microspheres.[49] Before injury, perfusion increased along a gravitational gradient in supine animals but was more evenly distributed in prone animals. After oleic acid injury, lung water increased dramatically, and perfusion once again increased gravitationally in supine animals with maximal perfusion in the dorsal region of the lung. In prone animals, however, perfusion was distributed preferentially to the nondependent dorsal regions, suggesting that the West model does not adequately explain perfusion in acute lung injury. Extravascular lung water was distributed evenly to all regions for both supine and prone animals, suggesting identical injury patterns.[49] In subsequent experiments, this group of researchers found gravity to be a minor determinant of regional perfusion under West zone 3 conditions, the condition presumably present in most, if not all, of the ARDS lung.[28]

It appears that prone positioning does not significantly affect the distribution of regional perfusion; that is, perfusion remains preferentially distributed to the dorsal lung regardless of position. If this is true, improvements in $\dot{V}/\dot{Q}$ must be the result of changes in the distribution of ventilation. As was discussed earlier, regional pleural pressure (P_{pl}) gradients are in fact lower in prone animals than in supine animals.[8, 9] Mutoh and colleagues demonstrated that the P_{pl} in the dependent lung regions of animals with acute lung injury becomes positive, presumably leading to airway collapse and atelectasis in those regions.[10] When compared with supine animals, prone animals had a much smaller gravitational gradient and a much less positive P_{pl} in the dependent portions of the lung. Therefore, when injured animals are turned prone, the dorsal (nondependent) regions are exposed to a lower P_{pl}, resulting in the opening of previously atelectatic lung. Because perfusion remains greatest in the dorsal lung, even in the prone position, intrapulmonary shunting decreases, leading to improved oxygenation.[49] Additional experimental evidence in oleic acid–injured dogs revealed that supine dogs had markedly diminished ventilation in the dorsal lung regions while maintaining perfusion to these areas, creating areas of shunt and low $\dot{V}/\dot{Q}$.[50] In contrast, prone animals demonstrated significantly improved ventilation in the well-perfused dorsal regions, with no marked effects on $\dot{V}/\dot{Q}$ in the ventral regions.[50]

Although there are no detailed physiologic studies of humans in the prone position, Gattinoni and associates used CT densitometry to demonstrate changes in ARDS subjects that are consistent with those measured in experimental animals.[11-13] They measured regional lung density using a gas/tissue ratio for single CT sections, usually taken at the base of the lung. For supine patients with ARDS, the regional inflation gradient decreased along the gravitational axis at a rate double that in the normal lung.[11] They theorized that the decreased regional inflation gradient is caused by increased P_{pl} gradients in patients with ARDS caused by increased lung weight due to edema. These results suggest that in supine patients with 0 positive end-expiratory pressure (PEEP), the increased P_{pl} gradient should result in complete collapse of the posterior half of the lungs. In prone patients, the gradient of regional inflation was more heterogeneous but reversed, leading to some collapse in the ventral lung zones with improved regional aeration in the dorsal lung (Fig. 16–4). The collapse in the ventral lung zones of prone positions was generally less than the dorsal collapse seen when the patients were prone.[11] Additional recent studies in humans with acute lung injury indicate that the chest wall compliance is improved significantly in the prone position, possibly also contributing to improved regional inflation and oxygenation.[17]

Acute Respiratory Distress Syndrome—Clinical Effects of Prone Positioning

Of the several clinical series on the use of prone positioning published since Bryan first proposed its use in patients with ARDS in 1974, few are prospective and none are randomized controlled trials.[17, 45-47, 51-59] Although flawed by its lack of randomized trials, the available published data outlined in Table 16–2 indicate that prone positioning results in improved oxygenation for most patients in whom it is tried. Although the magnitude of the response varies widely from marginal to dramatic, there is no adequate model predicting where a particular patient with ARDS will fall in the spectrum. Furthermore, patients' response times vary from immediate to several hours. As a result, very little is known about the optimal time period to maintain the prone position.

Patients respond to a return to a supine position after a trial of prone positioning in one of three ways. Some "prone-dependent" patients revert to their original supine oxy-

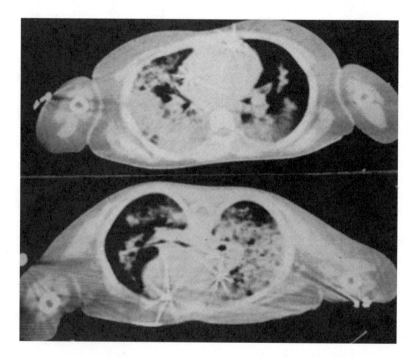

FIGURE 16–4
Chest tomographic images of prone and supine patient with adult respiratory distress syndrome (ARDS). Chest tomographic images of a patient with ARDS in the supine *(upper panel)* and prone *(lower panel)* positions. In the supine position, tissue densities predominate in the dorsal regions. After 15 minutes in the prone position, tissue densities are redistributed to the ventral lung regions. (Adapted with permission from Langer M, Mascheroni MD, Marcolin R: The prone position in ARDS patients. Chest 94:103–107, 1988.)

TABLE 16–2. Clinical Series Describing the Effect of Prone Positioning in Adult Respiratory Distress Syndrome

STUDY	NO. OF PATIENTS	NO. RESPONDING	pO$_2$ SUPINE (mm Hg)	pO$_2$ PRONE (mm Hg)
Piehl and Brown,[46] 1976	5	5	72 ± 13	106 ± 9
Douglas et al,[47] 1977	6	6	63 ± 10	138 ± 69
Faller et al,[51] 1988	3	3	103 ± 25	197 ± 29
Langer et al,[52] 1988	13	8	69 ± 8	111 ± 20
DuBois et al,[53] 1992	4	4	92 ± 37*	153 ± 5*
Brussel et al,[54] 1993	10	—	114 ± 47*	241 ± 92*
Albert,[55] 1993	9	7	63 ± 15	123 ± 121
Pappert et al,[56] 1994	12	7	98 ± 50	146 ± 95
Vollman and Bander,[57] 1996	15	9	86 ± 14	102 ± 33
Fridrich et al,[58] 1996	20	—	126 ± 9*	204 ± 19*
Chatte et al,[59] 1997	32	25	103 ± 28*	159 ± 59*
Pelosi et al,[17] 1998	16	12	103 ± 24	130 ± 33

*pO$_2$/FiO$_2$ ratio.
FiO$_2$, inspired oxygen concentration; pO$_2$, partial pressure of oxygen.

genation when returned to the supine position.[56, 58, 60] Others display reduced oxygenation that is still better than their original supine levels.[17, 51–54] Finally, some patients have even greater oxygenation levels than either previous supine or prone values.[61] Unfortunately, it is our experience that this third response is quite rare. To further cloud this issue, when the same patient is turned several times, the response to turning usually varies.[47, 58]

The mechanisms underlying the variable response to proning are not understood. It appears that position-induced differences in regional pleural pressures cause a steeper decrease in regional lung inflation in the supine position compared with the prone position. However, regional inflation patterns may be quite variable for individual patients.[61] There are, in fact, some patients for whom the decrease in regional inflation is steeper in the prone position than in the supine position. In these patients, oxygenation may deteriorate when the patient is placed in the prone position.[61] Recent data positively correlate improvement in oxygenation due to proning with the initial chest wall compliance.[17] Unfortunately, this study is quite small and has not yet been validated. Many questions remain about the effects of position on regional perfusion in patients with ARDS and whether these

changes are responsible for the failure of prone positioning to improve oxygenation in some patients.

Prone positioning has been associated with a number of complications. These range from skin breakdown to loss of airway.[46, 47, 54, 57, 59] The exact rate of complication is unknown, but it appears to be relatively low.[57–59]

Institutions use various methods for turning patients prone, including the use of commercial devices.[57] In our own experience, we have not found it necessary to use these devices. One simple proning technique employs five individuals for the turning procedure. One individual is assigned to the head of the bed to maintain the airway while four others, two on each side of the bed, move the patient to the edge of the bed and "logroll" the patient into the prone position. Additional people may be required for patients with multiple intravascular lines or chest tubes. Using this technique, the entire turning process generally is accomplished within a few minutes.

CONCLUSIONS

Body position has multiple effects on respiratory physiology and mechanics. These effects are important in the treatment of some conditions requiring mechanical ventilation. There is intriguing evidence that changes in body position may represent a supportive therapy for unilateral lung disease, some airway disease, and ARDS. Until good randomized prospective data become available, the prone position must be considered experimental in patients with ARDS. However, from the available data, it appears that placing patients in the prone position is relatively low risk and offers a reasonable chance of improving $\dot{V}/\dot{Q}$ matching and oxygenation. Hopefully, future randomized controlled trials will confirm the benefit of "position therapy" and reveal the underlying mechanisms for its effects, as well as its optimal duration.

REFERENCES

1. Marini JJ, Tyler ML, Hudson LD, et al: Influence of head-dependent positions on lung volume and oxygen saturation in chronic airflow obstruction. Am Rev Respir Dis 128:101–105, 1984.
2. Froese AB, Bryan AC: Effects of anesthesia and paralysis on diaphragmatic mechanics in man. Anesthesia 41:242–255, 1974.
3. Lumb AB, Nunn JF: Respiratory function and rib-cage contribution to ventilation in body positions commonly used during anesthesia. Anesth Analg 73:422–426, 1991.
4. Pelosi P, Croci M, Calappi E, et al: The prone positioning during general anesthesia minimally affects respiratory mechanics while improving functional residual capacity and increasing oxygen tension. Anesth Analg 80:955–960, 1995.
5. Cambell GS, Harvey RB: Postural changes in vital capacity with differential cuff pressures at the bases of the extremities. Am J Physiol 152:671–673, 1948.
6. Kaneko K, Milic-Emili J, Dolovich MD, et al: Regional distribution of ventilation and perfusion as a function of body position. J Appl Physiol 21:767–777, 1966.
7. Krugger JJ, Bain T, Patterson JL: Elevation gradient of intrathoracic pressure. J Appl Physiol 16:465–468, 1961.
8. Olson LE, Wardle RL: Pleural pressure as a function of body position in rabbits. J Appl Physiol 69:336–344, 1990.
9. Wiener-Kronish JP, Gropper M, Lai-Fook SJ: Pleural liquid pressure in dogs measured using a rib capsule. J Appl Physiol 59:597–602, 1985.
10. Mutoh T, Guest RJ, Lamm WJE, Albert RK: Prone position alters the effect of volume overload on regional pleural pressures and improves hypoxemia in pigs in vivo. Am Rev Respir Dis 146:300–306, 1992.
11. Gattinoni L, Pelosi P, Vitale G, et al: Body position changes redistribute lung computed-tomographic density in patients with acute respiratory failure. Anesthesiology 74:15–23, 1991.
12. Gattinoni L, D'Andrea L, Pelosi P, et al: Regional effects and mechanism of positive end-expiratory pressure in early adult respiratory distress syndrome. JAMA 269:2122–2127, 1993.
13. Pelosi P, D'Andrea L, Vitale G, et al: Vertical gradient of regional lung inflation in adult respiratory distress syndrome. Am J Respir Crit Care 149:8–13, 1994.
14. Navajas D, Farre R, Rotger M, et al: Effect of body position on respiratory impedence. J Appl Physiol 64:194–199, 1988.
15. Berger R, Burki NK: The effects of posture on total respiratory system compliance. Am Rev Respir Dis 125:262–263, 1982.
16. Behrakis PK, Baydur A, Jaeger MJ, et al: Lung mechanics in the sitting and horizontal positions. Chest 83:643–646, 1983.
17. Pelosi P, Tubiolo D, Mascheroni D, et al: Effects of prone position on respiratory mechanics and gas exchange during acute lung injury. Am J Respir Crit Care Med 157:387–393, 1998.
18. Mead J, Lindgren I, Gaenser EA: Mechanical properties of the lungs in emphysema. J Clin Invest 34:1005–1016, 1955.
19. Pedley TJ, Sudlow MF, Milic-Emili J: A non-linear theory of the distribution of pulmonary ventilation. Respir Physiol 15:1–38, 1972.
20. Roussos CS, Fixley M, Genest J, et al: Voluntary factors influencing the distribution of inspired gas. Am Rev Respir Dis 116:457–467, 1977.
21. Rheder K, Knopp JJ, Sessler AD: Regional intrapulmonary gas in awake and anesthetized-paralyzed prone man. J Appl Physiol 45:528–535, 1978.
22. West JB, Dollery CT: Distribution of blood flow and ventilation perfusion ratio in the lung, measured with radioactive CO_2.[15] J Appl Physiol 15:405–410, 1960.
23. West JB, Dollery CT, Naimark A: Distribution of blood flow in isolated lung; relation to vascular and alveolar pressures. J Appl Physiol 19:713–724, 1964.
24. Amis TC, Jones HA, Hughes JMB: Effect of posture on interregional distribution of pulmonary perfusion and VA/Q ratios in man. Respir Physiol 56:169–182, 1984.
25. Orphanidou D, Hughes JMB, Myers MJ, et al: Tomography of regional ventilation and perfusion using krypton 81m in normal subjects and asthmatic patients. Thorax 41:542–551, 1986.
26. Reed JH, Wood EH: Effect of body position on vertical distribution of pulmonary blood flow. J Appl Physiol 28:303–311, 1970.
27. Glenny RW, Robertson HT: Fractal properties of pulmonary blood flow: characterization of spatial heterogeneity. J Appl Physiol 69:532–545, 1990.
28. Glenny RW, Lamm WJE, Albert RK, et al: Gravity is a minor determinant of pulmonary blood flow distribution. J Appl Physiol 71:620–629, 1991.
29. Chevrolet JC, Martin JG, Flood R, et al: Topo-

graphical ventilation and perfusion during IPPB in the lateral position. Am Rev Respir Dis 118:847–854, 1978.

30. Mier-Jedrzejowicz C, Brophy C, Moxham J, et al: Assessment of diaphragmatic weakness. Am Rev Respir Dis 137:877–883, 1988.

31. Estenne M, DeTroyer A: Mechanism of the postural dependence in vital capacity in tetraplegic subjects. Am Rev Respir Dis 135:367–371, 1987.

32. McMichan JC, Michel L, Westbrook PR: Pulmonary dysfunction following traumatic tetraplegia: recognition, prevention and treatment. JAMA 243:528–531, 1980.

33. Sharp JT, Drutz WS, Moisan T, et al: Postural relief of dyspnea in severe chronic obstructive pulmonary disease. Am Rev Respir Dis 122:201–211, 1980.

34. Brenner BE, Abraham E, Simon RR: Position and diaphoresis in acute asthma. Am J Med 74:1005–1009, 1983.

35. Zack MB, Pontoppidan H, Kazemi H, et al: The effect of lateral positions on gas exchange in pulmonary disease: a prospective evaluation. Am Rev Respir Dis 110:49–55, 1974.

36. Dhainaut JF, Bons J, Bricard C, et al: Improved oxygenation in patients with extensive unilateral pneumonia using the lateral decubitus position. Thorax 35:792–793, 1980.

37. Remolina C, Khan AU, Santiago TV, et al: Positional hypoxemia in unilateral lung disease. N Engl J Med 304:523–525, 1981.

38. Ibanez J, Raurich JM, Abizanda R, et al: The effect of lateral positions on gas exchange in patients with unilateral lung disease during mechanical ventilation. Intensive Care Med 7:231–234, 1981.

39. Gillespie DJ, Rehder K: Body position and ventilation-perfusion relationships in unilateral pulmonary disease. Chest 91:75–79, 1987.

40. Dreyfuss D, Djedaini K, Lanore JJ, et al: A comparative study of the effects of almitrine bismesylate and lateral position during unilateral pneumonia with severe hypoxemia. Am Rev Respir Dis 146:295–299, 1992.

41. Winslow EH, Clark AP, White KM, et al: Effects of a lateral turn on mixed venous oxygen saturation and heart rate in critically ill adults. Heart Lung 19:557–561, 1990.

42. Shim C, Chun KJ, Williams MHJ, et al: Positional effects on the distribution of ventilation in chronic obstructive pulmonary disease. Ann Intern Med 105:346–350, 1986.

43. Gilespie DJ, Rehder K: Effect of positional change on ventilation-perfusion distribution in unilateral pleural effusion. Intensive Care Med 15:266–268, 1989.

44. Badr MS, Grossman JE: Positional changes in gas exchange after unilateral pulmonary embolism. Chest 98:1514–1516, 1990.

45. Bryan AC: Comments of a devil's advocate. Am Rev Respir Dis 110(suppl):143–144, 1974.

46. Piehl MA, Brown RS: Use of extreme position changes in acute respiratory failure. Crit Care Med 4:13–14, 1976.

47. Douglas WW, Rehder K, Beynen FM, et al: Improved oxygenation in patients with acute respiratory failure: the prone position. Am Rev Respir Dis 115:559–565, 1977.

48. Albert RK, Leasa D, Sanderson M, et al: The prone position improves arterial oxygenation and reduces shunt in oleic-acid-induced acute lung injury. Am Rev Respir Dis 135:628–633, 1987.

49. Wiener CM, Kirk W, Albert RK: Prone position reverses gravitational distribution of perfusion in dog lungs with oleic acid-induced injury. J Appl Physiol 68:1386–1392, 1990.

50. Lamm WJE, Graham MM, Albert RK: Mechanism by which the prone position improves oxygenation in acute lung injury. Am J Respir Crit Care Med 150:184–193, 1994.

51. Faller JP, Feissel M, Kara A, et al: La ventilation en procubitus dans les syndromes de detresse respiratoire aigue d'evolution severe. Presse Med 22:1154, 1988.

52. Langer M, Mascheroni MD, Marcolin R: The prone position in ARDS patients. Chest 94:103–107, 1988.

53. DuBois JM, Gaussorgues PH, Sirodot M, et al: Prone position dependency in severely hypoxic patients. Intensive Care Med 18(suppl):A18, 1992.

54. Brussel T, Hachenberg T, Roos N, et al: Mechanical ventilation in the prone position for acute respiratory failure after cardiac surgery. J Cardiothorac Vasc Anesth 7:541–546, 1993.

55. Albert RK: New ideas in the treatment of ARDS. In: Vincent JL (ed): Yearbook of Intensive Care and Emergency Medicine. Berlin: Springer-Verlag, 1993, pp 135–147.

56. Pappert D, Rossaint R, Slama K, et al: Influence of positioning on ventilation perfusion relationships in severe adult respiratory distress syndrome. Chest 106:1511–1516, 1994.

57. Vollman KM, Bander JJ: Improved oxygenation utilizing a prone positioner in patients with acute respiratory distress syndrome. Intensive Care Med 22:1105–1111, 1996.

58. Fridrich P, Krafft P, Hochleuthner H, et al: The effects of long-term prone positioning in patients with trauma-induced adult respiratory distress syndrome. Anesth Analg 83:1206–1211, 1996.

59. Chatte G, Sab JM, Dubois JM, et al: Prone position in mechanically ventilated patients with severe acute respiratory failure. Am J Respir Crit Care Med 155:473–478, 1997.

60. Marik PE, Iglesias J: A "prone dependent" patient with severe adult respiratory distress syndrome. Crit Care Med 25:1085–1086, 1997.

61. Gattinoni L, Pelosi P, Valenza F, et al: Patient positioning in acute respiratory failure. In: Tobin M (ed): Principles and Practice of Mechanical Ventilation, 1st ed. New York: McGraw-Hill, 1994, pp 1067–1076.

CHAPTER 17

Ventilator-Associated Pneumonia

Karen Welty-Wolf, MD

EPIDEMIOLOGY

INCIDENCE AND RISK FACTORS

MORBIDITY, MORTALITY, AND OTHER COSTS

PATHOGENESIS
Pulmonary Defenses Against Infection
Device-Related Infection Risk
Gastric Colonization

DIAGNOSIS

BRONCHOSCOPIC TECHNIQUES IN DIAGNOSIS
Bronchoscopic Methods
Interpretation of Quantitative Culture Results

MICROBIOLOGY

TREATMENT
Host Considerations
Empirical Therapy
Specific Therapy
Other Treatment Issues

PREVENTION
Infection Control
Reducing Gastric Colonization and Aspiration
Antibiotic Prophylaxis
Other Preventive Strategies

REFERENCES

KEY WORDS

antibiotics
aspiration
bronchoalveolar lavage

pneumonia
protected specimen brush

Pneumonia is a common and serious complication of mechanical ventilation, carrying an attributable mortality rate of approximately 30%.[1, 2] It is the most common of the nosocomial infections represented in intensive care units (ICUs) and is second only to urinary tract infections hospital-wide.[3, 4] Given the substantial impact of pneumonia on patient outcomes and hospital costs, nosocomial pneumonia has been a focus of clinical and epidemiologic study ever since the 1960s, when investigators first found a relationship between epidemic gram-negative pneumonia in hospitalized patients and contaminated reservoir nebulizers in respiratory therapy equipment.[5-7] The last decade has yielded a large volume of literature addressing diagnostic problems and treatment issues. Application of the information to clinical practice, however, has been hampered by the continuing lack of a readily applicable "gold standard" for diagnosis and an incomplete understanding of the pathogenesis of ventilator-associated pneumonia (VAP).

EPIDEMIOLOGY

Current knowledge about the epidemiology of nosocomial pneumonia in the ICU setting is derived from a variety of sources. Each of these sources contributes valuable information to our understanding of this problem, but the interpretation of epidemiologic data is limited by ongoing difficulties in the diagnosis of VAP and differences in patient populations between studies. At times, it has even been difficult to show a definitive risk for pneumonia from endotracheal intubation.[8] It has become more clear in recent years, however, that VAP in any given patient is a result of multiple factors that tilt the balance of the host–pathogen relationship toward active infection, and that the relative importance of these individual factors is not a constant from one patient to the next. The risk factors associated with VAP and their contributions to current concepts of the pathogenesis of VAP are discussed in the following section.

INCIDENCE AND RISK FACTORS

Nosocomial pneumonia is diagnosed in approximately 1% of patients admitted to acute care hospitals. The rate may be as much as 20-fold higher in patients on mechanical ventilation, although the reported incidence of VAP varies widely in epidemiologic studies.[9-13] The infection ratio (number of cases per 100 patients) in mechanically ventilated patients in these studies ranges from 8 to 54 cases per 100 ICU patients.[9, 14-32] Comparisons among these studies are confounded by several factors. The

ICU populations are very different, including medical, surgical, pediatric, and neurosurgical patients. Additionally, some studies did not restrict enrollment by duration of mechanical ventilation, thereby including patients with brief periods of assisted ventilation. Finally, surveillance data from the National Nosocomial Infection Surveillance (NNIS) system have shown that more accurate and reproducible data are collected when a time factor is included in the denominator and rates are expressed as a ratio per 1000 patient ventilator days.[33] NNIS incidence rates of VAP for different ICU types are shown in Table 17–1.

Several studies have attempted to distinguish specific risk periods that might help focus preventive efforts. Some have calculated an incremental risk of acquiring VAP at a relatively constant 1% to 3% per day.[21, 24] Others have found an increased incidence in patients ventilated for more than 5 days compared with patients ventilated for less than 5 days.[30] Still another group of investigators, looking at the onset of VAP rather than the incidence rate, found the rate of acquisition to be highest in the first 8 to 10 days after intubation, decreasing to a low rate thereafter.[9] This study suggested that VAP is an early event in the management of critically ill patients. The risk factors for developing pneumonia may be different, however, for patients developing pneumonia at different times during their ICU stay. Early-onset VAP, occurring within the first 5 days after intubation and ventilation, has been associated with a different set of organisms and is likely to be affected by events causing aspiration at the onset of respiratory failure or during intubation.[34, 35] Late-onset VAP may be influenced more by changes in the gastrointestinal environment.[36] These distinctions are important when evaluating preventive strategies that may be more appropriate for some patient subsets than others.

Apparent risk factors for nosocomial pneumonia in the mechanically ventilated patient include those found in the broader hospitalized patient population: chronic lung disease,[30] advanced age,[37] severe illness,[38] malnutrition,[39] immunosuppressive therapy,[40, 41] depressed level of conscious-

TABLE 17–1. Epidemiology of Ventilator-Associated Pneumonia (VAP) by Intensive Care Unit (ICU) Type, National Nosocomial Infection Surveillance Data

ICU	MEAN VAP RATE* (NO. OF UNITS)	VENTILATOR UTILIZATION†	PNEUMONIA AS % OF ALL REPORTED INFECTIONS (RANK)
Burn	24.1 (14)	0.30	25.9 (1)
Neurosurgical	18.3 (39)	0.37	29.8 (2)
Trauma	17.2 (16)	0.57	30.3 (1)
Surgical	14.5 (163)	0.45	31.4 (1)
Medical/Surgical	11.8 (185)	0.37	29.3 (1)
Coronary	10.2 (94)	0.18	23.7 (2)
Medical	8.9 (105)	0.47	28.0 (2)
Respiratory	6.7 (6)	0.49	30.6 (2)
Pediatric	5.8 (56)	0.47	19.6 (2)

From National Nosocomial Infection Surveillance Report: Data summary from October 1986–April 1997, issued May 1997. Am J Infect Control 25:477–487, 1997.
*(Number of VAP/Number of ventilator-days) × 1000.
†Number of ventilator-days/Number of patient-days.

ness,[13] and impaired ability to handle secretions or diminished airway reflexes.[34] Certain surgical groups also are at increased risk, including those undergoing upper abdominal or thoracic procedures.[8] Although only a few studies have applied multivariate analysis to groups of patients with nosocomial pneumonia associated with mechanical ventilation, their findings are consistent with theories on the pathogenesis of VAP. Findings from these studies are outlined in Table 17–2.

MORBIDITY, MORTALITY, AND OTHER COSTS

The costs of VAP have been measured in several ways, according to the impact on patient outcomes or healthcare resources. Crude mortality rates are dependent on the distribution of underlying diseases. The attributable mortality, defined as the percentage of deaths occurring in excess of that expected due to the underlying disease process, has been calculated at 27% in the general ICU.[1, 2] In selected groups, the attributable mortality may be much higher. In bone marrow transplant patients, for example, the excess mortality due to nosocomial pneumonia is as high as 62%.[42] Certain bacterial species, e.g., *Pseudomonas aeruginosa*

and *Acinetobacter* spp., are also associated with higher mortality rates,[1] as is the presence of secondary bacteremia.[43] The higher crude mortality in patients with selected gram-negative bacilli may be related to multiple antibiotic resistance in these organisms.[43] Other factors that have been associated with increased mortality due to VAP in multivariate analysis include the presence of an ultimately or rapidly fatal underlying illness, worsening of acute respiratory failure, shock, and inappropriate antibiotic therapy. In the latter analysis, mortality was lower in the postcardiac surgery ICU compared with other ICU types.[30] Another study found that supine positioning in the first 24 hours of mechanical ventilation was associated with increased mortality compared with semirecumbent positioning. Investigators were unable to determine the degree to which patient positioning was merely a marker for disease severity, i.e., hemodynamic instability.[38]

Measuring the impact of VAP on health care resources has been even more difficult. Studies have shown that pneumonia lengthens the duration of mechanical ventilation by 10 or more days[25] and increases ICU stay threefold.[44] The approximately 250,000 cases of nosocomial pneumonia that occur annually in the United States account for approximately 1.75 million excess hospital days and more than $1 billion in increased costs.[45] Similar calculations for the subset of patients on ventilators are not available but given the impact on length of stay, presumably much of this increased cost originates in the ICU.

PATHOGENESIS

The development of nosocomial pneumonia depends on both host and external factors. Some of the factors that determine whether pneumonia develops in the normal lung include the route of bacterial acquisition,[46, 47] the size of the inoculum,[48, 49] and the virulence of the organism. For example, experi-

ments have shown that animals given a bolus inoculation of 10^4 *Klebsiella* organisms become infected, whereas 10^9 *Staphylococcus aureus* organisms delivered via aerosol are cleared rapidly, leaving no pulmonary infection.[46, 47] The likelihood that a bolus inoculum will cause infection increases with the number of bacteria or the volume of the bolus.[48, 49] This becomes important when one considers that ventilated patients develop a variety of reservoirs that are potential sources of bolus aspiration. In addition, bacterial colonization increases in these patients because of changes in mucosal surfaces. This raises the potential for aspiration of innocula containing higher concentrations of bacteria from the orophar-

TABLE 17–2. Risk Factors for Pneumonia in the Intensive Care Unit (Multivariate Analyses)

SOURCE	Craven et al[19*]	Kollef[38*]	Torres et al[30*]	Rodriguez et al[64*]	Joshi et al[8]
POPULATION	Medical, surgical, cardiac	Medical, surgical, cardiothoracic	Medical, surgical, trauma, neurologic	Trauma	Medical, surgical
RISK FACTORS	Intracranial pressure monitor	Organ system failure index ≥ 3	Gastric aspiration	Blunt trauma	Nasogastric tube (1–6 d)
	Cimetidine	Age > 60 yrs	Reintubation	Emergent intubation	Upper abdominal/ thoracic surgery
	24-hr ventilator circuit changes	Prior antibiotics	COPD	Hypotension on admission	Recent bronchoscopy (2–5 d before)
	Fall–winter season	Supine head position in first 24 hrs	PEEP MV > 3 d	Head injury	
DIAGNOSTIC CRITERIA	Clinical (5 of 5 criteria)†	Clinical (radiograph + 3 of 3 clinical criteria or pathology, blood culture, or cavitation)	Clinical (radiograph + 2 of 3 criteria)	Clinical +PSB/ TTNA or histology	Clinical (4 of 4 criteria)

*Ventilated patients only.
†Requirement for new infiltrate effectively excluded patients with severe acute respiratory distress syndrome.
COPD, chronic obstructive pulmonary disease; MV, mechanical ventilation; PEEP, positive end-expiratory pressure; PSB, protected specimen brush; TTNA, transthoracic needle aspiration.

ynx or stomach. Pneumonia also may result from hematogenous spread or direct penetration from the pleural space or mediastinum, although these causes are less common. Respiratory equipment itself is no longer a common source of VAP in ICUs; pneumonia occurs rarely from the inhalation of bacteria via contaminated aerosols or direct inoculation into the airway by health care personnel.

Hospitalized patients are also compromised by a variety of underlying diseases that affect their local and systemic defense mechanisms. In addition to the risk factors noted in the previous section, other common medical conditions have measurable effects on various facets of the immune response. The presence of pulmonary edema fluid, for example, adversely affects alveolar macrophage function and the antibacterial functions of surfactant.[50, 51] An understanding of the lung's normal defenses against microbial invasion is crucial to attempts to manage and prevent pneumonia as a complication of mechanical ventilation. The lungs' normal defense mechanisms and the intrinsic and extrinsic factors predisposing to the development of VAP are discussed in detail in the following section.

Pulmonary Defenses Against Infection

The competence of local and systemic host defenses is crucial in determining whether infection will occur. The lung's unique role in gas exchange places it in constant contact with the outside environment, exposing the respiratory surfaces to more than 10,000 L per day of ambient air and an unending challenge by airborne pathogens and particulates. The normal bacterial load in the oropharynx (up to 10^7–10^{10} organisms per ml of saliva) presents an additional threat. **Aspiration** of oral secretions is a common event in healthy individuals, occurring in at least 45% of people during sleep.[52] The normal lung, therefore, is equipped with a variety of mechanisms, both physical and immunologic, to defend against infection from these sources. The upper airway includes important physical barriers that prevent large

innocula from reaching the lower airways, including the epiglottis and vocal cords. Coughing and continuous clearance by the ciliary epithelium also function to keep the lower airways relatively sterile. Airway secretions are an important part of the mucociliary clearance mechanisms. The secretions contain mucus and noncellular components of the immune system such as immunoglobulin A (IgA) and, in the smaller airways, IgG. Nonmucin components also include proteinase inhibitors, bactericidal enzymes such as lysozyme, and lactoferrin, which may chelate iron needed for bacterial growth. Bacteria that reach the alveolar surface encounter a local inflammatory cell population that includes alveolar macrophages and small numbers of lymphocytes and polymorphonuclear cells. Experimentally, a bacterial challenge introduced into the alveolar spaces is phagocytized by the resident macrophages within only about 30 minutes. Additional components of the epithelial lining fluid may function as nonimmune opsonins, including surfactant components and fibronectin.[53]

Device-Related Infection Risk

Instrumentation of the ICU patient is the most direct way in which normal defense mechanisms are breached. Although the relative contribution of equipment contamination has diminished, recognition of the problem was a major step in understanding the pathogenesis of pneumonia in hospitalized patients. Along with the rapid development of positive-pressure mechanical ventilation during the polio epidemics of the 1950s came the first reports of epidemic nosocomial pneumonia due to gram-negative bacilli.[54–56] A connection between the increased use of respiratory equipment and these infections was suspected, but the risk was not fully appreciated until autopsy studies at Parkland Memorial Hospital in Dallas documented a fourfold increase in gram-negative bacterial pneumonia. In these early ventilators, mainstream nebulizers were colonized by gram-negative bacteria, resulting in the production of bacterial aerosols that effectively delivered high innocula to the alveolar surface.[56]

Most ventilators currently in use have cascade humidifiers in which bacterial contamination is uncommon. Water temperature in this type of humidifier reaches 50° to 55°C, inhibiting the growth of most pathogenic bacteria, including *S. aureus* and gram-negative bacilli.[57] The degree of risk associated with the low-level contamination present in these systems is unclear, and they should not be changed more frequently than at 48-hour intervals if at all.[58] Bacteria contaminating not only humidification reservoirs but also ventilator circuit tubing most likely originate from the patient's own respiratory flora.[59, 60] Condensate collects in ventilator circuits at a rate of about 30 ml/hr (range 10–60 ml/hr) and is quickly colonized after circuit changes. One study found colonization of the tubing to be 33% as early as 2 hours after circuit change, increasing to 80% at 24 hours.[60] The highest levels of contamination are found closest to the patient (swivel adaptor, Y-junction, and proximal tubing).[60] Initial Centers for Disease Control and Prevention (CDC) recommendations called for daily ventilator circuit changes,[61] but subsequent randomized studies showed an increased risk of pneumonia in patients undergoing changes every 24 hours compared with every 48 hours[19] and no difference between patients whose circuits were changed every 48 hours compared with those without any routinely scheduled changes.[31]

Although no causal role in VAP has been demonstrated for tubing colonization, manipulating tubing that contains condensate with high bacterial concentration could lead to innoculation of the patient's airways by the fluid. This method has been used with good effect to produce pneumonia in experimental animals.[46] CDC guidelines published in 1994 recommend ventilator circuits be changed no more often than every 48 hours, but do not suggest any maximum time limit.[58] New developments in ventilator circuits address these problems by combining in-line filtration properties with heat–moisture exchange characteristics, although the heat and moisture exchanging filter (HMEF), or "artificial nose," currently in

use may not be optimal in all patients because of increases in dead space, circuit resistance, and insufficient humidification for some patients.[62] As of this writing there are insufficient data to determine whether these devices will affect VAP rates.[58, 63]

The endotracheal tube itself, both by its physical presence and by virtue of the insertion process, is a primary risk factor. Endotracheal intubation performed in an emergency setting has been associated with increased risk for nosocomial pneumonia,[64] and reintubation during mechanical ventilation is an independent risk factor by multivariate analysis.[30] The tube and cuff injure mucosal surfaces both at insertion and during respiratory effort.[65, 66] Autopsy studies show ciliary denudation along the insertion tract and at the site of cuff inflation,[65] damage that impairs mucociliary clearance and may increase adherence cababilities of some bacterial species.[67] Insertion of the tube may be accompanied by either gross or microscopic aspiration, which is a likely contributor to the increased risk of intubation in emergent settings. Once in place, biofilms form on the interior surface of endotracheal tubes. These films consist of polysaccharides, or glycocalyx, of both bacterial and patient origin. Bacteria can be seen embedded within this matrix via electron microscopy and have been cultured from patient tubes in amounts as high as 10^6 colony-forming units (CFUs)/cm. Particles may become dislodged from these biofilms by suction catheters or by the gas flow through a ventilator.[68, 69] Although the relative importance of such innocula in the pathogenesis of pneumonia in ICU patients is not known, such particles are more pathogenic than free bacteria under experimental conditions.[70] The space above the cuff of an endotracheal tube is another source of infectious innocula, tending to pool secretions that become heavily colonized with bacteria and are easily aspirated despite patency of the tracheal cuff.[71] Aspiration and epithelial damage are less likely with the high compliance cuffs used currently, although an incidence of aspiration of 20% to 40% is reported.[72, 73] The cough reflex, an important part of normal defenses, is also impaired,[74] and thickened or impacted secretions may be difficult to clear.

Obstruction of sinuses by nasally inserted tubes creates an additional reservoir for the growth of bacteria and other pathogens. Fluid accumulation in the sinuses is common in ventilated patients, with the highest rates of sinusitis found by radiography in those with nasal tubes and longer duration of endotracheal or gastric tube placement. In a group of 40 ventilated patients with normal initial sinus computed tomography (CT) scans, the incidence of radiologic sinusitis was 95.5% after 7 days of nasal gastric or tracheal intubation versus 22.5% in patients whose tubes were placed via the oral route. Approximately one third of the 133 patients in that study who underwent sinus aspiration had infectious sinusitis. The distribution of organisms closely approximated the epidemiology of VAP, with a predominance of gram-negative bacilli. *S. aureus,* streptococcal species, and *Candida albicans* were also seen in significant numbers. In this particular study there was a strong association between the development of infectious sinusitis and VAP, although it is not clear whether sinusitis is a true link in the pathogenesis of pneumonia or merely a result of shared risk factors.[75]

Not all the risk from respiratory devices is a direct result of physical trauma or the bypass of physical defenses. One of the primary indications for the initiation of assisted respiration is refractory hypoxemia. The endotracheal tube and mechanical ventilator permit the therapeutic administration of high inspired oxygen concentrations. The effects of hyperoxia on host defenses has not been explored clinically, but there are data from cell culture systems and animal experiments strongly suggesting that alveolar hyperoxia impairs host defenses through mechanisms such as decreasing tracheal mucus velocity and altering the function of macrophages and surfactant proteins.[76–78]

Gastric Colonization

The stomach, like the oropharynx and subglottic area, is an important reservoir for bacterial growth in ventilated patients. Unlike the upper airway, the stomach is ordinarily relatively sterile because of the secretion of acid. The resulting pH of 1 to 2 in a normal stomach effectively inhibits the growth of most human pathogens. Critically ill patients may lose this protective gastric acidity as a result of pharmacologic suppression of acid secretion, neutralization of acid via continuous enteral feeds, or intrinsic decrease in acidity. This last may occur chronically in the setting of advanced age or acutely from poor perfusion of the gastric mucosa during hemodynamic instability.[79, 80] In the absence of sufficient acid secretion, the stomach becomes a suitable environment for bacterial colonization. This has been shown by a number of studies and raises the possibility that the stomach may play an important role in the pathogenesis of VAP.[81–83]

Retrograde movement of bacteria has been a difficult concept to prove, however, and the relative contribution of the digestive tract to the development of VAP probably varies from patient to patient. Aerobic gram-negative bacteria colonize the upper gastrointestinal tract within a few days in ICU patients with gastric pH greater than 4, reaching concentrations as high as 10^8 CFUs/ml.[16, 82] In some studies, this is followed by colonization of the oropharynx and trachea and is associated with a higher rate of nosocomial pneumonia.[16] Any given sequence of colonization has not been demonstrated consistently, though, and in general the gastric-oropharyngeal-tracheal route has not been applicable to organisms like *P. aeruginosa,* which preferentially adheres to tracheal epithelium.[83, 84] Strategies that are designed to prevent pneumonia by blocking the gastric-to-pulmonary transmission of bacteria are discussed later in this chapter, although due to a lack of conclusive data they have not gained widespread acceptance.

DIAGNOSIS

The diagnosis of VAP has been plagued by the nonspecific nature of most clinical signs and symptoms, as well as a lack of sensitivity in patients with underlying diffuse lung disease. This continues to be true despite the advent of more invasive diagnostic techniques, although careful evaluation of bronchoscopic data over the past 10 years has made important contributions to the understanding of VAP. The histologic diagnosis of pneumonia is still considered by many to be the gold standard; it is this standard by which new diagnostic methods are usually evaluated.

The histologic features of pneumonia in the hospitalized patient include necrosis with abscess formation, focal hemorrhage, and vascular invasion. The lesion may be acquired hematogenously but usually is thought to be a descending infection via the airways or aspiration.[85] Other pathologic findings include bronchiolitis, although the clinical significance of this lesion is rarely addressed in the literature. Correlations between the histologic lesion of pneumonia and quantitative lung cultures have been made in both animals and humans. In studies of baboons, with either normal lungs or acute lung injury induced by oxygen or oleic acid aspiration, colony counts of $\geq 10^4$ CFUs/g of tissue correlated well with the presence of histologic foci of pneumonia. When lung tissue cultures yielded less than 10^4 CFUs/g, no pneumonia was seen.[86, 87] In an autopsy study in humans, this same quantitative correlation was found.[88] Bacterial count of 10^5 CFUs or more per milliliter of exudate also has been used as evidence of pneumonia.[89] These studies support the quantitative thresholds currently in use for bronchoscopic sampling methods.

Two large autopsy studies detailing the incidence of nosocomial pneumonia in patients with acute respiratory distress syndrome (ARDS) have been published. In the first, 75% of 98 patients had histologic evidence of pneumonia. In 54%, this was graded as moderate or severe. In 21%, pneumonia was the only histologic abnormality seen in the lung at autopsy, and half of these patients had both diffuse alveolar damage (DAD) and pneumonia.[85] The relationship between pulmonary infection and ARDS is complex, and the varying effects of infection on the evolution of DAD has been studied in animals. In a study of hamsters

with hyperoxic lung injury, *P. aeruginosa* was injected in different doses at different times during the exposure. The histologic features of infection differed depending on when during the development of acute lung injury the bacteria were inoculated.[87] In another study, 83 dying patients on mechanical ventilation underwent bedside pneumonectomy. A complete histologic evaluation of the lung was made, with 5- to 10-mm sections taken. Bronchiolitis or bronchopneumonia was seen in 72% of the patients. Bronchopneumonia, the dominant lesion, was more common in dependent lung areas. Only 28% of patients had no evidence of infection in the sectioned lung. The authors commented that the incidence of pneumonia could have been even higher if the contralateral lung had been examined. One important conclusion was that the focal nature of some bronchopneumonia and bronchiolitis could potentially lead to bronchoscopic sampling error, affecting the procedure's sensitivity, if this was used as the sole means of diagnosis.[90]

Because lung biopsy, either surgical or bronchoscopic, carries significant risk in mechanically ventilated patients, most pneumonia in the ICU is diagnosed using clinical data and microbiologic sampling techniques. These methods are employed variably and a thorough understanding of definitions used in pneumonia studies, as well as their strengths and limitations, is crucial to establishing an appropriate diagnosis. The NNIS system defines ventilator-associated pneumonia as pneumonia that develops during mechanical ventilation but was not present or incubating at the time ventilation was initiated. Pneumonia diagnosed through the first 48 hours after extubation or cessation of mechanical ventilation is included.[91] A number of clinical studies place an additional time constraint on the definition, disallowing any pneumonia that becomes evident within the first 48 hours after the onset of mechanical ventilation. Although the choice of 48 hours, or any similar time limit, is relatively arbitrary, it provides consistency for establishing trends and for comparing data on a national or international level. The epidemiologic use of these definitions does not preclude the possibility that VAP may develop 24 hours after the initiation of assisted ventilation, particularly if the innoculum is large, as when aspiration occurs during intubation. Likewise, pneumonia resulting from a small inoculum or an organism of low virulence may not become clinically apparent until more than 48 hours after cessation of ventilatory support.

The diagnostic criteria used by hospitals reporting to the NNIS system are published by the CDC and require either physical examination or radiographic findings of pneumonia along with one additional piece of evidence (Table 17–3).[92] This is a clinical diagnosis, based on active surveillance of laboratory data and patient records. The CDC has collected data via the NNIS system since 1970, shifting focus in 1986 to specific risk groups including the ICU. Epidemiologic data on nosocomial pneumonia originating with the NNIS system before that date reflect a hospital-wide population.[33] Recent work with invasive diagnostic methods has questioned the standards of clinical diagnosis on which much of the epi-

TABLE 17–3. Diagnostic Criteria for Ventilator-Associated Pneumonia in Adults

SOURCE	CDC/NNIS[92, 96]	CPIS[35]	Bronchoscopic PSB[93]	Bronchoscopic BAL[93]
CRITERIA	Two criteria: 1. Rales or dullness to percussion *and*: (a) new purulent sputum or (b) positive blood culture, or (c) pathogen from TTA, bronchial, brush, or biopsy OR 2. CXR with new or progressive infiltrate, consolidation, cavitation, or pleural effusion *and*: (a), (b), (c), or (d) isolation of virus or viral antigen or (e) diagnostic serology	Score > 6 (0–12 possible): 1. Temperature (°C): $\geq$36.5 and $\leq$38.4 (0 pt) $\geq$38.5 and $\leq$38.9 (1 pt) $\geq$39 or $\leq$36.0 (2 pt) 2. WBC $\geq$4K and $\leq$11K (0 pt) <4K or >11K (1 pt) plus band forms (1 pt) 3. Tracheal secretions: <14 + secretions (0 pt) $\geq$14 + secretions (1 pt) Plus purulence (1 pt) 4. PaO_2/FiO_2 (mm Hg): >240 or ARDS (0 pt) $\leq$240 and no ARDS (2 pt) 5. CXR: No infiltrate (0 pt) Diffuse/patchy infiltrate (1 pt) Focal infiltrate (2 pt) 6. ETA culture (0–3 + growth): No growth or $\leq$1 + pathogens (0 pt) >1 + of a pathogen (1 pt) plus same pathogen on Gram stain (1 pt)	PSB culture with any single bacterial isolate present in a quantity $\geq$ 10^3 CFUs/ml	Protected BAL culture with any single bacterial isolate present in a quantity $\geq$ 10^4 CFUs/ml OR Bacterial index $\geq$ 5
SENSITIVITY	68%	N/A	61–100%	70–100%
SPECIFICITY	97.8%	N/A	64–100%	70–100%

ARDS, acute respiratory distress syndrome; BAL, bronchoalveolar lavage; CDC, Centers for Disease Control and Prevention; CPIS, clinical pulmonary infection score; CXR, chest x-ray; ETA, endotracheal aspirate; FiO_2, inspired oxygen inspiration; NNIS, National Nosocomial Infection Surveillance (system); PaO_2, arterial oxygen pressure; PSB, protected specimen brush; TTA, transtracheal; WBC, white blood cell.

demiology in this field is based.[24, 88, 93–95] Despite these criticisms, NNIS data remain important for consistency, longevity, and national scope. A recent study performed by the CDC to evaluate the accuracy of these data found that prospective reporting of ICU-acquired pneumonia by the hospitals in the NNIS system had an 89% predictive value positive, with a sensitivity of 68% and a specificity of 97.8%.[96] This challenges the often-cited conclusion that the clinical diagnosis of pneumonia is plagued by lack of specificity.[24, 87, 92–94] An additional finding of this study was the poor positive predictive value (49%) when retrospective chart review alone was used "diagnostically."[96] This confirms the findings from a widely cited study by Andrews and associates in which a similar retrospective diagnosis of pneumonia had a sensitivity of 64% and a specificity of 80% when compared with autopsy findings.[97] Nevertheless, the relatively low sensitivity provides impetus for ongoing evaluation by the CDC to improve diagnostic surveillance in the area of nosocomial pneumonia.[96]

Most clinical studies of VAP use entry criteria based on radiographic and multiple clinical criteria. These generally include the presence of a new or progressive infiltrate on chest radiograph that otherwise is unexplained plus two or more of the following: fever, leukocytosis, purulent tracheal aspirates, and Gram stain findings in respiratory secretions. Positive blood or pleural fluid cultures or histologic evidence of pneumonia may substitute for clinical evidence of pulmonary infection.[8, 19, 25, 30, 38, 64] It appears likely that the application of these criteria overdiagnoses VAP in the general ICU population. Radiographic abnormalities are common in ventilated patients and may result from a wide variety of pathologic processes, including edema, hemorrhage, atelectasis, and acute lung injury. Because the chest radiograph is often an entry point triggering consideration of the diagnosis of VAP, these other entities must be distinguished from infection using supporting clinical data. Used alone, no radiographic finding has proved especially useful in diagnosing pneumonia in the ICU patient. A study correlating chest radiographs with autopsy evidence of pneumonia found that only the presence of air bronchograms correlated with pneumonia, although the positive predictive value was only 51%. In patients with ARDS, no radiographic signs were found to distinguish between patients with and without pneumonia.[98] When compared with invasive diagnostic methods, particularly **protected specimen brush** (PSB), some investigators have estimated that approximately two thirds of patients judged by clinical study criteria to have pneumonia in fact do not have pneumonia.[95]

Some investigators believe that the diagnosis of VAP should not be made in the absence of a positive quantitative culture from a PSB or bronchoalveolar lavage sample.[99] In their studies, the positive PSB culture has been used as a gold standard for the diagnosis of VAP (see Table 17–3).[24, 93, 100–102] However, many questions remain about the proper use and interpretation of these techniques. Whereas they may be useful in selected cases, they still are not appropriate for most ICUs. The diagnosis of nosocomial pneumonia for many remains a clinical one, although clinical practice often differs from published study criteria. One group of investigators developed a clinical pulmonary infection score (CPIS) using six clinical variables, weighted and combined into a final score between 0 and 12 (see Table 17–3). Using this simple system, the investigators found a good correlation between diagnosis based on bronchoalveolar lavage and CPIS results.[103] Although this scoring system is not used extensively, it approximates practical clinical decision-making more closely than many of the entry criteria in published clinical studies.

The application of diagnostic criteria can be difficult in the ICU because of the lack of specificity of any single sign or symptom. In the subgroup of ICU patients with ARDS, the diagnosis of pneumonia can be particularly elusive. In a 1981 autopsy series of 24 patients with ARDS, pneumonia was documented histologically in 14, for an incidence rate of 58%. Although the "clinical" suspicion for pneumonia was determined retrospectively, the investigators found that the diagnosis was suspected correctly in only 64% of the patients in whom pneumonia was present and was diagnosed in 20% without histologic evidence of lung infection.[97] This study is cited extensively to demonstrate the need for improved diagnostic methods and highlights the fact that available data are complicated by both overdiagnosis and underdiagnosis.

BRONCHOSCOPIC TECHNIQUES IN DIAGNOSIS

Bronchoscopic Methods

Although the role of bronchoscopy in the management of VAP requires further study before definitive recommendations can be made regarding its application in the ICU, the technique has become a standard part of the clinical investigation of pneumonia in some centers. As such, a detailed discussion of both the technical aspects and of the questions fueling ongoing controversy is warranted. Two methods have evolved for sampling the lung in patients undergoing mechanical ventilation, the PSB and **bronchoalveolar lavage** (BAL). Both are designed to obtain pulmonary secretions for culture in patients on even high levels of respiratory support. The goal of these techniques is twofold: (1) to improve the microbiologic diagnosis of pulmonary infection and (2) to increase the ability to distinguish infectious from noninfectious pulmonary processes in ventilated patients.

The methodology for obtaining uncontaminated samples of the lower airways using the PSB was developed in the late 1970s.[103] Initially applied to nonintubated patients, the technique uses a double-catheter system with an enclosed brush. Sterility of the system is maintained via a distal occluding polyethylene glycol plug until the catheter is positioned and the plug is ejected. This catheter design was shown to have a low incidence of contamination by upper airway secretions.[104, 105] Obtaining an adequate specimen is crucial if the results are to be used to decide whether treatment is to be given or withheld. Patients require sedation so that topical anesthetics are not needed. In some patients, short-acting paralytic agents may be required.[93] The use of lido-

caine administered through the suction port of the bronchoscope can lead to both false-positive and false-negative results. The injection of topical anesthetic can carry bacteria into the tracheobronchial tree and contaminate culture specimens.[93, 104] False-negative results may ensue if the concentration of lidocaine in the collected secretions reaches bacteriostatic levels.[106] The amount of lidocaine that can be used safely without effect on PSB culture results is not known.

Technical factors, such as suctioning through the bronchoscope, can also lead to contamination of the specimen. The endotracheal tube should be suctioned thoroughly before the procedure to decrease contact with secretions originating in the upper airway above the tube, in the endotracheal tube itself, or in the central airways. Suctioning during the procedure should be avoided until after the specimen is obtained.[93] After the bronchoscope is introduced, the tip is positioned in the desired location. This is generally the bronchus draining the area with new or progressing infiltrate seen on chest radiograph, although in patients with diffuse lung disease, it may be any (or all) segment(s) in which purulent secretions are seen.[93] The PSB within its protective cannula is advanced 2 to 3 cm out of the bronchoscope to free it from the secretions collected on the distal end of the scope. The inner cannula then is advanced slightly, ejecting the distal plug, and the brush is advanced into the desired subsegment. If purulent secretions are visualized, the brush is rotated in them. The brush is then retracted into the inner cannula, these are retracted into the outer cannula, and the entire system is withdrawn through the bronchoscope.[88, 93] Some investigators advance the brush to a wedge position to sample distal secretions,[24] although there is concern that this may cause sampling error and increase the risk for pneumothorax.[93] After a sample has been obtained, the distal segments of the two cannulae are wiped sequentially with 70% alcohol, cut with sterile scissors, and discarded. The brush is advanced and cut into a container with 1 ml diluent, usually either saline or Ringer's lactated solution. Specimens must be transported to laboratory facilities for quantitative bacterial culture within 15 minutes.[93, 105]

The handling of bronchoscopic specimens in the microbiology laboratory is not standardized, and several issues require further investigation.[105] Two methods may be used for quantitative cultures. Serial dilutions provide the most accurate quantitation but are labor intensive and are not available in every facility. Results are expressed as CFU/ml of sample. A simpler but less exact method is the calibrated loop method, similar to that used for urine culture. These results are reported as $\log^{10}$ colony count ranges.[105] Issues that remain unresolved involve the transportation of specimens and the limitations imposed by sample size. Delayed transport may necessitate a decrease in diagnostic threshold for quantitative cultures, in one study as much as 10-fold.[107] This may be in part due to the solutions chosen for diluent, which are deleterious to some bacteria (i.e., *Haemophilus influenzae, Streptococcus pneumoniae, Legionella* spp.).[108, 109] Anaerobes may also suffer under transport conditions because of oxygen exposure,[105] although they have been isolated with PSB in patients with lung abscess when careful culture techniques were used.[110] Because the volume of secretions sampled by the brush is small, approximately 0.001 ml,[103] direct microscopic examination of the sample may adversely affect quantitative results by decreasing the amount available for culture.[94] Stains not performed directly from the brush have low sensitivity[94, 111, 112]; therefore, there are no laboratory criteria for determining whether a sample obtained by PSB is adequate.[93] The small volume also may cause variations in sensitivity of the 10^3 cutoff proposed for quantitative culture results.[105] If additional studies are needed, such as viral or fungal cultures, the bronchoscopist must perform multiple brushings.

Other potential drawbacks of the PSB technique include the inherent risk of bronchoscopy to the critically ill ventilated patient. Even when high levels of oxygen were used, one study documented a mean decrease in arterial oxygen tension of 26% for fiberoptic bronchoscopy done using midazolam sedation in ventilated patients.[113] Cost is also a limitation in the use of the PSB, although if improved diagnosis led to more efficient use of antimicrobial therapy the cost–benefit ratio might tip in favor of the technique.[95] To address these criticisms, the catheter has been modified to allow undirected sampling. This method is not well studied but is reported to have comparable sensitivity.[114] It is not clear whether the loss of ability to direct catheter placement has a significant impact on the interpretation of culture results.[103, 107, 114]

Bronchoalveolar lavage was introduced as a diagnostic method and means of obtaining material for bacterial culture in response to the concerns raised because of small sample size from brushings. Lavage fluid samples an estimated 1 million alveoli,[115] and the larger volume of secretions collected is amenable to direct and immediate microscopic examination in addition to quantitative culture. The proper lavage technique is less well standardized than PSB methodology. Studies have used instilled volumes ranging from 100 to 240 ml.[116] The effect of variable dilution on interpretation of quantitative culture results has not been studied.[93] When initially evaluated, cultures obtained by BAL were characterized by excessive contamination by proximal airway flora introduced through the suction port[101, 117] and by difficulty in establishing an appropriate threshold for diagnosing pneumonia. The technique has been modified in a variety of ways to decrease the likelihood of contamination. One version uses a plugged double catheter such as that employed for the protected brush.[118] Another modification uses a protected balloon-tipped catheter.[94] Sensitivity and specificity of quantitative cultures reportedly are improved using these catheters, although confirmatory studies need to be done. Questions regarding the transport and handling of specimens are similar to those described previously for PSB specimens.

Interpretation of Quantitative Culture Results

The goal of these bronchoscopic techniques for sampling deep respiratory secretions is not just to obtain less contaminated culture material. They differ from other methods of culturing the lung because attempts have been made to define a specific *diagnostic* threshold based solely on quantitative results. It is important to remember, however, that these criteria have been studied primarily in a subset of ICU patients who met some clinical criteria for pneumonia, rather than in all ventilated patients. The techniques are not appropriate for screening purposes.

Criteria for interpretating results from PSB quantitative cultures are better defined than those for BAL cultures. Several studies have demonstrated that the presence of an organism in greater than 10^3 CFU/ml correlates highly with the presence of pneumonia diagnosed either by biopsy or by other means, although reported sensitivity and specificity of the cutoff for diagnosis of pneumonia varies (see Table 17–3).[88, 94, 95, 101, 107, 114, 117, 119–123] The PSB samples approximately 0.001 ml of secretions[103]; when diluted into 1 ml of transport medium, a bacterial concentration of 10^3 represents a level of 10^6 CFU/ml in pulmonary secretions. This correlates with the estimates of bacterial counts in sputum or tracheal aspirate specimens in acute pneumonia.[124, 125]

Although many clinical pneumonia studies currently use bronchoscopic methods for diagnosis as well as culture, the sensitivity and specificity of the techniques continue to be a source for controversy.[99, 126] Concerns over the use of strict cutoff points for the PSB include whether the small sample size is sufficient to rule out pneumonia in ventilated patients. One study found that more than one third of patients with borderline quantitative PSB cultures (between 10^2 and 10^3 CFU/ml) and persistent clinical suspicion for pneumonia meet quantitative culture criteria for VAP on subsequent sampling. Investigators could not determine whether the initial culture represented a false-negative result or a high level of colonization preceding the development of pneumonia.[127] The interpretation of any PSB result must also consider the fact that PSB cultures taken in patients recently started on antibiotics have a notable decrease in sensitivity,[88, 114, 117] although it has been ar-

gued that PSB might still be useful in ruling out superinfection in some patients.[128] Investigators have also attempted to correlate the results of follow-up PSB cultures with response to therapy for pneumonia, suggesting a role for the technique in optimizing antibiotic therapy.[128] These areas require additional investigations before recommendations can be made. The specificity of a 10^3 cutoff may also be a problem in certain types of patients. As many as half of patients with chronic bronchitis (but not pneumonia) who require mechanical ventilation for respiratory failure have PSB cultures on admission that exceed the cutoff used for nosocomial pneumonia in ventilated patients.[129]

The optimal diagnostic threshold for quantitative BAL cultures is controversial, in part because of the uncertain dilution of specimens. BAL has been estimated to recover 5 to 10 times the number of organisms obtained by PSB sampling,[117, 130] with a dilution factor of 10 to 100 (>1 ml in 10–100 ml lavage return).[131, 132] Although diagnostic thresholds ranging from 10^3 to 10^5 have been used in different studies, the most commonly cited figure is 10^4 CFU/ml.[94, 101, 102, 103, 117, 133] This represents 10^6 CFU/ml in the respiratory secretions, consistent with the cutoff used for PSB cultures. Reported sensitivity and specificity of this method using 10^4 CFU/ml to define pneumonia range from 70% to 100%. It can be argued that, given the polymicrobial nature of VAP, a cutoff point for a single organism does not fully represent the bacterial load present in the lung and is therefore diagnostically insensitive. Early studies in baboons expressed the results of BAL cultures as a "bacterial index" (BI), calculated by adding the $\log^{10}$ concentrations of each bacterial species isolated.[86] Although the BI correlated with tissue concentrations of bacteria, the results using BI in human studies have been less convincing.[101, 103, 117] If BAL is used to diagnose pneumonia in the clinical setting, a threshold of 10^4 CFU/ml of a single organism is preferred.[93]

Both PSB and BAL cultures have been compared with quantitative endotracheal aspirate (QEA) cultures in an animal model of VAP. As in human autopsy studies, the distribution of histologic pneumonia was heterogeneous. They also found that the bacterial load was distributed unevenly, and although it tended to correlate with pathologic findings, there was no quantitative threshold in PSB or BAL cultures that was useful for diagnosing pneumonia. Using standard cutoff points, PSB, BAL, and QEA had diagnostic sensitivities of 69%, 78%, and 100%, respectively. The specificity for all three techniques was less than 50%. In addition, PSB and BAL cultures were only 37% and 50% accurate in identifying the causative organisms.[134]

Information obtained from the direct examination of fluid from BAL specimens may eventually prove useful in the diagnosis of VAP. Samples can be screened for evidence of contamination; greater than 1% squamous epithelial cells was shown in one study to predict a level of contamination by oropharyngeal flora that affected quantitative culture results.[130] Specimens may be stained immediately and examined microscopically for bacteria and cells, providing evidence of the host response to organisms. The Gram stain has been reported to have a sensitivity of 100% and specificity of 88% to 100% in this setting and can assist in choosing empiric antibiotics.[94, 103] Intracellular bacteria have diagnostic significance and can be detected using a Wright-Giemsa stain.[94, 101, 103, 105, 119] Appropriate cutoffs for percentage of intracellular organisms that indicate pulmonary infection have not been defined. A combination of factors, including the number of intracellular and extracellular bacteria and the presence of elastin fibers, an indicator of parenchymal destruction by gram-negative bacteria, may prove to be the most sensitive microscopic test.[103, 105]

MICROBIOLOGY

There is little question that aerobic gram-negative bacilli comprise the largest group of organisms responsible for VAP, although the past two decades have seen a shift in the distribution of organisms isolated in epidemiologic and surveillance studies (Table 17–4). NNIS data provide a longitudinal view of organisms isolated from patients with nosocomial pneumonia, although patients other than those on mechanical ventilation are included to varying degrees during the different reporting periods. Data collected before 1986 reflect hospital-wide epidemiology. In subsequent data ICU populations are separated, although pathogens are included from all ICU patients, not just those on assisted ventilation. *P. aeruginosa* and *S. aureus* have been the most common organisms isolated from patients with pneumonia throughout this period although they have increased in frequency as well as in antimicrobial resistance.[34, 135, 136] Changes in the frequency of other gram-negative aerobes also reflect an increase in organisms with drug resistance. *Enterobacter* spp., which tend to develop resistance to beta-lactam **antibiotics,** have become more prevalent, whereas organisms such as *Escherichia coli,* which generally are still susceptible to these drugs, have become less common.[33, 135–138]

Like the NNIS data, studies using PSB and BAL cultures have shown a high incidence of resistant gram-negative isolates and *S. aureus.*[24, 100] *P. aeruginosa* and *Acinetobacter* spp. are the most commonly reported gram-negative bacilli and have been associated with prior exposure to antibiotics and a higher mortality.[24, 100] Other hospitals have reported a high incidence of *Enterobacter* spp.[139] These organisms are endemic to varying degrees in different ICUs as a result of local factors that include antibiotic prescribing patterns. *Enterobacter* spp. in particular have been associated with use of third-generation cephalosporins,[138, 139] although selection pressures have resulted in similar increases in resistance and infection with *Klebsiella* spp.[140, 141] Although the differences in organisms reported in studies using PSB may be partly due to improved culture methods that avoid contamination by bacteria colonizing the upper airways,[24, 43, 142] the last decade has brought real changes in the epidemiology of VAP coincident with widespread increases in resistant bacterial species.[136]

H. influenzae and pneumococcus, frequent causes of community-acquired pneumonia, are found in certain subsets of mechanically

TABLE 17–4. Microbiology of Pneumonia in the Intensive Care Unit (ICU)

SOURCE	NNIS[132]	NNIS[33]	NNIS[222]	Fagon et al[24]	Jimenez et al[25]	Rodriguez et al[64]
TIME SPAN	1980	1986–1997	1986–1994	1981–1985	1986	N/A
POPULATION	Hospital-wide	Multiple ICUs	Multiple neonatal ICUs	Medical/Surgical ICU (VAP)	Respiratory ICU (VAP)	Trauma ICU (VAP)
NO. OF EPISODES	N/A	42,363	6153	52	18	130
ISOLATES (%)	S. aureus (13)	P. aeruginosa (17.4)	S. aureus (16.7)	S. aureus (33)	P. aeruginosa (39)	S. aureus (28.5)
	P. aeruginosa (12)	S. aureus (17.4)	Coagulation-negative staphylococcus (16.5)	P. aeruginosa (31)	Acinetobacter spp. (33)	P. aeruginosa (23.8)
	K. pneumoniae (10)	Enterobacter spp. (11.4)	P. aeruginosa (11.7)	Acinetobacter spp., Proteus spp., streptococci* (15% each)	S. marcescens (17)	Enterobacter spp. (20)
	Enterobacter sp (9)	K. pneumoniae (6.7)	Enterobacter spp. (8.2)	M. catarrhalis, Haemophilus spp. (10% each)	Enterobacter spp., A. fumigatus (11% each)	H. influenzae (12.3)
	E. coli (9)	H. influenzae (4.9)	K. pneumoniae, E. coli (5.8% each)	E. coli, Corynebacteria spp. (8% each)	L. pneumophila (11%, Dx by TTNA only)	S. marcescens (10.8)
	P. mirabilis (6)		Group B streptococcus (5.7)		No organisms isolated (22)	
POLYMICROBIAL	N/A	N/A	N/A	40%	33%	30.7%
DIAGNOSTIC CRITERIA	CDC	CDC	CDC	PSB	Clinical + PSB/ TTNA or histology (3 of 9 at autopsy had previously unsuspected VAP)	Clinical (5 of 6 criteria)

*Nonpneumococcal.
CDC, Centers for Disease Control and Prevention; Dx, diagnosis; NNIS, National Nosocomial Infection Surveillance (system); PSB, protected specimen brush; VAP, ventilator-associated pneumonia.

ventilated patients, including those who have been intubated in the field as a result of head trauma.[143] These patients may aspirate at the time of intubation and develop pneumonia soon after ICU admission.[34, 35] These organisms are also more likely in patients who have not previously received antibiotics.[144, 145] Reports in ventilated patients using PSB cultures cite a 6% to 13% incidence of Haemophilus spp. that increases to approximately 20% in trauma patients.[24, 31, 143, 146] Both organisms are more likely to be found in patients who develop pneumonia early in the course of mechanical ventilation and whose endogenous mi-crobial flora has not experienced antibiotic selection pressures.[34–36]

S. aureus is also a significant pathogen, and although most epidemiologic studies do not report sensitivity patterns for the organisms isolated, resistant strains are likely to predominate in the ICU setting.[147] S. aureus is found commonly in patients after head trauma or neurosurgical procedures[143, 148–151] and in patients with medical risk factors, including chronic renal failure, diabetes mellitus, and intravenous drug abuse (Table 17–5).

Cultures for anaerobic bacteria have not been performed routinely in the NNIS studies, but careful cultures from transtracheal aspirates in a 1986 pneumonia study found anaerobes in 35% of cultures obtained.[152] This study was not limited to mechanically ventilated patients, however, and most recent microbiologic evaluations in this specific patient population have not found a high incidence of anaerobic flora.[24, 100] Anaerobes may play little part in the pathogenesis of VAP because of systemic alterations in the colonizing flora of critically ill patients, with decreases in the normal anaerobic bacterial load present in the oropharynx and gastrointestinal tract. The high inspired oxygen concentrations used in most intubated patients may suppress anaerobic growth even further. Another potential cause for the absence of anaerobes in studies using bronchoscopic diagnostic techniques is the difficulty in applying standard aerobic culture methods to more fastidious organisms. The importance of this factor is emphasized by a recent study in which cultures were performed with strict attention to both specimen transport and culture technique. Anaerobic bacteria were present in 23% of the 130 patients studied and usually were associated with aerobic organisms. Anaerobic bacteria were isolated with only slightly higher frequency in early as opposed to late VAP and were more likely in patients who were orotracheally intubated and had impaired consciousness or airway reflexes at the time of intubation. These patients were also younger, and their simplified acute physiologic scores were worse.[153] Given the available data, anaerobic bacteria are considered to be clinically important in situations in which gross aspiration is likely at the time of intubation and less so in patients on long-term mechanical ventilation.

Although community-acquired pneumonia (with the exception of aspiration pneumonia) is generally considered to be monomicrobial, an important result of the intensive evaluation given to bronchoscopic culture techniques is the recognition that nosocomial pneumonia is a polymicrobial infection in as many as 40% of culture-positive cases using PSB.[24, 100] This most often involves a combination of gram-negative aerobic bacilli, with or without gram-positive cocci

such as *S. aureus*.[25, 36] In autopsy series multiple organisms also have been cultured from the lungs of patients with VAP.

Although the frequency of other pathogens—including viruses, fungi, and intracellular bacteria—is not known, these organisms may be important pathogens, particularly in epidemic situations. Neonates and immunocompromised hosts are specific populations at risk. The diagnosis of viral pneumonia is pursued infrequently in ventilated patients because of low clinical suspicion, limitations of diagnostic techniques to differentiate asymptomatic shedding from actual disease, and lack of effective therapy.[154] In addition, traditional definitions of "nosocomial" are difficult to apply when incubation periods may extend well beyond 48 hours.[155] Respiratory viruses that have been implicated in ventilator-dependent patients include influenza, respiratory syncytial virus (RSV), parainfluenza, and adenovirus. These may cause outbreaks of pneumonia in ventilated patients in pediatric, neonatal, and bone marrow units and are associated with significant mortality.[156-160] In one pediatric/medical ICU, 45% of intubated patients had evidence of RSV infection, with an increased mortality noted in this group. Both community-acquired and nosocomial infection were found.[156] Adenovirus most often causes conjunctivitis and pharyngitis[161] but is also associated with sporadic pulmonary infection in mechanically ventilated patients.[157] It is probably an important pathogen in lung transplant patients as well and as such may be encountered in both medical and surgical ICUs.

The appearance of respiratory viruses may be sporadic or seasonal, as in the case of influenza and parainfluenza viruses, coinciding with community outbreaks. They may be transmitted through fomites or by contact with staff and visitors with mild or asymptomatic community-acquired illness. This is in contrast to bacterial VAP, in which aspiration is a more likely pathogenic mechanism, although epidemic bacterial VAP due to exogenous transmission is also reported.[160]

Cytomegalovirus (CMV), herpes simplex virus (HSV), and other viruses of the herpes group are important causes of pneumonia in immunocompromised patients. Most disease resulting from this group of viruses is due to reactivation of latent infection but may be newly acquired in the hospital as well. Reactivation of latent HSV may involve the lower respiratory tract, typically causing ulcerative tracheobronchitis, although parenchymal disease has been reported.[162, 163] Nosocomial acquisition, because it causes primary infection, is associated with more severe manifestations of disease.

Legionella spp. are well known causes of nosocomial pneumonia, found in approximately 3% to 10% of cases in some institutions.[164–169] One report showed an infection rate as high as 30% when hospital water systems were contaminated with the organism.[170] The likelihood of infection with *Legionella* is usually affected by the degree to which the bacterium is endemic in the local environment. *Mycoplasma pneumoniae* and *Chlamydiae pneumoniae* have only recently been recognized as respiratory pathogens. Diagnostic methods for these are not employed routinely, and until culture and identification techniques are more widely available, their relative importance in VAP will remain unclear.

Nosocomial fungal pneumonias are well documented in severely immunocompromised patients, but their true incidence in mechanically ventilated patients is unknown. In neutropenic patients, fungal pneumonia should be suspected in the presence of new infiltrates and positive cultures for *Aspergillus* spp. from any respiratory specimen, including nasal swabs. The diagnosis can be difficult to make, however, and open biopsy may be required to adequately rule it out in patients with prolonged neutropenia. *Candida* pneumonia in these patients may occur as a result of hematogenous spread of the organism and has a characteristic miliary pattern on chest radiographs. Evidence of metastatic infection to other organs, such as the retina, often can be found on physical examination. Most ICU patients do not fall into this group but may be relatively immune deficient in other ways. *Candida* spp. frequently are isolated from sputum and bronchoscopically obtained cultures in ventilated patients, al-

though histologic evidence of tissue invasion is rarely obtained. One study that carefully examined the significance of *Candida* spp. in respiratory specimens found that, although present in many ventilated non-neutropenic patients at autopsy (40%), *Candida* in culture did not predict tissue involvement in the lung. In that study, only 1 of 25 patients had histologically documented fungal pneumonia, and the incidence of candidal pneumonia was 8%.[171] Lung biopsy is not feasible in many ICU patients, and so the use of antifungal therapy in nosocomial pneumonia remains largely empiric, based on the presence of risk factors and a failure to respond to antibacterial therapy.

TREATMENT

Antimicrobial drugs, used singly or in combination, are the mainstay of therapy for nosocomial pneumonia. Unfortunately, there are relatively few data comparing different antibiotic regimens, despite the importance of nosocomial pneumonia and the tremendous costs of the drugs used to treat it. This is in part due to the difficulty with diagnosis, which hampers attempts to study the problem clinically. As a result, many of the underlying principles that guide antibiotic use in VAP are extrapolated from other patient populations, such as febrile neutropenics, or from epidemiologic studies in which comparisons of treatment modalities are often secondary. Although it is generally accepted that the use of one or more agents active against the pathogens involved leads to improved outcomes, at least one study has concluded that mortality in selected patient groups, such as those with ARDS, is not affected by using "appropriate" as opposed to "inappropriate" antibiotics.[172] Still other groups of investigators have found persistence of pathogens at autopsy despite use of drugs with in vitro activity.[173, 174] A few studies dealing specifically with pneumonia, however, have shown improved outcomes with the use of appropriate antibiotic therapy.[13, 174, 175]

Because patients with VAP are likely to have significant underlying lung pathology, it is unrealistic to expect antibiotic therapy to produce the cure rates seen in many other infections. The estimated attributable mortality rate of about 30% suggests that antimicrobials could at best decrease mortality by that amount. Other patients would be expected to die of their primary disease despite appropriate treatment.[176] Additional benefits might be incurred from the "appropriate" use of antimicrobial drugs, but these are more difficult to measure. They include a decreased prevalence of resistant bacteria and a decrease in the cost of ICU care. Whether an antimicrobial drug is judged appropriate is generally based on the results of sensitivity testing from the microbiology laboratory. Other factors, however, ensure that therapy is optimal. Issues to consider in choosing antibiotics can be thought of in terms of drug- and host-specific concerns. When initial empiric therapy is chosen, certain environmental factors become important as well.

Adequate drug delivery to the site of infection is a key principle of antimicrobial chemotherapy. Antibiotic penetration into lung tissues has been measured for most drugs that are used commonly for pneumonia, although it is not clear which drug levels are asociated with efficacy in respiratory infections.[177] In pneumonia, concentrations of drug in the epithelial lining fluid, macrophages, and neutrophils are likely to be especially relevant. Serum levels are also important when bacteremia is present.[177] Cephalosporins and other beta-lactam antibiotics do not enter cells, achieving levels in the extracellular space equal to those in the serum. Concentrations of these drugs in bronchial mucosal biopsy specimens are proportionate to the amount of extracellular space and are roughly 40% of serum levels. Levels of beta-lactam drugs decrease even further in the epithelial lining fluid.[177] The fluoroquinolones, in contrast, penetrate well into cells and across the pulmonary capillary epithelium, hence levels in both bronchial mucosa and epithelial lining fluid exceed serum levels.[177, 178] Macrolides and trimethoprim, which may be useful in selected cases, also penetrate well into lung tissues, although some macrolides (e.g., azithromycin) do not achieve high serum levels.[177] These two classes of drugs also concentrate within some inflammatory cells, such as macrophages and polymorphonuclear leukocytes.[177, 179] Aminoglycosides are too polar to penetrate readily into lung tissues and may be inactivated in the acid environment of a pulmonary infection.[177, 178] For these reasons, aminoglycosides are inappropriate monotherapy for pneumonia.

Proper dosing of different antibiotics also requires knowledge of bactericidal mechanisms. Beta-lactam drugs and vancomycin kill bacteria with time-dependent kinetics, based on the duration in which serum levels exceed the bacteria's minimal inhibitory concentration (MIC). The bactericidal effects of aminoglycosides and quinolones, in contrast, are concentration dependent. These drugs kill more effectively at higher concentrations, which is why poor aminoglycoside penetration into the lungs is such a significant factor in the choice of therapy for pneumonia. One advantage over beta-lactams, however, is the prolonged postantibiotic effect that allows for continued suppression of bacterial growth after serum levels fall below the organism's MIC. Of the beta-lactam drugs, only the carbapenems (such as imipenem and meropenem) have this feature. Attempts to circumvent the poor lung penetration of aminoglycosides include the use of aerosols and direct instillation via a catheter placed into the endotracheal tube.[180, 181] However, administration of aminoglycosides directly into the lung has not been studied adequately in the setting of VAP and should not be considered a viable alternative to the use of systemic therapy. All these individual pharmacokinetic profiles must be considered along with the MIC for specific organisms before appropriate drugs can be chosen.[182]

Host Considerations

Host considerations may dictate antibiotic choices via a need to minimize particular toxicities or avoid allergic reactions and drug interactions. Hypersensitivity to beta-lactam drugs is estimated to occur in 5% to 10% of the general population and may be a difficult factor to confirm or rule out in the critical care patient. For these patients, quinolones or aztreonam, a monobactam drug without significant cross-allergy, may be useful. Additive toxicity—particularly renal—is also a common concern in ICU patients being treated with aminoglycoside therapy. Although certain quinolones (ciprofloxacin), antipseudomonal penicillins (with or without beta-lactamase inhibitors), and later-generation cephalosporins and carbapenems share a spectrum of activity, none of these has shown consistent synergy in vitro, as is seen with the aminoglycosides. Because the in vitro synergy between beta-lactam drugs and aminoglycosides is supported by in vivo experience with pseudomonal infections, the risk–benefit balance may tilt toward continued use of this combination despite the presence of renal disease.[183] When aminoglycosides cannot be used, ciprofloxacin may be a reasonable substitute. Double beta-lactam coverage for gram-negative pathogens should be avoided unless specific testing is done. The results of in vitro synergy tests show that synergism, indifference, and antagonism all may occur in a somewhat unpredictable manner. Selection of resistance is an additional concern with beta-lactam combinations.[184]

Specific organ dysfunction, such as kidney or liver failure, also may limit the use of particular drugs because of the effects on drug metabolism and elimination. Trimethoprim-sulfamethoxazole is particularly difficult to administer in the setting of renal failure because of the differing and unpredictable effects on elimination of the two components and their metabolites, requir-

ing close monitoring of drug levels.[179] In choosing initial therapy, the clinician also must consider both the host and environmental factors that influence the nature of colonizing bacteria. Factors that predispose toward colonization with particular microorganisms are shown in Table 17–5.

Empirical Therapy

Initial therapy in patients with VAP is almost always empirical, based on endemic hospital flora, local sensitivity patterns, underlying diseases, and severity of illness. In 1995 the American Thoracic Society (ATS) published a consensus statement outlining initial treatment recommendations for the entire spectrum of hospital-acquired pneumonia, including VAP. Because the organisms implicated in VAP developing within the first 5 days after intubation are less likely to include *P. aeruginosa* or methicillin-resistant *S. aureus* (MRSA), ATS guidelines for early-onset VAP suggest empiric monotherapy with a nonpseudomonal second- or third-generation cephalosporin, a beta-lactam/beta-lactamase inhibitor combination, or, in the case of penicillin/cephalosporin allergy, a fluoroquinolone.[176] Aztreonam, a monobactam, is also valuable in patients allergic to penicillin, although its lack of activity against gram-positive organisms may require the addition of clindamycin, nafcillin, or vancomycin.

When risk factors for *Pseudomonas* and *S. aureus* are present, including both those

TABLE 17–5. Risk Factors for Colonization or Pneumonia with Specific Pathogens[139, 164, 176]

PATHOGEN	RISK FACTORS
S. aureus	Drug abuse, diabetes mellitus, chronic renal failure, coma, multiple trauma (especially neurologic trauma), recent influenza, atopy
Methicillin-resistant *S. aureus*	Same as *S. aureus* plus prior antibiotic therapy
P. aeruginosa, Acinetobacter spp., *Enterobacter* spp.	Prior antibiotic therapy, prolonged hospital or intensive care unit stay
Legionella spp.	High-dose steroids, endemic conditions
A. fumigatus	High-dose steroids, neutropenia, hospital construction
Anaerobes	Altered mental status, gross aspiration

noted in Table 17–5 or an onset of VAP more than 5 days after intubation, recommendations in the ATS review are to begin empirical treatment with combination therapy. Either an aminoglycoside or ciprofloxacin should be added to an antipseudomonal beta-lactam, and vancomycin should be given until cultures show that MRSA is not present.[178] In units with a high prevalence of *Enterobacter* spp, a cephalosporin never should be used alone because of the reports of in vivo beta-lactamase induction.[138] Optimal empirical therapy for *Enterobacter* consists of an antipseudomonal penicillin, for example, piperacillin, and an aminoglycoside. Given current patterns of resistance, tobramycin is preferred over gentamicin. In general, it is prudent to reserve the empirical use of selected antibiotics (e.g., carbapenems) for patients in whom pneumonia develops while they are being treated with other drugs.

Because most ICU patients seem to have risk factors for more resistant pathogens, the cornerstone of treatment for VAP traditionally has consisted of combination therapy with an aminoglycoside and a beta-lactam antibiotic. The rationale for a combination regimen is (1) to achieve broad spectrum coverage for empirical therapy, (2) to decrease the emergence of resistance during therapy, and (3) to provide synergy. In recent years, monotherapy for nosocomial pneumonia has become a possibility, with the development of agents having both extended gram-negative coverage and adequate lung penetration. These agents include the third-generation cephalosporins, carbapenems, ureidopenicillins, the beta-lactam/beta-lactamase inhibitor combinations, and fluoroquinolones. The choice of specific drugs in empirical regimens differs from one hospital to another and even among different ICUs in the same hospital. These choices should be based on a knowledge of endemic organisms and their sensitivity patterns in each ICU.

Specific Therapy

When specific pathogens are isolated, therapy should be narrowed to monotherapy when appropriate. This probably can be done safely after 2 to 3 days, even if the infecting pathogen is not isolated, as long as cultures do not show *P. aeruginosa, Acinetobacter* spp., *Enterobacter* spp., or MRSA.[185] Although oral agents with excellent absorption are currently available (i.e., ciprofloxacin) and have been used to complete therapy in hospitalized patients, they should be used with caution in critically ill patients who may have deficits in gastrointestinal function. Although antibiotics frequently are discussed in terms of a "course" of therapy, this is a particularly nonquantitative phrase when used in reference to nosocomial pneumonia. Duration of antibiotic therapy for VAP should be individualized because there are no prospective studies that address the issue. For most patients on mechanical ventilation, a minimum of 14 to 21 days is needed to decrease the risk of relapse. In patients with less severe pneumonia or pathogens such as *S. pneumoniae* or *H. influenzae* a shorter course of therapy may be sufficient. Features associated with delayed or incomplete resolution of nosocomial pneumonia include necrotizing gram-negative pneumonia, malnutrition, severe debilitation, and multilobar involvement or cavitation on chest radiograph.[176]

Defining an expected rate of resolution has been difficult. Because VAP occurs in a heterogenous group of patients, the natural history of the disease may vary with underlying disease conditions, bacterial virulence characteristics, antibiotic sensitivity patterns, and other patient factors. Improvement usually is not apparent in the first 48 to 72 hours after initiation of treatment and, unless specific microbiologic information is received or progressive deterioration is noted, antibiotic regimens should not be altered during this time.[176] In one study, fewer than 20% of patients with VAP had rapid improvement.[128] Reasons for failure to respond to therapy include incorrect diagnosis of pneumonia,[98] underlying disease conditions,[13, 30] bacterial resistance, unsuspected pathogens such as tuberculosis or *Pneumocystis carinii* pneumonia[176] and complications such as empyema. An apparent lack of response can also be seen as a result of drug fever or the presence of infection in other sites.[176] Sinus infection commonly coexists with VAP,[74] and in patients with ARDS, particular attention should be given to evaluating the abdomen for infection.[186]

Certain pathogens have proved especially difficult to eradicate[187, 188] and may be a cause for not responding to treatment. A retrospective study of *Pseudomonas* pneumonia in the ICU found that, of patients who survived the initial episode, half had recurrent disease despite what was considered to be adequate antibiotic therapy. The mortality rate of approximately 40% with the first episode increased to 60% by the end of the hospital stay in the entire group, largely because of additional deaths in the group of patients with recurrent *Pseudomonas* pneumonia.[187] Another group of investigators prospectively compared strains of *Pseudomonas* from patients with multiple episodes of VAP. Chromosomal fingerprinting showed that all but one of nine recurrent episodes were the result of persistence of the same organism that caused the original infection.[188] Whether a different approach to drug utilization might affect the incidence of recurrent pneumonia or long-term mortality rates is unknown.

Other Treatment Issues

These recommendations do not address the question of empirical therapy in the immunocompromised host, including patients with human immunodeficiency virus (HIV) infection, prolonged neutropenia, organ transplantation, and hematologic malignancies. Although bacterial infection is common in these patient groups as well, unusual pathogens such as *Aspergillus, Pneumocystis carinii,* and CMV occur with sufficient frequency that more extensive, and sometimes invasive, testing must be pursued. Little can be said regarding the role of antiviral therapy in the treatment of VAP. Acyclovir and ganciclovir are indicated for HSV and CMV, respectively. Most of these cases occur in a patient population with severe cellular immune dysfunction, although HSV has been seen in elderly patients with prolonged ventilation.[162, 163] Ribavirin and RSV immune globulin are approved for RSV pneumonia in children. Their efficacy in

adults with immune compromise due to bone marrow or solid organ transplants is not clear because there are no controlled trials, although they are being used more frequently in these settings.[189-191] There is no current therapy for adenovirus infection. Serious fungal pneumonia is best treated with amphotericin B, either standard or liposomal preparations. Although azole compounds with good in vitro activity are available, their use in the ICU has limited experience. In particular itraconazole, which is active against *Aspergillus* spp., is characterized by poor oral bioavailability in critically ill patients, and therapeutic drug levels are hard to achieve.[192] As yet, there is no parenteral formulation.

Although the pharmaceutical industry and others continue to develop new classes of antibiotics, resources have also been devoted to therapies that might remodulate the host response to infection. These immunomodulators include both passive and active immunization[193, 194] and monoclonal antibodies against bacterial cell wall components or host immune effector molecules, such as tumor necrosis factor.[195] Recombinant molecules designed to downregulate (interleukin-1 receptor antagonist, tumor necrosis factor receptor) or upregulate (interferon-gamma) the inflammatory response and therefore decrease tissue injury are also under study in animals and in human trials.[195, 196] To date, these interventions have not proved reproducibly effective, nor have they been shown to improve survival in ICU patients. Only one biologic modifier, filgrastrim (granulocyte colony-stimulating factor [G-CSF]), has been studied specifically in the setting of pneumonia, with results suggesting a decrease in complications in patients with severe community-acquired infection.[197]

PREVENTION

The prevention of VAP has been a significant challenge. Relatively few interventions have attained uniform clinical acceptance, despite a number of epidemiologic studies that have attempted to clarify the role of medical devices and bacterial reservoirs in the pathogenesis of pneumonia in these patients. Recommendations for the prevention of nosocomial pneumonia have been published by the CDC,[58] incorporating both epidemiologic evidence and expert consensus (Table 17–6). Several of the most important are discussed in detail below.

Infection Control

A national study conducted by the CDC in the 1970s found that the presence of a hospital-wide infection control and surveillance program, including at least one nurse per 250 hospital beds, was moderately effective in reducing rates of hospital-acquired pneumonia.[198] Although these data were not specific for ICU patients, the use of organized infection control is widely accepted as an important factor in reducing VAP rates. Surveillance data for bacterial pneumonia in ventilated patients should be expressed as a rate, for example, number of pneumo-

TABLE 17–6. Centers for Disease Control and Prevention Recommendations for Measures to Prevent Ventilator-Associated Pneumonia (VAP)*

	STRONGLY RECOMMENDED (STRONG EXPERIMENTAL AND EPIDEMIOLOGIC EVIDENCE)	STRONGLY RECOMMENDED (SUGGESTIVE EVIDENCE AND EXPERT CONSENSUS)	SUGGESTED (STRONG RATIONALE AND SUGGESTIVE EVIDENCE, MAY NOT APPLY TO ALL HOSPITALS)	UNRESOLVED ISSUE
EDUCATION AND SURVEILLANCE	Surveillance for pneumonia in ventilated patients with data on pathogens and susceptibility patterns No routine surveillance cultures of patients or equipment Staff education			
INTERRUPTION OF TRANSMISSION*	Handwashing, before and after contact with patients and respiratory devices (regardless of whether or not gloves are worn) Barrier precautions (wear gloves for handling secretions, change gloves and wash hands)	Change suction tubing and canisters between patients Use sterile water in suction catheter if re-entry planned Wear gowns when contact with respiratory secretions anticipated	Use of sterile single use catheter for open suction system	Closed vs. open system suctioning Sterile vs. clean gloves for suctioning

Table continued on following page

TABLE 17–6. Centers for Disease Control and Prevention Recommendations for Measures to Prevent Ventilator-Associated Pneumonia (VAP)* *Continued*

	STRONGLY RECOMMENDED (STRONG EXPERIMENTAL AND EPIDEMIOLOGIC EVIDENCE)	STRONGLY RECOMMENDED (SUGGESTIVE EVIDENCE AND EXPERT CONSENSUS)	SUGGESTED (STRONG RATIONALE AND SUGGESTIVE EVIDENCE, MAY NOT APPLY TO ALL HOSPITALS)	UNRESOLVED ISSUE
MODIFICATION OF HOST	Do not use systemic antibiotics for prophylaxis against VAP Pneumococcal vaccination in high-risk patients	Remove endotracheal and enteral tubes when possible Routine verification of feeding tube placement Assess GI motility and adjust feedings to avoid regurgitation Clear secretions above cuff before deflating or moving tube Elevate head of bed 30–45° if possible Postoperative pulmonary toilet, encourage deep cough	Stress ulcer prophylaxis that does not raise gastric pH Postoperative incentive spirometry or intermittent positive pressure breathing	Small bore tubes for enteral feeding Continuous vs. intermittent feedings Distal feeding tube placement Oro- vs. nasotracheal tube placement ET with port for suctioning of subglottic secretions SDD Acidification of gastric feedings Kinetic beds or continuous lateral rotational therapy

*See reference 58 for details regarding sterilization and maintenance of ventilators and respiratory therapy equipment.
ET, endotracheal tube; GI, gastrointestinal; SDD, selective digestive (tract) decontamination.

nias per 1000 ventilator days. Data in this format can be compared readily with NNIS benchmark rates or used to delineate trends within a given ICU. When interpreting surveillance data, remember that they may be affected by a number of factors, including changes in the intrinsic risk of the patient population (i.e., neutropenia, HIV infection), changes in case identification and surveillance techniques, and incomplete medical records.[136] Although routine surveillance cultures of patients or the environment are not recommended in the ICU,[58] the microbiology laboratory is an important source of information on both prevalence patterns for specific organisms and current microbial resistance patterns. These data can be used best if mechanisms are in place for frequent feedback to ICU practicioners.

Because ICU patients are most likely to become infected with endogenous flora, measures that decrease the rate of colonization with pathogenic bacteria are among the most important infection control procedures. Bacteria with increased resistance are harder to treat, increase expense, and are associated with increased mortality.[199] Strict attention to handwashing and barrier precautions when indicated can decrease the hand-to-hand transmission of resistant organisms. This remains a frequent mode of spread of these organisms despite recognition that good handwashing with antibacterial soap can cut transmission rates.[58] The other major means of acquiring resistant bacteria is through selection pressure. Prior antibiotic therapy may induce resistance in endogenous flora and is a well-described risk factor for pneumonia due to *Pseudomonas* and *Acinetobacter*.[24]

The impact of antibiotic choices reaches beyond individual patient outcomes. The decisions made daily in the ICU exert selection pressure on the local environment, favoring the emergence of organisms that are resistant to commonly used antibiotics. These organisms become endemic to a particular ICU and proceed to colonize even patients who may not have been treated previously with broad-spectrum antibiotics.

There are a number of examples in the literature that demonstrate this phenomenon on a local level as well as in response to national trends in antibiotic use. In one hospital, reporting in 1989, *Klebsiella pneumoniae* developed a specific substitution in beta-lactamase, which conferred transferable resistance to cefotaxime. This drug had been used heavily throughout the hospital.[140] Selection of a cephalosporin-resistant *Klebsiella* strain occurred in another hospital during attempts to eradicate an outbreak of aminoglycoside-resistant *Acinetobacter*. This prompted an institutional switch to imipenem use and resulted in re-emergence of the *Acinetobacter*, newly resistant to imipenem.[141] Resistance to cephalosporins has become widespread among *Enterobacter* spp. as well and may develop during therapy,[138] leading some to recommend that this class of drugs be avoided for specific therapy if *Enterobacter* is isolated, and for empiric therapy if this bacterial species is prevalent in a given setting.[138]

Perhaps the broadest spectrum antibiotic that has been in widespread use over the past decade is imipenem, a beta-lactam drug of the carbapenem class. These drugs are resistant to hydrolysis by the intrinsic chromosomal type I beta-lactamase that has become prevalent in gram-negative isolates

in hospitals. Several studies have shown a significant increase in imipenem resistance among *P. aeruginosa* isolates, more common in ICUs and in isolates from the respiratory tract.[200] The development of antimicrobial resistance, already a difficult clinical problem, eventually may outpace the rate at which new drugs enter the marketplace. The burden for delaying this crisis lies to a large extent on the ICU practitioner, as one of the primary users of antimicrobial agents.

Because of data showing that outbreaks of resistant organisms can be controlled through strict limits on antibiotic use,[141, 201] some have questioned whether these same principles could be applied to help prevent these outbreaks from occuring in the first place.[202] To this end, one institution published a study whereby the "default" empirical antibiotic used to treat suspected gram-negative infections in ventilated patients was switched from a third-generation cephalosporin (ceftazidime) to a fluoroquinolone (ciprofloxacin). Each drug was used preferentially for a 6-month period.[203] This has been referred to as "crop rotation,"[202] and, akin to the concept that diseases affecting corn will not persist if the field is planted in beans next year, the ultimate goal of such a schedule is to decrease that percentage of pneumonias that are caused by the spread of resistant and more virulent bacteria. This particular study was too limited in duration to show that such a strategy can have a long-term impact on pneumonia rates or the prevalence of resistant bacteria, but it added to data that show antibiotic choices can be made to effect specific changes in endemic ICU flora.

Reducing Gastric Colonization and Aspiration

Given the suggestion in some studies that the stomach is an important source of organisms for pneumonia, there have been a number of attempts to decrease the incidence of VAP by eradicating this reservoir. Most investigators have evaluated the effect of different regimens for stress ulcer prophylaxis, comparing agents that increase gastric pH, such as antacids and H_2 blockers, with sucralfate. These studies have produced conflicting results.[204–207] This is probably due to confounding factors such as differences in patient type and a potential antibacterial action of sucralfate. In addition, some of these studies did not record gastric pH, so that the effectiveness of acid suppression and the incidence of alkaline pH in sucralfate groups caused by intrinsic factors cannot be evaluated. There probably are subgroups of patients, such as those at risk for late-onset VAP, who might benefit from sucralfate for ulcer prophylaxis, but this point continues to be a source for debate.[36] Patient positioning has been cited as a potential risk for VAP, through an increased incidence of aspiration in the supine versus semirecumbant position.[208] The optimum method for feeding, with respect to enteral versus parenteral and stomach versus small bowel delivery, is not known, although it is logical to minimize gastric volume and preserve acidity by delivering enteral feeds directly to the small bowel.

Antibiotic Prophylaxis

Antibiotic prophylaxis has been a very successful means of infection control in the operative setting but has been much less useful in the ICU, where the period of risk extends over many days. Systemic prophylaxis for nosocomial pneumonia has proven uniformly unsuccessful. No difference was found in a 1959 study using chloramphenicol versus placebo,[209] and in a large ICU study 30 years later, no decrease in the incidence of early-onset pneumonia was found when patients underwent prophylaxis with either penicillin G or cefoxitin.[210] Topical prophylaxis, using aerosolized aminoglycosides and/or polymixin B, has been equally unsatisfactory.[211–214] The hazards of prophylactic antibiotics were well outlined in a study of aerosolized polymixin B in patients in a respiratory ICU, in which an initial decline in airway colonization and pneumonia rates was followed by the emergence of antibiotic resistance and an increase in pneumonia-related deaths.[211]

Selective decontamination of the digestive tract (SDD) was conceived as a means of selectively inhibiting colonization by gram-negative aerobic organisms through the use of nonabsorbable antibiotics given into the stomach and oropharynx. Some investigators have added a systemic antibiotic during the first few days of prophylaxis. Although a number of studies have shown a decrease in the incidence of pneumonia, this has not been a consistent finding, and there has been no impact on mortality, length of ICU stay, ventilator days, or overall antibiotic use.[215] Conceptually, this might have the same potential for encouraging the overgrowth of resistant pathogens, and this has been shown in several of the many studies in this area.[216–220]

Other Preventive Strategies

Recommended procedures for maintenance of respiratory equipment have been published by the CDC and therefore are not be discussed in detail here.[58] With current respiratory care methods, the ventilator itself is rarely believed to be the cause of pneumonia, despite rapid colonization by the patient's endogenous flora. One device-related source of bacterial innoculation that has not been addressed adequately, however, is the subglottic pool of secretions. Only a small number of patients have been studied to see whether systematic removal of these secretions can decrease the incidence of VAP.[71, 221] Further investigation is needed as specialized endotracheal tubes that allow suctioning of this area become more widely available. Another potential modification of the endotracheal tube is the use of new materials with decreased propensity for the development of biofilms.[176]

SUMMARY

The past two decades have seen significant progress in understanding the pathogenesis of and risks leading to the development of VAP. Although current diagnostic techniques remain somewhat lacking in sensitivity and specificity, the use of bronchoscopic culture methods has been a valuable research tool that should continue to help elucidate not only the microbiology but also the natural history of infection at all levels of the respiratory tract. One of the most significant concerns facing the ICU practitioner in the next decade is the increase in bacterial resistance. Because ICUs are a high-use area for antimicrobials, careful use of currently available drugs may have an impact on resistance patterns throughout hospitals. Finally, we can hope that strategies to enhance the host response to bacterial infections in the lung will become an invaluable addition to the armament for treating nosocomial pneumonia.

REFERENCES

1. Fagon JY, Chastre J, Hance AJ, et al: Nosocomial pneumonia in ventilated patients: a cohort study evaluating attributable mortality and hospital stay. Am J Med 94:281–288, 1993.
2. Leu HS, Kaiser DL, Mori M, et al: Hospital-acquired pneumonia: attributable mortality and morbidity. Am J Epidemiol 29:1258–1267, 1989.
3. Edwards J, Jarvis W: The distribution of nosocomial infections by site and pathogen in adult and pediatric intensive care units in the United States 1986. In: Final Program and Abstracts of the 3rd Decennial International Conference on Nosocomial Infections. Atlanta, GA: The Centers for Disease Control and the National Foundation for Infectious Diseases, 1990, abstract B19.
4. Horan TC, White JW, Jarvis WR, et al: Nosocomial infection surveillance: 1984. MMWR Morb Mortal Wkly Rep 35(1ss):17ss–29ss, 1986.
5. Remarz JA, Pierce AK, Mays BB, et al: The potential role of inhalation therapy equipment in nosocomial pulmonary infection. J Clin Invest 44:1834–839, 1965.
6. Pierce AK, Edmonson EB, McGee G, et al: An analysis of factors predisposing to gram-negative bacillary necrotizing pneumonia. Am Rev Respir Dis 94:309–315, 1966.
7. Pierce AK, Sanford JP, Thomas GD, et al: Long-term evaluation of decontamination of inhalation therapy equipment and the occurrence of necrotizing pneumonia. N Engl J Med 282:528–531, 1970.
8. Joshi N, Localio AR, Hamory BH: A predictive risk index for nosocomial pneumonia in the intensive care unit. Am J Med 91:135–142, 1992.
9. Langer M, Mosconi P, Cigada M, et al: Long-term respiratory support and risk of pneumonia in critically ill patients. Am Rev Respir Dis 140:302–305, 1989.
10. Wenzel, RP, Osterman CA, Hunting KJ: Hospital-acquired infections: II, infection rates by site, service and common procedures in a university hospital. Am J Epidemiol 104:645–651, 1979.
11. Cross AS, Roup B: Role of respiratory assistance in endemic nosocomial pneumonia. Am J Med 70:681–685, 1981.
12. Haley RW, Hoofon TM, Culver DH, et al: Nosocomial infections in U.S. hospitals 1975–1976: estimated frequency by selected characteristics of patients. Am J Med 70:947–959, 1981.
13. Celis R, Torres A, Gatell JM, et al: Nosocomial pneumonia: a multivariate analysis of risk and prognosis. Chest 93:318–324, 1988.
14. Bryant LR, Trinkle JK, Mobin-Uddin K, et al: Bacterial colonization profile with tracheal intubation and mechanical ventilation. Arch Surg 104:647–651, 1972.
15. Lareau SC, Ryan KJ, Diener CF: The relationship between frequency of ventilator circuit changes and infectious hazard. Am Rev Respir Dis 118:493–496, 1978.
16. Du Moulin GC, Hedley-White J, Paterson DG, et al: Aspiration of gastric bacteria in antacid-treated patients: a frequent cause of postoperative colonization of the airway. Lancet 1:242–245, 1982.
17. Mauritz W, Graninger W, Schindler I, et al: Keim-florain magensaft und bronchial sekret bei langzeitbeatmeten intensivpatienten. Anaesthesist 34:203–207, 1985.
18. Braun SR, Levin AB, Clark KL: Role of corticosteroids in the development of pneumonia in mechanically ventilated head trauma victims. Crit Care Med 14:198–201, 1986.
19. Craven DE, Kunches LM, Kilinsky V, et al: Risk factors for pneumonia and fatality in patients receiving continuous mechanical ventilation. Am Rev Respir Dis 133:792–796, 1986.
20. Rashkin MC, Davis T: Acute complications of endotracheal intubation: relationship to reintubation, route, urgency, and duration. Chest 89:165–167, 1986.
21. Ruiz-Santana S, Jiminez AG, Esteban A, et al: ICU pneumonias: a multi-institutional study. Crit Care Med 15:930–932, 1987.
22. Daschner F, Kappstein I, Schuster F, et al: Influence of disposable ("Conchapak") and reusable humidifying systems on the incidence of ventilator pneumonia. J Hosp Infect 11:161–168, 1988.
23. Daschner F, Kappstein I, Reuschenbach K, et al: Stress ulcer prophylaxis and ventilation pneumonia: prevention by antibacterial cytoprotective agents? Infect Control Hosp Epidemiol 9:59–65, 1988.
24. Fagon JY, Chastre J, Domart Y, et al: Nosocomial pneumonia in patients receiving continuous mechanical ventilation: prospective analysis of 52 episodes with use of a protected specimen brush and quantitative culture techniques. Am Rev Respir Dis 139:877–884, 1989.
25. Jimenez P, Torres A, Rodriguez-Roisin R, et al: Incidence and etiology of pneumonia acquired during mechanical ventilation. Crit Care Med 17:882–885, 1989.

26. Klein BS, Perloff WH, Maki DG: Reduction of nosocomial infection during pediatric intensive care by protective isolation. N Engl J Med 320:1714–1721, 1989.

27. Reusser P, Zimmerli W, Scheidegger D, et al: Role of gastric colonization in nosocomial infection and endotoxemia: a prospective study in neurosurgical patients on mechanical ventilation. J Infect Dis 160:414–421, 1989.

28. Deppe SA, Kelly JW, Thoi LL, et al: Incidence of colonization, nosocomial pneumonia, and mortality in critically ill patients using a Trach Care closed suction system versus an open-suction system: prospective randomized study. Crit Care Med 18:1389–1393, 1990.

29. Jacobs S, Chang RWS, Lee B, et al: Continuous enteral feeding: a major cause of pneumonia among ventilated intensive care unit patients. JPEN J Parenter Enteral Nutr 14:353–356, 1990.

30. Torres A, Aznar R, Gatell JM, et al: Incidence, risk, and prognosis factors of nosocomial pneumonia in mechanically ventilated patients. Am Rev Respir Dis 142:523–528, 1990.

31. Dreyfuss D, Djedaini K, Weber P, et al: Prospective study of nosocomial pneumonia and of patient and circuit colonization during mechanical ventilation with circuit changes every 48 hours versus no change. Am Rev Respir Dis 143:738–743, 1991.

32. Jarvis WR, Edwards JR, Culver DH, et al: Nosocomial infection rates in adult and pediatric intensive care units in the United States. Am J Med 91(suppl 3B):185S–191S, 1991.

33. National Nosocomial Infections Surveillance (NNIS) Report: Data summary from October 1986–April 1997, issued May 1997. Am J Infect Control 25:477–487, 1997.

34. Langer M, Cigada M, Mandelli M, et al: Early-onset pneumonia: a multicenter study in intensive care units. Intensive Care Med 13:342–346, 1987.

35. Pugin J, Auckenthaler R, Lew DP, et al: Oropharyngeal decontamination decreases incidence of ventilator-associated pneumonia: a randomized, placebo-controlled, double-blind clinical trial. JAMA 265:2704–2710, 1991.

36. Prod'hom G, Leuenberger P, Koerfer J, et al: Nosocomial pneumonia in mechanically ventilated patients receiving antacids, ranitidine, or sucralfate as prophylaxis for stress ulcer: a randomized controlled trial. Ann Intern Med 120:653–662, 1994.

37. Stevens RM, Teres D, Stallman JJ, et al: Pneumonia in an intensive care unit: a 30-month experience. Arch Intern Med 134:105–111, 1974.

38. Kollef MH: Ventilator-associated pneumonia: a multivariate analysis. JAMA 270:1965–1970, 1993.

39. Hanson LC, Weber DJ, Rutala WA, et al: Risk factors for nosocomial pneumonia in the elderly. Am J Med 92:161–166, 1992.

40. Gorensek MJ, Stewart RW, Keys TF, et al: A multi-variate analysis of risk factors for pneumonia following cardiac transplantation. Transplantation 46:860–865, 1988.

41. Hooton TM, Haley RW, Culver DH, et al: The joint association of multiple risk factors with the occurrence of nosocomial infection. Am J Med 70:960–970, 1981.

42. Pannuti C, Gingrich R, Pfaller MA, et al: Nosocomial pneumonia in patients having bone marrow transplant: attributable mortality and risk factors. Cancer 69:2653–2652, 1992.

43. Bryan CS, Reynolds KL: Bacteremic nosocomial pneumonia. Am Rev Respir Dis 129:668–671, 1984.

44. Craig CP, Connelly S: Effect of intensive care unit nosocomial pneumonia on duration of stay and mortality. Am J Infect Control 12:233–238, 1984.

45. Wenzel RP: Hospital-acquired pneumonia: overview of the current state of the art for prevention and control. Eur J Clin Microbiol Infect Dis 8:56–60, 1989.

46. Huber GL, La Force FM, Johansen WG Jr: Experimental models and pulmonary antimicrobial defenses. In: Brain JD, Proctor DF, Reird DL (eds): Respiratory Defense Mechanisms. New York: Marcel Dekker, 1997, p 983.

47. Berendt RF: Relationship of method of administration to respiratory virulence of *Klebsiella pneumoniae* for mice and squirrel monkeys. Infect Immunol 20:581–592, 1978.

48. Onofrio JM, Toews GB, Lipscombe MF, et al: Granulocyte-alveolar macrophage interaction in the pulmonary clearance of *Staphylococcus aureus*. Am Rev Respir Dis 127:335–341, 1983.

49. Toews GB, Gross GN, Pierce AK: The relationship of innoculum size to lung bacterial adherence and phagocytic cell response in mice. Am Rev Respir Dis 120:559–566, 1979.

50. Juers JA, Rogers RM, McCuredy JB, et al: Enhancement of the bactericidal capacity of alveolar macrophages by human "alveolar lining material." J Clin Invest 58:271–275, 1976.

51. LaForce FM: Effects of alveolar lining material on phagocytic and bactericidal activity of lung macrophages against *Staphylococcus aureus*. J Lab Clin Med 88:691–699, 1976.

52. Huxley EJ, Viroslav J, Grey WR, et al: Pharyngeal aspiration in normal subjects in patients with depressed consciousness. Am J Med 64:564–568, 1978.

53. Reynolds HY: Integrated host defense against infections. In Crystal RG, West JB (eds): The Lung: Scientific Foundations. Vol. 2. Philadelphia: JB Lippincott, 1991, pp 1899–1911.

54. Reinarz JA, Pierce AK, Mays BD, et al: The potential role of inhalation therapy equipment in nosocomial pulmonary infection. J Clin Invest 44:831–839, 1965.

55. Pierce AK, Edmonson EB, McGee G, et al: An analysis of factors predisposing to gram-negative bacillary necrotizing pneumonia. Am Rev Respir Dis 94:309–315, 1966.

56. Pierce AK, Sanford JT, Thomas GD, et al: Long-term evaluation of decontamination of inhalation

therapy equipment and the occurrence of necrotizing pneumonia. N Engl J Med 282:528–531, 1970.

57. Goularte TA, Manning M, Craven DE: Bacterial colonization in humidifying cascade reservoirs after 24 and 48 hours of continuous mechanical ventilation. Infect Control 8:200–203, 1987.

58. Tablan OC, Anderson LJ, Arden NH, et al: Guideline for prevention of nosocomial pneumonia. Infect Control Hosp Epidemiol 15:587–627, 1994.

59. Comhaire A, Lamy M: Contamination rate of sterilized ventilators in an ICU. Crit Care Med 9:546–548, 1981.

60. Craven DE, Goularte TA, Make BJ: Contaminated condensate in mechanical ventilator circuits: a risk factor for nosocomial pneumonia. Am Rev Respir Dis 129:625–628, 1984.

61. Simmons BP, Wong ES: Guideline for prevention of nosocomial pneumonia. Am J Infect Control 11:230–243, 1983.

62. Branson RD, Davis K, Campbell RS, et al: Prospective study of a new protocol utilizing heat humidification and hygroscopic condensor humidifyer. Chest 104:1800–1805, 1993.

63. Gallagher J, Strangeways JEM, Allt-Graham J: Contamination control in long-term ventilation: a clinical study using a heat- and moisture-exchanging filter. Anesthesia 42:476–481, 1987.

64. Rodriguez JL, Gibbons KG, Bitzer LG, et al: Pneumonia: incidence, risk factors, and outcome in injured patients. J Trauma 31:907–912, 1991.

65. Klainer AS, Turndof H, Wu WH, et al: Surface alterations due to endotracheal intubation. Am J Med 58:647–683, 1975.

66. Steen JA: Impact of tube design and material on complications of tracheal intubation. Probl Anesth 2:211–224, 1988.

67. Ramphal R, Small PM, Shands JW Jr, et al: Adherence of *Pseudomonas aeruginosa* to tracheal cells injured by influenza infection or by endotracheal intubation. Infect Immunol 27:614–619, 1980.

68. Sottile FD, Marrie TJ, Prough DS, et al: Nosocomial pulmonary infection: possible etiologic significance of bacterial adhesion to endotracheal tubes. Crit Care Med 14:265–270, 1986.

69. Inglis TJJ, Millar MR, Jones JG, et al: Tracheal tube biofilm as a source of bacterial colonization of the lung. J Clin Microbiol 27:2014–2018, 1989.

70. Cash HA, Woods DE, McCullough B, et al: A rat model of chronic respiratory infection with *Pseudomonas aeruginosa*. Am Rev Respir Dis 119:453–459, 1979.

71. Mahul PH, Auboyer C, Jospe R, et al: Prevention of nosocomial pneumonia in intubated patients: respective role of mechanical subglottic secretions drainage and stress ulcer prophylaxis. Intensive Care Med 18:20–25, 1992.

72. Grillo HC, Cooper JD, Geffin B, et al: A low-pressure cuff for tracheostomy tubes to minimize tracheal injury: a comparative clinical trial. J Thorac Cardiovasc Surg 62:898–907, 1971.

73. Spray SB, Zuidema GD, Cameron JL: Aspiration pneumonia: incidence of aspirations with endotracheal tubes. Am J Surg 131:701–703, 1976.

74. Gal TJ: How does tracheal intubation alter respiratory mechanics? Probl Anesth 2:191–200, 1988.

75. Rouby J-J, Laurent P, Gosnach M, et al: Risk factors and clinical relevance of nosocomial maxillary sinusitis in the critically ill. Am J Respir Crit Care Med 150:776–783, 1994.

76. Sackner MA, Rosen MJ, Wanner A: Effects of oxygen breathing and endotracheal intubation on tracheal mucus velocity of anesthetized dogs. Bull Physiopathol Respir 9:403–416, 1973.

77. Dedhia HV, Ma JY, Vallyathan V, et al: Exposure of rats to hyperoxia: alteration of lavagate parameters and macrophage function. J Toxicol Environ Health 40:1–13, 1993.

78. Minoo P, King RJ, Coalson JJ: Surfactant proteins and lipids are regulated independently during hyperoxia. J Am J Physiol 263:L291–L298, 1992.

79. Rigaud D, Chastre J, Accary JP, et al: Intragastric pH profile during acute respiratory failure in patients with chronic obstructive pulmonary disease: effects of ranitidine and enteral feeding. Chest 90:58–63, 1986.

80. McClelland RN, Shires GT, Prager M: Gastric secretory and splanchnic blood flow studies in man after severe trauma and hemorrhagic shock. Am J Surg 121:134–142, 1971.

81. Atherton ST, White DJ: Stomach as a source of bacteria colonizing respiratory tract during artificial ventilation. Lancet ii:968–969, 1978.

82. Hillman KM, Riordan T, O'Farrell SM, et al: Colonization of the gastric content in critically ill patients. Crit Care Med 10:444–447, 1982.

83. Donowitz GL, Page ML, Mileur BL, et al: Alteration of normal gastric flora in critical care patients receiving antacid and cimetidine therapy. Infect Control 7:23–6, 1986.

84. Neiderman MS, Mantovani R, Schoch P, et al: Patterns and routes of trancheobronchial colonization in mechanically ventilated patients: the role of nutritional status in colonization of the lower airway by *Pseudomonas* species. Chest 95:155–161, 1989.

85. Coalson JJ: The pathology of nosocomial pneumonia. Clin Chest Med 16:13–28, 1995.

86. Johanson WG Jr, Seidenfeld JJ, Gomez P, et al: Bacteriologic diagnosis of nosocomial pneumonia following prolonged mechanical ventilation. Am Rev Respir Dis 137:259–264, 1988.

87. Johanson WG Jr, Higuchi JH, Woods DE, et al: Dissemination of *Pseudomonas aeruginosa* during lung infection: role of oxygen-induced lung injury. Am Rev Respir Dis 132:358, 1985.

88. Chastre J, Viau F, Brun P, et al: Prospective evaluation of the protected specimen brush for the diagnosis of pulmonary infections in ventilated patients. Am Rev Respir Dis 130:924–929, 1984.

89. Bartlett JG: Invasive diagnostic techniques in pulmonary infections. In Pennington JE (ed): Respiratory Infections: Diagnosis and Management. 2nd ed. New York: Raven Press, 1989, p 52.

90. Rouby J-J, de Lassale EM, Poete P, et al: Nosocomial bronchopneumonia in the critically ill: histologic and bacteriologic aspects. Am Rev Respir Dis 146:1059–1066, 1992.
91. Horan TC, Emori TG: Definitions of key terms used in the NNIS system. Am J Infect Control 25:112–116, 1997.
92. Garner JS, Jarvis WR, Emori TG, et al: CDC definitions for nosocomial infections, 1988. Am J Infect Control 16:128–140, 1988.
93. Meduri GU, Chastre J: The standardization of bronchoscopic techniques for ventilator-associated pneumonia. Chest 102(suppl):557S–564S, 1992.
94. Meduri GU, Beals DH, Maijub AG, et al: Protected bronchoalveolar lavage: a new bronchoscopic technique to retrieve uncontaminated distal airway secretions. Am Rev Respir Dis 143:855–864, 1991.
95. Fagon JY, Chastre J, Hance AJ, et al: Detection of nosocomial lung infection in ventilated patients: use of a protected specimen brush and quantitative culture techniques in 147 patients. Am Rev Respir Dis 38:110–116, 1988.
96. Emori TG, Edwards JR, Culver DH, et al: Accuracy of reporting nosocomial infections in intensive-care-unit patients to the National Nosocomial Infections Surveillance system: a pilot study. Infect Control Hosp Epidemiol 19:308–316, 1998.
97. Andrews CP, Coalson JJ, Smith JD, et al: Diagnosis of nosocomial bacterial pneumonia in acute, diffuse lung injury. Chest 3:254–258, 1981.
98. Wunderink RG, Woldenberg LS, Zeiss J, et al: The radiologic diagnosis of autopsy-proven ventilator-associated pneumonia. Chest 101:458–463, 1992.
99. Chastre J, Fagon JY: Invasive diagnostic testing should be routinely used to managed ventilated patients with suspected pneumonia. Am J Respir Crit Care Med 150:570–574, 1994.
100. Torres A, de la Bellacasa JP, Xaubet A, et al: Diagnostic value of quantitative cultures of bronchoalveolar lavage and telescoping plugged catheters in mechanically ventilated patients with bacterial pneumonia. Am Rev Respir Dis 140:306–310, 1989.
101. Chastre J, Fagon JY, Soler P, et al: Diagnosis of nosocomial bacterial pneumonia in intubated patients undergoing ventilation: comparison of the usefulness of bronchoalveolar lavage and the protected specimen brush. Am J Med 85:499–506, 1988.
102. Chastre J, Fagon JY, Bornet M, et al: Comparison of the usefulness of bronchoalveolar lavage and the protected specimen brush for diagnosing nosocomial bacterial pneumonia. Am Rev Respir Dis 145:A542, 1992.
103. Pugin J, Auckenthaler R, Mili N, et al: Diagnosis of ventilator-associated pneumonia by bacteriologic analysis of bronchoscopic and nonbronchoscopic "blind" bronchoalveolar lavage fluid. Am Rev Respir Dis 143:1121–1129, 1991.
104. Wimberly N, Faling LJ, Bartlett JG: A fiberoptic bronchoscopy technique to obtain uncontaminated lower airway secretions for bacterial culture. Am Rev Respir Dis 119:337–343, 1979.
105. Baselski VS, El-Torky M, Coalson JJ, et al: The standardization of criteria for processing and interpreting laboratory specimens in patients with suspected ventilator-associated pneumonia. Chest 102(suppl):571s–579s, 1992.
106. Wimberly N, Willey S, Sullivan N, et al: Antibacterial properties of lidocaine. Chest 76:37–40, 1979.
107. Baughman RP, Thorpe JE, Stanek J, et al: Use of the protected specimen brush in patients with endotracheal or tracheostomy tubes. Chest 91:233–236, 1987.
108. Rein MF, Mandell GI: Bacterial killing by bacteriostatic saline solutions—potential for diagnostic error. N Engl J Med 298:794–795, 1973.
109. Edelstein PH, Meyer RD: Legionnaire's disease: a review. Chest 85:114–120, 1984.
110. Wimberly NW, Bass JB, Boyd BW, et al: Use of a bronchoscopic protected catheter brush for the diagnosis of pulmonary infections. Chest 5:556–562, 1982.
111. Pollock HM, Hawkins EL, Bonner JR, et al: Diagnosis of bacterial pulmonary infections with quantitative protected catheter cultures obtained during bronchoscopy. J Clin Microbiol 17:255–259, 1983.
112. Teague RB, Wallace RJ, Awe RJ: The use of quantitative sterile brush culture and Gram stain analysis in the diagnosis of lower respiratory tract infection. Chest 79:157–161, 1981.
113. Trouillet JL, Guiguet M, Gibert C, et al: Fiberoptic bronchoscopy in ventilated patients: evaluation of cardiopulmonary risk under midazolam sedation. Chest 97:927–933, 1991.
114. Pham LH, Brun-Buisson C, Legrand P, et al: Diagnosis of nosocomial pneumonia in mechanically ventilated patients: comparison of plugged telescoping catheter with the protected specimen brush. Am Rev Respir Dis 143:1055–1061, 1991.
115. Reynolds HY: Bronchoalveolar lavage. Am Rev Respir Dis 135:250–263, 1987.
116. Meduri GU, Baselski V: The role of bronchoalveolar lavage in diagnosing nonopportunistic bacterial pneumonia. Chest 100:179–190, 1991.
117. Torres A, de la Bellacasa JP, Xaubet A, et al: Diagnostic value of quantitative cultures of bronchoalveolar lavage and telescoping plugged catheters in mechanically ventilated patients with bacterial pneumonia. Am Rev Respir Dis 140:306–310, 1989.
118. Rouby JJ, Rosignon MD, Nicolas MH, et al: A prospective study of the protected bronchoalveolar lavage in the diagnosis of nosocomial pneumonia. Anesthesiology 71:679–685, 1989.
119. Chastre J, Fagon JY, Soler P, et al: Quantification of BAL cells containing intracellular bacteria rapidly identifies ventilated patients with nosocomial pneumonia. Chest 95:190S–192S, 1989.
120. Villers D, Derriennic M, Raffi F, et al: Reliability of the bronchoscopic protected specimen brush in

intubated and ventilated patients. Chest 88:527–530, 1985.

121. Lambert RS, Vereen LE, George RB: Comparison of tracheal aspirates and protected brush catheter specimens for identifying pathogenic bacteria in mechanically ventilated patients. Am J Med Sci 297:377–382, 1989.

122. Torres A, de la Bellacasa JP, Rodriguez-Roisin R, et al: Diagnostic value of telescoping plugged catheters in mechanically ventilated patients with bacterial pneumonia using the Metras catheter. Am Rev Respir Dis 138:117–120, 1988.

123. deCastro FR, Violan JS, Capuz BL, et al: Reliability of the bronchoscopic protected catheter bruch in the diagnosis of pneumonia in mechanically ventilated patients. Crit Care Med 19:171–175, 1991.

124. Salata RA, Lederman MM, Shlaes DM, et al: Diagnosis of nosocomial pneumonia in intubated, intensive care unit patients. Am Rev Respir Dis 135:426–432, 1987.

125. Bartlett JG, Finegold SM: Bacteriology of expectorated sputum with quantitative culture and wash techniques compared to transtracheal aspirates. Am Rev Respir Dis 117:1019–1027, 1978.

126. Neiderman MS, Torres A, Summer W: Invasive diagnostic testing is not needed routinely to manage suspected ventilator-associated pneumonia. Am J Respir Crit Care Med 150:565–569, 1994.

127. Dreyfuss D, Mier L, le Bourdelles G, et al: Clinical significance of borderline quantitative protected brush specimen culture results. Am Rev Respir Dis 147:946–951, 1993.

128. Montravers P, Fagon J-Y, Chastre J, et al: Followup protected specimen brushes to assess treatment in nosocomial pneumonia. Am Rev Respir Dis 147:38–44, 1993.

129. Fagon J-Y, Chastre J, Trouillet J-L, et al: Characterization of distal bronchial microflora during acute exacerbations of chronic bronchitis: use of the protected specimen brush technique in 54 mechanically ventilated patients. Am Rev Respir Dis 142:1004–1008, 1990.

130. Kahn FW, Jones JM: Diagnosing bacterial respiratory infection by bronchoalveolar lavage. J Infect Dis 155:862–869, 1987.

131. Rennard S, Basset G, Lecossier D, et al: Estimations of the absolute volume of epithelial lining fluid recovered by bronchoalveolar lavage using urea as an endogenous marker of dilution. J Appl Physiol 60:532–538, 1986.

132. Baughman RP, Bosken CH, Loudon RG, et al: Quantitation of bronchoalveolar lavage with methylene blue. Am Rev Respir Dis 128:266–270, 1983.

133. Guerra LF, Baughman RP: Use of bronchoalveolar lavage to diagnose bacterial pneumonia in mechanically ventilated patients. Crit Care Med 18:169–173, 1990.

134. Wermert D, Marquette C-H, Copin M-C, et al: Influence of pulmonary bacteriology and histology on the yield of diagnostic procedures in ventilator-acquired pneumonia. Am J Respir Crit Care Med 158:139–147, 1998.

135. Schaberg DR, Culver DH, Gaynes RP: Major trends in the microbial etiology of nosocomial infection. Am J Med 91(suppl 3B):72S–75S, 1991.

136. Emori TG, Gaynes RP: An overview of nosocomial infections, including the role of the microbiology laboratory. Clin Microbiol Rev 6:428–442, 1993.

137. Horan T, Culver D, Jarvis W, et al: Pathogens causing nosocomial infections. Antimicrob Newslett 5:65–67, 1988.

138. Chow JW, MJ Fine, DM Shlaes, et al: Enterobacter bacteremia: clinical features and emergence of antibiotic resistance during therapy. Ann Intern Med 115:585–590, 1991.

139. Flynn DM, Weinstein RA, Nathans C, et al: Patients' endogenous flora as the source of "nosocomial" Enterobacter in cardiac surgery. J Infect Dis 156:363–368, 1987.

140. Nicolas MH, V Jarleir, N Honore, et al: Molecular characterization of the gene encoding SHV-3 beta lactamase, responsible for transferable cefotaxime resistance in clinical isolates of Klebsiella pneumoniae. Antimicrob Agents Chemother 33:2096–2100, 1989.

141. Meyer KS, Urban C, Eagan JA, et al: Nosocomial outbreak of Klebsiella infection resistant to late-generation cephalosporins. Ann Intern Med 119:353–358, 1993.

142. Eason AL, Wunderink RG, Meduri GU, et al: Overrepresentation of gram-negative enterics in suspected ventilator-associated pneumonia. Chest 100:36s, 1991.

143. Rello J, Ausina V, Castela J, et al: Nosocomial respiratory tract infections in multiple trauma patients: influence of level of consciousness with implications for therapy. Chest 102:525–529, 1992.

144. Schleupner CJ, Cobb DK: A study of the etiologies and treatment of nosocomial pneumonia in a community-based teaching hospital. Infect Control Hosp Epidemiol 13:515–525, 1992.

145. Rello J, Ricart M, Ausina V, et al: Pneumonia due to Haemophilus influenzae among mechanically ventilated patients: incidence, outcome, and risk factors. Chest 102:1562–1565, 1992.

146. Rello J, Quintana E, Ausina V, et al: Incidence, etiology, and outcome of nosocomial pneumonia in mechanically ventilated patients. Chest 100:439–444, 1991.

147. Archibald L, Phillips L, Monnet D, et al: Antimicrobial resistance in isolates from inpatients and outpatients in the United States: increasing importance of the intensive care unit. Clin Infect Dis 24:211–215, 1997.

148. Braun SR, Levin AB, Clark KL: Role of corticosteroids in the development of pneumonia in mechanically ventilated head-trauma patients. Crit Care Med 14:198–200, 1986.

149. Reusser P, Zimmerli W, Scheidegger D, et al: Role of gastric colonization in nosocomial infections and endotoxemia: a prospective study in neurosurgical patients on mechanical ventilation. J Infect Dis 160:414–421, 1989.

150. Esperson F, Gabrielsen J: Pneumonia due to

Staphylococcus aureus during mechanical ventilation. J Infect Dis 144:19–23, 1981.

151. Rello J, Quintana E, Ausina V, et al: Risk factors for *Staphylococcus aureus* nosocomial pneumonia in critically ill patients. Am Rev Respir Dis 142:1320–1324, 1990.

152. Bartlett JG, O'Keefe P, Tally FP, et al: Bacteriology of hospital-acquired pneumonia. Arch Intern Med 146:868–871, 1986.

153. Dore P, Robert R, Grollier G, Rouffineau J, et al: Incidence of anaerobes in ventilator-associated pneumonia with use of a protected specimen brush. Am J Respir Crit Care Med 153:1292–1298, 1996.

154. Holladay RC, Campbell GD: Nosocomial viral pneumonia in the intensive care unit. Clin Chest Med 16:121–133, 1995.

155. Valenti WM, Hall CB, Douglas RG Jr, et al: Nosocomial viral infections: I, epidemiology and significance. Infect Control Hosp Epidemiol 1:133–137, 1981.

156. Guidry GG, Black-Payne CA, Payne DK, et al: Respiratory synsitial virus infection amount intubated adults in a university medical intensive care unit. Chest 100:1377–1384, 1991.

157. Pingleton SK, Pingleton WW, Hill RH, et al: Type 3 adenoviral pneumonia occurring in a respiratory care unit. Chest 73:554–555, 1978.

158. Suspected nosocomial influenza cases in an intensive care unit. MMWR 37:3–4, 1988.

159. Singh-Naz N, Willy M, Riggs N: Outbreak of parainfluenza virus types in a neonatal nursery. Pediatr Infect Dis J 9:31–33, 1990.

160. Maloney SA, Jarvis WR: Epidemic nosocomial pneumonia in the intensive care unit. Clin Chest Med 16:209–223, 1995.

161. Larsen RA, Jacobson JT, Jacobson JA, et al: Hospital-associated epidemic of pharyngitis and conjunctivitis caused by adenovirus (21/H21 + 35). J Infect Disease 154:706–709, 1989.

162. St. John RC, Pacht ER: Tracheal stenosis and failure to wean from mechanical ventilation due to herpetic tracheitis. Chest 98:1520–1522, 1990.

163. Sherry MK, Klainer AS, Wolff M, et al: Herpetic tracheobronchitis. Ann Intern Med 109:229–233, 1988.

164. Kirby BD, Snyder KM, Meyer RD, et al: Legionnaires' disease: report of 65 nosocomially acquired cases and review of the literature. Medicine 59:188–205, 1980.

165. Rudin JE, Wing EJ: A comparative study of *Legionella micdadei* and other nosocomial acquired pneumonia. Chest 86:675–680, 1984.

166. Parry MF, Stampleman L, Hutchinson JG, et al: Waterborne *Legionella bozemanii* and nosocomial pneumonia in immunosuppressed patients. Ann Intern Med 103:205–210, 1985.

167. Doebbeling BN, Ishak MA, Wade BH, et al: Nosocomial *Legionella micdadei* pneumonia: 10 years experience and a case-control study. J Hosp Infect 13:289–298, 1989.

168. Rhame FS, Streifel AJ, Kersey JH, McGlave PB: Extrinsic risk factors for pneumonia in the patient at high risk for infection. Am J Med 76(suppl):42–52, 1984.

169. Girod JC, Reichman RC, Winn WC Jr, et al: Pneumonia and nonpneumonic forms of legionellosis. Arch Intern Med 142:545–547, 1982.

170. Cordes LG, Wiesenthal DS, Gorman GW, et al: Isolation of *Legionella pneumophila* from hospital shower heads. Ann Intern Med 94:195–197, 1981.

171. El-Ebiary M, Torres A, Fabregas N, et al: Significance of the isolation of *Candida* species from respiratory samples in critically ill, non-neutropenic patients: an immediate postmortem histologic study. Am Rev Respir Dis 156:583–590, 1997.

172. Seidenfeld JJ, Pohl DF, Bell RC, et al: Incidence, site, and outcome of infections in patients with adult respiratory distress syndrome. Am Rev Respir Dis 134:12–16, 1986.

173. Chastre J, Fagon JY, Bornet-Lesco M, et al: Evaluation of bronchoscopic techniques for the diagnosis of nosocomial pneumonia. Am J Respir Crit Care Med 152:231–240, 1995.

174. Karnad A, Alvarez S, Berk SL: Pneumonia caused by gram-negative bacilli. Am J Med 79(1A):61–67, 1985.

175. Hilf M, Yu VL, Sharp J, et al: Antibiotic therapy for *Pseudomonas aeruginosa* bacteremia: outcome correlations in a prospective study of 200 patients. Am J Med 87:540–546, 1989.

176. Campbell GD Jr, Niederman MS, Broughton WA, et al: Hospital-acquired pneumonia in adults: diagnosis, assessment of severity, initial antimicrobial therapy, and preventive strategies. A consensus statement. Am J Respir Crit Care Med 153:1711–1725, 1995.

177. Honeybourne D: Antibiotic penetration into lung tissue. Thorax 49:104–106, 1994.

178. LaForce FM: Systemic antimicrobial therapy of nosocomial pneumonia: monotherapy versus combination therapy. Eur J Clin Microbiol Infect Dis 8:61–68, 1989.

179. Kucers A, Bennett NM: The Use of Antibiotics: A Comprehensive Review with Clinical Emphasis. Philadelphia: JB Lippincott, 1987.

180. Klastersky J, Carpentier-Meunier F, Kahan-Coppens L, et al: Endotracheally administered antibiotics for gram-negative bronchopneumonia. Chest 75:586–591, 1979.

181. Brown RB, Kruse JA, Counts GW, et al: Double-blind study of endotracheal tobramycin in the treatment of gram-negative bacterial pneumonia. Antimicrob Agents Chemother 34:269–270, 1990.

182. Craig W: Pharmacodynamics of antimicrobial agents as a basis for determining dosage regimens. Eur J Clin Microbiol Infect Dis 12:s6–s8, 1993.

183. Baltch AL, Smith RP: Combinations of antibiotics against *Pseudomonas aeruginosa*. Am J Med 79(suppl 1A):8–16, 1985.

184. Gutmann L, Williamson R, Kitzis M-D, et al: Synergism and antagonism in double beta-lactam combinations. Am J Med 90(suppl 5C):21–29, 1986.

185. Fink MP, Snydman DR, Niederman MS, et al:
Treatment of severe pneumonia in hospitalized
patients: results of a multicenter, randomized
double-blind trial comparing intravenous ciprofloxacin with imipenem-cilastin. Antimicrob
Agents Chemother 38:1309–1313, 1994.
186. Bell RC, Coalson JJ, Smith JD, et al: Multiple
organ system failure and infection in adult respiratory distress syndrome. Ann Intern Med
99:293–298, 1983.
187. Silver DR, Cohen IL, Weinberg PF: Recurrent
Pseudomonas aeruginosa pneumonia in an intensive care unit. Chest 101:194–198, 1992.
188. Rello J, Mariscal D, March F, et al: Recurrent
Pseudomonas aeruginosa pneumonia in ventilated patients: relapse or reinfection? Am J Respir Crit Care Med 157:921–916, 1998.
189. Aylward RB, Burdge DR: Ribavirin therapy of
adult respiratory syncytial virus pneumonitis.
Arch Intern Med 151:2303–2304, 1991.
190. Hall CB, McBride JT, Gala CL, et al: Ribavirin
treatment of respiratory syncytial viral infection
in infants with underlying cardiopulmonary disease. JAMA 254:3047–3051, 1985.
191. Win M, Mitchell D, Pugh S, et al: Successful therapy with ribavirin of late onset respiratory syncytial virus pnuemonitis complicating allogeneic
bone marrow transplantation. Clin Lab Hematol
13:29–32, 1992.
192. Lim SG, Sawyer AM, Sercombe J, et al: Short
report: the absorption of fluconazole and itraconazole under conditions of low gastric acidity. Ali-
ment Pharmacol Ther 7:317–321, 1993.
193. Polk HC Jr, Borden S, Aldrett JA: Prevention of
Pseudomonas respiratory infection in a surgical
intensive care unit. Ann Surg 177:607–615, 1973.
194. Intravenous Immunoglobulin Collaborative Study
Group: A prophylactic intravenous administration compared with core-lipopolysaccaride immune globulin in patients at high-risk of post
surgical infection. N Engl J Med 327:234–240,
1992.
195. Cross AS, Opal SM, Palardy JE, et al: The efficacy
of combination immunotherapy in experimental
Pseudomonas sepsis. J Infect Dis 167:112–118,
1993.
196. Jaffee HA, Buhl R, Mastrangeli A, et al: Organ
specific cytokine therapy: local activation of mo-
nonuclear phagocytes by delivery of an aerosol
of recombinant interferon-gamma to the human
lung. J Clin Invest 88:297–230, 1991.
197. Nelson S, Belknap SM, Carlson RW, et al: A randomized controlled trial of filgrastim as an adjunct to antibiotics for treatment of hospitalized
patients with community-acquired pneumonia.
CAP Study Group. J Inf Dis 178:1075–1080, 1998.
198. Haley RW, Culver DH, White JW, et al: The efficacy of infection surveillance and control programs in preventing nosocomial infections in US
hospitals. Am J Epidemiol 121:182–205, 1985.
199. Shlaes DM, Gerding DN, John JF, et al: Society
for Healthcare Epidemiology of America and
Infectious Diseases Society of America Joint Committee on the Prevention of Antimicrobial Resistance: guidelines for the prevention of antimicrobial resistance in hospitals. Clin Infect Dis
25:584–599, 1997.
200. Kahan FM, GL Drusano, ISS Study Group: Resistance of gram-negative organisms isolated from
ICU patients in four cities to beta-lactam antibiotics. Program Abst Proc 3rd Dec Int Conf Nosocomial Infect 1990:A66.
201. Gerding DN, Larson TA, Hughes RA, et al:
Aminoglycoside resistance and aminoglycoside
usage: ten years of experience in one hospital.
Antimicrob Agents Chemother 35:1284–1290,
1991.
202. Neiderman MS: Is "crop rotation" of antibiotics
the solution to a "resistant" problem in the ICU?
Am J Respir Crit Care Med 156:1029–1031, 1997.
203. Kollef MH, Vlasnik J, Sharpless L, et al: Scheduled change of antibiotic classes: a strategy to
decrease the incidence of ventilator-associated
pneumonia. Am J Respir Crit Care Med
156:1040–1048, 1997.
204. Tryba M: Sucralfate versus antacids or H2-antag-
onists for stress ulcer prophylaxis: a meta-analysis on efficacy and pneumonia rate. Crit Care
Med 19:942–949, 1991.
205. Cook DJ, Reeve BK, Scholes C: Histamine-2-re-
ceptor antagonist and antacids in the critically ill
population: stress ulceration versus nosocomial
pneumonia. Infect Control Hosp Epidemiol
15:437–442, 1994.
206. Cook DJ, Laine LA, Guyatt GH, et al: Nosocomial
pneumonia and the role of gastric pH: a meta-
analysis. Chest 100:7–13, 1991.
207. Martin LF, Booth FV, Kalstadt RG, et al: Continuous intravenous cimetidine decreases stress-re-
lated upper gastrointestinal hemorrhage without
promoting pneumonia. Crit Care Med 21:19–30,
1993.
208. Torres A, Serra-Batlles J, Ros E, et al: Pulmonary
aspiration of gastric contents in patients receiving mechanical ventilation: the effect of body position. Ann Intern Med 116:540–543, 1992.
209. Petersdorf RG, Merchant RK: A study of antibiotic prophylaxis in patients with acute heart failure. N Engl J Med 260:565–575, 1959.
210. Mandelli M, Mosconi P, Langer M, et al: Prevention of pneumonia in an intensive care unit: a
randomized, multi-center trial. Crit Care Med
17:501–503, 1989.
211. Klick JM, du Moulin GC, Headley-White J, et al:
Prevention of gram-negative bacillary pneumonia
using polymyxin aerosol as prophylaxis. J Clin
Invest 55:514–519, 1975.
212. Feeley TW, de Moulin GC, Headley-Whyte J, et
al: Aerosolized polymyxin and pneumonia in seriously ill patients. N Engl J Med 293:471–475,
1975.
213. Klastersky J, Huismans E, Weerts D, et al: Endotracheally administered gentamicin for the prevention of infections of the respiratory tract in
patients with tracheostomy: a double-blind study.
Chest 65:650–654, 1974.

214. Klastersky J, Hensgens D, Noterman J, et al: Endotracheal antibiotics for the prevention of tracheobronchial infections in tracheostomized, unconscious patients: a comparative study of gentamicin and aminosidin-polymyxin B combination. Chest 68:302–306, 1975.

215. Selective Decontamination of the Digestive Tract Trialists' Collaborative Group: Meta-analysis of randomised controlled trials of selective decontamination of the digestive tract. BMJ 307:525–532, 1993.

216. Brun-Buisson C, Legrand P, Rauss A, et al: Intestinal decontamination for control of nosocomial multi-resistant gram-negative bacilli: a study of an outbreak in an intensive care unit. Ann Intern Med 110:873–881, 1989.

217. Gastinne H, Wolff M, Delatour F, et al: A controlled trial in intensive care units of selective decontamination of the digestive tract with nonabsorbable antibiotics. N Engl J Med 326:594–599, 1992.

218. Rocha LA, Martin MJ, Pieta S, et al: Prevention of nosocomial infection in critically ill patients by selective decontamination of the digestive tract: a randomized double-blind, placebo-controlled study. Intensive Care Med 18:398–404, 1992.

219. Nau R, Rochel R, Mergerian H, et al: Emergence of antibiotic-resistent bacteria during selective decontamination of the digestive tract. J Antimicrob Agents Chemother 25:881–883, 1990.

220. Daschner F: Emergence of resistance during selective decontamination of the digestive tract. Eur J Clin Microbiol Infect Dis 11:1–3, 1992.

221. Valles J, Artigas A, Rello J, et al: Continuous aspiration of subglottic secretions in preventing ventilator-associated pneumonia. Ann Intern Med 122:179–186, 1995.

222. Gaynes RP, Edwards JR, Jarvis WR, et al: Nosocomial infections among neonates in high-risk nurseries in the United States. Pediatrics 98:357–361, 1996.

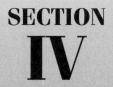

SECTION
IV

Specific Clinical Applications of Mechanical Ventilation

CHAPTER 18

Mechanical Ventilation Strategies for Parenchymal Lung Injury

Neil R. MacIntyre, MD

CAUSES OF PARENCHYMAL
LUNG INJURY
PATHOPHYSIOLOGY
GOALS OF MECHANICAL
VENTILATION TO PROVIDE
TOTAL VENTILATORY
SUPPORT IN PARENCHYMAL
LUNG INJURY
STRATEGIES FOR TOTAL
SUPPORT
Modes

Frequency–Tidal Volume
    Settings
Positive End-Expiratory
    Pressure/Inspired Oxygen
    Concentration
Inspiratory:Expiratory
    Timing
STRATEGIES FOR LESS
THAN TOTAL SUPPORT AND
WEANING
REFERENCES

KEY WORDS

acute respiratory distress
    syndrome
lung protective strategies

parenchymal lung injury
permissive hypercapnia
total ventilatory support

CAUSES OF PARENCHYMAL LUNG INJURY

Parenchymal lung injury describes disease processes that involve the air spaces and the interstitium of the lung. These processes can be diffuse or focal. Examples of diffuse processes include cardiogenic edema and interstitial pneumonias (e.g., interstitial fibrosis, interstitial pneumonias, viral syndromes, hypersensitivity reactions, sar-

coid, and idiopathic processes). **Acute respiratory distress syndrome** (ARDS) and acute lung injury (ALI) syndrome are also diffuse parenchymal injuries that have specific diagnostic criteria[1] (Table 18–1). ARDS and ALI can be divided further into lung-specific injuries (i.e., massive aspiration, bilateral pneumonias, drowning) and lung injuries as part of a systemic process, such as sepsis or pancreatitis (i.e., the lung is one of many organs affected by a diffuse in-

TABLE 18–1. Acute Respiratory Distress Syndrome and Acute Lung Injury Diagnostic Criteria

Acute-onset disease consistent with ALI/ARDS

$PaO_2/FiO_2 < 200$ (ARDS) < 300 (ALI)

Bilateral lung infiltrates on chest radiograph
Injury not reflecting cardiogenic edema (PCWP less than 18 if measured)

FiO₂, inspired oxygen concentration; PaO₂, arterial oxygen pressure; PCWP, pulmonary capillary wedge pressure.

flammatory response, the systemic inflammatory response syndrome [SIRS]). More focal parenchymal injuries include lobar pneumonias, regional aspiration, and lung contusions.

PATHOPHYSIOLOGY

Although the disease processes involved in parenchymal lung injury are clearly different, there are a number of important pathophysiologic similarities that relate to the management of mechanical ventilation. Specifically, all these disease processes have varying degrees of interstitial edema, alveolar flooding, surfactant dysfunction, and small airway dysfunction. These result in both mechanical and gas exchange abnormalities that must be addressed in a mechanical ventilation strategy.

In general, parenchymal injury produces stiff lungs and reduced lung volumes.[2, 3] Functional residual capacity thus is reduced, and the compliance curve is shifted to the right (Fig. 18–1). However, in all but the most diffuse diseases (e.g., cardiogenic edema), there can be marked regional differences in the degree of inflammation present and thus the degree of mechanical abnormalities that exist. This heterogeneity can have significant impact on the effects of a particular mechanical ventilation strategy. This is because delivered gases preferentially go to the regions with the highest compliance and the lowest resistance (i.e., the more normal regions) rather than to more affected regions. A "normal-sized"

tidal volume thus may be distributed preferentially to the healthier regions and may result in a much higher regional tidal volume and the potential for regional overdistension injury[4, 5] (Fig. 18–2). This is one of the rationales for using pressure-limited ventilation in severe parenchymal injury—it limits the maximal distension in all units to the set level, regardless of changes in regional lung mechanisms (see later discussion).

Parenchymal injury also can affect the airways, especially the bronchioles and alveolar ducts.[6] These narrowed and collapsible small airways can contribute to reduced regional ventilation to injured lung units. This also can lead to regions of air trapping, and it may be a factor in subsequent cyst formation during the healing phase.[7]

Gas exchange abnormalities in parenchymal lung injury are a consequence of the loss of lung volume and the maldistribution of ventilation, which result in ventilation-perfusion ($\dot{V}/\dot{Q}$) mismatching and shunts.[8] This can be made worse if there are concomitant pulmonary vascular abnormalities associated with the disease process. Also, the

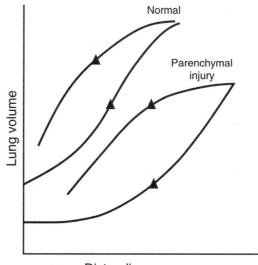

FIGURE 18–1
Static pressure volume curve in normal lungs and in lungs with parenchymal injury. Note that the lung with parenchymal injury has the curve shifted downward and to the right for a similar delivered tidal volume. This is a consequence of both alveolar collapse and reduced compliance.

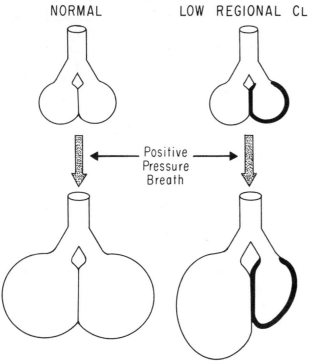

NORMAL   LOW REGIONAL CL

Positive Pressure Breath

FIGURE 18–2
Effects of a regional compliance abnormality on the distribution of a tidal breath. Note that in a lung with compliance inhomogeneities, a delivered tidal volume distributes to the region with the highest compliance. The resulting regional tidal volume may be sufficiently large to produce regional overdistension.

degree of $\dot{V}/\dot{Q}$ mismatch may change during the ventilatory cycle. Specifically, there may be low $\dot{V}/\dot{Q}$ relationships with inspiration and shunting during expiration if cyclical alveolar collapse occurs (Fig. 18–3). Because dead space ($\dot{V}/\dot{Q} = \infty$) is not a major manifestation of parenchymal lung disease unless there is very severe or end-stage injury, hypoxemia tends to be more of a problem than carbon dioxide (CO_2) clearance in parenchymal lung disease.

In parenchymal injury, severe hypoxemia coupled with direct vascular injury often leads to high pulmonary artery pressures. This can compound the gas exchange problem by overloading the right ventricle and reducing perfusion through the lung. The need for adequate right heart filling pressures must be balanced against the risk of worsening lung edema when fluid therapy[9] and ventilator pressures are adjusted.

GOALS OF MECHANICAL VENTILATION TO PROVIDE TOTAL VENTILATORY SUPPORT IN PARENCHYMAL LUNG INJURY

The overall goals in mechanical ventilatory support in parenchymal lung injury are to provide adequate gas exchange while minimizing any potential iatrogenic lung injury. Although many variables can be monitored during this process, clinical decisions generally involve balancing four important factors: arterial pH, arterial hemoglobin saturation (SaO_2), lung stretch, and lung exposure to oxygen[10] (Table 18–2). Put another way, the overall goal is to provide the best pH and SaO_2 for the least amount of unnecessary stretch and inspired oxygen concentration (FiO_2) exposure.

Ideally, the pH should be in the normal 7.35 to 7.45 range. However, lower pH levels from higher partial pressure of carbon dioxide (PCO_2) may be tolerated if they protect the lung from unnecessary stretch. Indeed, pH values as low as 7.10 to 7.20 have been reported as being tolerable by most patients in respiratory failure.[11] This correlates with PCO_2 greater than 80 torr in the acute situation. This willingness to accept a respiratory acidosis to prevent lung overstretch sometimes is referred to as **permissive hypercapnia**.[11, 12] Increases in CO_2 levels seem to be tolerated in increments of approximately 10 torr/hour.[11] However, allowing acidosis should be done with caution in patients with central nervous system

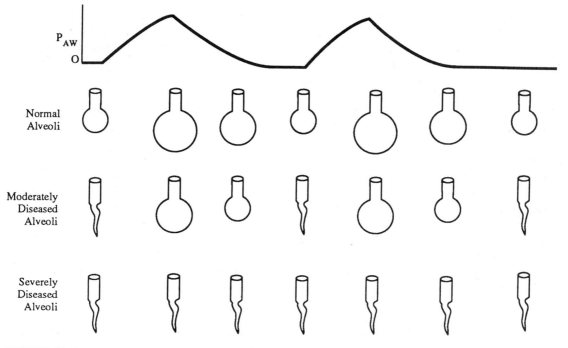

FIGURE 18–3
Degree of ventilation perfusion ($\dot{V}/\dot{Q}$) mismatch and shunt may depend on the phase of
ventilation.

(CNS) mass lesions (or mass effect) or in patients with unstable hemodynamics (pressor dependence or arrhythmias).[11]

Generally speaking, SaO_2 should be greater than 88% (PO_2 60–65 torr) to ensure adequate tissue oxygen unloading. Lower SaO_2 between 85% and 88%, however, may be tolerable if normal oxygen delivery (DO_2 of 300–400 ml/min/M^2) is maintained through manipulations of cardiac output and/or hemoglobin concentration. Regardless of DO_2, arterial PO_2 should be maintained above 55 torr to minimize reflex pul-

monary vasoconstriction and resultant pulmonary hypertension.[9]

The concept of stretch injury is discussed in more detail in Chapter 11. Simply put, however, the lung is subject to stretch injury in one of two ways: a shear stretch injury from repeated opening and closing of diseased alveoli and an overstretch injury induced by excessive distension at end inspiration from the combination of the delivered tidal stretch (tidal volume [V_T]) and baseline stretch positive end-expiratory pressure [PEEP]).[13] Addressing these two issues is

TABLE 18–2. Goals of Total Ventilatory Support

GOALS	KEY PARAMETER	KEY THRESHOLD
Ventilation/CO_2 clearance	pH	7.20–7.45
Oxygenation	SaO_2	> 88%
Avoid iatrogenic stretch injury	P_{PLAT}*	< 35 cm H_2O with adequate recruitment
Oxidant injury	FiO_2	< 0.6

*Also involves adequate recruitment. Lower and upper inflection points on a pressure–volume plot may be more appropriate future parameters.
CO_2, carbon dioxide; FiO_2, inspired oxygen concentration; P_{PLAT}, plateau pressure.

the concept behind **lung protective strategies**.

In general, the first goal is to provide enough PEEP to recruit the "recruitable" alveoli while simultaneously not applying so much PEEP that healthier regions are overdistended unnecessarily. The second goal is to avoid a PEEP/V_T combination that unnecessarily overdistends the lung at end inspiration, generally reflected by elevations in plateau pressure (end-inspiratory alveolar pressure) greater than approximately 35 cm H_2O.[14] Better estimates of lung mechanical properties might be obtained by static pressure–volume (PV) curves (see Fig. 18–1), and these might be enhanced further by using esophageal/pleural pressures to account for any chest wall abnormalities that may be present. Unfortunately, clinical monitors to easily and reliably make these static PV measurements are not widely available.

Oxygen toxicity is discussed in Chapter 8. Clinically, attempts usually are made to keep the inhaled oxygen concentration (FiO_2) to less than 0.5 to 0.6 in most situations. The exact FiO_2 at which oxygen becomes toxic is not clear, however.[15]

In summary, balancing these four clinical goals of pH, SaO_2, lung stretch, and FiO_2 constitutes the art of mechanical ventilation in parenchymal lung injury. Unfortunately, little data exist on the relative "toxicities" of the threshold values in Table 18–2.[10] Management of the very ill patient who is near or at all of these thresholds thus constitutes one of the greatest challenges of intensive care unit (ICU) medicine.

STRATEGIES FOR TOTAL SUPPORT

Modes

Generally, severe respiratory failure is managed during the acute phases with an assist/control (A/C) mode of ventilation. This ensures that all breaths have positive pressure supplied by the ventilator to provide virtually all the work of breathing. The assist capabilities of A/C ventilation allow the patient to trigger breaths. This may help in controlling CO_2 and improving patient comfort. If an inappropriate respiratory drive exists or patient triggering of assisted breaths is uncomfortable, sedation or paralysis or both may be needed such that only the control breaths of A/C ventilation are provided. However, unless the patient is grossly dys-synchronous with the ventilator despite every effort to make the assisted breaths comfortable, paralysis to eliminate muscle activity should be avoided.[16] Similarly, strategies that routinely employ paralysis and controlled ventilation to reduce oxygen consumption (VO_2) also should be avoided because the potential decrease in VO_2 is generally small and the risk of long-term myopathy is substantial.[17]

Choosing pressure- versus volume-targeted ventilation for **total ventilatory support** depends on the clinical situation. Volume-targeted ventilation (volume assist–control ventilation [VACV]) guarantees a certain V_T. This, in turn, gives the clinician control over minute ventilation and CO_2 clearance. Under these conditions, however, airway and alveolar pressures are dependent variables and increase or decrease depending on changes in lung mechanics or patient effort. Thus, sudden worsening of compliance or resistance can cause abrupt increases in airway and alveolar pressures. Pressure-targeted ventilation, conversely, does not guarantee volume but rather controls airway pressure. Volume is thus a dependent variable and changes as lung mechanics or patient efforts change. Sudden worsening of compliance or resistance with pressure-targeted ventilation results in a loss of volume. Pressure-targeted ventilation also has a variable decelerating flow waveform, which may improve gas mixing[18] and may interact with any patient efforts more synchronously[19] (see Chapter 9).

The choice of pressure- versus volume-targeted breaths depends on which feature is required for the clinical goal. Specifically, if CO_2 clearance is of primary concern and patient comfort and lung stretch are less important issues (e.g., mild lung injury with a cerebral mass lesion), volume-targeted ventilation is preferable. Conversely, if overdistension risk is high and/or patient synchrony is more of an issue than CO_2 clearance (e.g., severe ARDS with normal cardiac and neurologic function), pressure-targeted ventilation is probably the correct choice. There are several ventilator modes that offer pressure-targeting and volume-cycling features.[20] Although these modes do offer the decelerating waveform of pressure-targeted breaths and thus may help patient comfort and gas mixing, the volume guarantee means that pressure must increase if lung mechanics worsen. Thus, although these breaths in these modes have pressure-targeting features, they are not pressure limiting.

Frequency–Tidal Volume Settings

The tidal breath, in conjunction with the baseline pressure (see below), should be set in such a way that the plateau pressure is less than 35 cm H_2O (or some other index of overdistension does not occur). Generally, this involves V_T of 8 to 10 ml/kg,[10] although V_T as low as 5 to 6 ml/kg may be needed.[11, 12] Older strategies of using higher tidal volumes arose from a need to prevent atelectasis. Now that PEEP strategies are better understood and the risk of overdistension is better appreciated, this need has lessened.

The set ventilator frequency generally is used to control the CO_2. A reasonable starting point is a normal frequency of between 12 and 20 breaths per minute. Increasing the frequency increases minute ventilation and generally increases CO_2 clearance. At some point, however, air trapping develops because of inadequate expiratory times. Under these conditions, either minute ventilation starts to decrease (pressure-targeted ventilation) or airway pressures start to increase (volume-targeted ventilation) (see Fig. 6–16). In general, this begins to happen at breathing frequencies of approximately 35 breaths per minute, although it can occur at much lower frequencies if the inspiratory:expiratory (I:E) ratio is high or the time constant for lung emptying (resistance × compliance) is very high[21] (see Fig. 6–16).

Positive End-Expiratory Pressure/ Inspired Oxygen Concentration

The goal of PEEP therapy is to recruit "recruitable" alveoli while not overdistending

already patent alveoli (Fig. 7–8). As noted in Chapter 7, PEEP performs its recruitment action primarily by preventing the deflation and collapse of an alveoli opened by a tidal breath.[22] This may be enhanced by performing a volume recruitment maneuver consisting of 1 minute of PEEP values in the 25- to 40-cm H_2O range and then returning to an optimal setting, as described later. In determining the ultimate optimal setting, two basic approaches exist that use either mechanical criteria or gas exchange criteria.

Mechanical criteria involve assessments that attempt to ensure that PEEP recruits "recruitable" alveoli but does not overdistend alveoli already recruited. Two approaches have been reported:

1. Use pressure volume curves to set the PEEP/V_T combination between the upper and lower inflection points[23] (see Chapter 7). A modification of the conventional static approach uses a very slow inspiratory flow and then measures upper and lower inflection points from the resulting dynamic pressure volume curves[24] (see Fig. 6–4). As noted previously and in Chapter 6, using an esophageal pressure to account for chest wall mechanics enhances these techniques.

2. Use step increase in PEEP to determine the PEEP level that gives the best compliance.[25]

Gas exchange criteria to guide PEEP application involve several potential strategies. One approach is to do a PEEP titration curve (after a volume recruitment maneuver—see earlier discussion) to determine the lowest FiO_2 that can be achieved. Another approach is to use algorithms designed to provide adequate values for PaO_2 while minimizing FiO_2. An example is the PEEP/FiO_2 algorithm in Figure 18–4. Constructing a PEEP/FiO_2 algorithm is usually an empirical exercise in balancing SaO_2 with FiO_2 and depends on the clinician's perception of the relative "toxicities" of high thoracic pressures, high FiO_2, and low SaO_2.

In general, commonly used "operational" ranges for PEEP in parenchymal lung injury are 8 to 25 cm H_2O. However, some argue that, at least in the initial phases of lung injury, the range should be higher (e.g.,

OXYGENATION GOALS
Acceptable Oxygenation
$55 \leq PaO_2 \leq 80$ or
$88 \leq S_PO_2 \leq 95$

Use this if a patient's PEEP and FiO_2 are not compatible with the protocol scale and the $PaO_2 < 55$ or $SpO_2 < 88\%$. Find the box that corresponds to the current $PEEP/FiO_2$ settings. Make the change in PEEP or FiO_2 indicated in the box. The approved protocol $PEEP/FiO_2$ combinations are indicated by "*****".

For 12 ml/kg and 6 ml/kg patients*

	FiO_2 0.3	FiO_2 0.4	FiO_2 0.5	FiO_2 0.6	FiO_2 0.7	FiO_2 0.8	FiO_2 0.9	FiO_2 0.10
PEEP 5	*****	*****	↑ PEEP	↑ PEEP	↑ PEEP	↑ PEEP	↑ PEEP	↑ PEEP
PEEP 8	↑ FiO_2	*****	*****	↑ PEEP	↑ PEEP	↑ PEEP	↑ PEEP	↑ PEEP
PEEP 10	↑ FiO_2	↑ FiO_2	*****	*****	*****	↑ PEEP	↑ PEEP	↑ PEEP
PEEP 12	↑ FiO_2	↑ FiO_2	↑ FiO_2	↑ FiO_2	*****	↑ PEEP	↑ PEEP	↑ PEEP
PEEP 14	↑ FiO_2	↑ FiO_2	↑ FiO_2	↑ FiO_2	*****	*****	*****	↑ PEEP
PEEP 16	↑ FiO_2	↑ FiO_2	↑ FiO_2	↑ FiO_2	↑ FiO_2	↑ FiO_2	*****	↑ PEEP
PEEP 18	↑ FiO_2	↑ FiO_2	↑ FiO_2	↑ FiO_2	↑ FiO_2	↑ FiO_2	*****	*****
PEEP 20	↑ FiO_2	↑ FiO_2	↑ FiO_2	↑ FiO_2	↑ FiO_2	↑ FiO_2	↑ FiO_2	*****
PEEP 22–24	↑ FiO_2	↑ FiO_2	↑ FiO_2	↑ FiO_2	↑ FiO_2	↑ FiO_2	↑ FiO_2	***** Max. Rx.

*If $PaO_2 < 55$ or $SpO_2 < 95\%$ in low stretch patient with plateau pressure ≥ 30, increase FiO_2 in steps of 0.1 to 1.0 prior to any PEEP increase.
***** = approved $PEEP/FiO_2$ combination.

FIGURE 18–4
A positive end-expiratory pressure/fraction of inspired oxygen ($PEEP/FiO_2$) algorithm used in the National Institutes of Health ARDS Network mechanical ventilation protocol.

12–25 cm H_2O) and that a volume recruitment maneuver should be performed to ensure optimal recruitment.[23] With this approach, the patient would be weaned from PEEP only when the FiO_2 is 0.4 or less.

Inspiratory:Expiratory Timing

Setting the inspiratory time and the I:E ratio involves several considerations. The normal I:E ratio is roughly 1:2 to 1:4. This produces the most comfort and thus is the usual initial setting. Assessment of the flow graphic also should be done to ensure that an adequate expiratory time is present to avoid air trapping.

I:E prolongation beyond the physiologic range of 1:2 to 1:4 can be employed as an alternative to increasing PEEP to improve $\dot{V}/\dot{Q}$ matching in severe respiratory failure.[26, 27] Generally, inspiratory time prolongation is reserved for patients in whom the plateau pressure from the $PEEP/V_T$ combination has approached 35 cm H_2O and potentially toxic concentrations of FiO_2 are being employed without SaO_2 or DO_2 goals having been met. Inspiratory time prolongation has several important physiologic effects (see Chapter 7). First, a longer inspiratory time results in a longer alveolar-conducting airway gas-mixing time. Second, a longer inspiratory time can give slower filling alveolar units time to be ventilated and recruited. Finally, if expiratory time is inadequate for lung emptying, air trapping and intrinsic PEEP can develop (see Fig. 7–9). A number of studies have shown improved gas exchange as a consequence of longer inspiratory times,[26–28] but sorting out which physiologic mechanism is responsible is not easy. Indeed, long inspiratory times without air trapping have been shown in one study to improve PaO_2,[28] although others have argued that improved PO_2 occurs only as a consequence of intrinsic PEEP (PEEPi) development.[26, 27]

Several other aspects of long inspiratory

time strategies need to be considered when this technique is used. First, the development of air trapping has different effects on pressure- versus volume-targeted ventilation (see Fig. 6–14). Second, although long inspiratory times often are combined with pressure-controlled breaths to use the rapid initial flow pattern and the pressure limit feature, long inspiratory time strategies also have been used with volume-targeted breaths, generally by adding an inspiratory pause.[27] Third, long inspiratory time increases mean airway pressure and thus can reduce cardiac filling (see Chapter 10). Moreover, in the presence of air trapping, the mean alveolar pressure is higher than the mean airway pressure, making monitoring of intrathoracic pressure more difficult. Fourth, lengthening the I:E ratio beyond 1:1 is also quite uncomfortable and usually requires heavy sedation and/or paralysis.

One approach to using long inspiratory time strategies is given in Table 18–3. The rationale behind this approach is to use longer inspiratory times for their mixing and filling effects but not to produce PEEPi. This is because there is no evidence that PEEPi produces any greater improvement in $\dot{V}/\dot{Q}$ matching than extrinsic or applied PEEP. Moreover, PEEPi may be more pro-

nounced in lung regions with airway dysfunction and good compliance compared with the stiff alveolar regions that require recruitment. This contrasts with applied PEEP, which is distributed more homogeneously. Another reason to avoid air trapping and PEEPi with long inspiratory time strategies is their effects on the aforementioned desired ventilator settings.

It must be emphasized that no data exist that demonstrate improved outcome with long inspiratory time strategies. Clinical application thus is justified only on physiologic grounds. Because of this, and because of the potential problems noted previously, long inspiratory time strategies should be reserved only for very severe respiratory failure and should be applied only by clinicians skilled in monitoring ventilatory mechanics.

STRATEGIES FOR LESS THAN TOTAL SUPPORT AND WEANING

In less severe forms of parenchymal lung injury or during the recovery process, modes of partial support may be used. By definition, these modes provide some, but not all, of the work of breathing. Using partial support offers the advantage of lower ventilatory pressures and the ability to synchronize ventilatory support with patient efforts. Less lung stretch, cardiac compromise, and patient sedation requirements may result. Commonly used partial support modes include intermittent mandatory ventilation and pressure support/pressure assist. The use of these techniques, especially in the weaning process, are discussed in more detail in Chapter 20.

One other form of partial support that has been used primarily in less severe forms of parenchymal lung injury is airway pressure release ventilation (APRV). APRV is a variation of long inspiratory time ventilation and sometimes has been termed continuous positive airway pressure (CPAP) with release or upside down intermittent minute ventilation (IMV).[29] This ventilator strategy employs a pressure-targeted approach with long inflation phases and brief deflation phases. The inflation pressures, however, are more modest than those employed using

TABLE 18–3. Duke University Long Inspiratory Time Strategy

1. Consider only when conventional ventilator strategies with optimal PEEP have resulted in $P_{PLAT} > 35$ cm H_2O without producing acceptable PaO_2/FiO_2 values.
2. If in volume control, switch to pressure control with same delivered tidal volume, frequency, and inspiratory time (ti).
3. Increase T_i in 0.1- to 0.2-sec increments until either PaO_2/FiO_2 goals are achieved *or* air trapping develops.
4. When I:E ratio exceeds 1:1, patients may require sedation/paralysis.
5. Recognize that this approach has a physiologic rationale but that no studies to date have shown improved outcome as a consequence of it.

FiO₂, inspired oxygen concentration; I:E, inspiratory: expiratory; PaO₂, arterial oxygen pressure; PEEP, positive end-expiratory pressure; P_PLAT, plateau pressure.

total support strategies, and spontaneous breathing is permitted using a pressure relief mechanism during the inflation periods. The short deflation periods may or may not have a small amount of PEEP applied, and there may be some air trapping present. A more detailed comparison of APRV with other forms of partial support is summarized elsewhere in this book. The advantage to APRV is that it is a very simple approach to mechanical ventilatory support in the patient with parenchymal lung injury who does not need high-level total respiratory support as described previously. A disadvantage may be occasional patient discomfort.[29] Clinical data indicate the effectiveness of APRV as a partial support technique, but data do not exist that demonstrate superior outcomes.

OUTCOME OF PARENCHYMAL RESPIRATORY FAILURE

This outcome of patients with parenchymal lung injury requiring mechanical ventilation depends heavily on the cause of the injury and the severity of the injury (Table 18–4).[30–34] The cause of the lung injury is of particular importance. Specifically, in ARDS, the highest mortality is associated with lung injury as a manifestation of systemic injury. Depending on the numbers of other organs involved, mortality rates can approach 100% under these circumstances. Conversely, lung injury from a lung-only

TABLE 18–4. Mortality from Acute Lung Injury/Acute Respiratory Distress Syndrome

INVESTIGATOR (YEAR)	NO.	SURVIVAL RATE (%)
Ashbaugh et al[30] (1976)	12	34
Gillespie et al[31] (1986)		
No organ failures	20	60
Organ failures	60	19
Anzueto et al[32] (1996)	725	60
Milberg et al[34] (1995)		
1983	85	47
1993	89	64

process may be associated with a mortality rate of less than 30%. Initial oxygenation impairment is not a good predictor of mortality in ARDS, although persistence of lung injury is. There is some evidence that survival statistics of patients with ARDS actually may be improving.[34] If this is true, it probably is a reflection of better overall ICU management rather than any single new treatment modality.

Long-term outcome from parenchymal lung injury requiring mechanical ventilation is actually reasonable in survivors with ARDS. Long-term pulmonary function testing reveals good function, with near normal recovery in many of those patients.[35] Patients with chronic underlying lung disease (e.g., fibrosis), however, can have extended recovery periods and often never return to baseline function.

REFERENCES

1. Bernard GR, Artigas A, Brigham KL, et al: American–European consensus conference on ARDS. Am J Respir Crit Care Med 149:818–824, 1994.
2. Petty TL, Ashbaugh DG: The adult respiratory distress syndrome: clinical features, factors influencing prognosis, and principles of management. Chest 60:233–239, 1971.
3. Fulkerson WJ, MacIntyre NR: Pathogenesis and treatment of the adult respiratory distress syndrome. Arch Intern Med 156:29–38, 1996.
4. Gattinoni L, Pesenti A, Torresin A, et al: Adult respiratory distress syndrome profiles by computed tomography. J Thorac Imaging 3:25–30, 1988.
5. Gattinoni L, Pesenti A, Baglioni S, et al: Inflammatory pulmonary edema and PEEP: correlation between imaging and physiologic studies. J Thorac Imaging 3:59–64, 1988.
6. Pratt PC: Pathology of the adult respiratory distress syndrome. In: Thurlbeck WM, Abel MR (eds): The Lung: Structure, Function and Disease. Baltimore, MD: Williams and Wilkins, 1978, pp 43–57.
7. Pratt P, Vollmer R, Shelburne J, Crapo J: Pulmonary morphology in a multihospital collaborative extracorporeal membrane oxygenation project: I, light microscopy. Am J Pathol 95:191–214, 1979.
8. Wagner PD: Ventilation–perfusion relationships. Annu Rev Physiol 42:235–247, 1980.
9. Pinsky MR, Guimond JG: The effects of positive end-expiratory pressure on heart-lung interactions. J Crit Care 6:1–15, 1991.
10. Slutsky AS: ACCP consensus conference: mechanical ventilation. Chest 104:1833–1859, 1993.
11. Fiehl F, Perret C: Permissive hypercapnia—how permissive should we be? Am J Respir Crit Care Med 150:1722–1737, 1994.

12. Hickling KG, Walsh J, Henderson S, Jackson R: Low mortality rate in adult respiratory distress syndrome using low-volume, pressure-limited ventilation with permissive hypercapnia: a prospective study. Crit Care Med 22:1568–1578, 1994.

13. Vincent JL: The relationship between oxygen demand, oxygen uptake and oxygen supply. Intensive Care Med 16:s145–s148, 1990.

14. Kolobow T, Moretti MP, Fumagalli R, et al: Severe impairment in lung function induced by high peak airway pressure during mechanical ventilation. Am Rev Respir Dis 135:312–315, 1987.

15. Jenkinson SG: Oxygen toxicity. New Horiz 1:504–511, 1993.

16. Hansen-Flashen J, Brazinsky S, Bassler C, Lanken PN: Use of sedating drugs and neuromuscular blockade in patients requiring mechanical ventilation for respiratory failure. JAMA 266:2870–2875, 1991.

17. Raps EC, Bird SJ, Hansen-Flashen J: Prolonged muscle weakness after neuromuscular blockade in the ICU. Crit Care Clin 10:799–813, 1994.

18. Abraham E, Yoshihara G: Cardiorespiratory effects of pressure controlled ventilation in severe respiratory failure. Chest 98:1445–1449, 1990.

19. MacIntyre NR, McConnell R, Cheng KC, Sane A: Pressure limited breaths improve flow dys-synchrony during assisted ventilation. Crit Care Med 25:1671–1677, 1997.

20. MacIntyre NR, Gropper C, Westfall T: Combining pressure limiting and volume cycling features in an interactive mechanical breath. Crit Care Med 22:353–357, 1994.

21. Marini JJ, Crooke PS: A general mathematical model for respiratory dynamics relevant to the clinical setting. Am Rev Respir Dis 147:14–24, 1993.

22. American Association for Respiratory Care: Positive end expiratory pressure—state of the art after 20 years. Respir Care 33:417–500, 1988.

23. Amato MB, Barbas CSV, Medeivos DM, et al: Effect of a protective-ventilation strategy on mortality in the acute respiratory distress syndrome. N Engl J Med 338:347–354, 1998.

24. Servillo G, Svantesson C, Beydon L, et al: Pressure–volume curves in acute respiratory failure: automated low flow inflation vs occlusion. Am J Respir Crit Care Med 155:1629–1636, 1997.

25. Suter PM, Fairley HB, Isenberg MD: Optimum end-expiratory pressure in patients with acute pulmonary failure. N Engl Med 292:284–289, 1975.

26. Cole AGH, Weller SF, Sykes MK: Inverse ratio ventilation compared with PEEP in adult respiratory failure. Intensive Care Med 10:227–232, 1984.

27. Tharratt RS, Allen RP, Albertson TE: Pressure controlled inverse ratio ventilation in severe adult respiratory failure. Chest 94:755–762, 1988.

28. Armstrong BW, MacIntyre NR: Pressure controlled inverse ratio ventilation that avoids air trapping in ARDS. Crit Care Med 23:279–285, 1995.

29. Chiang AS, Steinfeld AS, Gropper C, MacIntyre NR: Demand flow airway pressure release ventilation as a partial ventilatory support mode. Crit Care Med 22:1431–1437, 1994.

30. Ashbaugh DG, Bigelow DB, Petty TL, Levine BE: Acute respiratory distress in adults. Lancet 2:319–323, 1967.

31. Gillespie DJ, Marsh HMN, Divertie MB, Meadows JA: Clinical outcome of patients requiring prolonged (> 24 hrs) mechanical ventilation. Chest 90:364–382, 1986.

32. Anzueto A, Baughman RP, Guntapalli KK, et al: Aerosolized surfactant in adults with sepsis induced ARDS. N Engl J Med 334:1417–1421, 1996.

33. Montgomery AB, Stager MA, Carrico CJ, Hudson LD: Causes of mortality in patients with ARDS. Am Rev Respir Dis 132:485–489, 1985.

34. Milberg JA, Davis DR, Steinberg KP, Hudson LD: Improved survival of patients with ARDS:1983–1993. JAMA 273:306–309, 1995.

35. Ingbar DH, Matthew RA: Lung function in survivors. Crit Care Clin 2:377–380, 1986.

CHAPTER 19

Mechanical Ventilation Strategies for Obstructive Airway Disease

Neil R. MacIntyre, MD

CAUSES OF RESPIRATORY FAILURE DUE TO AIRFLOW OBSTRUCTION

PATHOPHYSIOLOGY OF AIRFLOW OBSTRUCTION

GOALS OF MECHANICAL VENTILATION IN PROVIDING TOTAL SUPPORT IN RESPIRATORY FAILURE DUE TO AIRFLOW OBSTRUCTION

MECHANICAL VENTILATION SETTINGS AND STRATEGIES IN AIRFLOW OBSTRUCTION REQUIRING TOTAL MECHANICAL VENTILATOR SUPPORT

Mode Selection
Tidal Volume/Frequency/ Inspiratory Time
Positive End-Expiratory Pressure/Inspired Oxygen Concentration

PARTIAL VENTILATORY SUPPORT IN LESS SEVERE AIRFLOW OBSTRUCTION AND DURING WEANING

REFERENCES

KEY WORDS

air trapping
low-density gases

obstructive lung disease
permissive hypercapnia

CAUSES OF RESPIRATORY FAILURE DUE TO AIRFLOW OBSTRUCTION

Airflow obstruction is a manifestation of a number of disease processes.[1] Among the most common of these are asthma and chronic obstruction pulmonary disease (COPD). Less common causes include bronchiectasis, cystic fibrosis, brochiolititis, and other processes involving the small and large airways of the lung. Acute respiratory failure from acute exacerbation of airflow obstruction is a common occurrence in these diseases.[1] Causes for these acute exacerbations include infection (both bacterial and viral), environmental stresses (e.g., allergens, toxins, dusts), cardiac abnormalities, and systemic inflammatory processes. Of these, infection is by far the most common. In patients with airway disease, respiratory failure is often the end result of a progressive worsening of airflow obstruction over several days. In the asthmatic patient, respiratory failure also can occur very rapidly, with acute bronchospasm and mucous plugging in an "asthma sudden death" syndrome.[2]

PATHOPHYSIOLOGY OF AIRFLOW OBSTRUCTION

Respiratory failure from airflow obstruction is a direct consequence of critical increases in airway resistance. Airway narrowing and increased resistance lead to two important mechanical changes. First, the increased pressures required for airflow may overload respiratory muscles, producing a "ventilatory pump failure" with spontaneous minute ventilation inadequate for gas exchange. Second, the narrowed airways create regions of lung that cannot properly empty and return to their normal "resting volume." This sometimes is called **air trapping** and produces elevated end-expiratory pressures (intrinsic positive end-expiratory pressure [PEEP] or auto-PEEP). These regions of overinflation put inspiratory muscles at a substantial mechanical disadvantage,[3, 4] which further worsens respiratory muscle function. Overinflated regions also may compress more healthy regions of the lung, impairing ventilation-perfusion ($\dot{V}/\dot{Q}$) matching. Regions of air trapping and intrinsic PEEP also function as a threshold load to trigger mechanical breaths[5] (see later discussion).

There are several gas exchange abnormalities in worsening airflow obstruction.[1, 2] First, minute ventilation decreases because of respiratory **muscle overload**. Although there may be a transient hyperventilation due to dyspnea in the asthmatic, worsening respiratory failure in **obstructive lung disease** generally is characterized by decreasing minute ventilation as respiratory muscles fatigue in the face of airflow obstruction. The result is termed *hypercapneic respiratory failure*. Second, as noted previously, regional lung compression and regional hypoventilation produce $\dot{V}/\dot{Q}$ mismatch that results in progressive hypoxemia. Alveolar inflammation and flooding, however, are not characteristic features of respiratory failure due to pure airflow obstruction, and thus shunts are less of an issue than in parenchymal lung injury. Third, overdistended regions of the lung coupled with underlying emphysematous changes in some patients result in capillary loss and increasing dead space. This wasted ventilation further compromises the ability of the respiratory muscles to supply an adequate ventilation for alveolar gas exchange. Fourth, hypoxemic pulmonary vasoconstriction coupled with chronic pulmonary vascular changes in some airway diseases overload the right ventricle, further decreasing blood flow to the lung and making the dead space larger.

GOALS OF MECHANICAL VENTILATION IN PROVIDING TOTAL SUPPORT IN RESPIRATORY FAILURE DUE TO AIRFLOW OBSTRUCTION

In general, the overall goals of ventilatory support in respiratory failure due to airflow obstruction are similar to overall goals in other forms of respiratory failure (i.e., providing adequate gas exchange while minimizing lung injury (see Table 18–2). There are, however, several considerations that are particularly important in the patient with airflow obstruction. First, ventilatory muscle overload and fatigue are common manifestations of respiratory failure in obstructed patients. Therefore selecting modes that initially provide substantial muscle unloading is particularly important (see subsequent considerations of modes and settings).

Second, the presence of very narrowed airways can result in very high peak airway pressures. Moreover, the development of intrinsic PEEP can further increase the inflation pressures delivered by a mechanical ventilator[2, 6] (Fig. 19–1). These pressures, in the setting of heterogeneous regional airflow characteristics, can result in transient overinflation of less obstructed regions in a pendelluft effect (Fig. 19–2). Lung stretch injury, described in more detail in Chapter 11, is the result. Although a plateau pressure greater than 35 cm H_2O is a useful marker for risk of lung stretch injury, clinicians also must be aware that high peak airway pressures, even in the presence of acceptable plateau pressures, may transiently subject regions of the lung to periods of overdistension injury because of this pendelluft effect.[2, 5] Reducing tidal volumes as much as possible is therefore desirable, and decreasing pH and increasing partial pres-

sure of carbon dioxide (PCO_2) is usually an acceptable tradeoff. As noted in Chapter 18, respiratory acidosis seems to be well tolerated in patients without severe cardiac or central nervous system (CNS) difficulties.[6–8] Letting the PCO_2 increase 10 torr per hour and accepting pH values in the 7.10 to 7.20 range thus would seem reasonable if airway and alveolar presures can be kept lower (**permissive hypercapnia**).

Third, although V̇/Q̇ mismatching does occur in acute airflow obstruction, shunts are less of a problem and thus oxygenation usually can be maintained reasonably well without having to use toxic levels of inspired oxygen concentration (FiO_2). Thus, the role of expiratory pressure (applied PEEP) to recruit alveoli in respiratory failure from obstructive disease is less than in parenchymal disease. Moreover, additional expiratory pressure in the face of already overdistended lung regions may only serve to further overdistend them. As discussed subsequently and in Chapter 9, one clinical situation in which applied PEEP can offer benefit in patients with obstructed lung disease is when intrinsic PEEP produces an imposed inspiratory triggering threshold during patient-triggered breaths.

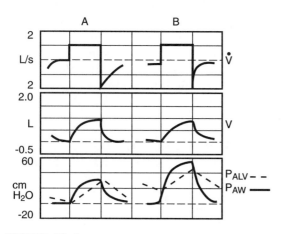

FIGURE 19–1
Effects of airflow obstruction and air trapping (intrinsic positive end-expiratory pressure [PEEP]) or airway pressure during constant tidal volume positive pressure ventilation. Depicted are air flow *(top panel),* volume *(middle panel),* and airway (P_{AW}) and alveolar (P_{ALV}) pressures *(lower panel).* In breath A, there is neither airway obstruction nor intrinsic PEEP. Alveolar pressures thus are equal at end expiration, and the airway-alveolar pressure gradient during inspiration is small. In breath B, there is marked airway obstruction and intrinsic PEEP. Alveolar pressures thus are greater than airway pressure at end expiration, and the airway-alveolar pressure gradient during inspiration is large. In this example, the 30 cm H_2O increase in end-inspiratory peak pressure from breath A to breath B is the result of both the increase in baseline alveolar pressure (20 cm H_2O) and the increases in the flow resistive airway-alveolar pressure (10 cm H_2O).

MECHANICAL VENTILATION SETTINGS AND STRATEGIES IN AIRFLOW OBSTRUCTION REQUIRING TOTAL MECHANICAL VENTILATOR SUPPORT

Mode Selection

As noted previously, substantial muscle unloading generally is required in the initial management of patients with airflow obstruction, and thus assist/control (A/C) ventilation is often indicated. Both pressure-targeted (pressure assist–control [PACV]) and volume-targeted (volume assist–control [VACV]) modes are effective in this regard. PACV offers very high initial flows that vary with patient efforts. This can help keep the inspiratory time short (and thus, expiratory time long) and, if patient triggering is occurring, may synchronize with patient efforts more easily than set flows.[9] Pressure-

NORMAL   HIGH REGIONAL RAW

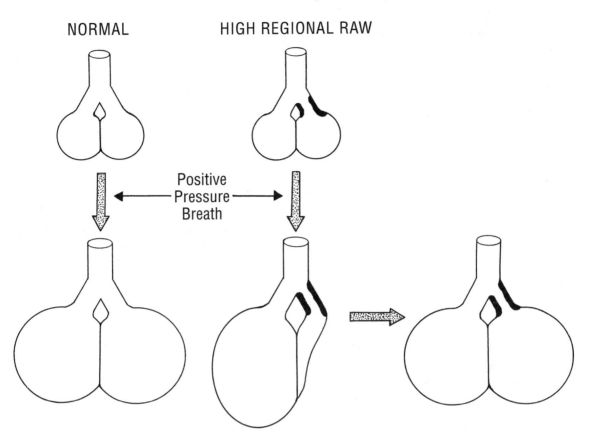

FIGURE 19–2
Regional overdistension and pendelluft effect from heterogeneous distribution of airway properties.

limited breaths also impose an absolute pressure limit on the airway. If this is set at 35 cm H_2O or below, the risk of overdistension injury is conceivably less. Pressure-targeted breaths, however, do not offer the volume guarantee of volume-targeted breaths. As in the management of parenchymal lung injury (see Chapter 18), the choice of pressure-versus volume-targeted breaths generally involves determining the most important management goal. Specifically, if CO_2 clearance is believed to be more important than overdistension protection or synchrony, VACV should be the choice. In contrast, if overdistension protection or synchrony is deemed more important than CO_2 clearance, PACV should be the choice.

Tidal Volume/Frequency/Inspiratory Time

The tidal volume should be set as low as possible in accordance with CO_2 goals to keep maximal alveolar pressures (plateau pressures) at less than 35 cm H_2O. This may mean tidal volume settings in the 6- to 8-ml/kg range.

Inspiratory time settings should be adequate for comfort and avoidance of unnecessarily high peak (i.e., flow resistive) pressures (e.g., 0.7–1.0 sec). However, when setting inspiratory time, clinicians must take into account frequency (and thus the inspiratory:expiratory [I:E] ratio) as they attempt to balance alveolar ventilation needs with the high risk of air trapping. As discussed in Chapter 6, air trapping is dependent on three factors: patient respiratory system mechanical properties (best expressed in this context by the time constant, which is the product of compliance × resistance), the total minute ventilation, and the I:E ratio.[10] As any of these factors increase, the risk of air trapping increases (see Fig. 6–16). Given the high time constants in obstructive airway disease (resulting from generally high resistance and often high compliance units), the risk of air trapping is high. The clinical challenge thus is to reduce the total ventilation and I:E ratio as much as possible to minimize this risk. As noted previously, the tradeoff often is an increasing level of CO_2. This, plus patient dyspnea from small tidal volume and/or air trapping, may require substantial amounts of sedation. In extreme cases, it may be necessary to paralyze the patient to prevent "fighting" with the ventilator and the generation of high airway pressures.[11] An additional consequence of air trapping and resulting high intrathoracic pressures may be compromised right ventricular function (see Chapter 10). Care must be taken to ensure that adequate vascular filling pressures are present to optimize right ventricular function under these circumstances.

Other considerations in the management of acute severe airflow obstruction include the use of anesthetic gases[12] to reduce airway muscle tone in refractory bronchospasm. Another strategy is the use of mixtures of low-density gases (80:20, 70:30, or 60:40 helium:oxygen) mixtures[13] to reduce patient inspiratory work and to facilitate lung emptying (recall that driving pressure decreases and/or flow increases through a tube as gas density decreases). If a helium:oxygen gas mixture is used, remember that many flow sensors must be recalibrated to account for the change in gas density. Finally, in management of patients with airflow obstruction on a ventilator, techniques to deliver bronchodilator aerosols through the ventilator circuitry must be employed. This generally involves in-line circuit nebulizers, although metered dose inhalers with inspiratory circuit-holding chambers are also effective.[14] Because endotracheal tubes significantly reduce aerosol delivery, doses usually are increased three- to fourfold (or even aerosolized continuously) to ensure adequate drug effectiveness.[14] Assessment of airway pressures (peak to plateau gradients) or flow–volume patterns can be used to monitor bronchodilator effectiveness. See Chapter 15 for further discussion on aerosol delivery during mechanical ventilation.

Positive End-Expiratory Pressure/ Inspired Oxygen Concentration

As noted previously, because alveolar inflammation, flooding, and collapse are not major features of acute respiratory failure from airflow obstruction, PEEP is generally not necessary. Moreover, because applied PEEP can further overdistend obstructed regions, it probably should be avoided unless clear regions of atelectasis or alveolar edema exist. FiO_2 adjustments generally can be maintained below 0.6 in these patients to deliver adequate oxygenation. As described in more detail subsequently and in Chapter 9, applied PEEP may help patient triggering of assisted breaths in the setting of high levels of intrinsic PEEP.

PARTIAL VENTILATORY SUPPORT IN LESS SEVERE AIRFLOW OBSTRUCTION AND DURING WEANING

Partial ventilatory support modes (i.e., modes supplying only part of the work of breathing) are appropriate in the patient with less severe airflow obstruction and with nonfatigued ventilatory muscles, especially during the weaning process (see Chapter 20). Commonly used modes include volume-targeted intermittent mandatory ventilation (IMV), pressure support and pressure assist (patient-triggered, pressure-targeted, time-cycled breaths). In patients with airflow obstruction, the presence of air trapping and high levels of muscle loading can markedly increase the sense of dyspnea and make it difficult to properly synchronize ventilator breath triggering, flow delivery, and breath cycling with patient demand.

During ventilator breath triggering by the patient with airflow obstruction, a particularly important problem encountered is the inspiratory threshold load imposed by intrinsic PEEP.[5] This is discussed in more detail in Chapter 9. Simply stated, however, the intrinsic PEEP must be overcome by the inspiratory muscles before airway pressure and flow change to produce a signal to the ventilator that a patient breath is desired. This is manifested clinically by a patient who appears to be contracting the inspiratory muscles but in whom the ventilator detects no activity. An esophageal balloon often can be helpful in detecting this phenomenon (see Fig. 9–4). Judicious amounts of extrinsic PEEP in the airway help equilibrate this trapped pressure with pressure throughout the ventilator circuitry. This allows for less effort on the part of the patient to trigger the ventilator[15–17] (see Fig. 9–4). Using an esophageal pressure measurement, proper PEEP application under these circumstances can be shown to be as high as 70% to 80% of the measured intrinsic PEEP. Up to this level, the applied PEEP only affects circuit and airway pressures—not alveolar pressures. Applied PEEP greater than this, however, appears to begin elevating alveolar pressures and thus becomes counterproductive because regional overdistension develops in less obstructed regions.[16, 17] If an esophageal balloon is not available, trial and error can be used to provide applied PEEP to effect this triggering load. Clinically, one would add small increments (e.g., 2–5 cm H_2O) and watch the patient response. If successful, the patient effort to trigger the breaths should become less as the appropriate level of PEEP is provided. Increasing dyspnea and other signs of increasing intrathoracic pressure (e.g., decreasing blood pressure, worsening of clinical signs of hyperinflation)

suggest that excessive PEEP is being provided.

Patient–ventilator flow and cycle synchrony also can be problematic in patients with airflow obstruction. As in other patients receiving assisted ventilation, pressure-targeted breaths with their variable flow (and initial flow adjustments)[9, 18] often synchronize better with an active ventilatory drive than a fixed flow breath. However, in patients having airflow obstruction, this same increased ventilatory drive can cause excessive triggering of assisted breaths that can worsen air trapping, especially if a large tidal volume is supplied. Lungs hyperinflated from air trapping and large tidal volumes also can cause expiratory muscle activity during breath delivery.[19] Careful adjustments of inspiratory pressure, volume, and timing therefore must be done to ensure proper assisted breath synchrony. Indeed, in some cases, judicious use of sedation to blunt the ventilatory drive may be necessary to achieve these goals.

Finally, partial ventilatory support can be supplied successfully to patients with acute airflow obstruction using a noninvasive mask system (see Chapter 29). Generally, these systems use pressure-targeted breaths, and they can be used either to prevent intubation in acute disease or to facilitate postextubation management. Indeed, some of the strongest data supporting the use of mask ventilation come from studies on patients with acute airflow obstruction.[20]

TABLE 19–1. Mortality for Patients with Obstructive Airway Diseases Requiring Mechanical Ventilation

AUTHOR (YEAR)	TYPE OF PATIENT	NO.	SURVIVAL RATE (%)
Westerman et al[21] (1979)	Asthma	39	90
Zimmerman et al[22] (1993)	Asthma	69	94
Witek et al[23] (1985)	COPD	11	81
Gillespie et al[24] (1986)	COPD	54	77
Senoff et al[25] (1995)	COPD	170	
APACHE III <30			97
APACHE III 40–60			72
APACHE III >75			45

APACHE, Acute Physiology and Chronic Health Evaluation; COPD, chronic obstructive pulmonary disease.

OUTCOMES OF RESPIRATORY FAILURE IN OBSTRUCTED DISEASE

The **outcome** of patients with acute airflow obstruction on mechanical ventilators depends on whether the underlying acute airflow obstruction can be reversed. In general, the outcome of patients with asthma is quite good, although there is a certain mortality associated with even the best management of status asthmaticus[21, 22] (Table 19–1). This mortality is the result of intractable airflow inflammation and mucous secretion that cannot be overcome by medications and mechanical support. Long-term survivors of mechanical ventilation for asthma, however, generally have respiratory function very similar to their baseline.

In contrast to patients with asthma, mortality is substantial in patients with COPD who are receiving mechanical ventilation[23, 24] (although it is still better than in patients with acute lung injury/ acute respiratory distress syndrome) (Table 19–1). Like asthmatic patients, COPD survivors tend to gradually return to baseline lung function. Interestingly, in a recent large multicenter study, the need for mechanical ventilation did not influence outcome in patients with COPD admitted to an intensive care unit.[25] However, the risk for rehospitalization and reintubation for patients with COPD is increased markedly after an episode of respiratory failure requiring mechanical ventilation.[25]

REFERENCES

1. American Thoracic Society: Standards for the diagnosis and care of patients with chronic obstructive pulmonary disease. Am J Respir Crit Care Med 152:578–621, 1995.
2. Fromm RE, Varon J: Acute exacerbations of obstructive lung disease. Postgrad Med 95:101–106, 1994.
3. Tobin MJ: Respiratory muscles in disease. Clin Chest Med 9:263–286, 1988.
4. Annat GJ, Viale JP, Dereymez CP, et al: Oxygen cost of breathing and disphragmatic pressure–time index: measurement in patients with COPD during weaning with pressure support ventilation. Chest 98:411–414, 1990.
5. Pepe PE, Marini JJ: Occult positive end-expiratory pressure in mechanically ventilated patients with airflow obstruction. Am Rev Respir Dis 126:166–170, 1982.
6. Pierson D, Kacmarek R: PEEP therapy: state of the art. Respir Care 33:450–525, 1988.
7. Darioli R, Perret C: Mechanical controlled hypoventilation in status-asthmaticus. Am Rev Respir Dis 129:385–387, 1984.
8. Fiehl F, Perret C: Permissive hypercapnia—how permissive should we be? Am J Respir Crit Care Med 150:1722–1737, 1994.
9. MacIntyre NR, McConnell R, Cheng KC, Sane A: Pressure limited breaths improve flow dys-synchrony during assisted ventilation. Crit Care Med 25:1671–1677, 1997.
10. Marini JJ, Crooke PS: A general mathematical model for respiratory dynamics relevant to the clinical setting. Am Rev Respir Dis 147:14–24, 1993.
11. Hansen-Flaschen J, Brazinsky S, Bassles C, Lanken PV: Use of sedating drugs and neuromuscular blockade in patients requiring mechanical ventilation for respiratory failure. JAMA 266:2870–2875, 1991.
12. Rosseel P, Lauwers LF, Baute L: Halothane treatment in life threatening asthma. Intensive Care Med 11:241–246, 1985.
13. Kass JE, Castriotta RJ: Heliox therapy in acute severe asthma. Chest 107:757–760, 1995.
14. AARC–ARCF Consensus Group: Aerosol therapy. Respir Care 36:916–971, 1991.
15. MacIntyre NR, McConnell R, Cheng KC: Applied PEEP reduces the inspiratory load of intrinsic PEEP during pressure support. Chest 111:188–193, 1997.
16. Gay PC, Rodarte JR, Hubmayr RD: The effects of positive expiratory pressure on isovolume flow and dynamic hyperinflation in patients receiving mechanical ventilation. Am Rev Respir Dis 139:621–626, 1989.
17. Smith TC, Marini JJ: Impact of PEEP on lung mechanics and work of breathing in severe airflow obstruction. J Appl Physiol 65:1488–1499, 1988.
18. MacIntyre NR, Ho LI: Effects of initial flow rate and breath termination criteria on pressure support ventilation. Chest 99:134–138, 1991.
19. Jubran A, Van de Graaff WB, Tobin MJ: Variability of patient ventilator interactions with pressure support ventilation in patients with chronic obstructive pulmonary disease. Am J Respir Crit Care Med 152:129–136, 1995.
20. AARC–ARCF Consensus Group: Non-invasive mechanical ventilation. Respir Care 42:364–425, 1997.
21. Westerman DE, Benatar SR, Potgieter PD, Ferguson AD: Identification of the high risk asthmatic patient. Am J Med 66:565–572, 1979.
22. Zimmerman JL, Dellinger RP, Shah AN, et al: Endotracheal intubation and mechanical ventilation in severe asthma. Crit Care Med 21:1727–1736, 1993.
23. Witek TJ, Schachter EN, Dean NL, Beck GJ: Mechanically assisted ventilation in a community hospital. Arch Intern Med 145:235–239, 1985.

24. Gillespie DJ, Marsh HMN, Divartie MB, Meadows JA: Clinical outcome of patients requiring prolonged (> 24 hrs) mechanical ventilation. Chest 90:364–382, 1986.

25. Senoff MG, Wagner DP, Wagner RP, Zimmerman JE, Knauss WA: Hospital and 1 year survival of patients admitted to ICUs with acute exacerbation of COPD. JAMA 274:1852–1857, 1995.

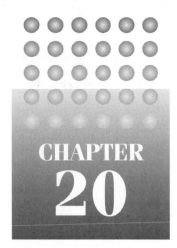

CHAPTER 20

Weaning Mechanical Ventilatory Support

Neil R. MacIntyre, MD

WHY ARE
DISCONTINUATION AND
WEANING STRATEGIES
IMPORTANT?

WHEN SHOULD
VENTILATOR
DISCONTINUATION BE
CONSIDERED?

MANAGING THE NOT-YET-
READY-TO-BE-
DISCONTINUED PATIENT ON
THE VENTILATOR
Aggressiveness/Fatigue

Synchrony and Load
  Characteristics
Characteristics of Patient
  Loads

COMPARING THE
DIFFERENT APPROACHES

CAN WEANING BE
AUTOMATED?

PUTTING TOGETHER A
REASONABLE APPROACH
TO WEANING

REFERENCES

KEY WORDS

flow synchrony
muscle fatigue
partial ventilatory support

ventilator dependence
ventilator discontinuation
weaning

Removing a patient from mechanical ventilation has been termed "liberation," "removal," "discontinuation," "withdrawal,"
and, most commonly, "weaning." Precision
is needed when discussing this process because two distinct concepts are involved.
First is the process of permanent removal
from the ventilator, often with removal of
the artificial airway (i.e., extubation). This
is done in patients fully capable of supporting ventilation on their own. Second is the
process of gradual reduction in the level of
support, often accomplished by using grad-

ual reductions in a mode providing partial
ventilatory support. This is done in patients
capable of doing some, but not all, of the
necessary ventilation. The term **ventilator
discontinuation** should be used for the
first process whereas the term **weaning**
should be reserved for the second process.

In general, patients recovering from rapidly reversing ventilatory insufficiency/fail-
ure (e.g., recovery from anesthesia, drug
overdose, or asthma attack) can be discontinued promptly from the ventilator. In contrast, weaning often is performed in pa-

tients with slowly resolving lung processes in the hope that if the patient performs some comfortable level of ventilatory work, it will accelerate muscle recovery, avoid unnecessary ventilator pressures, and require less sedation for ventilator–patient synchrony.

WHY ARE DISCONTINUATION AND WEANING STRATEGIES IMPORTANT?

The process of ventilator discontinuation and weaning can constitute up to 40% of the time a patient is on a ventilator.[1, 2] Therefore, proper ventilatory management during these processes are crucial. Clearly, ventilator management should be aimed at getting the patient off ventilator support as rapidly as possible. Delayed discontinuation from mechanical ventilatory support exposes patients to unnecessary risks of infection, stretch injury, sedation needs, airway trauma, and costs.[3] Weaning and discontinuation must be done with proper caution and monitoring, however, because premature withdrawal has its own problems. These include loss of airway protection, cardiovascular stress, suboptimal gas exchange, and muscle overload and fatigue.[3] Muscle overload and fatigue are of particular concern because it may take 24 hours or more of muscle rest (i.e., reintubation and high levels of mechanical support) to recover fatigued ventilatory muscles.[4]

WHEN SHOULD VENTILATOR DISCONTINUATION BE CONSIDERED?

In general, when a patient's underlying respiratory disease begins to stabilize and reverse, consideration for ventilator discontinuation should begin. Specific criteria are given in Table 20–1.

When a patient meets Table 20–1 criteria, an assessment for discontinuation potential is appropriate. This usually involves a number of measurements during spontaneous breathing with little or no ventilator assistance (e.g., t-piece trial or using either 1–5 cm H_2O continuous positive airway pressure

TABLE 20–1. Criteria for Consideration of Ventilator Discontinuation

Underlying disease stable or improving
$PaO_2/FiO_2 \geq 200$
$PEEP \leq 10$ cm H_2O
Reliable respiratory drive
Stable cardiovascular status with minimal ionotropes and pressors

FiO_2, inspired oxygen concentration; PaO_2, arterial oxygen pressure; PEEP, positive end-expiratory pressure.

[CPAP] or 5–7 cm H_2O of pressure support from the ventilator[5-8] [Table 20–2]).

Some of the factors in Table 20–2 are readily obtained (e.g., vital capacity [VC], minute ventilation [MV], frequency/tidal volume [f/V_T] ratio, muscle force generated during 20 seconds of effort against a closed airway maximum inspiratory force [MIF], and patient observations). Ventilator discontinuation is more likely if the MV is ≤ 15 L/min, the VC is greater than 10 ml/kg, the f/V_T ratio is less than 105, and the MIF is more negative than -25 cm H_2O.[5, 6]

TABLE 20–2. Criteria to Predict Discontinuation Success

MECHANICAL FACTORS	MV < 15 L/min MIF < −25 cm H_2O VC > 10 ml/kg f/V_T <105 Work < 5 joules/min (exclusive of endotracheal tube work) PTI < 0.15
INTEGRATED FACTORS	CROP index > 13[7] Weaning score based on compliance, resistance, V_D/V_T, $PaCO_2$ and f/V_T < 3[8] Weaning index (PTI × MV for $PaCO_2$ of 40/V_T) < 4[33] Neural network[13]
PATIENT ASSESSMENT	Lack of: Dyspnea Accessory muscle use Abdominal paradox Agitation/anxiety/ tachycardia

f, frequency; MV, minute ventilation; $PaCO_2$, partial pressure of carbon dioxide; PTI, pressure–time index; VC, vital capacity; V_D, dead-space volume; V_T, tidal volume.

Other parameters in Table 20–2 require more sophisticated measurements. For instance, an esophageal balloon to measure esophageal pressure (P_{ES}, an estimate of pleural pressure) is necessary to assess patient muscle loads.[8] Muscle loads can be expressed as either work or pressure–time products (PTPs) per breath (work $= \int P_{ES} \cdot V_T$, PTP $= \int P_{ES} \cdot T_i$).[9–12] These indices of muscle load can be expressed with respect to time (i.e., work/min), to ventilation (i.e., work/liter) or to maximum muscle strength (i.e., PTP/MIF). As work/minute or work/liter approaches normal values (5 joules/min or 0.5 joules/L), ventilation discontinuation becomes more likely. Multiplying the PTP/MIF by the inspiratory time fraction (T_i/T_{tot}) results in the pressure–time index (PTI), which can be a useful predictor of fatigue (PTI > 0.15 predicts fatigue).[11]

Integrated factors also have been employed. The CROP index multiplies dynamic compliance by PaO_2/PAO_2 (arterial oxygen pressure/alveolar partial pressure of oxygen) by MIF and divides this product by respiratory rate. A CROP index greater than 13 predicts weaning success.[7] Other integrated scores incorporate P_{ES} load calculations[8] and may use neural networks.[13] Important clinical assessment criteria include subjective dyspnea, accessory muscle use, diaphoresis, tachycardia, abdominal paradox, and subjective comfort.

Analyses of receiver–operator characteristics (ROC curves) have shown none of these indices alone to be 100% sensitive and specific in predicting discontinuation success.[7] Indeed, a spontaneous breathing trial of up to 1 hour with simple observations of f/V_T, dyspnea, and accessory muscle use is probably the easiest and most reliable guide to decide the likelihood of ventilator discontinuation.[7] This procedure probably should be done daily in all patients meeting the criteria in Table 20–1 but who, for whatever reason, were not permanently discontinued from the ventilator the previous day. As several studies have shown,[1, 2, 14] spontaneous breathing trials with simple clinical observations often reveal that a patient actually may be ready for successful ventilatory discontinuation, even though other traditional assessments may not seem to support it.

The decision to perform subsequent artificial airway removal after ventilator discontinuation depends on additional considerations. First, artificial airway removal must be done only in patients with the ability to protect the airway. Second, the risk of potential recurrence of acute respiratory failure and thus ventilator need also must be assessed before removing the artificial airway.

MANAGING THE NOT-YET-READY-TO-BE-DISCONTINUED PATIENT ON THE VENTILATOR

Patients who meet criteria in Table 20–1 but who either cannot meet the discontinuation criteria (Table 20–2) or who fail discontinuation pose an important management challenge. A first step in addressing this issue is to determine the reasons for failure. Common causes for failed discontinuation and continued ventilator dependence are: (1) respiratory drive failure involving inability of the patient to generate a reliable respiratory drive because of central nervous system (CNS) injury or drugs[15]; (2) oxygenation failure involving rapid hemoglobin desaturation from loss of expiratory pressure and/or inspired oxygen concentration (FiO_2); (3) cardiovascular failure involving dysrhythmias and/or hypotension from catechol release, edema formation, or coronary hypoxemia due to loss of ventilatory support[16]; and (4) muscle failure involving muscle overload from abnormal respiratory system impedances in the setting of weakened, fatigued, or metabolically disturbed muscles.[9, 17–22] A particular clinical venue may be the site of one form of failure more commonly than others (e.g., coronary care units may see more cardiac problems, neurologic units may see more respiratory drive failures). In intensive care units in which respiratory diseases are treated predominantly, the most common cause of **ventilator dependence** is muscle load exceeding muscle capabilities.[23]

Once a cause of ventilator dependence has been established, a management plan can be developed. This plan first must focus on the cause of the ventilator dependency (e.g., improving respiratory drive, improving cardiac function, or improving gas exchange). However, managing the ventilator and the patient ventilator loads also can be important in developing and maintaining optimal ventilator muscle function. Two fundamental approaches to this exist: (1) near total rest with assist/control (A/C) ventilation or (2) various modes of partial support. Modes of partial support generally involve either intermittent support (intermittent mandatory ventilation [IMV]) or partial support of every breath (pressure support: PS and pressure assist: PA). These are described in Figure 20–1 and Table 20–3.

The conceptual advantages to near total rest with A/C ventilation are twofold. First, **muscle fatigue** risk is minimized with high-level support. Second, management requires no decision-making other than the daily spontaneous breathing trials for dis-

continuation assessment. Both of these conceptual advantages require that the A/C mode be applied synchronously. Specifically, the trigger, the flow delivery, and the cycling criteria of the A/C breaths must be synchronized properly to any patient effort (see Chapter 9). Otherwise, high levels of imposed muscle loading can develop, which can increase the risk of fatigue. Proper ventilator settings (including consideration of pressure-targeted A/C) are thus crucial, and sedation may be required to reduce imposed loads from dys-synchrony.

There are several advantages to **partial ventilatory support**. First, a more gradual withdrawal may be tolerated better than periods of sudden total withdrawal, especially in patients who have been on a ventilator for a prolonged period or who may have an impaired cardiovascular system. Second, less pressure is applied to the

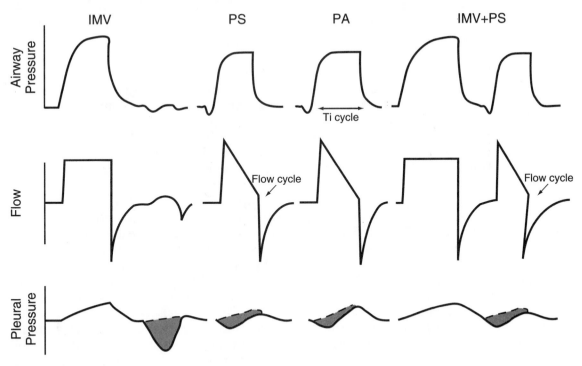

FIGURE 20–1

Airway pressure flow and pleural pressure patterns of commonly used modes of partial support. The shaded area reflects patient contribution to the work of breathing. The left panel is intermittent mandatory ventilation (IMV) with volume assist-control breaths alternating with spontaneous unassisted breaths. The second panel is pressure support (PS), in which a patient-triggered, pressure-targeted, flow-cycled breath provides partial support of the patient effort. The third panel is pressure assist (PA), in which a patient-triggered, pressure-targeted, time-cycled breath provides partial support of patient effort. The last panel depicts a combination of IMV and PS.

TABLE 20–3. Modes of Partial Support

MODE	DESCRIPTION	INITIAL SETTINGS	SUPPORT WEANED BY
IMV	Set number of volume- or pressure-targeted A/C breaths interspersed with spontaneous breaths (up to 10 cm H_2O PS during those breaths sometimes given to compensate for endotracheal tube resistance)	Mimic volume or pressure A/C ventilation settings with mandatory breath rate slightly below total A/C ventilation	Reduce number of mandatory breaths*
PS or PA	Inspiratory pressure delivered with every effort. PS terminates by flow, PA terminates on a set time	Use pressure support mode for PS; use pressure A/C with rate set to 0 for PA, mimic plateau pressure, and inspiratory time of A/C ventilation	Reduce inspiratory pressure level†
IMV + PS	Combine IMV with > 10 cm H_2O PS	As with IMV, except that PS is set between 10 cm H_2O and plateau pressure A/C ventilation	Reduce both IMV mandatory breath rate and PS level

*Mandatory minute ventilation can automate this according to total minute ventilation.
†Can be automatically set by tidal volume (V_T).
A/C, assist-control; IMV, intermittent mandatory ventilation; PA, pressure assist; PS, pressure support.

thorax with partial support than with total support and thus, there is potentially less risk of lung stretch injury and cardiovascular compromise. Third, muscle recovery may be enhanced using partial support. This is a complex and controversial issue. Fatigued muscles need rest for recovery, but prolonged inactivity clearly can produce atrophy.[9, 24–26] An optimal balance may be to provide these types of patients with a near normal muscle load using a comfortable, nonfatiguing level of partial support.

In using modes of partial support to optimize muscle recovery, three issues must be considered: (1) proper balancing of aggressiveness versus fatigue; (2) patient–ventilator synchrony; and (3) characteristics of patient muscle loads.

Aggressiveness/Fatigue

When partial support modes are used, regular assessment and adjustments are mandatory for two reasons. First, weaning cannot be accomplished unless ventilatory support is reduced. This must be done carefully, however, because too prompt a reduction may precipitate fatigue. Protocols to regularly assess patients and adjust support loads accordingly are thus a vital part of any weaning strategy with partial support. Indeed, much of the variability in reported weaning studies likely was the result of variability in assessment and adjustment strategies.[1, 2] Proper weaning strategy aggressiveness might be inferred by the reintubation rate (i.e., percentage of patients who are extubated but need to be reintubated in 24–48 hours) of a particular unit. If the reintubation rate is very low (i.e., <5%), one might wonder whether weaning practices are too cautious. In contrast, if the reintubation rate is very high (i.e., >15%), one might wonder whether weaning practices are excessively aggressive.

Synchrony and Load Characteristics

During partial support weaning techniques, patients must interact with the ventilator flow delivery system. Important issues on triggering, flow delivery, and breath cycling interactions are covered in Chapter 9. During weaning, patient–ventilator synchrony is crucial in minimizing unnecessary sedation, minimizing unnecessary muscle work, and providing appropriate rest for sleep. As discussed in Chapter 9, patient–ventilator synchrony enhancement with pressure-targeted breaths is the rationale behind pressure support and pressure assist weaning strategies.[27–29]

Characteristics of Patient Loads

Muscle loads are characterized both by total load involved (work or PTP, see Chapter 6) and by load characteristics (i.e., the pressure–volume relationship, Fig. 20–2).[12, 27, 30, 31] Load quantity already has been discussed, and the goal of weaning is to aggressively reapply tolerable but not fatiguing loads. Load characteristics, however, also may be important. Specifically, distortion of work characteristics to a high-pressure/low-volume load is clearly less efficient (i.e., work/oxygen consumption falls) and probably more readily induces fatigue.[12, 23] Thus, a similar level of work performed on a lung with abnormal compliance and/or resistance using unassisted spontaneous breaths with high-pressure/low-volume characteristics (IMV approach) may be more fatiguing than a reconfigured patient breath using pressure-targeted breaths that "normalize" the pressure–volume relationship (PS/PA approach) (see Fig. 20–2). This is another rationale for using pressure-targeted breaths as a primary partial support technique.[27]

COMPARING THE DIFFERENT APPROACHES

Two large trials have been performed comparing t-piece/ACV, IMV and stand-alone PS approaches to weaning[1, 2] (Table 20–4). As seen in Table 20–4, one found PS to be superior and one found t-piece/ACV to be superior in patients requiring substantial ventilatory support for more than several days. There is obvious difficulty in drawing general conclusions from these studies be-

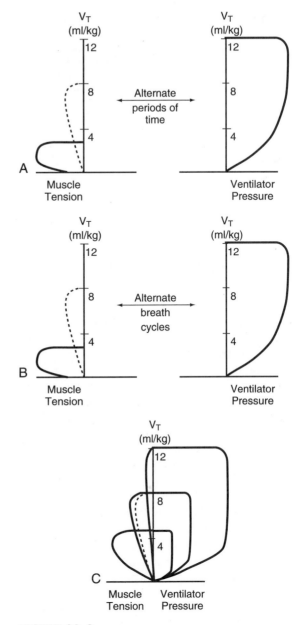

FIGURE 20–2
Pressure-volume diagrams illustrating the configuration of patient work during various forms of partial support. Patient effort (muscle tension) is directed leftward, ventilator-delivered pressure is directed rightward. The dotted line represents a normal pressure-volume work configuration. In these examples, respiratory disease has produced impedance changes that have reconfigured patient work to a high pressure-low volume pattern (solid lines). With t-piece breathing (A) and intermittent mandatory ventilation (IMV) (B), patient work remains in this abnormal configuration during the spontaneous breaths. With pressure-targeted partial support (C), ventilator assistance with every breath reconfigures patient effort to a more normal pressure-volume pattern.

TABLE 20–4. Weaning Success Using Different Ventilator Strategies

| STUDY | % PATIENTS REMAINING ON VENTILATOR | |
	Day 5	Day 10
Esteban trial[1]		
IMV	70	44
t-piece	44	16
PS	61	38
Brochard trial[2]		
IMV	66	54
t-piece	60	41
PS	47	24

IMV, intermittent mandatory ventilation; PS, pressure support.

cause the way in which these modes were used in each study was so different. For example, the Esteban study[1] had very aggressive t-piece weaning rules that not only produced a faster weaning rate than the more conservative Brochard t-piece weaning rule[2] but also produced an almost fourfold increase in the rate of reintubation. There are important messages from both of these studies, however. First, weaning strategy clearly can affect outcome. Indeed, depending on strategy, weaning time could increase severalfold in both of these two controlled studies. Second, a weaning strategy must be aggressive. This can be frequent discontinuation assessments, frequent protocol-driven reduction in partial support, or both. Third, fatigue potential needs to be monitored carefully to minimize the risk of overaggressiveness. Finally, both studies demonstrated that substantial numbers of patients thought to be ventilator dependent could be discontinued safely from the ventilator after successfully passing a spontaneous breathing trial. These observations, coupled with more recent reports on weaning protocols,[14, 32] re-emphasize the importance of frequent (e.g., daily) assessments for discontinuation potential.

CAN WEANING BE AUTOMATED?

A number of newer ventilators supply certain feedback features that theoretically may be helpful in the weaning process (Table 20–5). An inherent problem in all of these, however, is that the input variable for machine decision-making is currently only a single variable, either minute ventilation or tidal volume. As noted previously, many other variables (including clinical assessment), seem far more important in aggressive weaning than these two, and thus the potential utility of these current approaches seems limited. Indeed, the weaning process actually might be *delayed* if an inappropriately high minute ventilation or tidal volume is set as the target-weaning variable using the currently available approaches listed in Table 20–5.

PUTTING TOGETHER A REASONABLE APPROACH TO WEANING

Once a patient reaches the criteria in Table 20–1, daily consideration for discontinua-

TABLE 20–5. Automated Weaning Approaches

MODE	STRATEGY	WEANING ACCOMPLISHED BY
Mandatory minute ventilation	Adjusts IMV rate to ensure minimum minute ventilation	IMV rate decreased if MV maintained
Volume support	Adjust PS level to ensure minimum V_T	PS level reduced if V_T maintained
Volume-assured pressure support/pressure augmentation	Provides a backup flow/V_T to the PS breath	PS level reduced by clinician while machine provides "safety net" V_T

IMV, intermittent mandatory ventilation; PS, pressure support; V_T, tidal volume.

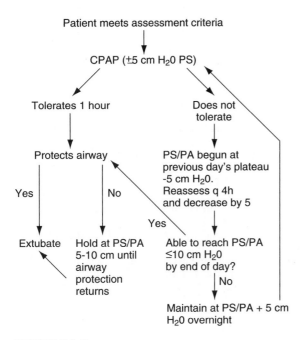

FIGURE 20–3
A proposed weaning strategy. CPAP, continuous positive airway pressure; PA, pressure assist; PS, pressure support.

tion must be given. Although many indices can help predict successful discontinuation, a short CPAP, low-level PS or spontaneous breathing trial using some of the simple assessment criteria in Table 20–2 is probably the best indication. Patients who may be capable of ventilator discontinuation can be identified in this manner.

Patients in whom this trial fails are probably best served by a weaning protocol rather than A/C ventilation rest for the aforementioned reasons. In designing the protocol, the approach to assessment/adjustment is probably more important than the actual partial support mode used. However, three considerations in selecting mode may be important. First, pressure-targeted modes do offer improved **flow synchrony** and more physiologic muscle loading than do flow-limited volume-targeted breaths alternating with spontaneous breaths. Second, combining two modes of support, such as IMV and substantial pressure support, may unnecessarily complicate the weaning process (i.e., two types of support must be adjusted to be aggressive). Third, if a backup mandatory breath rate is desired,

adding a breath rate to PA (i.e., pressure assist/control) or using a minimum minute ventilation backup mode is often more comfortable than supplying irregular patterns of support with modes such as IMV.

Once the weaning process has begun, regular assessment and adjustment are mandatory to provide weaning that is both aggressive and safe. A proposed scheme is given as Figure 20–3.

As shown in Table 20–4, the weaning strategy can have profound effects on ventilator length of stay in patients. Keys to successful weaning are appropriate aggressiveness (i.e., frequent assessments/adjustments), maximal patient comfort, and proper muscle loading.

REFERENCES

1. Esteban A, Frutos F, Tobin MJ, et al: A comparison of four methods of weaning from mechanical ventilation. N Engl J Med 332:345–350, 1995.
2. Brochard L, Ramos A, Benito S, et al: Comparison of these methods of gradual withdrawal from ventilatory support during weaning from mechanical ventilation. Am J Respir Crit Care Med 150:896–903, 1994.
3. Fulkerson WJ, MacIntyre NR: Problems in Respiratory Care: Complications of Mechanical Ventilation. Philadelphia: JB Lippincott, 1991.
4. Laghi F, D'Alfonso N, Tobin MJ: Pattern of recovery from diaphragmatic fatigue over 24 hours. J Appl Physiol 79:539–546, 1995.
5. Sahn SA, Lakschminarayan MB: Bedside criteria for the discontinuation of mechanical ventilation. Chest 63:1002–1005, 1973.
6. Morganroth ML, Morganroth JL, Nett LM, et al: Criteria for weaning from prolonged mechanical ventilation. Arch Intern Med 144:1012–1016, 1984.
7. Yang K, Tobin MJ: A prospective study of indexes predicting outcome of trials of weaning from mechanical ventilation. N Engl J Med 324:1445–1450, 1991.
8. Gluck EH: Predicting eventual success or failure to wean in patients receiving long term mechanical ventilation. Chest 110:1018–1024, 1996.
9. Tobin MJ: Respiratory muscles in disease. Clin Chest Med 9:263–286, 1988.
10. Collett PW, Perry C, Engel LA: Pressure time product, flow, and oxygen cost of resistive breathing in humans. J Appl Physiol 58:1263–1272, 1985.
11. Bellemare F, Grassino A: Effect of pressure and timing or contraction on human diaphragm fatigue. J Appl Physiol 53:1190–1195, 1982.
12. MacIntyre NR, Leatherman NE: Mechanical loads on the ventilatory muscles: a theoretical analysis. Am Rev Respir Dis 139:968–973, 1989.

13. Ashutosh K, Hyukjoon L, Mohan CK, et al: Prediction criteria for successful weaning from respiratory support. Crit Care Med 20:1295–1301, 1992.
14. Ely EW, Baker AM, Dunagan DP, et al: Effect on the duration of mechanical ventilation of identifying patients capable of breathing spontaneously. N Engl J Med 335:1864–1869, 1996.
15. Argov Z, Mastaglia FL: Disorders of neuromuscular transmission caused by drugs. N Engl J Med 301:409–413, 1979.
16. Lemaire F, Teboul JL, Cinotti L, et al: Acute left ventricular dysfunction during unsuccessful weaning from mechanical ventilation. Anesthesiology 69:171–179, 1988.
17. Hussain SNA, Simkus T, Roussos C: Respiratory muscle fatigue: a cause of ventilatory failure in septic shock. J Appl Physiol 58:2033–2040, 1985.
18. Roussos CS, Macklem PT: Diaphragmatic fatigue in man. J Appl Physiol 43:189–197, 1977.
19. Agusti AGN, Torres A, Estopa R, Agustividal A: Hypophosphatemia as a cause of failed weaning: the importance of metabolic factors. Crit Care Med 12:142–143, 1984.
20. Molloy DW, Dhingra S, Solven F, et al: Hypomagnesemia and respiratory muscle power. Am Rev Respir Dis 129:497–498, 1984.
21. Bark H, Heimer D, Chaimowitz C, Mostoslowski M: Effect of chronic renal failure on respiratory muscle strength. Respiration 54:151–163, 1988.
22. Pingleton SK, Harmon GS: Nutritional management in acute respiratory failure. JAMA 257:2094–2099, 1987.
23. MacIntyre NR, Ho L: Weaning mechanical ventilatory support. Anesth Rep 3:211–215, 1990.
24. Auzueto A, Peters JI, Tobin MJ, et al: Effects of prolonged controlled mechanical ventilation on diaphragmatic function in healthy adult baboons. Crit Care Med 25:1187–1190, 1997.
25. Marini JJ: Exertion during ventilator support: how much and how important? Respir Care 31:385–387, 1986.
26. Roussos CS, Macklem PT: The respiratory muscles. N Engl J Med 307:786–797, 1982.
27. MacIntyre NR: Weaning from mechanical ventilatory support: volume-assisting intermittent breaths versus pressure-assisting every breath. Respir Care 33:121–125, 1988.
28. Brochard L, Harf A, Lorino H, et al: Pressure support prevents diaphragmatic failure during weaning from mechanical ventilation. Am Rev Respir Dis 139:513–521, 1989.
29. MacIntyre NR, McConnell R, Cheng KC, Sane A: Pressure limited breaths improve flow dys-synchrony during assisted ventilation. Crit Care Med 25:1671–1677, 1997.
30. McGregor M, Becklake MR: The relationship of oxygen cost of breathing to respiratory mechanical work and respiratory force. J Clin Invest 40:971–980, 1961.
31. Leith DE, Bradley M: Ventilatory muscle strength and endurance training. J Appl Physiol 41:508–516, 1976.
32. Kollef MH, Shapiro SD, Silver P, et al: A randomized controlled trial of protocol directed vs physician directed weaning from mechanical ventilation. Crit Care Med 25:567–574, 1997.
33. Jabour ER, Rabil DM, Truwit JD, Rochester DF: Evaluation of a new weaning index based on ventilatory endurance and the efficiency of gas exchange. Am Rev Respir Dis 144:531–537, 1991.

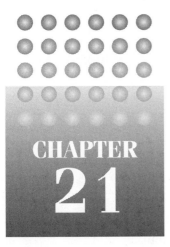

Long-Term Mechanical Ventilation

Neil R. MacIntyre, MD
Janice Thalman, BS, RRT
Robert B. Campbell, RRT

VENTILATOR-DEPENDENT PATIENTS: CAUSES AND OUTCOMES

NONINVASIVE VERSUS INVASIVE APPLICATION OF POSITIVE PRESSURE VENTILATION

VENTILATORS FOR LONG-TERM USE
Volume Targeted
Pressure Targeted

VENTILATOR MANAGEMENT STRATEGIES
Scenario 1: Category 1 Patients with Potentially Reversible Disease Requiring the Ventilator for Life Support

Scenario 2: Category 2 Patients with Irreversible Lung Disease Requiring Mechanical Ventilation for Life Support
Scenario 3: Category 1 or 2 Patients Requiring Only Intermittent (Nocturnal) Requirements for Ventilatory Support

THE ROLE OF COMPREHENSIVE REHABILITATION IN THE LONG-TERM VENTILATOR-DEPENDENT PATIENT

KEY WORDS

extended care facilities
assessments for ventilator withdrawal
mechanical ventilation outcome

ventilator dependence
weaning units

TABLE 21-1. Diseases Associated with Ventilator Dependence in Category 1 Patients (%)

	SCHEINHORN ET AL, 1994	GRACEY ET AL, 1995
Acute lung disease	32	1
Chronic lung disease	24	13
Postoperative	23	63
Other	15	23

VENTILATOR-DEPENDENT PATIENTS: CAUSES AND OUTCOMES

Long-term ventilator-dependent patients are often defined as those who require mechanical ventilatory support for at least 6 hours/day for more than 21 to 30 days.[1-5] These patients usually fall into one of two categories: category 1, an episode of reversible acute respiratory failure that has not fully resolved; or category 2, irreversible progression of an underlying chronic respiratory process.

Category 1 patients are typically those who are recovering from pneumonia, acute respiratory distress syndrome (ARDS), acute exacerbation of chronic respiratory disease (e.g., chronic obstructive pulmonary disease [COPD]), or prolonged respiratory problems after surgery. After 3 to 4 weeks of intensive care and mechanical ventilatory support, in most of these patients the underlying disease has either resolved or they have died. The need for ventilatory support beyond 30 days in such patients usually indicates serious residual lung injury that may take months (if ever) to resolve. Data from two "weaning units" give a representation of the distribution of these types of patients (Table 21-1).[1, 6, 7]

The prevalence of category 1 patients is largely unknown because many are cared for in acute care hospitals. Indeed, in calendar year 1998, 7% of ventilated patients at Duke University Hospital (800 inpatient beds) received ventilatory support for more than 20 days, and 4% received support for more than 30 days. This, coupled with the fact that weaning units admit 50 to 150 patients per year,[1, 6, 7] suggests that the number of category 1 patients in the United States is substantial. When cared for in specially designed centers, the outcome for category 1 patients is remarkably good in terms of weaning from **ventilator dependence** (Table 21-2). This probably is because many category 1 patients merely need a more prolonged ventilatory support period to recover enough lung function to be liberated from the ventilator. However, subsequent mortality in category 1 patients removed from the ventilator is variable and probably depends heavily on underlying lung function (see Table 21-2).[1, 6-11]

Category 2 patients generally have neuromuscular diseases or progressive pulmo-

TABLE 21-2. Outcome of Category 1 Patients Managed in a Weaning Unit Over 1 Year

	SCHEINHORN ET AL, 1997	GRACEY ET AL, 1995
No.	1026	132
Discharged/weaned	569 (54%)	103 (78%)
Ventilator dependent	159 (15%)	16 (12%)
Died in unit	298 (29%)	13 (10%)
Alive for discharge	728 (71%)	119 (90%)
Alive at 1 yr postdischarge	253 (25%)	97 (74%)

nary diseases (e.g., interstitial fibrosis) with inexorable deterioration of their respiratory function and escalation of mechanical ventilation needs (Table 21–3).[2, 3, 5, 12] In these patients, what often begins as intermittent support becomes nocturnal support, then full-time support. Category 2 also includes category 1 type patients who are never able to be weaned successfully from the ventilator. The prevalence of category 2 ventilator-dependent patients is growing. In the United States in 1983, there were an estimated 6800 such patients.[5, 13] By 1990, that estimate had nearly doubled,[5, 14] and by 1997, it had increased to more than 17,000.[2] Financial and social factors are shifting the venues of care for category 2 patients.[15–17] In the 1980s, most of these patients were cared for in acute care hospitals, whereas **extended care facilities** and home are the most common sites in the 1990s.[5] Mortality in category 2 patients depends heavily on the nature of the underlying disease.

NONINVASIVE VERSUS INVASIVE APPLICATION OF POSITIVE PRESSURE VENTILATION

There are two basic ways to provide positive pressure ventilation long term: through a mask system and through a tracheostomy. Noninvasive mask systems offer the advantage of not requiring an invasive artificial airway.[18–20] Noninvasive systems, however, can be cumbersome and do not provide adequate airway protection. Long-term noninvasive strategy thus should be reserved for patients who do not need the ventilatory

support for more than 12 hours a day (i.e., patients requiring ventilatory support only at night) and in patients who have adequate airway protection. See Chapter 29 for more detailed discussions of noninvasive positive pressure ventilation.

A tracheostomy is indicated for long-term mechanical ventilation patients who either need more than nocturnal support or who do not tolerate the mask or who have difficulty protecting the airway. Tracheostomy tube design features are summarized in Tables 21–4 through 21–6.[21]

VENTILATORS FOR LONG-TERM USE

Ventilators designed for long-term use can be either volume targeted or pressure targeted.[22]

Volume Targeted

Generally, volume-targeted ventilators are very simple devices that supply fixed flow (usually sine wave) breaths over a limited range of tidal volumes. Spontaneous breathing also is allowed, although the patient-triggering mechanisms are usually less sensitive and less responsive than current-generation intensive care unit (ICU) ventilators. This can lead to significant patient discomfort in patients with active ventilatory drives.[23] If positive end-expiratory pressure (PEEP) is required, an external PEEP valve usually is needed. These devices are often portable (i.e., can be moved with the patient), have some sort of built-in compres-

TABLE 21–3. Diseases Associated with Category 2 Ventilator Dependence

DISEASE	% OF CATEGORY 2 PATIENTS
Cervical trauma	14
Muscular dystrophy	14
Chronic lung disease	13
Polio	10
Amyotrophic lateral sclerosis	6
Other (33 diagnoses)	43

From Adams AB, Shapiro R, Marini JJ: Changing prevalence of chronically ventilator-assisted individuals in Minnesota: increases, characteristics, and the use of noninvasive ventilation. Respir Care 43:643–649, 1998.

TABLE 21–4. Tracheostomy Tube Design Features

FEATURE	COMMENTS
Cuffs	Cuffed tubes offer some airway protection and minimize air lead; uncuffed tubes allow phonation and are less traumatic
Fenestrations	Fenestrations allow phonation when inner cannula removed, also provide for low resistance for spontaneous breathing
Length	Goal is to have tracheostomy tube tip in mid trachea (may require custom-built tubes for those with very thick necks)
Inner cannula	Allows for cleaning without removal of entire tracheostomy
Speaking valves	In spontaneously breathing patients, these permit inspiration through the tracheostomy but then force expiration around uncuffed tube or through fenestrations for phonation
Buttons	These are plugs to maintain tracheostomy sites after tube is removed

TABLE 21–5. Tracheostomy Tube Materials

TUBE MATERIAL	COMMENT
Silver-Jackson	Durable, long lasting, and inner cannula easy to clean; rigidity, however, is potentially traumatic, and tissue irritation can develop from oxidation
Natural and synthetic rubber	Not good for long term because it is affected by a variety of cleaning solutions and gases; additives also can injure tissue
Polyvinyl chloride	Not good for long term because it degrades thermally and can react with sterilizing agents
Nylon	Rigid, lightweight, easy to clean, and nontoxic
Silicone	Durable and flexible, hydrophobic and biocompatible ("tissue friendly"); probably material of choice

TABLE 21–6. Tracheostomy Tube Cuff Features

FEATURE	COMMENTS
Compliance	High-volume, low-pressure cuffs conform better to tracheal anatomy and produce less pressure injury (generally kept below 20–25 cm H_2O inflation pressure)
Pressure relief valve	Valve prevents intracuff pressure >25 cm H_2O
Lanz cuff equalization	Cuff attached to external reservoir balloon; cuff self fills to equalize pressure
Fome cuff	Cuff filled with soft material that conforms to tracheal anatomy
Tight to shaft	Outer diameter of the tracheostomy tube can be expanded with air inflation to effect seal

sor, and may have optional supplemental oxygen (O_2). The advantages to these devices are that they generally are inexpensive, simple to use, and reliable. In addition, neuromuscular patients often can use these volume-targeted breaths to stack them and facilitate coughing. The disadvantage is that it is not always easy to synchronize the fixed-flow pattern to active patient demands. In addition, when this type of ventilator is used with a mask interface, variable mask leaks can significantly affect delivered volume.

Pressure Targeted

Pressure-targeted devices also can be relatively simple to operate and usually can deliver ventilator-controlled (i.e., pressure-targeted, time-cycled breaths) as well as two types of patient-triggered breaths: pressure support breaths (pressure targeted, flow cycled) or pressure assist breaths (pressure targeted, time cycled). When using pressure-targeted, flow-cycled breaths (i.e., pressure support) with a mask system, the inevitable leak must be accounted for by the ventilator to avoid inappropriately long inspiratory times. Expiratory pressure capabilities may be integral on some of these systems but may require external PEEP valves on others. When compared with ICU ventilators, the maximal pressures generated by these devices are usually less. The advantage to these pressure-targeted devices is that they usually synchronize with patients' efforts more easily than do the fixed-flow devices, especially if there are vigorous efforts.[24, 25] The disadvantage to these systems is that a volume guarantee is not provided with each breath (although more complex ICU-style ventilators can provide minimum volume "safety nets.")[26]

For category 1 patients, substantial ventilatory support may be needed initially, whereas more comfortable interactive modes may be required subsequently during the weaning process. For this reason, volume- and pressure-targeted ICU equivalent ventilators generally are used in these patients initially. As weaning progresses and ventilatory support needs decrease, however, simpler long-term devices with pres-

sure-targeted interactive capabilities (i.e., pressure support/pressure assist) may be used.

For category 2 patients requiring substantial support with little or no patient–ventilator interactions, control ventilation or assist/control ventilation can be provided with simple long-term volume or pressure-targeted devices. However, category 2 patients who require only intermittent support (i.e., nocturnal) and who can interact with the gas delivery system may be supported better with pressure support/pressure assist systems attached to a mask or a tracheostomy. The need for a backup rate (capability of controlled mechanical breaths in the event of patient apnea or bradypnea) depends on the clinical situation in these types of patients.

Required monitoring capabilities of long-term ventilators depend on the level of support being provided.[22] High-pressure relief is required in all devices. However, additional monitors and alarms to detect ventilator failure, ventilator disconnection, minute ventilation, flow patterns, and gas concentrations should be required only if these devices are used for life support (i.e., virtually 24-hour usage in a patient in whom ventilator malfunction could result in serious injury or death). If the devices are used only intermittently, these types of monitors and alarms still may be desirable but are not mandatory.[22]

There are other issues regarding long-term devices. Although compressors use room air (which is partially humidified), supplemental O_2 may be dry. Thus, the need for additional humidification depends on the clinical situation.[27] Because room air often is used, a simple heat and moisture exchanger (HME) is usually adequate if humidification is believed to be needed. However, HMEs can interfere with the sensing function of some of these ventilators. Caregivers in the long-term situation also need to be familiar with airway care issues such as tracheostomy care, suctioning, circuit maintenance, and aerosol delivery.

VENTILATOR MANAGEMENT STRATEGIES

Depending on the clinical situation, different management strategies are required.

Following are suggested approaches to three clinical scenarios: category 1 patients with potentially reversible respiratory failure requiring the ventilator for life support; category 2 patients with irreversible disease requiring full ventilatory support to sustain life; and category 1 or 2 patients with ventilatory insufficiency requiring only partial support (e.g., nocturnal support).

Scenario 1: Category 1 Patients with Potentially Reversible Disease Requiring the Ventilator for Life Support

The focus on these types of patients is to provide them with comfortable levels of ventilatory support with an eye toward gradually reducing the support (see Chapter 20). Clinical observations such as subjective comfort, dyspnea, and the patient's ventilatory pattern (especially the frequency tidal volume relationship[28]) should guide the level of support. A crucial part of management is to have frequent (even as often as daily) assessment to see how close the pa-

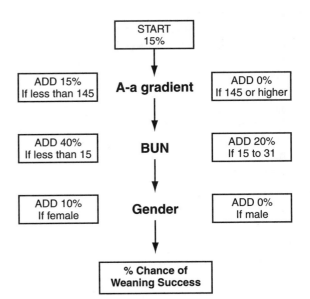

FIGURE 21–2
Predictive values of weaning success from a large ventilator weaning unit. (Reproduced with permission from Scheinhorn DJ, Hassenpflug M, Artinian BM, et al: Predictors of weaning after 6 weeks of mechanical ventilation. Chest 107:500–505, 1995.)

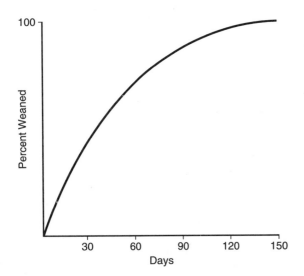

FIGURE 21–1
Time course of weaning success in those eventually weaned in a large ventilator weaning unit. (Adapted from Scheinhorn DJ, Chao DC, Stem-Hassenpflug M, et al: Post-ICU mechanical ventilation: treatment of 1,123 patients at a regional weaning center. Chest 111:1654–1659, 1997.)

tient is to being able to breathe without the ventilator.[29] Because these types of patients usually have active ventilatory drives, modes of support that provide comfortable muscle unloading are desirable. Thus, pressure-targeted breaths with variable flow are generally preferable to volume-targeted modes with fixed flows.[25] In the initial phases of weaning, ventilatory support usually is needed for 24 hours a day. Therefore, mask applications are generally not appropriate. However, as weaning progresses and the need for ventilatory support becomes only intermittent, tracheostomy removal and mask applications may become reasonable. Low-level PEEP may be useful for atelectasis prevention, and supplemental O_2 can be provided as needed. Generally, if weaning is to be successful, it will occur within the first 6 months (Fig. 21–1).[7] Predictors of weaning success from a large regional weaning center are depicted in Figure 21–2.[28] Multidisciplinary teams with a rehabilitation focus are crucial in optimizing a patient's chance at being removed from the ventilator under these circumstances (see below).

Scenario 2: Category 2 Patients with Irreversible Lung Disease Requiring Mechanical Ventilation for Life Support

These types of patients require substantial ventilatory support, and this is best provided with an assist-control mode (either volume or pressure targeted) with appropriate mandatory rate backup and disconnect alarms. Flow settings and inspiratory:expiratory timing is generally set to mimic the normal 1:2 to 1:3 ratio. The clinical focus is to ensure that blood gases are maintained and that any assisting that is done by the patient is comfortable. Low levels of PEEP may be useful for atelectasis prevention. Inspired oxygen concentration (FiO_2) may be supplemented as needed to keep arterial hemoglobin saturation adequate. Unsupported spontaneous breaths or attempts at weaning usually are not indicated in these types of patients. Mask applications are generally not suitable under these conditions because continuous ventilatory support is required.

Scenario 3: Category 1 or 2 Patients Requiring Only Intermittent (Nocturnal) Ventilatory Support

These patients generally can support ventilatory function during much of the day but use a ventilator at night to unload the ventilatory muscles. In the category 1 patient, this level of support may represent the "bridge" between 24-hour support and total liberation from the ventilator. In the category 2 patient, this level of support may be a permanent requirement or may be a step in the gradually increasing need for ventilatory support as the underlying disease worsens. Mask interfaces may be useful under these intermittent support circumstances, although tracheostomies commonly are employed. In this clinical scenario, the focus is on providing a level of support that is both comfortable to the patient and that provides some degree of unloading of the ventilatory muscles. Pressure-targeted modes such as

pressure support or pressure assist are ideally suited for this. Low levels of PEEP may be helpful in either reducing atelectasis potential or in reducing the inspiratory triggering load imposed by intrinsic PEEP in patients with airflow obstruction[30] (see Chapter 19). The goals of this form of support are not necessarily to normalize daytime arterial blood gases. Instead, outcome assessment should focus on functional status and quality of life.

THE ROLE OF COMPREHENSIVE REHABILITATION IN THE LONG-TERM VENTILATOR-DEPENDENT PATIENT

Comprehensive rehabilitation refers to the process of providing multiple integrated services designed to maximize a patient's functional status.[13, 30, 31] Disciplines involved in this process for long-term ventilator-dependent patients include physical therapy, psychology, nutrition, patient education, and occupational therapy, along with the respiratory care team. It is beyond the scope of this chapter to discuss how each member of this "team" can contribute. Nevertheless, note that ventilator management in these patients is not an isolated process and that the "whole" patient should be considered. Indeed, one of the reasons that **weaning units** often have better success at ventilator liberation than traditional ICUs is that the weaning unit provides a much more comprehensive rehabilitative plan of management, including weaning techniques and assessments for ventilator withdrawal.

Rehabilitative plans must be individualized. For the patient with potentially reversible category 1 disease, rehabilitative efforts must focus on improving respiratory function, nutrition, psychological function, and the like to facilitate ventilator weaning. In contrast, for the patient with category 2 irreversible disease, these rehabilitative efforts must focus on maximizing quality of life for the patient permanently attached to a ventilator. Healthcare professionals and family caregivers need to interact closely to provide these comprehensive rehabilitation services.

REFERENCES

1. Gracey DR, Naessens JM, Viggiano RW, et al: Outcome of patients cared for in a ventilator-dependent unit in a general hospital. Chest 107:494–499, 1995.
2. Adams AB, Shapiro R, Marini JJ: Changing prevalence of chronically ventilator-assisted individuals in Minnesota: increases, characteristics, and the use of noninvasive ventilation. Respir Care 43:643–649, 1998.
3. Adams AB, Whitman J, Marcy T: Surveys of long-term ventilatory support in Minnesota: 1986 and 1992. Chest 103:1463–1469, 1993.
4. O'Donohue WJ, Giovannoni RR, Goldberg AI, et al: Long-term mechanical ventilation: Guidelines for management in the home and at alternate community sites: Report of Ad Hoc Committee, Respiratory Care Section, American College of Chest Physicians. Chest 90(suppl):1S–37S, 1986.
5. ACCP Consensus Conference, Mechanical ventilation beyond the intensive care unit. Chest 113(suppl):289S–344S, 1998.
6. Scheinhorn DJ, Artoinian BM, Catlin JL: Weaning from prolonged mechanical ventilation: the experience at a regional weaning center. Chest 105:534–539, 1994.
7. Scheinhorn DJ, Chao DC, Stern-Hassenpflug M, et al: Post-ICU mechanical ventilation: treatment of 1,123 patients at a regional weaning center. Chest 111:1654–1659, 1997.
8. Gracey DR, Viggiano RW, Naessens JM, et al: Outcomes of patients admitted to a chronic ventilator-dependent unit in an acute-care hospital. Mayo Clin Proc 67:131–136, 1992.
9. Gracey DR, Naessens JM, Krishan I, Marsh HM: Hospital and post-hospital survival in patients mechanically ventilated for more then 29 days. Chest 101:211–214, 1992.
10. Spicher JE, White DP: Outcome and function following prolonged mechanical ventilation. Arch Intern Med 147:421–425, 1987.
11. Elpern EH, Larson R, Douglass P, et al: Long-term outcomes for elderly survivors of prolonged ventilator assistance. Chest 96:1120–1124, 1989.
12. Goldberg AI: Outcomes of home care for life-supported persons: long term oxygen and prolonged mechanical ventilation. Chest 109:595–596, 1996.
13. Make B, Gilmartin M: Care of the ventilator-assisted individual in the home and alternative and community sites. In: Hodgkin JE, Connors GL, Bell CW (eds): Pulmonary Rehabilitation: Guidelines to Success, 2nd ed. Philadelphia: JB Lippincott, 1993 pp 359–391.
14. Milligan S: AARC and Gallup estimate numbers and costs of caring for chronic ventilator patients. AARC Times 15:30–36, 1991.
15. Wagner DP: Economics of prolonged mechanical ventilation. Am Rev Respir Dis 140(Pt 2):S14–S18, 1989.
16. Bach JR, Intintola P, Alba AS, Holland IE: The ventilator-assisted individual: cost analysis of institutionalization vs. rehabilitation and in-home management. Chest 101:26–30, 1992.
17. Kurek CJ, Cophen IL, Lambrinos J, et al: Clinical and economic outcome of patients undergoing tracheostomy for prolonged mechanical ventilation in New York state during 1993: analysis of 6,353 cases under diagnosis-related group 483. Crit Care Med 25:983–988, 1997.
18. Bach JR, Alba AS, Shin D: Management alternatives for post-polio respiratory insufficiency: assisted ventilation by nasal or oral-nasal interface. Am J Phys Med Rehab 68:264–271, 1989.
19. Hill NS, Bach JR: Non-invasive mechanical ventilation. Respir Care Clin North Am 2:1–352, 1996.
20. AARC Consensus Group: Non-invasive positive pressure ventilation. Respir Care 42:364–369, 1997.
21. Branson RD, Hess D, Chatburn R: Respiratory Care Equipment, 2 ed. Philadelphia: Lippincott Williams and Wilkins, 1999, pp 172–173.
22. AARC Consensus Group: Essentials of a mechanical ventilator. Respir Care 37:998–1008, 1992.
23. Marini JJ, Rodriguez RM, Lamb V: The inspiratory workload of patient initiated mechanical ventilation. Am Rev Respir Dis 134:902–909, 1986.
24. Lofaso F, Brochard L, Hang T, et al: Home versus intensive care pressure support devices: experimental and clinical comparison. Am J Respir Crit Care Med 153:1591–1599, 1996.
25. MacIntyre NR, McConnell R, Cheng KC, Sane A: Pressure limited breaths improve flow dyssynchrony during assisted ventilation. Crit Care Med 25:1671–1677, 1997.
26. Branson RD, MacIntyre NR: Dual control modes of mechanical ventilation. Respir Care 41:294–305, 1996.
27. Branson RD, Peterson BD, Carson KD: Humidification: current therapy and controversy. Respir Care Clinics North Am 3:1–270, 1998.
28. Scheinhorn DJ, Hassenpflug M, Artinian BM, et al: Predictors of weaning after 6 weeks of mechanical ventilation. Chest 107:500–505, 1995.
29. Yang KL, Tobin MJ: A prospective study on indexes predicting the outcome of trials of weaning from mechanical ventilation. N Engl J Med 324:1445–1450, 1991.
30. Ely EW, Baker AM, Dunagan DP, et al: Effects of duration of mechanical ventilation of identifying patients capable of breathing spontaneously. N Engl J Med 335:1864–1869, 1996.
31. MacIntyre NR, Cheng KC, McConnell R: Applied PEEP during pressure support reduces the inspiratory threshold load of intrinsic PEEP. Chest 111:188–193, 1997.

Mechanical Ventilation During Transport and Cardiopulmonary Resuscitation

Richard D. Branson, BA, RRT
Jay A. Johannigman, MD
Robert S. Campbell, RRT

VENTILATION DURING CARDIOPULMONARY RESUSCITATION
Standards for Ventilation and Devices
Lung Compliance After Cardiac Arrest

TECHNIQUES OF EMERGENCY VENTILATION
Expired Air Resuscitation
Cricoid Pressure
Disease Transmission
Barrier Devices
Mouth-to-Mask

BAG-VALVE DEVICES
Description
Bag-Valve Device Performance
Ventilation Efficacy
Delivered Oxygen Concentration

Non-rebreathing Valve Performance
OXYGEN-POWERED BREATHING DEVICES
Description
Assessment
Ventilator-to-Mask Ventilation

TRANSPORT OF THE MECHANICALLY VENTILATED PATIENT
Why Transport?
Preparation
Equipment
Characteristics of a Ventilator for Intrahospital Transport
Physiologic Effects and Risks of Transport

KEY WORDS

American Heart Association (AHA) Device Classification System
bag-valve resuscitator

barrier device
cricoid pressure
expired air resuscitation
gas consumption

gastric insufflation
oxygen-powered breathing device
Sellick maneuver

Ventilation in emergency care and transport represents a significant challenge to the health care team. The need for rapidly available, rugged, light-weight ventilation devices is crucial to success in both cases. Training and preparation are also important to ensure appropriate application of devices and retention of skills. In this chapter, ventilatory support during cardiopulmonary resuscitation (CPR) and mechanical ventilation during transport are discussed.

VENTILATION DURING CARDIOPULMONARY RESUSCITATION

Ventilatory support during CPR can be accomplished using an array of methods and devices. These include **expired air resuscitation** (EAR), including mouth-to-mouth (MO–MO) and mouth-to-mask (MO–MA) resuscitation, and the use of mechanical ventilators. Appropriate application of these techniques depends on the clinical situation, rescuer training, and availability of equipment.

Standards for Ventilation and Devices

Several agencies have published recommendations for the use and evaluation of emergency ventilation devices. These include the American Heart Association (AHA), the Emergency Care Research Institute (ECRI), the American Society of Testing and Materials (ASTM), and the International Standards Organization (ISO).[1–9] Of these, the AHA provides standards for the depth and timing of ventilation as well as device characteristics.[1] The remaining agencies suggest standards for rate and volume but are more focused on the testing of devices.

Current AHA recommendations for adults include a frequency (f) of 10 to 12 breaths per minute with a tidal volume (V_T) of 0.8 to 1.2 L and an inspiratory time of 1.5 to 2.0 seconds. This corresponds with an inspiratory flow of 30 to 40 L/min.[1] The use of longer inspiratory times and slower flows is recommended to prevent **gastric insufflation**.[10, 11] ISO and ASTM standards suggest a V_T of 0.6 L and an f of 12 breaths per minute.

According to AHA guidelines,[1] all devices used for ventilation can be classified according to a scale. The **AHA device classification** follows and is referred to during device descriptions.

Class I   A therapeutic option that is usually indicated, always is acceptable, and is considered useful and effective.

Class II   A therapeutic option that is acceptable, is of uncertain efficacy, and may be controversial.

   Class IIa A therapeutic option for which the weight of evidence is in favor of its usefulness and efficacy.

   Class IIb A therapeutic option that is not well established by evidence but may be helpful and probably is not harmful.

Class III   A therapeutic option that is inappropriate, is without scientific supporting data, and may be harmful.

Lung Compliance After Cardiac Arrest

Changes in compliance and resistance after cardiopulmonary arrest have been attributed to pulmonary aspiration, pulmonary venous congestion, effects of chest compressions, and pulmonary embolism.[12–14] Fillmore and colleagues made comparisons of arterial blood gases (ABGs) to postmortem lung weights and found that the lightest lungs were associated with the best ABGs.[12]

Ornato and associates measured ventilation during CPR and estimated pulmonary compliance during cardiac arrest to be 0.022 L/cm H_2O, or about one quarter of normal lung compliance.[15] More recently, Davis and colleagues evaluated lung compliance in the

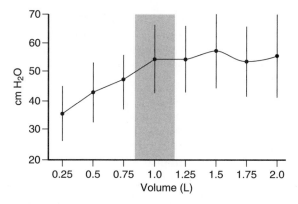

FIGURE 22–1
Mean pulmonary compliance of 25 patients after cardiac arrest.

emergency department after cardiac arrest.[16] Twenty-five patients requiring CPR because of cardiac arrest were studied immediately after discontinuation of CPR. A super-syringe technique was used to construct compliance curves.

Data from the study are shown in Figure 22–1. The mean compliance was 0.051 L/cm H_2O, a value more than twice that reported by Ornato and associates. These findings have implications for future emergency ventilation research and interpretation of previous studies. The use of longer inspiratory times and slower flows during CPR is, in part, related to the suspected low lung compliance (0.02 L/cm H_2O). Based on findings that lung compliance is twice that previously reported, ventilation strategies might be modified.

Another variable affecting delivered V_T is esophageal opening pressure. Because airway pressure is increased to deliver volume in the face of increased pulmonary impedance, gastric insufflation results. Based on work by Ruben and associates, esophageal opening pressure is approximately 20 cm H_2O.[10]

TECHNIQUES OF EMERGENCY VENTILATION

Expired Air Resuscitation

Description

EAR includes MO–MO, MO–MA, and mouth-to-nose ventilation. MO–MO ventila-

tion is the oldest method of EAR, with origins in biblical times.[17] MO–MO ventilation is accomplished by the rescuer's placing his or her mouth over the victim's mouth while maintaining an open airway. While observing the victim's chest, the rescuer should watch the chest rise and fall, listen for air escaping during exhalation, and feel the exhaled air flow. During EAR, a V_T of 0.8 to 1.2 L should be delivered over a period of 1.5 to 2.0 seconds, 10 to 12 times per minute. This results in a minute ventilation (V_E) of 8.0 to 14.6 L/min and an inspiratory:expiratory (I:E) ratio of 1:1.5 to 1:2.

Assessment

MO–MO ventilation has been recommended for basic life support (BLS) since 1974. The major advantages of MO–MO are availability, ease of use, universal application, large reservoir volume (the delivered volume is limited only by the rescuer's vital capacity, which is 3 to 4 times the necessary V_T), and the fact that no equipment is necessary.

Numerous publications have shown that MO–MO is effective in providing AHA-recommended tidal volumes, regardless of lung compliance.[18-23] Johannigman and colleagues[23] found that MO–MO was superior to MO–MA, bag-valve mask (BVM), and ventilator-to-mask ventilation with respect to delivered V_T (Fig. 22–2). However, it was also associated with the greatest amount of gastric insufflation.[23] The increase in gastric insufflation is related to the ability of the rescuer to deliver a larger, more forceful volume when pulmonary impedance is increased.

Other data provided by Johannigman and colleagues[23] demonstrate that at normal lung compliance, gastric insufflation during MO–MO ventilation is low (Fig. 22–3). This is in agreement with work by Melker and Banner.[24]

Disadvantages of MO–MO ventilation include low delivered oxygen concentration (FDO_2), gastric insufflation, unpleasantness of the task, fear of the possibility of disease transmission, and actual disease transmission.

During EAR, FDO_2 is approximately 16 to 18%, allowing for an alveolar oxygen ten-

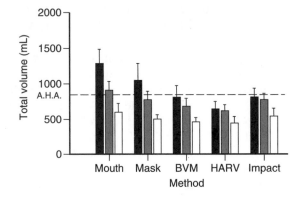

FIGURE 22-2
Delivered tidal volume of five methods of
ventilation. (From Johannigman JA, Branson RD,
Davis K, Hurst JM: Techniques of emergency
ventilation: a model to evaluate tidal volume,
airway pressure, and gastric insufflation. J Trauma
31:93–98, 1991.)

sion of 52 to 76 mm Hg, assuming a barometric pressure of 747 mm Hg and partial
arterial pressure of carbon dioxide ($PaCO_2$)
of 40 mm Hg. This range of arterial oxygen
pressure (PaO_2) is associated with an oxygen saturation of approximately 90. During
MO–MO, FDO_2 can be increased by increasing inspired oxygen concentration (FiO_2) of
the rescuer. Hess and colleagues evaluated
the change in FDO_2 when the rescuer was
wearing a nasal cannula with oxygen flows
of 6 L/min and 10 L/min.[25] They found an
FDO_2 of 16% during EAR, 27% at an oxygen
flow of 6 L/min, and 31% at an oxygen flow
of 10 L/min. Hess and colleagues suggested
that in the absence of other devices, oxygen
breathing by the rescuer is a viable method
of delivering adequate V_T and elevated
FDO_2.

In a lung model study, Rottenberg and
associates found an FDO_2 of 18% during
EAR and an FDO_2 of 32% when the rescuer
was breathing oxygen via a nasal cannula
at 10 L/min.[26] They also evaluated the role
of oral inspiration of oxygen via the supply
tubing at 15 L/min. With this technique, the
rescuer places the connecting tubing between his or her lips and inspires just before
ventilating the mannequin. Lastly, rescuers
breathed air from a manually triggered demand valve. The demand valve is placed
between the rescuer's lips and the manual

trigger activated. In this instance, the rescuers were essentially ventilating themselves with 100% oxygen via the demand
valve before ventilating the mannequin.
Breathing oxygen from the supply tubing
allowed an FDO_2 of 37% and inspiring from
the demand valve provided an FDO_2 of 78%.
The authors concluded that patients at risk
for cardiac arrest could have oxygen "on
hand" in the home to allow family members
to use supplemental oxygen during resusci-
tative efforts. They likewise suggested having oxygen available in high-risk areas,
such as swimming pools.

Both these studies make reasonable comments about the potential usefulness of increasing rescuer FiO_2 to increase FDO_2.
However, it is more than likely that wherever oxygen is available, other methods of
ventilation—for example, MO–MA, or
BVM—probably will be available. In the
study by Rottenberg and associates, it is
unclear why, if the rescuer has a demand
valve, he or she does not use it to ventilate
the patient. These data do prove, however,
that FDO_2 can be increased by increasing
rescuer FiO_2.

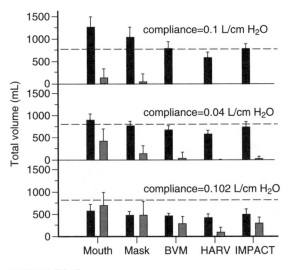

FIGURE 22-3
Comparison of delivered tidal volume versus
gastric insufflation. Dashed line represents
American Heart Association (AHA) minimum
volume of 800 ml. (From Johannigman JA, Branson
RD, Davis K, Hurst JM: Techniques of emergency
ventilation: a model to evaluate tidal volume,
airway pressure, and gastric insufflation. J Trauma
31:93–98, 1991.)

Cricoid Pressure

Gastric insufflation with the potential sequelae of pulmonary aspiration is a problem whenever ventilation via an unprotected airway is attempted. Using less forceful inspirations, longer inspiratory times, and smaller tidal volumes are effective strategies in limiting gastric insufflation.[24]

Another technique to prevent gastric insufflation is the use of **cricoid pressure,** often referred to as the **Sellick maneuver.**[27] Sellick described this method in 1961 as a method to prevent regurgitation during induction of anesthesia and endotracheal intubation. By pushing down on the cricoid membrane, the esophagus is collapsed against the cervical vertebrae. In children, cricoid pressure has been shown to prevent gastric insufflation during mask ventilation up to a peak inspiratory pressure of 40 cm H_2O.[28] Vanner and associates found that a cricoid force of 40 newtons increased esophageal opening pressure to a mean of 38 torr in anesthetized adults.[29]

Cricoid pressure is a fairly simple technique, but it is not without complications. If excessive pressure is applied, the trachea can also be collapsed, causing complete airway obstruction. There are also reports of gastric rupture occurring when the patient regurgitates during application of cricoid pressure.[30, 31]

Disease Transmission

Concern about disease transmission has become a major issue regarding MO–MO resuscitation.[32–37] Ornato and colleagues found that 40% of basic cardiac life support (BCLS) instructors, including health care workers, public service workers, and lay persons, would hesitate to perform MO–MO for fear of contracting a disease.[32]

Additional surveys have found that although many BCLS providers say that they would perform MO–MO on a stranger (97%), only half (44%) would do CPR on a patient known to or suspected to have AIDS.[33] Link and associates found that 48% of medical residents employed in New York City hospitals reported a moderate to major

concern about contracting AIDS from a patient.[34]

The AHA has addressed the issue of infection risk during CPR.[1, 35] When a patient is known to be "high risk," recommendations regarding ventilation techniques include the following: (1) rescuers who have an infection that may be transmitted by blood or saliva or believe that they have been exposed to such an infection should not perform MO–MO if other methods are available (e.g., MO–MA or BVM); (2) individuals have a duty to respond to the CPR needs of high-risk patients using MO–MA ventilation of adequate design to BVM device and should be trained in their use; and (3) early intubation should be encouraged when equipment and trained professionals are available.[35]

The effect of these suggestions on bystander CPR has been debated.[36, 37] Bystander CPR is primarily performed by family members and public health service personnel.[1] In the latter case, equipment designed to obviate the need for MO–MO contact is available. In the former, the caregiver is knowledgeable of the patient's health history and is quite frequently a relative. The issue then may be more academic than practical.

There remains, however, a reluctance on the part of many people to perform MO–MO resuscitation. Although the risk of infection is small, there are reports of possible cases of infection after CPR. These include infection with *Mycobacterium tuberculosis*,[38] meningococcus,[39] herpes simplex virus,[40–42] shigella,[43] and salmonella.[44]

In essence, health care policy has added to the confusion on this issue. Although the risk of infection is reported to be very low, and the risk of human immunodeficiency virus (HIV) transmission even smaller, recommendations are made that devices to prevent MO–MO contact be available in high-risk areas.[35, 45] The city of New York has even made the availability of infection control equipment for CPR in public places mandatory.[46]

Debate about the true risk of infection from performing CPR may be futile. The unpleasantness of the task of MO–MO breathing (contact with vomitus, blood, and the like) and even the minute possibility of infection mandate that we develop cost-effective, readily available, safe, and efficacious alternatives to MO–MO breathing.

Barrier Devices

Description

A **barrier device** is a flexible sheet that typically contains a valve or filter that separates the rescuer from the patient (Fig. 22–4). Barrier devices are, quite frankly, a disposable version of the "handkerchief" recommended by Waters as a protective device some 50 years ago.[47] Barrier devices are sometimes called face shields but should not be confused with face masks. An effective barrier device should have the following characteristics:

- Have universal application—conform to the anatomy of patients of all sizes and shapes.
- Be small, lightweight, and easy to carry.
- Have minimal air flow resistance.
- Prevent cross-infection (victim to rescuer and vice versa).
- Resist tearing.

Assessment

Few evaluations have been made on the safety and efficacy of barrier devices. Anecdotal reports of the ability of barrier devices to prevent movement of HIV-infected broth[48, 49] have been published. A mannequin study found that use of a barrier device allowed similar ventilation as MO–MO ventilation without a barrier device.[50] In a 1985 health devices report, barrier devices were believed to be inferior to face masks with respect to creating an effective seal on the face.[8] There is also some concern that barrier devices may slip if the patient's face is wet and that during prolonged resuscitation efforts, the plastic sheet may tear away from the central valve.[51, 52]

More recently, Rossi and colleagues compared MO–MA, mouth-to-tube, and mouth-to-barrier device methods of ventilation in the laboratory.[53] Using a motorized calibra-

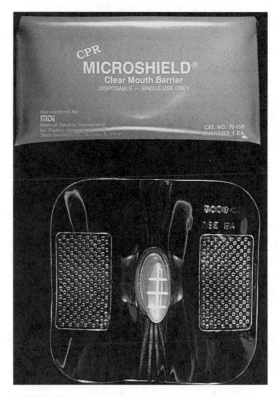

FIGURE 22–4
Barrier device used for cardiopulmonary resuscitation.

tion syringe, they delivered a tidal volume of 1.0 L to a mannequin and test lung. Inspiratory and expiratory pressures and valve leakage were measured. Rossi and colleagues concluded that resistance to air flow was excessive in several of the devices tested. This has been confirmed by Simmons, who found that the MicroSHIELD device created 17 cm H_2O back pressure at a flow of 50 L/min.[54]

Simmons and coworkers also compared volume delivered to a mannequin using MO–MO with three barrier devices.[55] They reported a volume of 1.0 L using MO–MO, 0.25 L using the Kiss of Life, 0.75 L using the MicroSHIELD, and 0.64 L using the Res-Cue Key. The reasons for these disparities are unclear.

If anything can be said definitely about barrier devices, it is that more research is necessary to determine their safety and efficacy. The AHA considers barrier devices as class IIb (acceptable, possibly helpful).

Mouth-to-Mask

Description

MO–MA ventilation devices can be as simple as a face mask or include a face mask, oxygen inlet, non-rebreathing valve (NRV) extension tube, filter, and mouth piece (Fig. 22–5). Both devices can be used effectively, but the latter incorporates components that help protect the rescuer and patient from cross-contamination.

Desirable characteristics of an MO–MA device include a clear, soft mask capable of making an effective seal with the patient's face; an oxygen inlet nipple; an NRV that diverts expired flow away from the rescuer; low-flow resistance; no back leak; and a filter with low-flow resistance that is not adversely affected by humidity or vomitus. Dead space should be considered in pediatric applications. In adults, a dead space of less than 200 ml is acceptable.

Assessment

MO–MA ventilation was shown to be an effective method of ventilation as early as 1954 by Elam and colleagues.[56] Safar and McMahon described the first MO–MA device (Laerdal pocket mask) in 1958,[57] and Safar described the role of oxygen supplementation in 1974.[58] The technique of MO–MA ventilation has been recommended for more than a decade by the AHA as the method of choice before endotracheal intubation unless a rescuer with experience

with BVM is present. Despite the use of the mask, proximity of the rescuer to the victim continues to be the major deterrent to widespread use of MO–MA ventilation.

MO–MA ventilation has been shown to be superior to BVM ventilation in a number of studies.[18-23, 59-62] Hess and Baran found higher volumes were provided with MO–MA compared with BVM by one rescuer using a mannequin and a test lung.[19] In this study, mean delivered volume with MO–MO was 0.73 L, with MO–MA was 0.6 L, and with BVM was 0.3 L. When two people used the BVM device, one to hold the mask seal and one to squeeze the bag, delivered volumes increased to 0.58 L. Interestingly, the authors found no difference in performance of any of these techniques related to operator experience. This is contrary to the AHA statement concerning the use of BVM if an experienced user is present. Hess and Baran's work suggests that even with experience, BVM by a single rescuer is inadequate.[19] Seidelin and colleagues agreed, recommending that ventilation should be provided by MO–MA until a third rescuer arrives to allow two-person BVM.[22]

Johannigman and colleagues[23] found that MO–MA ventilation consistently provided higher tidal volumes than BVM or ventilator-to-mask ventilation. At normal compliance, 0.1 L/cm H_2O, Johannigman and colleagues found that MO–MO, MO–MA, BVM, and ventilator-to-mask techniques provided adequate tidal volumes with little to no gastric insufflation (see Fig. 22–3). At a compliance of 0.04 L/cm H_2O, which is

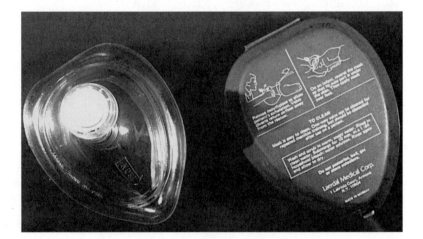

FIGURE 22–5
Mouth-to-mask resuscitation device.

near the value measured clinically, they found that MO–MO ventilation provided the largest tidal volumes but also produced gastric insufflation equivalent to 50% of the tidal volume. MO–MA ventilation produced similar tidal volumes but with approximately half the gastric insufflation of MO–MO. Johannigman and colleagues made a further plea for early use of MO–MA during single-rescuer CPR.[23]

Studies by Sainsbury and associates[18] and Lawrence and Sivaneswaran[20] also have demonstrated the superiority of MO–MA compared with BVM. More recently, Thomas and colleagues evaluated MO–MA ventilation using a mannequin[59] and in anesthetized patients.[60, 62] The authors had anesthesia residents provide MO–MA or BVM ventilation, both with an oxygen flow of 15 L/min, to 30 subjects (ASA class I or II) requiring general anesthesia. Residents were given "brief tuition" by the investigators and used a Laerdal pocket mask or Laerdal silicone resuscitator for ventilation. During a 4-minute period, airway pressure, carbon dioxide, and oxygen concentrations were measured. The authors found that BVM provided a mean FDO_2 of 0.95 and mean delivered carbon dioxide ($FDCO_2$) of 0.05. MO–MA yielded a mean FDO_2 of 0.54 and mean $FDCO_2$ of 0.14. Despite the higher $FDCO_2$, mean expired CO_2 was equivalent between the groups, suggesting no adverse effect on CO_2 removal. Arterial oxygen saturation as measured by pulse oximetry was also equal between the two ventilation methods.

Thomas and Weber also suggested using MO–MA during two-rescuer CPR but with an alternative strategy.[59] Rather than having one rescuer provide ventilation while the other performs compressions, they suggested that one rescuer hold the mask and provide airway control (head-tilt, chin-lift) while the second rescuer provides both ventilation and compressions. During conventional two-rescuer CPR, tidal volume was lower and respiratory rate was higher than during modified CPR. Although the compression rate was slowed during modified CPR, the delivered tidal volume was significantly improved. The authors postulated that reducing the ventilation:compression

ratio from 1:5 to 2:15 would increase the number of compressions while maintaining gas exchange by virtue of the larger tidal volume.

One of the disadvantages related to use of MO–MA is the inability to increase FDO_2. Safar demonstrated an FDO_2 of 0.54 using MO–MA at a tidal volume of 1.0 L, frequency of 12 beats/min, and oxygen flow of 15 L/min.[58] In an effort to increase FDO_2, Johannigman and Branson[63] recommended placing the oxygen inlet valve of the MO–MA device above the NRV and allowing the rescuer to inspire from the continuous oxygen flow during patient expiration. This so-called "inhalation technique" was compared with conventional MO–MA ventilation in a mannequin and lung model to determine the effect on FDO_2. Oxygen flows of 5 L/min, 10 L/min, and 15 L/min were used. Figure 22–6 demonstrates the increase in FDO_2 seen with the inhalation technique. Interestingly, at a flow of 15 L/min, mean FDO_2 was 0.43, not far from that originally reported by Safar.[58] Using the inhalation technique, FDO_2 was increased to a mean of 0.71. Johannigman and Branson also noted that increasing oxygen flow was associated with increased delivered tidal volume.[63] This is particularly evident at high oxygen flows, in which rescuer expiratory effort is

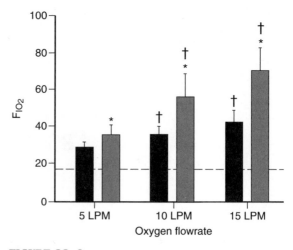

FIGURE 22–6

FDO_2 at different oxygen flows using standard and inhalation technique. (From Johannigman JA, Branson RD: Oxygen enrichment of expired gas for mouth to mask resuscitation. Respir Care 36:99–103, 1991.)

supplemented by the oxygen flow. At an oxygen flow of 15 L/min and inspiratory time of 1.5 seconds, an additional 375 ml of oxygen (250 ml/sec) is added to the rescuer's effort. The authors cited previous work demonstrating the superiority of MO–MA ventilation and suggested that oxygen supplementation using the inhalation technique might represent the ventilatory method of choice in early CPR before endotracheal intubation.

Stahl and associates studied five MO–MA devices and evaluated the FDO_2 delivered to a test lung at two combinations of frequency and tidal volume (500 ml $\times$ 20 breaths/min and 90 ml $\times$ 12 breaths/min).[64] A ventilator was used to keep rate and volume constant while oxygen flow to the MO–MA device was varied from 2 L/min to 14 L/min in 2-L increments. The devices performed similarly, with the limiting factor being dead-space volume of the mask. As dead-space volume increased, so did FDO_2. The authors recommended that during MO–MA ventilation, (1) high oxygen flows be used (14 L/min) and (2) slow inspirations be used.

Thomas and colleagues studied the effects of increasing oxygen flow to the Laerdal pocket mask.[65] Using a recording mannequin, the authors had 24 volunteers provide MO–MA ventilation for 90 seconds with oxygen flows of 5 L/min, 10 L/min, 15 L/min, and 20 L/min. Similar to previous work, Thomas and colleagues found that as oxygen flow increased, inspired CO_2 decreased and tidal volume was enhanced. The authors recommended that if MO–MA is used, a flow of 20 L/min is preferable.

Palmisano and colleagues evaluated the effect of supplementary oxygen flow on MO–MA ventilation in a pediatric model.[66] They demonstrated an FDO_2 of 0.50 with an oxygen flow of 5 L/min when tidal volume was 100 ml and frequency was 20 beats/min. Increasing oxygen flow to 15 L/min served to increase FDO_2 to 0.60 but also increased delivered volume to 221 ml, a 121% increase. The authors also pointed out the adverse effects of the ill-advised attempt of introducing oxygen flow below the non-rebreathing valve. In this case, high flows interfere with function of the NRV.

Hess and colleagues have compared MO–MA devices and found considerable variability in device performance.[67] Hess and colleagues attributed differences in device performance to design characteristics. Specifically, they suggest differences are the result of: (1) ability of the mask to fit the face and achieve a seal; (2) resistance to flow through the NRV; and (3) size and shape of the mask, which either aids or hinders the rescuer's grip.

MO–MA ventilation, when combined with supplemental oxygen, is arguably the safest, most effective method of ventilatory support in the unintubated patient when one rescuer is present. Resistance to use of MO–MA devices may be related to rescuer proximity to the patient with the attendant fears of disease transmission and the unpleasantness of the task. MO–MA also may appear unsophisticated when compared with BVM. Another issue may be related to a hindering of communication of the rescuer performing MO–MA ventilation.

BAG-VALVE DEVICES

Description

Bag-valve resuscitators consist of a self-inflating bag, an oxygen reservoir, and an NRV (Fig. 22–7). The operator ventilates the patient by squeezing the self-inflating bag, which forces air into the NRV and to the patient. The self-inflating bag typically is made of a resilient material, such as rubber, silicone, or polyvinylchloride. Most self-inflating bags have a volume of approximately 2.0 L for adults. When the operator releases the bag, it returns to its resting inflated position. During re-expansion, the bag fills with room air via a one-way valve on the rear of the bag or with oxygen from an oxygen reservoir. Oxygen reservoirs usually are classified as "tube" or "bag" reservoirs based on their construction and appearance. During the exhalation phase, the patient's expired air is directed away from the self-inflating bag to ambient by the NRV. NRVs have numerous designs, including duck-bill valves, spring-disk valves, spring-ball valves, diaphragm valves, and leaf valves.

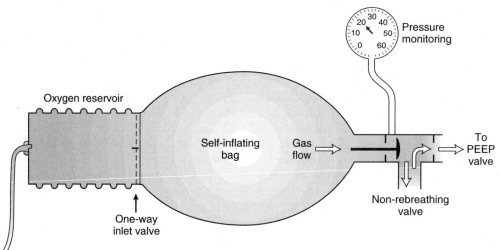

FIGURE 22–7
Schematic of a manual resuscitator.

An ideal self-inflating resuscitator would have the following characteristics:[68]

1. Volume delivery—Bag volume should be twice the volume to be delivered, and construction should allow the operator to deliver 800 ml while squeezing the bag with one hand.

2. FDO_2—An FDO_2 of 0.85 to 1.0 should be available for CPR. The reservoir should be lightweight and unobtrusive.

3. Self-inflating bag characteristics—The construction of the bag should allow rapid refill so that faster respiratory rates can be provided as required. The bag should not require gas flow to inflate, and the material used for construction should allow the operator a "feel" for patient impedance characteristics.

4. Non-rebreathing valve—The NRV should prevent any back leak of patient expired gases into the self-inflating bag, have a low resistance to inspiratory and expiratory flow (< 5 cm H_2O pressure decrease at 50 L/min), and possess a minimum dead space (< 30 ml for adults). The NRV should be transparent to allow detection of vomitus or other obstructions and perform effectively at high-oxygen flows.

5. Pressure relief valve—Adult resuscitators should not have a pressure relief valve. Pediatric devices should use a 35- to 40-cm H_2O pressure relief valve, which may be overridden if required.

6. Options—For selected situations, the bag-valve device should allow attachment of a spirometer to measure expired volumes, a positive end-expiratory pressure (PEEP) valve and a tap for monitoring airway pressure with an aneroid manometer.

7. Construction—The resuscitator bag should be lightweight, easily held in one hand, easy to disassemble, easy to clean, and impossible to reassemble improperly. The device should be rugged and able to perform in adverse conditions of temperature.

Bag-Valve Device Performance

The performance of bag-valve devices has been the subject of significant interest.[69] Controversy regarding BVM use is presented below.

Ventilation Efficacy

Numerous studies have evaluated the ability of rescuers to provide ventilation to models using BVM. Uniformly, results have shown that one-rescuer BVM is ineffective.[19, 21–24, 60, 70, 71] These reports suggest diminished volume delivery resulting from the inability of a single rescuer to use one hand to hold the mask securely while maintaining airway patency (head-tilt, chin-lift) and squeezing the bag with the other hand. Results from these studies vary widely, with a minimum value reported by Hess and Baran[19] of 300 ml up to 700 ml reported by Seidelin and colleagues.[22] Even with the wide variability in results, it can easily be concluded that BVM by one rescuer is typically ineffective.

Several suggestions have been made to improve ventilation provided by BVM. Cummins and associates and Barnes and Adams have evaluated the face and thigh squeeze, or so-called FATS, technique.[72, 73] This method is used in prehospital care to increase delivered volume. The rescuer kneels and places the victim's head between his or her knees. One hand holds the mask and provides the head-tilt/chin-lift by pulling up on the mandible. The remaining hand squeezes the bag against the rescuer's thigh in an attempt to maximize bag deflation.

Increasing volume delivery during BVM also can be accomplished by using two rescuers.[74] Similarly, when two hands are used to squeeze the bag, tidal volume is enhanced. Hess and Baran[19] found that delivered volume almost doubled when using two-person BVM and two-hand compression of the bag (from 300 to 580 ml). Practically speaking, in the prehospital setting, it is unlikely to have the luxury of two rescuers to perform ventilation.

Other factors affecting BVM performance include mask design,[75] respiratory impedance,[76] hand size,[77, 78] and volumetric feedback.[79] In general, a soft, pliable, inflatable sealing mask improves the face-to-mask seal and increases tidal volume. As pulmonary compliance decreases or resistance increases, delivered volume decreases, and larger hands are associated with larger tidal volumes. Volumetric feedback improves volume delivery by allowing the rescuer to get a feel for adequate volume delivery.

Branson and colleagues recorded breath-by-breath volumes during bag-valve–endotracheal tube ventilation during CPR in the emergency department.[80] These results showed mean tidal volumes during CPR were 571 ml at a frequency of 24 breaths/min. Mean peak airway pressures were 41 cm H_2O, and the average inspiratory time was 1.1 seconds. These values are considerably different from AHA guidelines and suggest that some type of volume or frequency monitor might improve the efficiency of bag-valve ventilation.

Delivered Oxygen Concentration

Numerous reports have evaluated the ability of resuscitators to deliver a desired FDO_2.[81-90] According to ASTM[8] and ISO,[9] FDO_2 should be 0.85 with an oxygen reservoir in use and an oxygen flow of 15 L/min. The AHA recommends an FDO_2 of 1.0 or "the highest possible oxygen concentration should be administered as soon as possible to all patients with cardiac or respiratory arrest."[1] This recommendation seems to be prudent, but no studies have proved that an FDO_2 of 1.0 is superior to an FDO_2 of 0.50. In fact, it could be speculated that an FDO_2 of 1.0 might accentuate reperfusion injury. The required, safe FiO_2 during CPR is a matter of some controversy and requires some sound scientific investigation for clarification.

Cases with an FDO_2 of less than 0.85 have been reported with bag-valve devices and are related to high minute ventilation, insufficient reservoir volume, and ambient temperatures < 0°C.[81-90] Most current resuscitator designs are capable of delivering a minimum FDO_2 of 0.85 during CPR.

Non-rebreathing Valve Performance

The NRV is the heart of the resuscitation bag. According to the ASTM, the NRV should resist breakage, function in the presence of vomitus, allow flows of up to 30 L/min without sticking, and continue to function at extremes of temperature (−18–+50°C).[8]

Studies of NRV competence in the presence of vomitus have shown adequate performance in most cases.[81-90] Several devices have failed at low temperatures when condensation freezes the valve's components.[90] Reports have also shown that many devices fail the "drop test" of falling 1 m to a concrete floor.[87-90]

Back leak through an NRV should be minimal to prevent rebreathing, and most devices produce few problems with valve incompetence. Several cases of NRV failure caused by misassembly have been reported, which underscores the need for operator vigilance.[91]

Hess and Simmons found that resistance to flow of NRV in adult resuscitators was variable.[92] They found three devices that exceeded the 5-cm H_2O back pressure standard at a flow of 50 L/min specified by the ASTM.[8] Hess and Simmons suggested that the increased flow resistance of some NRVs could prolong expiration and cause air-trapping, which might lead to barotrauma or further impediment to ventilation. They also suggested that NRVs with high flow resistance might contribute to fatigue of the rescuer squeezing the bag.

Spontaneous breathing through the NRV of resuscitators has been an area of some controversy.[93, 94] Hess and colleagues evaluated the imposed work of breathing created during simulated spontaneous breathing via the NRV of 11 disposable resuscitators.[95] They found that both inspiratory and expiratory work of breathing was elevated. Imposed work of breathing increased with the application of PEEP and with increased patient flow demand. Measurements of work in this study were quite high (up to 2.0 J/L) and represent a 10- to 100-fold increase compared with the imposed work of common intensive care ventilators.[95] Hess et al recommended that the practice of allowing spontaneous breathing via disposable resuscitator bags be abandoned.

Bag-valve mask ventilation remains the most popular method of ventilatory support by BLS providers in the field.[96] Many factors previously discussed allow BVM to be used extensively despite the plethora of evidence suggesting its inefficiency. Effort in the area of provider education may be the answer to problems with BVM, rather than introduction of new ventilatory techniques.

OXYGEN-POWERED BREATHING DEVICES

Description

Oxygen-powered breathing devices (OPDs) are frequently called demand valves. Both the ASTM and the ISO have created standards for OPDs.[8, 9] A typical OPD consists of a demand valve that can be manually triggered or patient triggered (Fig. 22–8). The OPD is connected to a 50-psig source of gas and connects to the patient via a standard 15/22-mm connector. During manual activation of the demand valve, the operator depresses the actuator, allowing flow to travel to the patient. According to the ASTM standard, this flow should be restricted to 40 L/min to prevent

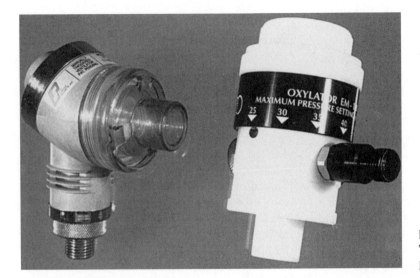

FIGURE 22–8
Two manually triggered oxygen-powered breathing devices.

excessive ventilation and gastric distension. Modern OPDs also limit the available airway pressure via a pressure-limiting valve and limit the length of inspiratory time. In the latter case, inspiration is terminated after 3 seconds, even if the operator continues to depress the actuator. During spontaneous breathing, the demand valve is pressure-triggered and allows a flow of up to 100 L/min for patient demand.

Assessment

The history of OPDs indicates problems with the devices. A number of studies have shown failure of the pressure-limiting devices within the OPD and subsequent high airway pressure (> 100 cm H_2O).[97–99] Pradis and Caldwell have reported a case of pneumocephalus resulting from OPD-to-mask ventilation caused by excessive airway pressures.[98] Much of this work was done before limiting flow during manual ventilation to 40 L/min.

More recently, Menegazzi and colleagues evaluated the use of the OPD in a model, providing ventilation via OPD to mask and OPD to endotracheal tube.[100, 101] Using a mannequin system similar to that developed by Johannigman and colleagues,[23] Menegazzi and colleagues found no difference in delivered tidal volumes between BVM and OPD-to-mask. They did, however, report significantly increased gastric insufflation with BVM. This difference was attributed to the high inflation pressures and flows that can be developed during BVM compared with the fixed steady flow of 40 L/min provided by the OPD. Menegazzi and Winslow[100] suggested that OPD-to-mask ventilation was superior to BVM in preventing gastric insufflation in this model. They did, however, suggest that clinical studies be performed before widespread use of the OPD.

Mesezzo and associates compared the OPD with a bag-valve device for ventilation of a model via an endotracheal tube. They found similar delivered tidal volumes at all levels of compliance tested. Additionally, they reported a higher airway pressure with the bag-valve device compared with the OPD (31 cm H_2O vs. 13 cm H_2O at normal lung compliance). These authors suggested that the lower airway pressures were caused by the fixed 40-L/min inspiratory flow and that demand valve ventilation through an endotracheal tube may be preferable.[101] One limitation of the OPD is the inability of the rescuer to detect patient compliance.

The history of the OPD is a major limitation to its adoption. However, devices that meet the ASTM standard can probably be used safely and effectively. Clinical studies of the OPD in the field are necessary before widespread use can be recommended. The AHA rates the OPD as class II.

Ventilator-to-Mask Ventilation

Description

Transport ventilators for prehospital care and CPR are typically machine-triggered, volume-limited, time-cycled devices.[102, 103] They are typically simple, having one or two controls, providing only one mode, no PEEP, and strictly a 1.0 FiO_2. The AHA has suggested that automatic transport ventilators meeting the following criteria are class I devices:

- Have a lightweight connector with a standard 15/22-mm connector;
- Have a lightweight (2–5 kg), compact, rugged design;
- Operate in all environmental conditions and extremes of temperature;
- Have a peak pressure limit of 60 cm H_2O with an option of 80 cm H_2O;
- Have an audible alarm when the peak pressure limit is exceeded;
- Have minimal **gas consumption**;
- Have minimum gas compression volume in the circuit;
- Deliver an FiO_2 of 1.0;
- Have an inspiratory time of 2.0 seconds for adults and 1.0 second for children with corresponding peak inspiratory flow rates of 30 L/min and 15 L/min, respectively; and
- Have at least two respiratory frequency settings.[1]

Additionally, the AHA lists desirable features, which include a pressure manometer, separate rate and volume controls, and a low-pressure alarm.

Our group previously has published descriptions of prehospital ventilators and desirable characteristics.[103] These are similar to those listed by the AHA, and descriptions follow.

Operational Characteristics

All ventilators used in prehospital care should be time or volume cycled. Modified pressure-cycled devices have been used by skilled clinicians, although their general use is discouraged. Constant flow rate ventilators are preferred, but nonconstant flow ventilators can be used successfully. Inspiratory flow rate and tidal volume should be affected minimally by changes in airway resistance and lung–thorax compliance ($< 10\%$ change). Ideally, gas consumption to power the ventilator's system components should be zero. Low-level gas consumption (< 5 L/min) is acceptable but decreases the ventilator's operating time.

Portability

Size and weight are the chief concerns. Orientation of controls and handles for carrying the device are also important. Generally, a weight less than 4 kg is considered desirable.

Power Source

Ventilators that require pneumatic and electronic power sources require compressed oxygen and a direct current power source (battery); thus, *two* perishable power sources are necessary. There are tradeoffs, however, with these two types of ventilators. Electronically powered ventilators provide more precise control of variables and do not consume gas during operation. Either type of ventilator is thus adequate.

Ease of Operation

Operation of the ventilator should be as simple as possible with the minimum number of controls. Each control should be labeled as to function, effects, and possible hazards. When possible, a diagram of the circuit and its proper connection to the patient should be printed on the side or back panel of the ventilator. Ventilators used in prehospital care *do not* need a variable FiO_2, continuous positive airway pressure (CPAP), or a variety of ventilatory modes. In our study of prehospital ventilatory support, 95% of patients remained apneic during transport. Addition of a demand-flow valve adds size and weight to the ventilator and can also increase gas consumption. Some transport ventilators position the demand-flow valve on the endotracheal tube. This can result in inadvertent extubation or kinking of the tube because of the weight of the demand-flow valve. As stated previously, independent control knobs for tidal volume and ventilator rate should be available. An important, and often overlooked, feature is the "manual inhalation" control push button. This allows the operator to control ventilator rate and tidal volume manually, independent of the ventilator's settings, in special situations. This control is also helpful during auscultation of breath sounds to confirm proper endotracheal tube placement.

Assembly and Disassembly

The ventilator breathing circuit and exhalation valve should be simple, and incorrect assembly should be impossible. Likewise, high-pressure hoses from the gas source to the ventilator and from ventilator to patient should not be interchangeable such that misassembly can occur. If a valve is used to control the flow of inspiratory and expiratory gases (such as an NRV), it should be easily cleaned of vomitus, blood, and secretions.

Safety

The number of safety devices is limited by the small size of transport ventilators. A high-pressure relief valve, which vents gas to the atmosphere at a preselected peak inflation pressure (PIP) (typically 60–80 cm H_2O for adults and 30–40 cm H_2O for children), should be required on transport ventilators. Activation of the high-pressure limit should be signaled by a visual or audible alarm to alert the operator. The ventilator also should have an antiasphyxia valve. If gas or electric power supplies are exhausted, the patient should be able to breathe ambient air without excessive resistance. Battery-powered ventilators should be equipped with a "low battery" signal that indicates when 1 hour of power remains. Loss of oxygen power supply to a transport ventilator should activate audible or visual alarms, or both.

Durability

Extremes of temperature and humidity should not adversely affect the operation of transport ventilators. These ventilators should be capable of operating at a moment's notice, even after prolonged periods of storage, and should be able to withstand rough treatment and still operate properly. Occasionally, transport ventilators are used in hazardous environments and should, therefore, have protective cases that can withstand erosion by chemicals or other foreign substances.

Maintenance

Preventive maintenance should be performed periodically by the manufacturer or a trained technician. Routine maintenance should be minimal.

Breathing Valve

One distinct feature incorporated in ventilators used in prehospital care is a breathing or inhalation/exhalation valve mechanism. This valve is connected to the ventilator by corrugated or high-pressure tubing and directs inspiratory and expiratory gases to and from the patient. The valve may be simple, such as an NRV, or it can be complicated. Some of these valves may house an NRV, a pressure-limiting valve, a demand-flow valve, and an antiasphyxia valve. As a result, several connecting ports on these breathing valves are required to accommodate additional valves. The connecting ports should have different inside and outside diameters such that improper connection cannot occur. Resistance to inhalation and exhalation should be low (< 3 cm H_2O/L/sec).

The weight of the breathing valve should be minimal (< 0.3 kg) because heavy or awkward valves can cause kinking of the endotracheal tube or accidental extubation. Also, this valve should be easy to clean.

Assessment

Evaluations of the ability of transport ventilators to deliver adequate tidal volumes have been published.[104–107] These studies, however, typically deal with a model of an intubated patient. We have presented data regarding use of transport ventilators in the prehospital environment, but also only in intubated patients.[96]

Johannigman and colleagues[23] found that a transport ventilator with an adjustable flow control delivered more consistent tidal volumes than BVM. The ventilator provided smaller tidal volumes than MO–MO or MO–MA ventilation but had significantly less gastric insufflation than either of those techniques.[19] A ventilator with a fixed flow provided smaller tidal volumes.

Greenslade compared volumes delivered to a mannequin with MO–MO, MO–MA, BVM, and ventilator-to-mask ventilation during one-rescuer CPR.[108] This fascinating study had rescuers perform CPR in the back of a moving ambulance with each ventilation technique. Greenslade found that MO–MO allowed the largest minute ventilation and most successful number of compressions per minute. Use of the ventilator and manual resuscitator resulted in the smallest minute ventilation and lowest number of compressions. He recommended that MO–MA be used in unintubated patients and that ventilators be reserved for intubated patients. Greenslade further suggested that "keeping ambulance speed below 30 mph and using oxygen supplemented mouth to mask ventilation . . . appear to offer the best chance of success in unintubated patients receiving one-operator CPR."[108]

We agree with Greenslade and would recommend that BLS squads perform oxygen-supplemented MO–MA until endotracheal intubation is performed, after which time bag-valve, OPD, or ventilator work effectively. One advantage of the ventilator is that it frees up a rescuer to perform other tasks. A disadvantage is the loss of "feel" for pulmonary compliance.

We are also puzzled by the AHA recommendation for a ventilator with a fixed flow of 30 L/min. Because the ventilator most often is used in intubated patients, there is no advantage to a slow inspiratory flow. In fact, the slow inspiratory flow creates two distinct disadvantages:

1. It makes it impossible to make up for leaks around a mask if used in an unintubated patient,
2. If a higher frequency is desired (e.g., for head injury), air-trapping may result because of insufficient expiratory time.

It is our contention that, although a fixed flow setting may be useful, the ventilator should have a provision for increasing flow.

TRANSPORT OF THE MECHANICALLY VENTILATED PATIENT

Why Transport?

Critically ill patients in the intensive care unit (ICU) frequently require diagnostic testing or therapeutic procedures that cannot be performed at bedside. These include computed tomography (CT) scans, angiography, and magnetic resonance (MR) imaging. When transportation is deemed necessary, every effort should be made to "take the ICU with the patient." This includes taking the appropriate personnel and providing for ventilation, care, and monitoring similar to those provided in the ICU.

Preparation

Ensuring a safe and uneventful transport begins long before any movement actually occurs. In elective situations, patience is the operative word. Time taken before transport to stabilize hemodynamics, oxygenation,

and ventilation is well spent. Electrolyte abnormalities should be corrected and the necessary invasive monitoring devices (arterial line, pulmonary artery catheter, intracranial pressure monitor) placed and secured.

Although a special transport team is deemed necessary for interhospital transport, intrahospital transport can best be accomplished by personnel familiar with the patient. The type and number of personnel should be commensurate with the degree of support required and the severity of patient illness.[109] Our ICU guidelines require that a physician, a respiratory care practitioner (RCP), and a nurse attend the transport of any mechanically ventilated patient. We also find it useful in many cases to enlist orientees and students to assist in physically moving the patient and equipment to and from the destination. Smith and colleagues[110] have published guidelines (Table 22–1) for accompanying staff based loosely on the therapeutic intervention scoring system (TISS).[111] This system allows for as few as two attendants (one nurse and one transporter) for transporting stable patients, and up to three attendants (one physician, one RCP, and one nurse) for critically ill patients. These guidelines were developed at a teaching hospital and therefore may not apply to community hospitals, where physicians are not as readily available. In these instances, if the patient's physician is unavailable, an in-house physician should be contacted and be available in case of an emergency. Typically, the attending physician in the emergency room fills this role.

Once the personnel are assembled, delineation of roles and responsibilities should be established. The nurse or physician should be in a position to observe the electrocardiographic (ECG) monitor and reach intravenous (IV) pumps to manipulate pharmacologic agents. The RCP should be positioned at the head of the bed to ensure adequate control of the airway and provide ventilatory support. As always, the "team approach" is essential for a safe, successful transport.

Equipment

Equipment for transport must be similar to that used in the ICU in terms of perfor-

TABLE 22–1. Staff Who Must Accompany and Remain With Patients Who Must Leave the Intensive Care Unit (ICU)*

Purpose: In recognizing the need to observe closely ICU patients during periods of time when the patient must be outside the ICU for studies or procedures, the following guidelines are established.

TYPE OF PATIENT	STAFF WHO MUST ACCOMPANY AND REMAIN WITH THE PATIENT UNTIL RETURN TO ICU
Stable patient with only an IV line	Staff to be determined by head nurse and ICU director
Stable patient with arterial line only	RN
Patient on ventilator	RN and RT
Patient with pulmonary artery catheter or any vasoactive drips	RN and resident†
Patient with arterial line, ventilator, and pulmonary artery catheter	RN, resident,† and RT
Any unstable patient	RN, resident,† and RT

IV, intravenous; RN, registered nurse; RT, respiratory therapist.

*If appropriate staff cannot be assembled to accompany the patient, the patient's attending physician should be contacted. The attending physician will decide whether the patient can be transported safely without the specified staff or whether the study should be cancelled. The attending physician will indicate his or her decision in the form of an order.

†For patients managed by the medical residents, one of the unit residents must accompany the patient. For patients managed by the surgical resident, a resident from the primary surgical service must accompany the patient. A medical student may not substitute for the RN or a resident.

From Smith J, Flemming S, Cernaianu A: Mishaps during transport from the intensive care unit. Crit Care Med 18:278-281, 1990.

mance, yet be portable, small, lightweight, and rugged. Of course compromises must be made, and complexity often gives way to simplicity for the sake of size and reliability. The following items are essential for inhospital transport of the mechanically ventilated patient (Table 22–2).

Portable Monitor

A portable ECG monitor capable of monitoring two pressure channels should accompany all patients. This allows continuous monitoring of heart rate, rhythm, and arterial blood pressure. The second pressure channel may be used for patients with a pulmonary artery catheter or those who need intracranial pressure monitoring. The monitor should be small and lightweight but provide a display large enough and bright enough to be seen from 8 to 10 feet away. This is particularly important when the patient is isolated from the caregivers, as occurs during a CT scan. The monitor should have its own rechargeable power supply that continuously charges while connected to AC power. A typical transport takes approximately 80 minutes,[110, 112, 113] 10 to 20 minutes of which are spent in transit to the respective destinations. Based on these figures, a portable monitor should be capable of operating at least 2 hours without recharging. When possible, the monitor should be powered by a permanent AC power supply while the patient is stationary. We currently use a Siemens Sirecust 630 portable monitor. The Sirecust 630 weighs 12 kg, and its dimensions are 21 cm W × 13 cm H × 10.5 cm L. This monitor has two pressure channels, provides a continuous display of ECG, heart rate, systolic, diastolic, and mean blood pressures, can display temperature, and is also capable of operating a noninvasive blood pressure (NIBP) cuff. High and low alarms for each monitored parameter can be set, silenced, or disabled by the operator.

Monitoring blood pressure noninvasively during transport is essential when the patient lacks arterial access. However, recent work by Runcie and associates demonstrates that NIBP underestimates systolic blood pressure by 13 to 21% and overestimates diastolic pressure by 5 to 27% during transport when compared with direct measurement.[114, 115] These inaccuracies have been ascribed to movement of the patient or simply the difference between the two techniques in a heterogeneous group of critically ill patients.[115, 116] In any event, trends are to be followed. Whenever direct measurement of arterial blood pressure is precluded, intermittent manual oscillometric values should be ascertained.

TABLE 22–2. Essential Equipment for Transport of the Mechanically Ventilated Patient

EQUIPMENT	CAPABILITY
Portable monitor	ECG; 2 pressure channels for monitoring arterial blood pressure and pulmonary artery pressures or intracranial pressure
Portable ventilator or self-inflating bag	IMV and/or AMV; PEEP; PEEP compensation of the demand valve; disconnect alarm; manual breath control; separate frequency and tidal volume controls; low gas consumption
Airway maintenance	Laryngoscope; endotracheal tubes 6–9 mm; ID curved and straight laryngoscope blades; oral and nasal airways; stylet; Magill forceps; batteries; tape
Drug box	Epinephrine; sodium bicarbonate; atropine; calcium chloride; IV fluids—D$_5$W and lactated Ringer's solution; IV tubing; other drugs currently being delivered in the ICU—sedatives, paralytic agents, vasoactive agents, and antiarrhythmics
Infusion pumps	Must operate reliably from an internal battery
Stethoscope	Auscultation of breath and heart sounds; measurement of blood pressure

AMV, assisted mechanical ventilation; D$_5$W, 5% dextrose (in water); ECG, electrocardiogram; ICU, intensive care unit; ID, internal diameter; IMV, intermittent mechanical ventilation; IV, intravenous; PEEP, positive end-expiratory pressure.

Ventilator

Ventilatory support during transport has been the subject of several recent investigations.[117–119] Hurst and associates,[117] Gervais and colleagues,[118] and Braman and coworkers[119] all have demonstrated that manual ventilation with a self-inflating bag during transport can lead to unintentional respiratory alkalosis. In each of these studies, episodic hypotension and cardiac dysrhythmias were associated with this rapid change in acid–base status. Gervais and colleagues demonstrated that hyperventilation could be avoided if tidal volume (V$_T$) and minute ventilation (V$_E$) were monitored with a portable spirometer.[118] All three studies suggest that use of a transport ventilator avoids unintentional hyperventilation and is superior to manual ventilation during transport.

Weg and Haas recently reported that manual ventilation of critically ill patients during transport can be accomplished without detriment.[120] They compared blood gases and pH values obtained while patients were being manually ventilated to values obtained while patients were mechanically

ventilated in the ICU. In their group of 20 patients, only one was found to have acute respiratory alkalosis (pH increased 0.13 units and PaCO$_2$ decreased 9 mm Hg). However, in their report, there was a tendency for pH to increase and PaCO$_2$ to decrease during periods of manual ventilation. They also had one patient who had an increase in PaCO$_2$ of 13 mm Hg. Weg and Haas concluded that use of a transport ventilator is unnecessary and expensive. However, the reality of transport cannot guarantee this, and interoperator variability is inevitable.[121] Therefore, we consider that use of a transport ventilator or a system allowing delivered V$_T$ to be measured is the preferred method of ventilatory support during transport. A typical transport ventilator is shown in Figure 22–9.

Characteristics of a Ventilator for Intrahospital Transport

Operational Characteristics

Ideally, the transport ventilator should be capable of operating in both the intermittent mandatory ventilation (IMV) and assisted mechanical ventilation (AMV) modes. However, a single mode may be acceptable if most patients are managed in the ICU with that technique. There should be separate controls for respiratory frequency (f) and V_T, and the delivered V_T should be within 10% of set V_T regardless of PIP. A continuously adjustable FiO_2 is generally unnecessary in adults in whom 100% O_2 is acceptable. Infants at risk for developing retrolental fibroplasia (RLF) should be ventilated with the appropriate FiO_2. It should be remembered that delivery of a precise FiO_2 requires an air tank and air-oxygen blender, thus increasing the cost, complexity, weight, and size of transport system. Alternatively, some transport ventilators use Venturi systems that entrain room air to decrease FiO_2 and increase oxygen source life.[122, 123] The application of PEEP/CPAP should be possible, and a demand valve, able to compensate for elevated baseline pressures, should be available if IMV is used. A basic alarm system, consisting of a low-pressure/disconnect and high-pressure alarm, also must be included.

Portability

Size and weight are chief concerns for transport ventilators. A weight less than 5 kg is desirable, and the ventilator's dimensions should make it easy to mount it or lay it on the bed. Orientation of controls should be in a single plane and inadvertent movement of dials difficult.

Power Source

Pneumatically powered and operated ventilators have been considered preferable to those requiring electronic control.[116] The reasoning has suggested that if two power sources are required, the likelihood of failure is doubled with a device requiring both gas and electric (battery) supplies. As usual, there are tradeoffs with each type of ventilator. Although pneumatic ventilators require only one power source, they often consume gas for operation, depleting the gas source more quickly. Conversely, although an electronically controlled device has the possibility of battery failure, these ventilators generally provide more precise control of

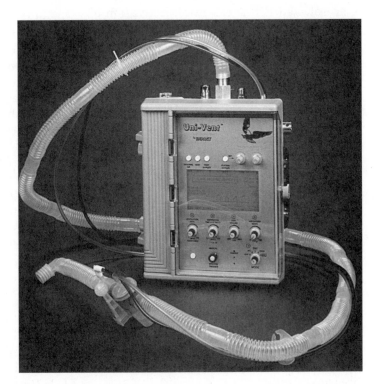

FIGURE 22–9
A typical transport ventilator (Impact 754, Impact Medical, West Caldwell, NJ).

settings, are less likely to be affected by fluctuations in source gas pressure, and do not consume as much gas during operation. Both types have been used successfully.[117–119, 124, 125]

Gas Consumption

Under ideal circumstances, all gas leaving the oxygen cylinder is delivered to the patient. However, pneumatic and fluidic logic circuits often consume gas to control inspiration and expiration. In some cases, gas is also consumed by pneumatic components of electronically controlled ventilators.[124] Gas consumption is defined as gas used by the ventilator for operating circuits or valves, which is exhausted into the atmosphere and not delivered to the patient. Acceptable levels of gas consumption are less than 5 L/min.

Safety

The number and complexity of safety devices are limited by the small size of transport ventilators. A high-pressure relief valve that vents gas into the atmosphere at a preselected PIP is essential. Activation of the high-pressure limit should be signaled by a visual or audible alarm to alert the operator. An antiasphyxia valve that allows the patient to breathe from ambient air in the event of gas source failure is also desirable. Battery-powered ventilators should be equipped with a "low-battery" signal that indicates when 1 hour of power remains. Loss of oxygen power to the ventilator also should result in an audible or visual alarm.

Durability

Transport ventilators should be built to withstand the harsh treatment given them during movement. Control knobs should be protected to keep them from being broken off or cracked. If the ventilator is accidentally dropped from the bed, it should withstand the shock and continue operating. If it fails after impact, it should fail closed (no gas delivery) or open to ambient air (no pressure rise).

Ease of Operation

A delicate balance between operational flexibility and simplicity must be maintained. Most transport ventilators have controls for V_T and f. Additional controls should include mode selection, inspiratory time or I:E, alarm settings, PEEP (if applicable), and a manual breath control. Sensitivity should be preset at a minimum level or should be clinician adjustable.

Ancillary Equipment for Ventilators

All ventilators require a self-contained oxygen supply source. Both compressed gas cylinders and liquid systems can fulfill this need. Intrahospital transport usually is accomplished with an E cylinder or two E cylinders yoked together. This provides 630 L and 1260 L of gas, respectively. We routinely use two E cylinders and whenever possible operate the ventilator from stationary sources at the destination. For longer transports, an H cylinder containing 6900 L may be required. Although the H cylinder provides a substantially larger supply of gas, it is 152 cm in height and weighs 68 kg, and an additional member of the transport team is required just to move it. Movement of a cylinder of this size must be accomplished carefully because of potential dangers should it fall from an upright position.

Liquid oxygen systems can provide 860 cubic feet of gaseous oxygen for every cubic foot in the liquid stage. However, most liquid systems cannot operate at 50 psig, which is necessary for proper ventilator operation. Additionally, should liquid oxygen be spilled, its extremely low temperature may result in thermal injury.[125]

Humidification is frequently overlooked during transport of ventilated patients.[126] This is in part the result of the impracticality of transporting the patient with the humidifier used in the ICU. The logistics and dangers of transporting an electrically powered, position-dependent, water-filled device are exasperating. However, some humidification should be used because delivery of anhydrous medical gases to the tracheobronchial tree can cause tissue damage in less than 30 minutes.[127] A passive humidification device, or "artificial nose," may be used. These devices collect the patient's own respired heat and moisture and return them during the following inspiration. Artificial noses are not as efficient as heated humidifiers but are particularly suited for use during transport.[128] Use of an artificial nose may result in a progressive increase in breathing-circuit resistance, and the patient should be monitored for signs of respiratory distress.[129] Also, premoistening an artificial nose is inadvisable. It does not improve efficiency and serves only to further increase the flow resistance of the device.

Airway Maintenance Equipment

Airway management is a primary concern during transport and frequently is the responsibility of the RCP. During movement of the patient, the possibility of disconnecting or pulling out tubes (e.g., endotracheal, IV) is increased. Therefore, movement of the patient should be done slowly, with one member of the team solely responsible for maintaining the airway in place. This member should also lead the team in deciding when movement should take place so that movement is coordinated and efficient. This is usually accomplished by counting down from 5 and coordinating movement on the count of 1. While away from the ICU, the transport team should carry all the necessary supplies for airway management (see Table 22–2). The patient's endotracheal tube should be secured. Our practice is to use adhesive tape to hold endotracheal tubes in place. We have not found it necessary to carry a cricothyrotomy tray with the team because in extreme emergencies it can be brought quickly to the patient by surgeons capable of performing the procedure.

Infusion Pumps

Continuous delivery of fluids and pharmacologic agents should not be interrupted during transport. Infusion pumps can be easily attached to IV poles and are usually capable of operating for several hours on internal batteries. These devices should have alarms to warn of infusion problems and should be as small and lightweight as possible. When the patient is receiving enteral nutrition, we usually elect to discontinue feeding during transport.

Drug Box

A drug box with all pharmacologic agents necessary to manage emergency situations should accompany the team. Additionally, extra IV fluids, IV tubing, and other drugs currently being delivered should be available.

Stethoscope

The stethoscope is essential equipment for all members of the team. Without fancy electronics, it can detect the quality or presence of breath sounds and heart sounds and can assist in the manual measurement of blood pressure. Frequent use of the stethoscope is recommended to ensure patient safety.

Additional Equipment

In selected cases, it may be advantageous for the transport team to carry a pulse oximeter and a defibrillator. Pulse oximetry can detect inadequate oxygen saturation before overt clinical signs.[130] However, if an FiO_2 of 1.0 is used, the incidence of hypoxemia during transport is low.[131] If an oximeter is used, it should have its own battery, be relatively insensitive to motion, and, like all other equipment, be as small and lightweight as possible.

A defibrillator may be necessary when transferring patients with known cardiac disease. In some cases, the defibrillator may be part of the ECG monitor, in which case additional equipment is unnecessary. The defibrillator should have its own power supply and meet size and weight requirements.

Physiologic Effects and Risks of Transport

The detrimental physiologic effects and risks of intrahospital transport have been described by several authors. However, there is difficulty in comparing results because some reports consider ECG lead disconnection a complication of transport, whereas others consider only physiologic changes.

Taylor and colleagues described their experience transporting 50 patients with acute cardiac disease.[131] All patients had continuous ECG monitoring and a defibrillator accompanied every trip. Forty-two of 50 patients were noted to have arrhythmias during transport, and of these, 22 were considered life-threatening, requiring immediate treatment. The average length of transport in this survey was 57 minutes. The authors noted that transportation also resulted in an increase in heart rate but no consistent change in blood pressure. No patient died during transport. Taylor and colleagues concluded that ECG monitoring of these patients was essential, and they speculated that patient movement in and of itself may predispose the patient to arrhythmias.

Waddell published results of a prospective trial of patient transport in 1975.[132] He studied 55 patients transported to and from the ICU during a 5-month period and reported that "one patient a month suffered major cardiorespiratory collapse or death as a direct result of movement." In one instance, movement resulted in renewed bleeding from a pelvic fracture and death. In two cases, movement was associated with cardiac arrhythmia and hypotension, and in one case, airway obstruction occurred. In the second part of his study, Waddell demonstrated that 70 postoperative patients could be moved without incident. Waddell recommended that critically ill patients should be moved only when absolutely necessary and that preparation and stabilization of the patient were essential to limit adverse effects.

Ehrenwerth and associates retrospectively studied 204 critically ill patients transported to the ICU and identified only three instances in which the transport process resulted in morbidity.[133] They concluded that critically ill adults could be transported safely.

Insel and colleagues described the cardiovascular changes during transport of patients after major surgery from the operating room to the ICU.[134] They recorded heart rate and blood pressure: preoperatively, at 30 minutes, at 15 minutes, and immediately before transport; in the elevator; on arrival; and 30 minutes after arrival at their destination. They demonstrated that cardiovascular instability was common during transport and attributed most of the changes to the emergence from anesthesia. Additionally, they reported cases of hypotension, hypertension, and ventricular fibrillation before or just after arrival at the ICU. Insel and colleagues stated that "transport itself has little hemodynamic impact."

Rutherford and Fisher studied 49 patients during transport from a medical ICU.[135] They classified patients into three groups according to level of support required: (1) ECG monitoring only, (2) invasive hemodynamic monitoring plus ECG, and (3) mechanical ventilation or pharmacologic cardiovascular support plus ECG and invasive monitoring. They observed a 45% incidence of life-threatening complications during transport, including five episodes of systolic blood pressure less than 80 mm Hg, four episodes of respiratory distress, three disconnections of central venous lines, and two dysrhythmias requiring pharmacologic intervention and cardioversion. Rutherford and Fisher concluded that "transport should be kept to an absolute minimum."[135]

In 1987, separate studies by Braman and associates[119] and Gervais and colleagues[118] demonstrated the adverse effects of unintentional hyperventilation during transport, as previously discussed. However, Braman and associates also reported other complications during transport. In two instances, ventilator malfunction was associated with a deterioration in patient condition. This was caused by battery failure and disconnection of the oxygen source. Five patients demonstrated significant hypotension, one had bradycardia, and one had premature ventricular contractions (16/min). In this study, an LP-6 ventilator was used for ventilation during transport. It is unclear whether any adverse effects were related to the increased work of breathing seen with this ventilator in the IMV mode.[136] Braman and associates also suggested that "tests be kept to a minimum" and that improvements in ventilatory support "may substantially reduce the risk for serious complications."[119]

Indeck and colleagues prospectively evaluated the risk, cost, and benefits of 103 transports to and from the ICU.[112] They defined complications as a change in oxygen saturation greater than 5%, a change in blood pressure of 20 mm Hg for longer than 5 minutes, a change in heart rate of 20 beats/min for longer than 5 minutes, and a change in respiratory frequency greater than 5 breaths/min for more than 5 minutes. During these transports, they recorded 113 significant physiologic changes. Most changes occurred in blood pressure (46/113), followed by heart rate (24/113), respiratory rate (23/113), and oxygen saturation (20/113). Indeck and colleagues also documented whether the test being performed outside the ICU altered patient management. They concluded that in their series, 76% of tests resulted in no change in patient treatment. Although no patient died or had significant morbidity, Indeck and colleagues suggest that "the decision to transport must be weighed carefully in the face of a > 76% chance that the result will not alter management."[112]

Smith and colleagues prospectively studied 125 patients requiring intrahospital transport for "mishaps" related to transport.[110] Although most of these mishaps seem inconsequential (ECG lead disconnect), the 14% incidence of monitor power failure is disturbingly high. This study demonstrated that one-third of all transports are associated with mishaps in various degrees. However, no patient died during transport.

The diverse opinions and findings by the previous authors leave questions regarding the safety and efficacy of transport. We recently completed a prospective cohort study of 100 transports.[113] Using the method of Indeck and colleagues,[112] we monitored the patient during transport, as well as a control patient remaining in the ICU with a similar APACHE (Acute Physiology and Chronic Health Evaluation) II score. We found the incidence of physiologic complications and equipment failures to be similar in the two groups (71 vs. 64 and 5 vs. 4, respectively). We also monitored ABGs and found no differences during transport compared with ICU blood gases. Our study demonstrates that the "mishaps" and "complications" often attributed to transport are experienced by critically ill patients in the ICU as well. This suggests that the nature of the patient's illness is more important than the act of transport.

REFERENCES

1. Guidelines for cardiopulmonary resuscitation and emergency cardiac care. JAMA 268:2171–2302, 1992.
2. Emergency Care Research Institute: Manually operated resuscitators. Health Devices 1:13–17, 1971.
3. Emergency Care Research Institute: Manual resuscitators. Health Devices 8:133–146, 1979.
4. Emergency Care Research Institute: Gas-powered resuscitators. Health Devices 8:24–38, 1978.
5. Emergency Care Research Institute: Gas-powered pulmonary resuscitators. Health Devices 18:362–363, 1989.
6. Emergency Care Research Institute: Pulmonary resuscitators. Health Devices 17:348–354, 1988.
7. Emergency Care Research Institute: Exhaled air pulmonary resuscitators (EAPR's) and disposable manual pulmonary resuscitators (DMPR's). Health Devices 18:333–352, 1989.
8. American Society of Testing Materials: Standard Specifications for Minimum Performance and Safety Requirements for Resuscitators Intended for Use with Humans. Designation F 920-85. Philadelphia: ASTM, 1985.
9. International Standards Organization: International Standard ISO 8382:1988(E): Resuscitators Intended for Use with Humans. New York: American National Standards Institute, 1988.
10. Ruben H, Knudsen EJ, Carugti G: Gastric insufflation in relation to airway pressure. Acta Anaesthesiol Scand 5:107–114, 1961.
11. Melker RJ: Recommendations for ventilation during cardiopulmonary resuscitation: time for a change? Crit Care Med 13:882–883, 1985.
12. Fillmore SJ, Shapiro M, Killip J: Serial blood gas studies during cardiopulmonary resuscitation. Ann Intern Med 72:465–470, 1970.
13. Gilston A: Clinical and biochemical aspects of cardiac resuscitation. Lancet 2:1039–1043, 1965.
14. Himmelhoch SR, Dekker A, Gazzaniga AB, Like AA: Closed-chest cardiac resuscitation: a prospective clinical and pathological study. N Engl J Med 270:118–122, 1964.
15. Ornato JP, Bryson BL, Donovan PJ, et al: Measurement of ventilation during cardiopulmonary resuscitation. Crit Care Med 11:79–82, 1983.

16. Davis K, Johannigman JA, Johnson RC, Branson RD: Lung compliance following cardiac arrest. Acad Emerg Med 2:874–878, 1995.
17. 11 Kings 4:31–35 The Bible, King James Version.
18. Sainsbury DA, Davis R, Walker MC: Artificial ventilation for cardiopulmonary resuscitation. Med J Aust 141:509–511, 1984.
19. Hess D, Baran C: Ventilatory volumes using mouth-to-mouth, mouth-to-mask, and bag-valve-mask techniques. Am J Emerg Med 3:292–296, 1985.
20. Lawrence PJ, Sivaneswaran N: Ventilation during cardiopulmonary resuscitation: which method? Med J Aust 143:443–446, 1985.
21. Harrison RR, Maull KI, Keenan RL, Boyan CP: Mouth-to-mask ventilation: a superior method of rescue breathing. Ann Emerg Med 11:74–76, 1982.
22. Seidelin PH, Stolarek IH, Littlewood DG: Comparison of six methods of emergency ventilation. Lancet 2:1274–1275, 1986.
23. Johannigman JA, Branson RD, Davis K, Hurst JM: Techniques of emergency ventilation: a model to evaluate tidal volume, airway pressure, and gastric insufflation. J Trauma 31:93–98, 1991.
24. Melker RJ, Banner MJ: Ventilation during CPR: two-rescuer standards reappraised. Ann Emerg Med 14:397–402, 1985.
25. Hess D, Kapp A, Kurtek W: The effect of delivered oxygen concentration of the rescuer's breathing supplemental oxygen during exhaled gas ventilation. Respir Care 30:691–694, 1985.
26. Rottenberg EM, Dzwonczyk R, Reilley TE, Malone M: Use of supplemental oxygen during bystander-initiated CPR. Ann Emerg Med 23:1027–1030, 1994.
27. Sellick BA: Cricoid pressure to control regurgitation of stomach contents during induction of anesthesia. Lancet 2:404–406, 1961.
28. Moynihan RJ, Brock-Utne JG, Archer JH, et al: The effect of cricoid pressure on preventing gastric insufflation in infants and children. Anesthesiology 78:652–656, 1993.
29. Vanner RG, O'Dwyer JP, Pryle BJ, Reynolds F: Upper oesophageal sphincter pressure and the effect of cricoid pressure. Anesthesia 47:95–100, 1992.
30. Ralph SJ, Wareham CA: Rupture of the oesophagus during cricoid pressure. Anaesthesia 46:40–41, 1991.
31. Barker SJ, Karagianes T: Gastric barotrauma: a case report and theoretical considerations. Anesth Analg 64:1026–1028, 1985.
32. Ornato JP, Hallagan LF, McMahon SB, Rostafinski A: Attitudes of BCLS instructors about mouth to mouth resuscitation during the AIDS epidemic. Ann Amerg Med 19:151–156, 1990.
33. Pane GA, Salness KA: A survey of participants in a mass CPR training course. Ann Emerg Med 16:1112–1116, 1987.
34. Link RN, Feingold AR, Charap MH, et al: Concerns of medical and pediatric house officers about acquiring AIDS from their patients. Am J Public Health 78:455–459, 1988.
35. American Heart Association: Supplemental guidelines: Risk of infection during CPR training and rescue. JAMA 262:2714–2715, 1989.
36. Fluck RR, Sorbello JG: Mouth to mouth resuscitation by lay rescuers—should they or shouldn't they? Respir Care 35:831–832, 1990.
37. Durbin CG: Mouth to mask resuscitation by lay rescuers—will they or won't they? Respir Care 35:832–834, 1990.
38. Heilman KM, Muscheheim C: Primary cutaneous tuberculosis resulting from mouth to mouth respiration. N Engl J Med 273:1035–1036, 1965.
39. Feldman HA: Some recollections of the meningococcal disease. JAMA 220:1107–1112, 1972.
40. Hendricks AA, Shapiro EP: Primary herpes simplex infection following mouth to mouth resuscitation. JAMA 243:257–258, 1980.
41. Finkelhorn RS, Lampman JH: Herpes simplex infection following cardiopulmonary resuscitation. JAMA 243:650, 1980.
42. Harris MJ, Wendel RT: Transmission of herpes simplex during cardiopulmonary resuscitation. Compr Ther 10:15–17, 1984.
43. Todd MA, Bell JS: Shigellosis from cardiopulmonary resuscitation. JAMA 243:331, 1980.
44. Ahmad F, Senadhira DC, Charters J, Acquilla S: Transmission of salmonella via mouth-to-mouth resuscitation. Lancet 335:787–788, 1990.
45. Mamby SA: A plea for CPR equipment in public places. N Engl J Med 322:1161, 1990.
46. Hodgin L: New law in the Big Apple mandates CPR infection control equipment. Occup Health Saf 61:56–58, 1992.
47. Waters RM: Simple methods for performing artificial respiration. JAMA 123:559–561, 1943.
48. Don Michael A, Forrester JS: Mouth to mouth ventilation: the dying art. Am J Emerg Med 10:156–161, 1992.
49. Lightsey DM, Shah PK, Forrester JS, Don Michael A: A human immunodeficiency virus resistant airway for cardiopulmonary resuscitation. Ann J Emerg Med 10:73–77, 1992.
50. Rossi R, Ahnefeld FW: Expired air resuscitation in emergency situations with Ambu-Life key. Notfallmedizin 16:3–7, 1990.
51. Baskett PJF: Advances in cardiopulmonary resuscitation. Br J Anaesth 69:182–193, 1992.
52. Westfall MD: Kiss of life mask: evaluation or opinion? (Letter) Am J Emerg Med 10:616, 1992.
53. Rossi R, Lindner KH, Ahnefeld FW: Devices for expired air resuscitation. Prehospital Disaster Med 8:123–126, 1993.
54. Simmons M: Resistance to flow through the valves of three face shield CPR barrier devices. Respir Care 39:1068, 1994.
55. Simmons M, Deao D, Moon L: Bench evaluation: three face shield barrier devices. Respir Care 40:618–623, 1995.
56. Elam JO, Brown ES, Elder JD Jr: Artificial respiration by mouth-to-mask method. N Engl J Med 250:749–754, 1954.
57. Safar P, McMahon M: Mouth to airway emergency artificial respiration. JAMA 166:1459–1461, 1958.

58. Safar P: Pocket mask for emergency artificial ventilation and oxygen inhalation. Crit Care Med 2:273–276, 1974.

59. Thomas AN, Weber EC: A new method of two-resuscitator CPR. Resuscitation 26:173–176, 1993.

60. Thomas AN, O'Sullivan K, Hyatt J, Barker SJ: A comparison of bag mask and mouth mask ventilation in anaesthetized patients. Resuscitation 26:13–21, 1993.

61. Tolley PM, Watts J, Hickman JA: Comparison of the use of the laryngeal mask and face mask by inexperienced personnel. Br J Anaesth 69:320–321, 1992.

62. Thomas AN, Bergesio R, Hyatt J, Barker SJ: Mouth mask ventilation: use of a pall ultipor breathing system and effect of mask design (abstract). Br J Anaesth 69:527P–528P, 1992.

63. Johannigman JA, Branson RD: Oxygen enrichment of expired gas for mouth to mask resuscitation. Respir Care 36:99–103, 1991.

64. Stahl JM, Cutfield GR, Harrison GA: Alveolar oxygenation and mouth to mask ventilation: effects of oxygen insufflation. Anaesth Intensive Care 20:177–186, 1992.

65. Thomas AN, Hyatt J, Chen JL, Barker SJ: The Laerdal pocket mask: effects of increasing supplementary oxygen flow. Anaesthesia 47:967–971, 1992.

66. Palmisano JM, Moler FW, Galura C, et al: Influence of tidal volume, respiratory rate, and supplemental oxygen flow on delivered oxygen fraction using a mouth to mask ventilation device. J Emerg Med 11:685–689, 1993.

67. Hess D, Ness C, Oppel A, Rhoads K: Evaluation of mouth to mask ventilation devices. Respir Care 34:191–195, 1989.

68. Hess DR: Manual and gas powered resuscitators. In: Branson RD, Hess DR, Chatburn RL (eds): Respiratory Care Equipment. Philadelphia: Lippincott Williams and Wilkins, 1999, pp 187–202.

69. Barnes TA: Emergency ventilation techniques and related equipment. Respir Care 37:673–694, 1992.

70. Elling R, Politis J: An evaluation of emergency medical technicians ability to use manual ventilation devices. Ann Emerg Med 12:765–768, 1983.

71. Giffen PR, Hope CE: Preliminary evaluation of a prototype tube-valve-mask ventilator for emergency artificial ventilation. Ann Emerg Med 20:262–266, 1991.

72. Cummins RO, Austin D, Graves JR, et al: Ventilation skills of emergency medical technicians: a teaching challenge for emergency medicine. Ann Emerg Med 15:1187–1192, 1986.

73. Barnes TA, Adams G: Ventilatory volumes using mouth to mouth, bag-valve-mask, and pocket face mask (abstract). Respir Care 36:1292, 1991.

74. Jesudian MC, Harrison RR, Keenan RL, Maull KI: Bag-valve-mask ventilation: two rescuers are better than one: preliminary report. Crit Care Med 13:122–123, 1985.

75. Stewart RD, Kaplan R, Penrock B, Thompson F: Influence of mask design on bag-mask ventilation. Ann Emerg Med 14:403–406, 1985.

76. Hess D, Goff G: The effects of two-hand versus one-hand ventilation on volumes delivered during bag-valve ventilation at various resistances and compliances. Respir Care 32:1025–1028, 1987.

77. Augustine JA, Seidel DR, McCabe JB: Ventilation performance using a self-inflating anesthesia bag: effect of operator characteristics. Am J Emerg Med 5:267–270, 1987.

78. Hess D, Goff G, Johnson K: The effect of hand size, resuscitator brand, and use of two hands on volumes delivered during adult bag-valve ventilation. Respir Care 34:805–810, 1989.

79. Powers WE: Evaluation of a training method that uses volummetric feedback with bag-valve-mask ventilation techniques (abstract). Respir Care 33:942–943, 1988.

80. Branson RD, Davis K, Johnson RC, et al: Manual ventilation during cardiopulmonary resuscitation (abstract). Respir Care 39:1068, 1994.

81. Priano L, Ham J: A simple method to increase FDO_2 of resuscitator bags. Crit Care Med 6:48–49, 1978.

82. Fitzmaurice MW, Barnes TA: Oxygen delivery performance of three adult resuscitation bags. Respir Care 25:928–933, 1980.

83. LeBovet L: 1980 assessment of eight adult manual resuscitators. Respir Care 25:1136–1142, 1980.

84. Barnes TA, Watson MW: Oxygen delivery performance of four adult resuscitation bags. Respir Care 27:139–146, 1982.

85. Barnes T, Watson M: Oxygen delivery performance of old and new designs of the Laerdal, Vitalograph, and AMBU adult manual resuscitators. Respir Care 28:1121–1128, 1983.

86. Phillips GD, Showronski GA: Manual resuscitators and portable ventilators. Anaesth Intensive Care 14:306–313, 1986.

87. Campbell TP, Stewart RD, Kaplan RM, et al: Oxygen enrichment of bag-valve-mask units during positive-pressure ventilation: a comparison of various techniques. Ann Emerg Med 17:232–235, 1988.

88. Barnes TA, Potash R: Evaluation of five disposable operator powered adult resuscitators. Respir Care 34:254–261, 1989.

89. Barnes TA, McGarry W: Evaluation of ten disposable manual resuscitators. Respir Care 35:960–968, 1990.

90. Barnes TA, Stockwell DL: Evaluation of ten manual resuscitators across an operational temperature range of −18EC to 50EC. Respir Care 36:161–172, 1991.

91. Munford BJ, Wishaw KJ: Critical incidents with non-rebreathing valves. Anaesth Intensive Care 18:560–563, 1990.

92. Hess D, Simmons M: An evaluation of the resistance to flow through the patent valves of twelve adult manual resuscitators. Respir Care 37:432–438, 1992.

93. Mills PJ, Baptiste J, Preston J, Barnes GM: Man-

ual resuscitators and spontaneous ventilation: an evaluation. Crit Care Med 19:1425–1431, 1991.

94. Stemp LI: Manual resuscitators and spontaneous ventilation—an evaluation (letter). Crit Care Med 20:1496, 1992.

95. Hess D, Hirsch C, Marquis-D'amico C, Kacmarek R: Imposed work and oxygen delivery during spontaneous breathing with adult disposable manual ventilators. Anaesthesiology 81:1256–1263, 1994.

96. Johannigman JA, Branson RD, Johnson DJ, et al: Out-of-hospital ventilation: bag-valve device versus transport ventilator. Acad Emerg Med 2:719–724, 1995.

97. Osborn HH, Kayen D, Horne H, Bray W: Excess ventilation with oxygen powered resuscitators. Am J Emerg Med 2:408–413, 1984.

98. Pradis IL, Caldwell EJ: Traumatic pneumocephalus: a hazard of resuscitators. J Trauma 19:61–63, 1979.

99. Fasi TH, Lucas BG: An evaluation of some mechanical resuscitators for use in the ambulance service. Ann R Coll Surg Engl 62:291–293, 1980.

100. Menegazzi JJ, Winslow HJ: In-vitro comparison of bag-valve-mask and the manually triggered oxygen powered breathing device. Acad Emerg Med 1:29–33, 1994.

101. Mesezzo VN, Lukitsch K, Menegazzi J, Mosesso J: Comparison of delivered volumes and airway pressures when ventilating through an endotracheal tube with bag valve versus demand valve. Prehosp Disaster Med 9:24–28, 1994.

102. Branson RD: Intrahospital transport of critically ill mechanically ventilated patients. Respir Care 37:775–795, 1992.

103. Branson RD, McGough EK: Transport ventilators. In: Banner MJ (ed): Problems in Critical Care: Positive Pressure Ventilation. Philadelphia: JB Lippincott, 1990, pp 254–274.

104. Nolan JP, Baskett JF: Gas-powered and portable ventilators: an evaluation of six models. Prehosp Disaster Med 7:25–34, 1972.

105. McGough EK, Banner MJ, Melker RJ: Variations in tidal volume with portable transport ventilators. Respir Care 37:233–239, 1992.

106. Campbell RS, Davis K, Johnson DJ, Porembka D: Laboratory and clinical evaluation of the Impact 750 portable ventilator. Respir Care 37:29–36, 1992.

107. Johannigman JA, Branson RD, Campbell RS, Hurst JM: Laboratory and clinical evaluation of the MAX transport ventilator. Respir Care 35:952–959, 1990.

108. Greenslade GL: Single operator cardiopulmonary resuscitation in ambulances. Anaesthesia 46:391–394, 1991.

109. Smith IV, Flemming S, Bekes CE: Written policy and patient transport from the intensive care unit (letter). Crit Care Med 15:1162, 1987.

110. Smith I, Flemming S, Cernaianu A: Mishaps during transport from the intensive care unit. Crit Care Med 18:278–281, 1990.

111. Keene AR, Cullen DJ: Therapeutic intervention scoring system: update 1983. Crit Care Med 11:1–8, 1983.

112. Indeck M, Peterson S, Smith J, Brotman S: Risk, cost and benefit of transporting ICU patient for special studies. J Trauma 28:1020–1025, 1988.

113. Hurst JM, Davis K Jr, Johnson DJ, et al: Cost and complications during in-hospital transport of critically ill patients: a prospective study (abstract). J Trauma 31:1717, 1991.

114. Runcie CJ, Reeve W, Reidy J, Dougall JR: A comparison of measurements of blood pressure, heart rate and oxygenation during inter-hospital transport of the critically ill. Intensive Care Med 16:317–322, 1990.

115. Runcie CJ, Reeve WG, Reidy J, Dougall JR: Blood pressure measurement during transport. Anaesthesia 45:659–665, 1990.

116. Gallagher TJ, Melker RJ: Transport of the critically ill/injured patient. In: Civetta JM, Taylor RW, Kirby RR (eds): Critical Care. Philadelphia: JB Lippincott, 1988, pp 1579–1588.

117. Hurst JM, Davis K, Branson RD, Barrette RR: Comparison of blood gases during transport using two methods of ventilatory support. J Trauma 29:1637–1640, 1989.

118. Gervais HW, Eberle B, Konietzke D, et al: Comparison of blood gases of ventilated patients during transport. Crit Care Med 15:761–764, 1987.

119. Braman SS, Dunn SM, Amico C, Millman RP: Complications of inter-hospital transport in critically ill patients. Ann Intern Med 107:469–473, 1987.

120. Weg JG, Haas CF: Safe intra-hospital transport of critically ill ventilator dependent patients. Chest 96:631–635, 1989.

121. Adams KS, Branson RD, Hurst JM: Variabilities in delivered tidal volume and respiratory rate during manual ventilation (abstract). Respir Care 31:986, 1986.

122. Branson RD, McGough EK: Transport ventilators. In: Banner MJ (ed): Positive Pressure Ventilation. Philadelphia: JB Lippincott, 1990, pp 254–274.

123. Park GR, Manara AR, Bodenham AR, Moss CJ: The pneuPAC ventilator with new patient valve and air compressors. Anaesthesia 44:419–424, 1989.

124. Johannigman JA, Branson RD, Campbell RS, Hurst JM: Laboratory and clinical evaluation of the MAX transport ventilator. Respir Care 35:952–959, 1990.

125. Campbell RS, Davis K Jr, Johnson DJ, Hurst JM: Laboratory and clinical evaluation of the UniVent 750 portable ventilator. Respir Care 37:29–36, 1992.

126. Shelly MP, Park GR, Warren RE: Portable lung ventilators: the potential risk from bacterial colonisation. Intensive Care Med 12:328–331, 1986.

127. Chalon J, Loew DAY, Malebranche J: Effect of dry anesthetic gases on the tracheobronchial epithelium. Anesthesiology 37:338–343, 1972.

128. Branson RD, Hurst JM: Laboratory evaluation of moisture output of seven airway heat and moisture exchangers. Respir Care 32:741–747, 1987.

129. Ploysonsang Y, Branson RD, Rashkin MC, Hurst JM: Pressure flow characteristics of commonly used heat–moisture exchangers. Am Rev Respir Dis 138:675–678, 1988.

130. Adams KS, Branson RD, Hurst JM: Monitoring oxygenation with oximetry during transport. Respir Manage Nov/Dec:63–69, 1987.

131. Taylor JO, Landers CF, Chulay JD, et al: Monitoring high-risk cardiac patients during transportation in hospital. Lancet 2:1205–1208, 1970.

132. Waddell G: Movement of critically ill patients within hospital. Br Med J 2:417–419, 1975.

133. Ehrenwerth J, Sorbo S, Hacker A: Transport of critically ill adults. Crit Care Med 14:543–547, 1986.

134. Insel J, Weissman C, Kemper M, et al: Cardiovascular changes during transport of critically ill and postoperative patients. Crit Care Med 14:539–542, 1986.

135. Rutherford WF, Fisher CJ: Risks associated with in-house transportation of the critically ill (abstract). Clin Res 34:414, 1986.

136. Kacmarek RM, Stanek KS, McMahon KM, Wilson RS: Imposed work of breathing during synchronized intermittent mandatory ventilation provided by five home care ventilators. Respir Care 35:405–414, 1990.

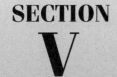

SECTION V

Specialized Techniques and Future Therapies

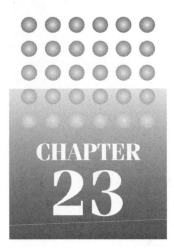

Assessing Innovations in Mechanical Ventilation

Neil R. MacIntyre, MD

INNOVATION CLAIMS AND
TYPES OF EFFICACY
TESTING
Engineering and Clinical
   Performance Assessment
Physiologic Assessment
Clinical Outcome
   Assessment

SELECTING THE
APPROPRIATE EFFICACY
ASSESSMENT STRATEGY
REFERENCES

KEY WORDS

end points
engineering assessment

Food and Drug
   Administration

Although the current generation of mechanical ventilators generally provides safe and effective support of gas exchange, significant performance limitations still exist.[1] The most important of these include the following:

1. Adequate gas exchange may not always be maintained in the sickest of patients.

2. Lung injury from both overdistension and under-recruitment can develop even with the best of management strategies.

3. Patient–ventilator dys-synchrony during assisted or supported modes can lead to the need for sedation and paralysis.

4. The endotracheal tube/ventilator circuitry exposes the patient to infection risks.

5. Elevated intrathoracic pressures can impair cardiac filling and reduce cardiac output.

6. The cost of mechanical ventilatory support, both in terms of equipment as well as professional expertise, can be substantial.

Innovations are needed to address all these issues.

Innovations in mechanical ventilation can come from both new engineering designs and new applications of existing designs. Examples of new engineering designs range from simple features, such as flow triggering and inspiratory pressure slope adjustors, to completely new approaches to ventilatory support, such as high-frequency ventilation and liquid ventilation. Examples of new applications include inverse-ratio ventilation, stand-alone pressure support ventilation, and applied expiratory pressure (positive end-expiratory pressure [PEEP]) to reduce the inspiratory triggering load induced by air trapping in obstructive lung disease. Regardless of the type of innovation, the claimed benefit for the innovation (by either the manufacturer or the clinician) needs to be verified through efficacy assessment.[2, 3] This process is the focus of this chapter.

INNOVATION CLAIMS AND TYPES OF EFFICACY TESTING

An innovation is designed to provide a benefit. This benefit constitutes the "claim" of the manufacturer or clinician-innovator. This claim can be of three general types:

1. **Engineering**. A claim of engineering benefit states that the innovation improves technical performance, ease of operation, or cost of operation.
2. **Physiologic**. A claim of physiologic benefit states that the innovation improves a physiologic parameter such as gas exchange or patient work.
3. **Outcome**. A claim of outcome benefit states that the innovation improves an important clinical outcome.

Because efficacy must be assessed according to the claim, efficacy assessment can be engineering, physiologic, or outcome focused. These different approaches differ in their cost, complexity, and relationship to the actual innovation's function (Tables 23–1 and 23–2) and are discussed in more detail in the following sections.

Engineering and Clinical Performance Assessment

Engineering assessment involves specific evaluation of an innovation's performance in a testing laboratory using computer or mechanical models. With this approach, engineering specifications can be validated and reliability can be established. A **clinical** performance evaluation has a similar function because it is focused on the specific performance characteristics of the innovation in the clinical setting. Subjective impressions of the innovation also can be determined. This form of evaluation is inexpensive and innovation specific but does not provide information to evaluate any substantial clinical benefits. Clinical efficacy can only be inferred from this form of assessment. Unanticipated safety issues also cannot be assessed.

Physiologic Assessment

This type of testing involves a variety of clinical parameters that can be assessed readily as the innovation is applied and used. Examples relative to mechanical ventilation include gas exchange, respiratory mechanics, patient work, and cardiovascu-

TABLE 23–1. Efficacy Assessment Criteria

ASSESSMENT CRITERIA	ASSESSMENT COST/ COMPLEXITY	ASSESSMENT RESULTS PREDICT CLINICAL OUTCOME	ASSESSMENT RESULTS ARE DIRECTLY ATTRIBUTED TO THE INNOVATION'S FUNCTION
Engineering, clinical technical performance	Low	No	Yes—by definition
Physiologic	Moderate	Outcome effect is inferred	Yes—if criteria are focused on expected benefits
Clinical outcome	High	Yes—by definition	Maybe—a technical innovation may have limited impact on overall clinical outcome in complex patients

TABLE 23–2. Examples of Types of End Points for Efficacy Assessment in Mechanical Ventilation

ENGINEERING ASSESSMENT

- Valve performance (sensitivity, responsiveness)
- Monitor accuracy
- Flow capabilities
- Ease of operation
- Noise
- Durability
- Cost of operation

PHYSIOLOGIC ASSESSMENT

- Ventilation (total, alveolar, dead space)
- Gas exchange
- Cardiac function (filling, contractility)
- Respiratory system mechanics
- Muscle function (drive, work, pressure–time products)
- Air trapping (intrinsic PEEP)

CLINICAL OUTCOME ASSESSMENT

- Overall survival, long-term survival
- Ventilator days, ICU days, hospital days
- Days alive off ventilator
- Incidence of important complications (barotrauma, pneumonia)

ICU, intensive care unit; PEEP, positive end-expiratory pressure.

lar function. Specific parameters usually are based on anticipated mechanisms of benefit or potential risk. Ideally, these **end points** also should have some reasonable link to outcome (outcome "surrogate").[4, 5] These types of assessment are generally more expensive to do as clinical protocols are required. Any effect on clinical outcome, however, only can be inferred from the physiologic parameters. Moreover, long-term safety issues cannot be addressed.

Clinical Outcome Assessment

With this type of testing longer periods of time are used to see if an innovation actually affects an important clinical outcome. The advantage of this type of assessment is that an important clinical outcome can be strong justification for implementation of an innovation. Outcome assessments, however,

are complex and expensive because they usually involve randomized clinical trials.[6–8] In designing such trials, several considerations are important. First, an appropriate end point must be chosen. Because mechanical ventilation is primarily a support technique, mortality may not be an appropriate end point (i.e., mortality usually is influenced most by the underlying disease, not by a support system such as a ventilator strategy). Ventilator-free days, intensive care unit (ICU) length of stay, and days to ventilator removal clearly are more focused, clinically relevant outcome end points for a mechanical ventilation innovation. Second, an appropriate study population is required. For instance, if an innovation is designed to reduce overdistension and under-recruitment injury, study populations at risk for these problems should be selected. In this example, it would make no sense to study a "lung-protective" strategy in a population having only mild lung injury that could be managed easily with low levels of ventilatory support. Third, an appropriate sample size is important in designing any outcome study. Specifically, it is crucial to "power" the study properly by considering what the control group outcome and the impact of the innovation are likely to be. Only in this way can a sample size be chosen so that a significant benefit that actually exists is not missed because the study population was too small.[9]

SELECTING THE APPROPRIATE EFFICACY ASSESSMENT STRATEGY

Two important factors must be considered in choosing an efficacy assessment strategy: the incremental risk of the innovation and the incremental cost of the innovation. Clinicians and regulators particularly are concerned about the incremental risks. Specifically, the higher the potential risk of the innovation, the greater the need for a claim of outcome benefit and an appropriate outcome assessment.[10, 11] Conversely, payers particularly are concerned about the cost of the innovation. From this perspective, the higher the cost of the innovation, the greater the need for a claim of outcome benefit and appropriate outcome assessment.[12-14] Table 23–3 summarizes these different perspectives.

In the United States, the **Food and Drug Administration** (FDA) is the major regulatory body having, since 1976, responsibility for ensuring medical device safety and effi-

TABLE 23–3. Different Perspectives of Efficacy Assessment

FROM THE MANUFACTURER'S PERSPECTIVE

- Efficacy criteria required for regulators, payers, and clinicians are often unclear (i.e., What needs to be demonstrated?).
- Regulatory process is viewed as overly cautious and slow.
- Establishing efficacy is a costly portion of innovation development.

FROM THE REGULATORY AGENCY'S PERSPECTIVE

- Federal mandates for ensuring public protection from harmful devices requires more regulation and a less speedy approval process.
- Mechanical ventilation innovations are increasingly complex—especially microprocessor systems and software.
- Efficacy criteria for medical devices are not well established (i.e., Which devices need only engineering tests or 510K review, and which devices need physiologic or clinical outcomes tests or premarket application review?).
- Federal funding to perform an increasingly complex task is shrinking.

FROM THE CLINICIAN'S PERSPECTIVE

- Claims by an innovation's advocate may not be supported by appropriate levels of efficacy assessment (i.e., physiologic claims are made from engineering tests and outcome claims are made from physiologic tests); clinicians must realize that the freedom to use devices beyond established applications must be balanced by safety, liability, and reimbursement concerns.
- Manufacturers, regulators, and payers can be perceived as being too slow in making innovations possible.

FROM THE PAYER'S PERSPECTIVE

- Cost analyses of innovations rarely are done.
- Definitions of "beneficial" cost-effectiveness to justify reimbursement do not exist for mechanical ventilation innovations.

cacy.[15] The FDA's charge is to ensure that the manufacturer's claim of efficacy (and safety) is supported by appropriate efficacy assessment. The manufacturer's marketing and advertising claims can be only those judged by the FDA to be supported by appropriate efficacy assessment. There are actually two regulatory processes that the FDA uses to do this: (1) the premarket notification (often referred to as a "510K" procedure) or (2) the premarket application (PMA). The relatively simple 510K process is used for innovations that are judged "substantially equivalent" to devices on the market before 1976. Risks and efficacy of the new device generally are assumed to be "substantially equivalent" to the previous device. Any additional claims of benefit must be substantiated by the appropriate efficacy assessment for that claim. In contrast, the PMA is a more complex and rigorous assessment of an innovation judged not "substantially equivalent" to a pre-1976 device. The PMA process is actually much more akin to the new drug approval process used by the FDA. To date, only the high-frequency ventilator has undergone a PMA evaluation in the field of mechanical ventilation.

From this regulatory (and clinical) view point, innovations generally are judged from a risk/benefit perspective—that is, the claimed benefit must be commensurate with the risk. Thus, a claim of an engineering benefit coupled with a proper engineering assessment would be appropriate for a low-risk innovation to be judged acceptable. In contrast, a claim of an outcome benefit coupled with a confirming outcome assessment would be necessary for a high-risk innovation to be judged acceptable. Payers view efficacy assessment from a different perspective. In general, payers do not even consider an innovation until risk/benefit issues have been judged favorable. The payers instead must focus on the cost/benefit of a regulatory and clinically approved innovation. Indeed, it is this cost/benefit assessment that may well determine the innovation's reimbursement potential and, thus, its likelihood to actually be used.[16] From this reimbursement perspective, low-cost innovation might be justified by only demon-

| | | Incremental cost increase (payer issues) | | |
		Minor	Moderate	Major
Incremental risk increase (regulatory/ clinician issues)	Minor	Level I	Level II	Level III
	Moderate	Level II	Level II	Level III
	Major	Level III	Level III	Level III

FIGURE 23-1

Proposed scheme for efficacy assessment based on risk and cost. Level I = engineering end points. Level II = physiologic (intermediate) end points. Level III = clinical outcome end points. (Reprinted with permission from American Association for Respiratory Care Consensus Group: Assessing innovations in mechanical ventilatory support. Respir Care 40:928-932, 1995.)

strating engineering advantages, subjective preferences, clinical experience, or even theoretical considerations. However, an expensive innovation, although it satisfies regulatory risk/benefit concerns with only engineering or physiologic assessment, often is required by payers to have favorable clinical outcome data to justify its widespread application.

The approach to efficacy assessment thus depends largely on risk and cost of the innovation as well as the perspective of the group interest in the innovation. Figure 23-1 summarizes a proposed efficacy assessment scheme based on these concepts.

CONCLUSIONS

Efficacy assessment is required for all innovations to satisfy clinical, regulatory, liability, and reimbursement concerns. Efficacy assessment can be done in a variety of ways using a variety of criteria that can range from the simple and inexpensive engineering test to the very complex and expensive randomized clinical trial. The purpose of efficacy assessment is to validate a claim of benefit. This claim for the innovation becomes the basis for the ultimate "marketing" of the innovation, either by the manufacturer or by the clinical innovator. Efficacy assessment for a claim that an inexpensive device has a "faster response time" needs only an engineering test to validate it, whereas a claim that an expensive innovation "reduces mortality" would need a clini-

cal trial. In selecting the appropriate claim and the assessment required, risk and cost must be considered. Risk/benefit assessment must be used to evaluate the claim for regulatory and liability concerns. Cost/benefit assessment must be used to evaluate the claim for payer concerns.

REFERENCES

1. MacIntyre NR: Mechanical ventilation: the next 50 years. Respir Care 43:490-493, 1998.
2. American Association for Respiratory Care Consensus Group: Assessing innovation in mechanical ventilatory support. Respir Care 40:928-932, 1995.
3. Health Care Technology Institute: The dialogue of device innovation: an overview of the medical technology innovation process. Geigle and Associates, November 1993.
4. Terrin ML: Efficient use of endpoints in clinical trials: a clinical perspective. Stat Med 9:155-160, 1990.
5. Boisal JP, Colletti JP, Moleur P, Haugh M: Surrogate endpoints; a basis for a rational approach. Eur J Clin Pharmacol 43:235-244, 1992.
6. Dellinger RP: Clinical trials in ARDS. New Horiz 1:584-592, 1993.
7. Terrin ML: Efficient use of endpoints in clinical trials: a clinical perspective. Stat Med 9:155-160, 1990.
8. Dellinger RP: Clinical outcome endpoints and assessment of mechanical ventilation and points. Respir Care 40:975-979, 1995.
9. Rubenfeld GD: Study design: statistical and methodologic considerations. Respir Care 40:980-986, 1995.
10. FDA: Potential harm is key to significant risk decisions. Devices Diagn Lett 13:1-2, 1986.
11. Sherertz RJ, Stead SA: Medical devices: significant risk vs non-significant risk. JAMA 272:955-956, 1994.

12. Anderson G, Steinberg E: To buy or not to buy: technology aquisition under prospective payment. N Engl J Med 311:182–185, 1984.

13. Kane NM, Manowkian PD: The effect of the Medicare prospective payment system on the adoption of new technology. N Engl J Med 321:1378–1382, 1989.

14. Trajtenberg M: Economic Analysis of Product Innovation: The Case of CT Scanners. Cambridge, MA: Harvard University Press, 1990.

15. Kessler DA, Pape SM, Sundwall DN: The federal regulation of medical devices. N Engl J Med 317:357–366, 1987.

16. Tengs TO, Adams ME, Pliskin JS, et al: Five hundred life saving interventions and their cost effectiveness. Risk Anal 15:369–389, 1995.

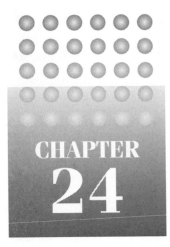

CHAPTER 24

Modifications on Conventional Ventilation Techniques

Robert R. McConnell, Jr., BA, RRT

AIRWAY PRESSURE RELEASE VENTILATION
Description/Rationale
Data
Recommendations
INDEPENDENT LUNG VENTILATION
Description/Rationale
Data
Recommendations
PROPORTIONAL ASSIST VENTILATION
Description/Rationale
Data
Recommendations

TRACHEAL GAS INSUFFLATION
Description/Rationale
Data
Recommendations
MODIFICATIONS FOR HYPERBARIC CHAMBERS AND MRI SCANNERS
MRI–Compatible Ventilators
Hyperbaric Chamber–
  Compatible Ventilators
REFERENCES

KEY WORDS

airway pressure release ventilation
hyperbaric oxygen therapy

independent lung ventilation
proportional assist ventilation
tracheal gas insufflation

Conventional positive pressure ventilation provides respiratory support through periodic lung inflations, often in conjunction with expiratory pressure applications. Additional features usually include patient interactive capabilities (patient breath triggering and patient flow control), various feedback control systems (intermittent mandatory ventilation [IMV], mandatory minute ventilation [MMV]), and sophisticated monitoring and alarm systems. In the past several years, some variations to this basic strategy have been proposed. Two of the more important are discussed in separate chapters (see high-frequency ventilation in Chapter 25 and partial liquid ventilation in Chapter 27). Several other modifications or variations to conventional strategies, however, also deserve comment and are reviewed in this chapter: **airway pressure release ventilation** (APRV), **independent lung ventilation** (ILV), **proportional assist ventilation** (PAV), and **tracheal gas insufflation** (TGI). Two other technical modifications of conventional ventilation that address the application of positive pressure ventilation in the hyperbaric environment and the magnetic resonance imaging scanner also are discussed.

AIRWAY PRESSURE RELEASE VENTILATION (APRV)

Description/Rationale

APRV (also known as BIPAP in Europe) is a respiratory support pattern that provides a moderately high (i.e., 15–25 cm H_2O) level of continuous (baseline) airway pressure that is interspersed with brief deflation (release) periods (Fig. 24–1).[1–3] Alveolar recruitment is maintained by the baseline pressure application while ventilatory support is provided through two mechanisms. First, the periodic brief (< 1.5 sec, generally 8–12/min) deflations provide some level of bulk flow gas transport. Second, spontaneous (i.e., unsupported/unassisted) ventilation is permitted during both the baseline and the release phases. This unique airway pressure pattern of APRV has been described variously as "continuous positive airway pressure (CPAP) with release," "pressure-controlled inverse-ratio ventilation with spontaneous ventilation," and "upside down IMV." The proposed advantages to APRV are that the prolonged duration of baseline pressure application maintains effective alveolar recruitment and that ventilatory support can be provided without additional positive airway pressure. Under these circumstances, maximal airway and alveolar pressures never exceed the baseline pressure setting.

There are several limitations to APRV. First, APRV does not supply total support (i.e., spontaneous breaths are required for adequate carbon dioxide [CO_2] clearance). Comparisons of APRV therefore should be made with other forms of partial support (i.e., IMV or pressure support) rather than assist/control (A/C) modes. Second, airflow obstruction can significantly impair APRV ventilation effectiveness because CO_2 elimination depends on adequate emptying and filling of the lung during the brief release phase. Third, although the deflation (release) phase is brief, short time-constant lung regions may have the potential to collapse (de-recruit) during these deflations. Fourth, APRV can impact patient comfort adversely because: (1) the spontaneous efforts may not necessarily coincide with the timing of the pressure release leading to imposed loading and (2) even if spontaneous breathing is not impeded, the pattern of mechanical ventilation can be perceived as abnormal by the patient and can precipitate agitation.

APRV can be provided in two general ways: a simple continuous flow with release valves[2, 3] or microprocessor control of a conventional ventilator.[1] The continuous-flow APRV system must include five principal elements: a flow generator, a humidifier system, a threshold resistor expiratory valve, a pressure release valve, and a timer. The continuous flow of gas must meet the patient's peak flow demands and therefore should provide at least 100 L/min of flow at a prescribed inspired oxygen concentration (FiO_2). The pressure release valve is located in the expiratory limb. When this valve is closed, the high gas flow exits through the resistor expiratory valve, creating the baseline pressure. At the preset interval, the timer opens the pressure release valve. The airway pressure decreases abruptly to the set release pressure and the lung volume decreases passively as the pressure is released, thus effecting the elimination of CO_2 from the lung. When the set release time elapses, the pressure resistor valve is closed and the airway pressure level increases quickly to the original set baseline level, resulting in the re-establishment of baseline lung volume. Microprocessor control of flow and pressure can accomplish a similar pattern. With microprocessor control, spontaneous breaths can come either from a continuous flow gas source or from a demand valve. Currently in the United States, only one

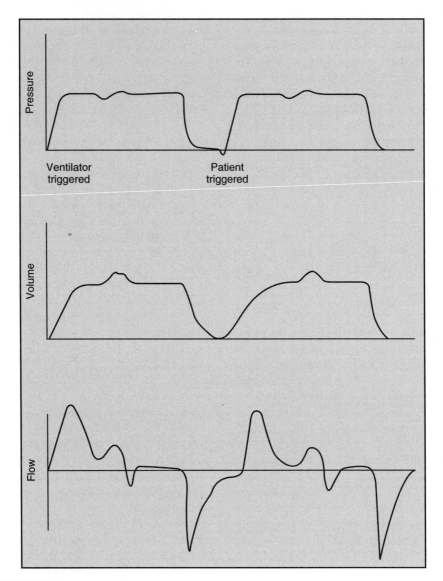

FIGURE 24–1
Schematic depiction of airway pressure, volume, and flow during airway pressure release
ventilation (APRV). Note that spontaneous unassisted breathing is permitted throughout
the ventilatory cycle. (Reprinted with permission from Chang AA, Steinfeld A, Gropper C,
et al: Demand-flow airway pressure release ventilation as partial ventilatory support mode:
comparison with synchronized intermittent mandatory ventilation and pressure support
ventilation. Crit Care Med 22:1431–1437, 1994.)

manufacturer provides microprocessor-
based APRV as a mode of ventilation, the
Drager Evita and Drager Dura (North
American Drager, Telford, PA). Pending
U.S. Food and Drug Administration (FDA)
approval, Nellcor Puritan-Bennett (Carlsbad, CA) soon may release APRV on a model
of their newest generation of mechanical
ventilators.

Data

There have been a number of small studies
of APRV in both animal and human subjects. Stock and associates[2, 3] demonstrated
in oleic acid–injured canines similar gas exchange and hemodynamic function on APRV
or conventional ventilation. They also
showed that APRV airway pressures did not

exceed the CPAP level before APRV. Additionally, with similar minute ventilation, the resultant partial pressure of CO_2 ($PaCO_2$) with APRV was lower, suggesting less physiologic dead space. In work with swine, Smith and Smith[4] showed that intrapulmonary venous admixture, arterial oxyhemoglobin saturation, and oxygen delivery were maintained adequately with APRV without hemodynamic compromise.

Most of the studies in humans have been done on patients with acute lung injury (ALI). These studies have shown that similar ventilation and oxygenation can be achieved at a lower peak airway pressure (P_{AW}) without hemodynamic compromise when compared with conventional strategies.[1, 4–8] Moreover, Sydow's data[7] suggested that there may have been a progressive alveolar recruitment over time with APRV. Chang and colleagues[1] compared APRV with other forms of partial support (i.e., IMV and pressure support ventilation [PSV]) and showed that APRV provided lower peak P_{AW} and comparable mean P_{AW} and gas exchange at similar levels of ventilatory support. However, Chang also reported that there was some patient dys-synchrony and discomfort when APRV was used.

Recommendations

Studies done thus far have shown that APRV is a safe and effective ventilatory support technique for use in the treatment of ALI or acute respiratory distress syndrome (ARDS). When set up as a total support technique (i.e., no spontaneous ventilation occurring), APRV is essentially pressure-controlled inverse-ratio ventilation (see Chapter 2). The uniqueness of APRV is thus as a partial support technique in less severe forms of lung injury. In this role, peak P_{AW} is generally lower with APRV, but whether this is important in only mild/moderate injury and whether it is worth the potential patient discomfort remains to be seen. Certainly one potential advantage to a continuous-flow APRV system is its simplicity as a stand-alone ventilatory support device.

INDEPENDENT LUNG VENTILATION (ILV)

Description/Rationale

ILV is a method by which the gas flow to each lung is effectively separated mechanically by either two small endotracheal tubes (ETs) or one specially designed double-lumen ET (Fig. 24–2). The rationale for separation can be either anatomic or physiologic. Anatomic reasons include massive hemoptysis, pulmonary alveolar proteinosis, and interbronchial aspiration. Physiologic reasons for lung separation include unilateral lung disease, single-lung transplant, and bronchopleural fistula.

The common thread for use of ILV is asymmetric lung disease that requires substantially different support strategies (especially positive end-expiratory pressure [PEEP]). ILV should be considered when the tidal volume–PEEP combination beneficial for one lung is detrimental to the other. For example, whole-lung PEEP application in an emphysematous patient with severe unilateral pneumonia might result in the uninjured lung units being overexpanded and underperfused, with the injured lung being underexpanded and overperfused. The goal of ILV in these circumstances is to isolate the right and left lungs for the purpose of applying aggressive PEEP lung recruitment in one lung and lower PEEP application in the other. Management of patients with ILV creates a number of potential problems, one being the confusion that can arise from having different goals for two separate lung units. For this reason, each ventilator should be labeled clearly as to its control relationship (master vs. slave) and designated right versus left lung clearly on the ventilator.

Before the mechanical ventilator methods are described, the types of devices needed to mechanically separate the right and left lungs first must be discussed. The Carlens double-lumen (endotracheal) tube (DLT), introduced in 1949, was the first available device designed to separate the lungs. Since then, other devices have been developed to separate the right and left lungs for one of two broad purposes: obstruct one lung (i.e.,

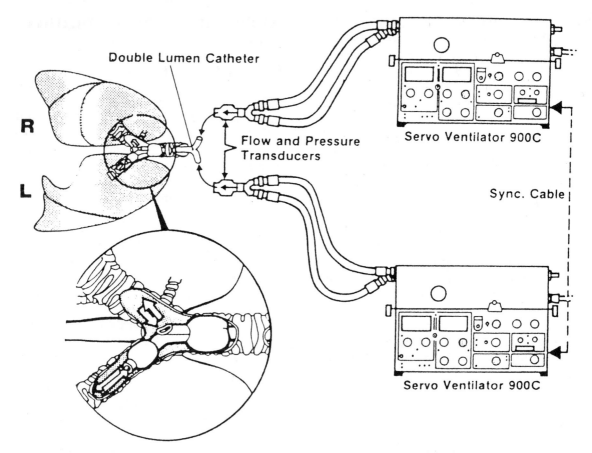

FIGURE 24-2
Setup of an independent lung ventilation system using two synchronized ventilators attached to separate lumens of a double-lumen endotracheal tube. (Reprinted with permission from Siegel JH, Stoklosa JC, et al: Quantification of asymmetric lung pathophysiology as a guide to the use of simultaneous independent lung ventilation in posttraumatic and septic adult respiratory distress syndrome. Ann Surg 202:425–439, 1985.)

to control hemoptysis) or provide the capability to ventilate the two lungs differently. Devices for each purpose are discussed separately.

When intentional obstruction of an airway is indicated to protect normal lung from insult by focal processes such as massive hemoptysis, several devices and strategies are available. These include cuffed rubber bronchial blockers, embolectomy balloons, pulmonary artery catheters, or other specially designed plastic tubes. In some cases, all that is required is to intubate the main stem bronchus of the unaffected side. The Fogarty embolectomy catheter is the most widely used endobronchial blocker. It usually is passed through a normal ET with the

tip of the catheter angled at 30° to help direct it into the correct main stem bronchus. A fiberoptic bronchoscope can be inserted through the ET with the catheter to assist with positioning. The balloon then is inflated until occlusion of the bronchus occurs. The disadvantage of using the Fogarty occlusion techniques is that they do not afford access to the affected lung and therefore prevent ventilation and pulmonary hygiene.

An alternative occlusion strategy is the Univent catheter. This device was first described by Inoue and associates[9] in 1982 and consists of an ET with an extra exterior lumen, 2 mm in internal diameter, in the anterior portion of the tube. Although the lumen is small, it does allow for a special blocking device that passes through the small lumen and can be positioned up to 8 cm beyond the ET. The Univent has several advantages over the Fogarty catheter. Because the device is attached to the main ET, displacement is less likely. Moreover, suctioning, pulmonary lavage, oxygen insufflation, and even high-frequency ventilation can be provided through the Univent tube to the occluded lung.

If substantial ventilatory support is required for both lungs during ILV, a larger DLT is required. Current versions are made of nontoxic polyvinyl chloride with high-volume, low-pressure cuffs. Generally, one lumen is longer than the other, which allows it to be inserted into a mainstem bronchus (both left and right mainstem designs are available). The more proximal lumen thus opens into the trachea for ventilating the other lung. Because each lumen is less than half the diameter of a regular ET, suctioning and bronchoscopy are difficult. Available DLTs include: Sher-I-Bronch (Sheridan of Kendall Australia, North Ryde, Sydney, Australia); BronchoCath and BronchoCath II (Mallinckrodt Medical, St Louis, MO); Rusch (Wailbilngen, Germany); Portex single use (Portex, Keen, NH); and Phoenix single-use Robertshaw, (Promedica, Preston, Lancashire, UK).

The challenge in using the DLT is in placement of, positioning, and securing the tube. At least two authors[10, 11] recommend that a DLT should be placed routinely using bronchoscopy. Although many may find this unnecessary, a bronchoscope may improve safety and may decrease procedure time. Once placed, the DLT may have a tendency to migrate. Distal migration potentially could block a mainstem bronchus, creating further collapse or atelectasis. A more recent sigmoid-shaped cuff with a right mainstem angle may help reduce this. Proximal migration may compromise the ability to do ILV. Because of this, pressures and volumes from each lung should be monitored carefully during ILV.

Ventilator managment during ILV depends on the clinical goals for each lung. A single conventional ventilator can be used in circumstances in which one lung needs conventional support while the other is managed with a T tube, CPAP system, or a high-frequency ventilator. ILV, however, usually involves different PEEP, tidal volume, FiO_2, pressure targets, and/or flow settings customized for each lung. This generally involves two separate ventilators, each attached to one of the lumens of the DLT. However, there also has been successful ILV with a single ventilator when using a specialized selective ventilation distribution circuit (SVDC). The SVDC was one of the first devices described for ILV. It uses a single circuit adapted at the wye with an additional wye that adapts to the two lumens of a DLT. A variable-flow resistance device is used in the inspiratory limb of the uninjured lung.[12] By varying the set resistance, the proportion of the tidal volume delivered to the injured lung or to the uninjured lung can be varied. Because there are separate expiratory limbs, each with its own PEEP device, PEEP to each lung can be modified individually and according to the severity of injury or need. Yamamura and colleagues[13] have described a one-piece SVDC device for use in anesthesia, but there has been no testing of this device in the critical care setting. Problems associated with SVDC include (1) there are limitations of independent ventilation parameters, (2) the additional adapters needed can be a source for leaks, and (3) rapid changes in the compliance or resistance of either lung alter tidal volume delivery.

When two ventilators are used, rate synchrony can be achieved by mechanically or electronically linking the two machines. Currently, several manufacturers (Siemens Medical Systems, Schamburg, IL; Drager, Lubeck, Germany; and J.H. Emerson Co., Cambridge, MA) have systems capable of synchronizing. Given the continued use of microprocessors, it should be possible to link electronically other ventilators in a master/slave fashion in the future. The major disadvantages to synchronization of two ventilators for ILV is in dedicating two ventilators for one patient and the required space for two ventilators in a patient room. The latter can be tempered somewhat by stacking one ventilator on top of the other.

However, the cart used must be sturdy and stable for the added height and weight.

Two unconnected (i.e., asynchronous) ventilators also can provide ILV. Asynchronous ventilators once were thought to compromise the cardiovascular system and cause substantial discomfort. There has been evidence reported by Hillman and Barber[14] however, that there are no adverse effects with asynchronous ILV compared with standard ventilation and that there may be a benefit to cardiovascular function in the resultant reduction in lung volume and decrease in mean airway pressure. If the patient has adequate respiratory drive, both ventilators might be set in an assist or support mode of ventilation[15] such as pressure assist, pressure support, or volume assist. As long as the patient effort is recognized equally for both lungs by appropriate sensitivity settings, both lungs will inflate simultaneously. If, however, there is need for a mandatory respiratory rate, there is evidence to suggest that asynchronous inflation of the individual lung units is not detrimental as long as they are not 180° out of phase.[16]

Data

Much of the literature available on ILV relates to case studies detailing the accounts of various asymmetric lung processes and how ILV was applied to the particular circumstances. These include reports of two cases of unilateral pulmonary contusion,[17] a bronchopulmonary fistula managed with a variable-resistance valve and a single ventilator,[18] and the treatment of unilateral pulmonary edema after a single-lung transplant for primary pulmonary hypertension.[19]

It also is well documented that the most common complications involve migration or displacement of the tube or device used to isolate the two lung units. Because of this, it is reasonable to have ready at hand equipment such as a fiberoptic bronchoscope to replace or reposition the artificial airway under direct visualization. Another reported complication is regional overinflation because of inappropriate tidal volume settings for an individual lung.

One of the most complete descriptions of the use of ILV in the management of asymmetric lung pathophysiology is found in the work of Siegel and associates.[20] Included in this report is a detailed description of two Servo 900Cs (Siemens Medical Systems, Schamburg, IL) synchronized by electronically linking the devices. Moreover, these authors also describe the use of a computer-based system through which the respiratory mechanics of each lung unit can be monitored independently.

Recommendations

ILV provides the opportunity to provide different ventilatory support strategies to the right and left lung in the setting of asymmetric lung disease. The safe use of ILV is dependent on the available resources and the clear establishment of the management goals for each lung. Besides the commitment of equipment, consideration should be given to the level of intensive care required to safely administer ILV. ILV should not be attempted unless there is adequate monitoring, ongoing assessment, and the availability of experienced personnel to respond to management and emergencies.

PROPORTIONAL ASSIST VENTILATION (PAV)

Description/Rationale

PAV is an interactive ventilatory support mode that provides patient-triggered breaths in which flow and volume delivery are controlled by clinician-set "gains" placed on sensed patient effort.[21-23] With PAV, increases in patient effort result in increased flow, volume, and airway pressure. In contrast, with pressure-targeted breaths, increases in patient effort result in increased flow and volume but constant airway pressure (Fig. 24–3). The conceptual benefit to PAV is enhanced flow synchrony during interactive breaths. The downside of PAV is that proper flow and volume gain settings

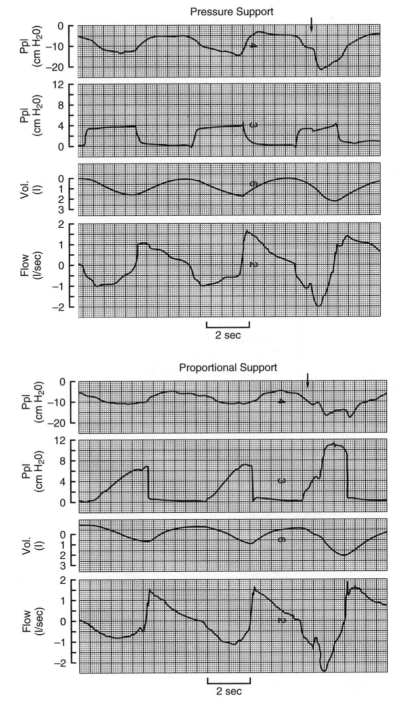

FIGURE 24–3
Effect of increasing patient effort during pressure support *(top)* and during proportional assist *(bottom)*. At arrow, patient pulls with increased effort as reflected by a more negative deflection in the pleural pressure tracing. With pressure support, airway pressure remains constant while flow and volume increase. In contrast, with proportional assist, airway pressure also increases and the delivered flow and volume are even greater. (Reprinted with permission from Younes M, Puddy A, Roberts D, et al: Proportional assist ventilation: results of an initial clinical trial. Am Rev Respir Dis 145:121–129, 1992. © American Lung Association.)

are not easy to set and, indeed, setting the gains too high may result in excessive flows and volumes being delivered.

An effective PAV system requires sensitive patient flow monitors and responsive flow delivery systems. These can be electronically or microprocessor linked. The flow and volume gain settings by the clinician are usually a proportion of the patient's total elastic and resistive load. Mathematically, these gain settings are expressed as K1 (cm H_2O/L) and K2 (cm H_2O/L/sec), respectively. Applied transpulmonary pressure during PAV thus is expressed as:

$$P_{APPL} = K1 \times \text{elastance} \times V + K2 \times \text{resistance} \times \dot{V}$$

where P_{APPL} is the sum of the pressure developed by the respiratory muscles (P_{MUS}) and the pressure supplied by the ventilator (P_{AW}) (i.e., $P_{APPL} = P_{MUS} + P_{AW}$); V is the inspiratory volume; and $\dot{V}$ is the inspiratory flow.

As of this writing, only prototype PAV ventilators exist, and most of the following reported data have come from the Winnipeg system designed by Younes and associates.[21] Development of PAV capabilities for both invasive and noninvasive (i.e., mask) applications is under way.

Data

Bigatello and colleagues[22] used a lung model to study the muscle-unloading effects of PAV. This model produced a sine wave spontaneous flow pattern, and the "ventilatory drive" was varied by adjusting the tidal volume from 0.2 to 1.2 L. By adjusting the flow and volume gains accordingly, the model illustrated the muscle-unloading effects of PAV.

Much of the theoretical and early clinical data have been produced by Younes.[23] This group has proposed flow and volume gain settings based on calculated resistance and elastance measurements. The goal with this approach is to allow clinicians to select a desired percent unloading of these two components of ventilatory muscle loading. Using their device in patients, this group has demonstrated that PAV is a comfortable form of ventilatory support and that this approach to proportional unloading behaves as predicted.

Navalesi and colleagues[24] studied PAV in eight patients with acute respiratory failure. They also demonstrated that the flow gain provided unloading from resistive loads and that the volume gain provided unloading from the elastance loads.

Ranieri and associates[25] compared PAV and pressure support (PS) at two levels of support in 12 mechanically ventilated patients. These patients had stimulation of their ventilatory drive by the addition of dead space into the circuit. The induced hypercapnia increased tidal swings of the esophageal pressure and pressure–time product during both PAV and PS, but these were greater with PS. An interesting finding was that with PS, the compensatory mechanism with induced hypercapnia was patient breathing frequency, whereas with PAV, tidal volume increased in response to hypercapnia without an increase in respiratory rate. They concluded that the compensatory strategy to increase minute ventilation during PSV requires more muscle effort and creates more patient discomfort than with PAV.

Ranieri and associates[26] also described what they referred to as "runaway" effect in PAV. This phenomenon can occur under two conditions. First, a leak in the system can result in an apparent excessive flow and volume demand, which elicits even further flow and volume delivery from PAV. Second, flow and volume gains in excess of those required by passive resistance and elastance of the patient can produce a similar excess delivery of flow and volume by PAV. This underscores the need to closely monitor the respiratory mechanics and patient status during PAV, and systems in development need to have appropriate safeguards.

Recently, PAV has been studied as a noninvasive approach to support using nasal or face masks. Effectiveness has been demonstrated in patients in acute respiratory failure[27] and in patients with chronic obstructive pulmonary disease (COPD).[27-30]

Recommendations

PAV is an interesting approach to improving patient ventilator synchrony during interactive mechanical ventilatory support. In small studies, PAV seems to be effective in unloading ventilatory muscles. For general clinical application, however, clinicians need easy ways to assess resistance and elastance loads and the development of management algorithms that supply appropriate gains to the flow and volume signal. Although the idea of amplifying the patient effort has merit, there remains concern about inappropriate adjustments that do not train or challenge the patient's ability or that result in "runaway breathing." It remains to be seen whether controls and systems that address these issues can be incorporated into future ventilators.

TRACHEAL GAS INSUFFLATION (TGI)

Description/Rationale

TGI is a technique whereby a low flow (e.g., 6–10 L/min) of fresh gas is delivered to the distal end of the ET through a small-diameter catheter. This flow can be either continuous (i.e., throughout the ventilatory cycle) or delivered only during exhalation. The primary purpose of TGI is to flush the upper airway with fresh gas during exhalation, thereby reducing functional dead space. TGI also may improve gas mixing because of the turbulent flow created at the tip of the catheter. TGI typically is delivered through either a stand-alone catheter or a catheter imbedded in the ET wall positioned just above the carina. By improving CO_2 removal, TGI may lessen the tidal volume requirement and thus serve to reduce maximal distending pressures in patients at risk for lung stretch injury. Although a number of prototype TGI catheters are in the development stage, none have been approved by the FDA for use in the United States.

With continuous TGI flow systems, the TGI flow is added to the ventilator's delivered flow. Under these circumstances, the ventilator must interact properly with the additional flow to ensure that the desired airway pressures and volumes are delivered. Imanaka and colleagues[31] developed a lung model to look at the effect of TGI on two commonly used modes of support: pressure assist-control ventilation (PACV) and volume assist-control ventilation (VACV). As expected, during PACV, TGI flow during inspiration reduced ventilator flow delivery as the ventilator strove to maintain the inspiratory pressure target. However, the TGI flow added to this reduced ventilator flow resulted in a constant tidal volume. In contrast, during VACV, TGI flow during inspiration added to the set ventilator flow delivery such that both tidal volume and peak airway pressure increased.

At higher levels of TGI flow, there is a concern that there may be some interference with assisted breath triggering. Hoyt and associates[32] showed that this is especially true in patients with weak effort. Also, increased expiratory resistance is associated with higher flow rates. This may require monitoring of tracheal PEEP when TGI is in use. Finally, gas supplied to the TGI circuit should be preblended to the same FiO_2 as ventilator gas.

Data

The use of TGI to increase elimination of CO_2 has been well documented in the literature. Kalfon and colleagues[33] showed in mechanically ventilated patients that TGI (what they termed *expiratory washout*) reduced $PaCO_2$ and increased pH. They also showed that TGI can significantly increase tracheal PEEP and mean airway pressure (thereby reducing cardiac filling). Adjustments in applied PEEP (perhaps with tracheal pressure monitoring) and the use of a pressure relief valve are thus important to maintain desired airway pressures during TGI.[34]

One of the largest clinical studies with TGI comes from Barnett and associates.[35] This prospective study over a 5-year period collected data on 68 trauma patients with ARDS. The results showed improvement in $PaCO_2$ (from 72 ± 5 to 59 ± 5 torr) and pH (from 7.25 ± 0.03 to 7.33 ± 0.03) despite a reduced tidal volume (from 7.9 ± 0.6 ml/kg to 7.2 ± 0.6 ml/kg) and minute ventilation (from 13 ± 1 to 11 ± 1 L/min) ($P < 0.05$).

The position of the catheter relative to the carina and whether a straight or inverted catheter is more effective has been addressed by several authors. Nahum and colleagues[36] have shown that the best CO_2 clearance occurs with the catheter placed 1 cm above the carina. A typical initial setting for the flow is between 4 to 6 L/min,[37] but this should be titrated to either arterial PCO_2 or to an end-tidal exhaled CO_2 concentration approaching zero (Fig. 24–4). Nahum and colleagues[38, 39] also demonstrated

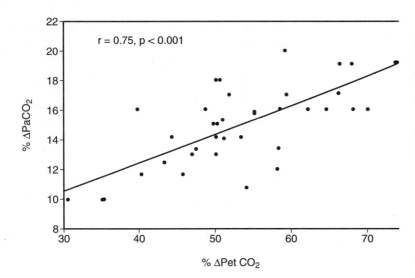

FIGURE 24–4
Relationship between reduction in end tidal CO_2 ($P_{et}Co^2$) concentrations using tracheal gas insufflation *(horizontal axis)* and reductions in arterial PCo_2 *(vertical axis)*. (Reprinted with permission from Kuo PH, Wu HD, Yu CJ, et al: Efficacy of tracheal gas insufflation in acute respiratory distress syndrome with permissive hypercapnia. Am J Respir Crit Care Med 154[3 Pt 1]:612–616, 1996. © American Lung Association.)

that the straight catheter is more effective, probably because dead-space washout is the most prominent mechanism. However, they also concluded that some CO_2 elimination occurs as a result of turbulence around the tip of the straight catheter. In contrast to this, Kolobow and associates'[40] work with a "reverse thruster" system (intratracheal ventilation [ITPV]) in sheep showed good CO_2 clearance with only minimal increases in tracheal PEEP. Moreover, this catheter also appeared to improve secretion clearance in 14 sheep using 5 ml/hr of saline added to the TGI gas flow.[41]

TGI also has been used in conjunction with APRV (see first section of chapter) to enhance CO_2 clearance. Okamato and colleagues[42] showed that TGI plus APRV was more effective at maintaining normocarbia than either IPPV or APRV alone in a canine restrictive-thorax model with and without pulmonary edema.

TGI usage also has been reported in other potential clinical settings. Miro and associates[43] used TGI in a canine model with methacholine-induced bronchospasm and showed improved CO_2 elimination without any evidence of hyperinflation or hemodynamic instability. In clinical trials of partial liquid ventilation (see Chapter 27), the elevated $PaCO_2$ created by the rapid instillation of perflubron may be decreased with the use of TGI.[44] TGI also has been reported as useful in high-frequency oscillatory ventilation (HFOV) and in reducing intracran-

ial pressure resultant from permissive hypercapnia.[45–47]

TGI has not been evaluated as extensively in infants as in adults. Animal research suggests that TGI may reduce the risk of ventilation-induced lung disease in the newborn.[48] Given the size of the neonatal ET, a TGI catheter could impose a significant increase in airway resistance. To address this, Danan and colleagues[49] described a technique of TGI in newborns using a specially designed ET with capillaries molded into the wall that produce TGI dead-space washout without the need for a tracheal catheter. Further use of TGI in newborns is contingent on future development of appropriate delivery systems.

Recommendations

Reduction (or elimination) of dead space has conceptual appeal in a number of circumstances, especially during mechanical ventilatory support when appropriate CO_2 elimination requires unacceptably high ventilation pressures. TGI is designed to flush the ET during exhalation to provide dead-space reduction. There are important TGI–ventilator interactions involving breath triggering, tidal volume size, peak airway pressure generation, and increases in tracheal PEEP that need to be addressed before TGI can be used safely. In addition, optimal catheter positioning and TGI flow rates for different clinical situations are not yet clear.

MODIFICATIONS FOR HYPERBARIC CHAMBERS AND MAGNETIC RESONANCE IMAGING SCANNERS

Although many transport versions of mechanical ventilators are available for the purpose of maintaining ventilatory support in many specialized diagnostic or therapeutic areas, two such areas that can have profound effects on the operation of mechanical ventilators are the magnetic resonance imaging (MRI) scanner and the hyperbaric chamber. The MRI scanner incorporates a very large electromagnet that attracts any ferrous material in close proximity. Besides the possibility of equipment involuntarily moving toward the magnet or scanner (or in the case of small metal objects, becoming projectile), components of the mechanical ventilator may fail to operate properly in this environment. Additionally, electronic components can be affected by the magnetic field developed around the scanner. This applies not only to the ventilator, but to the monitors as well. The hyperbaric oxygen (HBO) chamber uses high barometric pressures and high oxygen concentrations. In addition to the possible effect of barometric pressure changes on the accuracy and operation of the mechanical ventilator, the oxygen-rich environment is an inherent fire risk.

Magnetic Resonance Imaging– Compatible Ventilators

Equipment used in the MRI scanner must be free of ferrous materials and electronics. This requires that ventilators operate on either fluidic or pneumatic principles. Most ventilators of this type are pressure limited and time cycled. Although this does severely limit the choice of ventilators, some specific brands have been tested and have functioned well in the MRI scanner. These include the Monaghan 225 (Monaghan Medical Corp., Syracuse, NY), the Biomed IC2A (Biomed Medical Devices, Guilford, CT),

and the Omnivent (Allied Health Care, St. Louis, MO). A disconnect monitoring device, or high–low airway pressure detection device, also should be included in the setup, whether incorporated in the ventilator or as an add-on. The Tau monitor (Core-M Medical Products, Allston, MA) is one that is known to be compatible with the MRI scanner. Although manufacturers should have information on compatibility, MRI facilities should test ventilators and monitoring equipment before allowing their use in the scanner.

Hyperbaric Chamber–Compatible Ventilators

Hyperbaric oxygen therapy can be provided through either monoplace or multiplace chambers. Mechanical ventilator requirements are different in these two environments.

In the monoplace chamber, a single patient is exposed to the hyperbaric environment, with most of the support equipment outside. In this type of chamber, there is less chance of spark because all electrical components and mechanically moving parts are outside the hyperbaric environment. Generally, the chamber is compressed with a high level of oxygen (100%), except where mechanical ventilation is used.

Boyle's law should be considered to understand how mechanical ventilators are affected under monoplace hyperbaric conditions. Boyle's law states that an enclosed volume of gas will change in proportion to the pressure exerted on it. For example, if 1 L of gas from an externally controlled ventilator is introduced into a monoplace chamber, the volume will be compressed to 0.5 L at 2 atmospheres absolute (ATA), 0.333 L at 3 ATA, and so forth. In addition, the required airway pressures to drive gas into a thorax with an elevated external pressure will be accordingly higher. Therefore, the availability of ventilators for use in monoplace hyperbaric chambers is very limited. A specific ventilator that can be used in the Sechrist monoplace chamber, for example, is the Sechrist 500HC ventilator (Sechrist Industries, Anaheim, CA).[50] This ventilator is a time-cycled, pressure-limited device that is adapted specially to compensate for volume changes related to pressure changes during compression and decompression of the chamber. Manufacturers of monoplace chambers should provide information about available ventilators that can be used with their devices.

The other type of hyperbaric chamber is the multiplace chamber, a larger chamber that allows for more than one person's inhabitation, sometimes interconnected to other chambers of similar size. This design can be more efficient and cost-effective, as when treating groups of patients. An additional benefit lies in the ability for physicians, nurses, or respiratory therapists to reside in the chamber with the patient(s) during their treatment, affording hands-on care of patients.

The multiplace chamber usually is not pressurized with 100% oxygen. Instead, the ambient level is kept at 21% (room air) while the patient is treated with either a ventilator circuit or hood containing the appropriate FiO_2. This lower ambient oxygen level in the chamber reduces much of the risk of fire, but any spark is still a potential hazard, and oxygen levels can increase in the chamber under some circumstances. Therefore, minimizing moving parts, electrical components, and anything that may spark is critical. There are other safety considerations as well: first, oxygen should not be allowed to flow freely inside the case housing the ventilator or into the chamber. Second, all electrical devices used in the chamber should be flushed continuously with nitrogen[51] to lessen the chance that oxygen might come in contact with electrical interfaces. If any device incorporates a battery, a gel cell battery is suggested, when possible, because it is known to be less hazardous under pressurized conditions.

Any ventilator used in the multiplace chamber should be tested for the effect of high ambient pressure on the delivered volume, pressure, or other operating features of the ventilator, such as rate control. Another consideration is the effect of pressure on electronic controls. In particular, if "touch pad" controls are a feature of the ventilator or any other equipment, make certain that there is not an air interface between the touch pad and the control. Under hyperbaric conditions, any air present might pressurize and inadvertently activate a control.

Ventilators successfully used in the multiplace chamber include the Bird Mark 7 (Bird Corp., Palm Springs, CA), Monaghan 225, Penlon Oxford (Penlon Corp., Abingdon, UK), Servo 900B and 900C (Siemens Medical Systems, Schamburg, IL).[52] Of these mentioned, only the Siemens ventilator is powered electrically. If this device is to be used, it must be checked carefully and shielded for possible electrical hazards. The pneumatically driven, pressure-limited, time-cycled ventilators mentioned previously for use in MRI may have some appeal for use in hyperbarics. Their only drawback may be in their lack of versatility and optional modes.

During all forms of hyperbaric therapy, ET and tracheostomy tube cuffs must be filled with water.[52] Sterile water or saline in the cuff, unlike air, does not change volume under pressure. Air in the cuff has the potential for rupturing the cuff, resulting in potential damage to the trachea and loss of a closed system for mechanical ventilation. It is also general practice in many hyperbaric chambers to perform a myringotomy to prevent the potential rupture of the ear drum under pressure changes.

REFERENCES

1. Chang AA, Steinfeld A, Gropper C, et al: Demand-flow airway pressure release ventilation as partial ventilatory support mode: comparison with synchronized intermittent mandatory ventilation and pressure support ventilation. Crit Care Med 22:1431–1437, 1994.
2. Stock CS, Downs JB: Airway pressure release ventilation: a new approach to ventilatory support during acute lung injury. Respir Care 32:517–520, 1987.
3. Stock MC, Downs JB: Airway pressure release ventilation. Crit Care Med 15:462–466, 1987.
4. Smith RA, Smith DB: Does airway pressure release ventilation alter lung function after acute lung injury? Chest 107:805–808, 1995.
5. Garner W, Downs JB: Airway pressure release ventilation (APRV): a human trial. Chest 94:779–781, 1988.
6. Cane RD, Peruzzi WT: Airway pressure release ventilation in severe acute respiratory failure. Chest 100:460–463, 1991.

7. Sydow M, Burchardi H, Ephrain E, et al: Long-term effect of two different ventilatory modes on oxygenation in acute lung injury. Am J Respir Crit Care Med 149:1550–1556, 1994.
8. Rasanen J, Cane RD, Downs JB, et al: Airway pressure release ventilation during acute lung injury: a prospective multicenter trial. Crit Care Med 19:1234–1241, 1991.
9. Inoue H, Shotsu H, Ogawa J, et al: New device for one lung anesthesia: endotracheal tube with removeable blocker. Thorac Cardiovasc Surg 83:940–941, 1982.
10. Charan NB, Carvalho CG, Hawk P, et al: Independent lung ventilation with a single ventilator using a variable resistance valve. Chest 107:256–260, 1995.
11. Benumof JL: The position of a double-lumen tube should be routinely determined by fiberoptic bronchoscopy. Cardiothorac Vasc Anesth 7:513–514, 1993.
12. Shinnick JP, Freedman AP: Bronchofiberscopic placement of a double-lumen endotracheal tube. Crit Care Med 10:544–545, 1982.
13. Yamamura T, Furumido H, Saito Y: A single-unit device for differential lung ventilation with only one anesthesia machine. Anesth Anal 4:1017–1020, 1985.
14. Hillman KM, Barber JD: Asynchronous independent lung ventilation (AILV). Crit Care Med 8:390–395, 1980.
15. Schmitt HJ, Mang H, Kirmse M: Unilateral lung disease treated with patient-triggered independent-lung ventilation: a case report. Respir Care 39:906–911, 1994.
16. Branson RD, Hurst JM, DeHaven CB: Synchronous independent lung ventilation in the treatment of unilateral pulmonary contusion: a report of two cases. Respir Care 29:361–367, 1984.
17. Branson RD, Hurst JM, Davis K Jr: Alternative modes of ventilatory support. Probl Respir Care 2:48–60, 1989.
18. Carvalho P, Thompson WH, Riggs R, et al: Management of bronchopleural fistula with a variable-resistance valve and a single ventilator. Chest 111:1452–1454, 1997.
19. Badesch DB, Zamora MR, Jones S, et al: Independent ventilation and ECMO for severe unilateral pulmonary edema after SLT for primary pulmonary hypertension. Chest 107:1766–1770, 1995.
20. Siegel JH, Stoklosa JC, Borg U, et al: Quantification of asymmetric lung pathophysiology as a guide to the use of simultaneous independent lung ventilation in posttraumatic and septic adult respiratory distress syndrome. Ann Surg 202:425–439, 1985.
21. Younes M, Puddy A, Roberts D, et al: Proportional assist ventilation: results of an initial clinical trial. Am Rev Respir Dis 145:121–129, 1992.
22. Bigatello L, Nishimura M, Imanaka H, et al: Unloading of the work of breathing by proportional assist ventilation in a lung model. Crit Care Med 25:267–272, 1997.
23. Younes M: Proportional assist ventilation: a new approach to ventilatory support (theory). Am Rev Respir Dis 145:114–120, 1992.
24. Navalesi P, Hernandez P, Wongsa A, et al: Proportional assist ventilation in acute respiratory failure: effects on breathing pattern and inspiratory effort. Am J Respir Crit Care Med 154:1330–1338, 1996.
25. Ranieri VM, Grasso S, Mascia L, et al: Effects of proportional assist ventilation on inspiratory muscle effort in patients with chronic obstructive pulmonary disease and acute respiratory failure. Anesthesiology 86:79–91, 1997.
26. Ranieri VM, Giuliani R, Mascia L, et al: Patient–ventilator interaction during acute hypercapnia: pressure-support vs. proportional assist ventilation. J Appl Physiol 81:426–436, 1996.
27. Dolmage T, Goldstein RS: Proportional assist ventilation and exercise tolerance in subjects with COPD. Chest 111:948–954, 1997.
28. Bianchi L, Foglio K, Pagani M, et al: Effects of proportional assist ventilation on exercise tolerance in COPD patients with chronic hypercapnia. Eur Respir J 11:422–427, 1998.
29. Ambrosino N, Vitacca M, Polese G, et al: Short-term effects of nasal proportional assist ventilation in patients with chronic hypercapnic respiratory insufficiency. Eur Respir J 10:2829–2834, 1997.
30. Gutheil T, Pankow W, Becker H, et al: Work of breathing in noninvasive proportional assist ventilation in patients with respiratory insufficiency. Medizinische Klinik 92(Suppl 1):85–89, 1997.
31. Imanaka H, Kacmarek RM, Ritz R, et al: Tracheal gas insufflation-pressure control versus volume control ventilation: a lung model study. Am J Respir Crit Care Med 153:1019–1024, 1996.
32. Hoyt JD, Marini JJ, Nahum A: Effect of tracheal gas insufflation on demand valve triggering and total work during continuous positive airway pressure ventilation. Chest 110:775–783, 1996.
33. Kalfon P, Rao GS, Gallart L, et al: Permissive hypercapnia with or without expiratory washout in patients with severe acute respiratory distress syndrome. Anesthesiology 87:6–17, discussion 25A–26A, 1997.
34. Gowski DT, Delgado E, Miro AM, et al: Tracheal gas insufflation during pressure-control ventilation: effect of using a pressure relief valve. Crit Care Med 25:145–152, 1997.
35. Barnett CC, Moore FA, Moore EE, et al: Tracheal gas insufflation is a useful adjunct in permissive hypercapnic management of acute respiratory distress syndrome. Am J Surg 172:518–521; discussion 521–522, 1996.
36. Nahum A, Ravenscraft SA, Adams AB, et al: Distal effects of tracheal gas insufflation: changes with catheter position and oleic acid lung injury. J Appl Physiol 81:1121–1127, 1996.
37. Kuo PH, Wu HD, Yu CJ, et al: Efficacy of tracheal gas insufflation in acute respiratory distress syndrome with permissive hypercapnia. Am J Respir Crit Care Med 154(3 Pt 1):612–616, 1996.
38. Nahum A, Ravenscraft SA, Nakos G, et al: Effect of catheter flow direction on CO_2 removal during

tracheal gas insufflation in dogs. J Appl Physiol 75:1238–1246, 1993.

39. Nahum A, Ravenscraft SA, Nakos G, et al: Tracheal gas insufflation during pressure-control ventilation: effect of catheter position, diameter, and flow rate. Am Rev Respir Dis 146:1411–1418, 1992.

40. Kolobow T, Powers T, Mandava S, et al: Intratracheal pulmonary ventilation (ITPV): control of positive end-expiratory pressure at the level of the carina through the use of a novel ITPV catheter design. Anesth Analg 78:455–461, 1994.

41. Trawoger R, Kolobow T, Cereda M, et al: Clearance of mucus from endotracheal tubes during intratracheal pulmonary ventilation. Anesthesiology 86:1367–1374, 1997.

42. Okamato K, Kishi H, Choi H, et al: Combination of tracheal gas insufflation and airway pressure release ventilation. Chest 111:1366–1374, 1997.

43. Miro AM, Hoffman LA, Tasota FJ, et al: Tracheal gas insufflation improves ventilatory efficiency during metacholine-induced bronchospasm. J Crit Care 12:13–21, 1997.

44. Meszaros E, Ogawa R: Continuous low-flow tracheal gas insufflation during partial liquid ventilation in rabbits. Acta Anaesthesiol Scand 41:861–867, 1997.

45. Dolan S, Derdak S, Solomon D, et al: Tracheal gas insufflation combined with high-frequency oscillatory ventilation. Crit Care Med 24:458–465, 1996.

46. Belghith M, Fierobe L, Brunet F, et al: Is tracheal gas insufflation an alternative to extrapulmonary gas exchange in severe ARDS? Chest 107:1416–1419, 1995.

47. Levy B, Bollaert PE, Nace L, et al: Intracranial hypertension and adult respiratory distress syndrome: usefulness of tracheal gas insufflation. J Trauma 39:799–801, 1995.

48. Bermath MA, Henning R: Tracheal gas insufflation reduces requirements for mechanical ventilation in a rabbit model of respiratory distress syndrome. Anaesth Intensive Care 25:15–22, 1997.

49. Danan C, Dassieu G, Janaud JC, et al: Efficacy of dead-space washout in mechanically ventilated premature newborns. Am J Respir Crit Care Med 153:1571–1576, 1996.

50. Kindwall EP, Goldman RW: Hyperbaric Medicine Procedures. Milwaukee: St Luke's Medical Center, Aurora Health Care, 1988.

51. Moon R, Camporesi E: Clinical applications of hyperbaric oxygen. Probl Respir Care 4:182–184, 1991.

52. Janin KK: Textbook of Hyperbaric Medicine, 2nd ed. Seattle: Hogrefe and Huber Publishers, 1996.

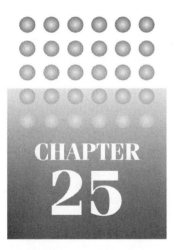

High-Frequency Ventilation

Neil R. MacIntyre, MD

DEFINITIONS AND RATIONALES

DEVICES
Jets
Oscillators

MECHANISM OF GAS TRANSPORT

APPLICATIONS

COMPLICATIONS

REFERENCES

KEY WORDS

---

convective gas transport
jets
lung-protective strategy

noncovective gas transport
oscillators

DEFINITIONS AND RATIONALES

Usual approaches to mechanical ventilatory support generally attempt to duplicate the normal bulk flow ventilatory pattern (i.e., tidal volumes and rates in the physiologic range) in conjunction with elevations in baseline pressures and inspired oxygen concentration (FiO_2). Unfortunately, in diseased lungs, these strategies may not always provide adequate carbon dioxide (CO_2) removal and oxygen (O_2) delivery, or they may require the production of very high alveolar pressures, which can be deleterious to both the lung and the cardiovascular system. An alternative approach to ventilatory support that has generated a great deal of interest over the past decade is high-frequency ventilation (HFV).[1, 2] Broadly speaking, HFV is defined as mechanical ventilatory support using higher-than-normal breathing frequencies. For purposes of this discussion, however, only those techniques that utilize breathing frequencies severalfold higher than normal (i.e., > 100 breaths/min in the adult and > 300 breaths/min in the neonate/pediatric patient) are considered. When these frequencies are used, tidal volumes are usually much smaller than normal (and may be less than anatomic dead space) and airway pressure swings are consequently less. The frequency–tidal volume product during HFV, however, is generally much higher than during conventional ventilation.

There are two general reasons for considering HFV. First, the smaller tidal pressure swings, coupled with appropriate baseline

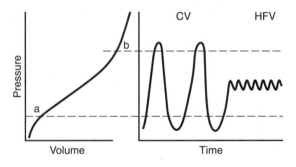

FIGURE 25-1

Conceptual rationale for high-frequency ventilation (HFV). Left panel is a static pressure-volume plot in a hypothetical patient. Points "a" and "b" represent alveolar recruitment pressure and overinflation pressure, respectively (so-called lower and upper inflection points). Right panel illustrates how a high-frequency ventilator with intrinsic positive end-expiratory pressure (PEEP) and smaller tidal pressure swings might be expected to ventilate between inflection points more readily than conventional ventilation (CV) with applied PEEP.

pressure elevations, create a conceptually ideal **lung-protective strategy.** Specifically, the combination of applied and intrinsic positive end-expiratory pressure (PEEP) provides alveolar recruitment, and the smaller tidal pressure swings prevent overdistension. Ventilation thus occurs between upper and lower inflection points on a static pressure volume curve (Fig. 25–1), the presumed ideal mechanical range for positive pressure ventilatory support (see Chapters 6 and 18). Second, in addition to better alveolar recruitment, the rapid flow pattern may enhance gas mixing and improve ventilation–perfusion ($\dot{V}/\dot{Q}$) matching.

DEVICES

Delivery of gas at the frequencies being considered is generally impossible for conventional ventilators with their standard valves and circuits. Different systems therefore must be used, and these usually consist of either **jets** or **oscillators** (Table 25–1).

Jets

High-frequency jets (Fig. 25–2) operate on the principle of a nozzle or injector that creates a high velocity "jet" of gas directed into the lung.[4, 5] These injectors are usually only 1 to 3 mm in diameter and can be placed in one of several locations in the ventilator circuit/patient airway (Fig. 25–2). Generally, the further down the airway that the injector is placed, the less is the functional dead space. Jet injectors also can entrain gas from an additional fresh gas source to increase delivered tidal volume. Because of the inertia of jetted gas, exhalation valves and cuffed airway tubes are unnecessary (although they can be used to manipulate mean and baseline airway pressures). Exhalation with jet ventilation is

TABLE 25-1. High-Frequency Ventilation Devices (Jets and Oscillators) vs. Conventional Ventilation

	JETS	OSCILLATORS	CONVENTIONAL
Frequencies available	up to 600 b/min	300–3000 b/min	2–60 b/min
Target delivered volumes	<or> than V_D	<V_D	≫V_D
Expiration	Passive	Active	Passive
Baseline pressure manipulated by	Extrinsic PEEP valve	Bias flow	Extrinsic PEEP valve
Potential for intrinsic PEEP	+ + +	+ +	+
Necessary f × V_T product for effective VA	≫Conventional	≫Conventional	—
Peak airway pressures	<Conventional	<Conventional	—
Mean airway pressures	<or>Conventional*	<or>Conventional*	—

*Standing waves can create high alveolar/airway pressure relationships near lung resonance frequencies.
f, frequency; PEEP, positive end-expiratory pressure; VA, alveolar ventilation; V_D, dead-space volume; V_T, tidal volume.

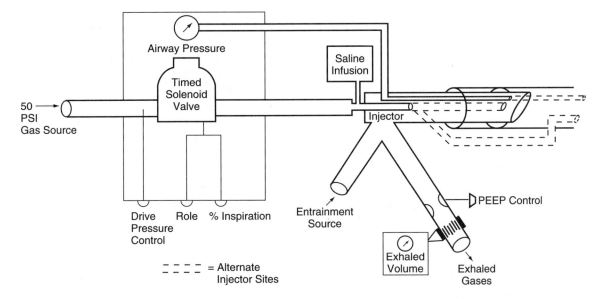

FIGURE 25–2

Schematic diagram of a jet ventilator for delivering high-frequency ventilation. Source gas is supplied to a controlling valve, which then provides jet pulses at the desired pressure, inspiratory duration, and frequency. The delivered pulse may be injected into the distal endotracheal tube or directly into tracheal catheters. In addition, injected pulses can be augmented through entrainment (as shown). Exhalation is passive and does not need an expiratory valve. Positive expiratory pressure can be applied, if desired, in the exhalation circuit. Airway pressure must be measured distal to the jet injector for accuracy. (Reprinted with permission from Tobin M: Principles and Practice of Mechanical Ventilation. New York: McGraw-Hill, 1994.)

passive (i.e., due to lung recoil). With a jet ventilator, the clinician usually has control over rate, inspiratory time, jet "drive pressure," and the expiratory pressure. The ultimately delivered jet volume, however, depends on a number of factors (Fig. 25–3), including the set drive pressure, the injector diameter, the inspiratory time, the endotracheal tube size (the more narrow the tube, the smaller the volume), the presence of an entrainment gas, and the development of air trapping ("intrinsic" PEEP).[1–6]

Monitoring actual volume delivery with flow sensors during jet HFV is difficult because the system is often open (see Fig. 25–2), and entrainment often is occurring. External chest impedance bands are an alternate approach but must have appropriate frequency response characteristics to be accurate. Peak and mean airway pressures must be monitored several centimeters distal to the jet nozzle to get representative values for the proximal airway.[4, 5] It must be appreciated, however, that at high frequencies (especially near lung resonant frequencies), alveolar pressures can be considerably *higher* than proximal airway pressures because of the development of standing waves.[7] In addition, air trapping from short expiratory times may not be detected in proximal airway sensors.[6] Ventilation parameters with jets usually are set according to pressure monitoring, visual inspection of chest movement, and arterial blood gases. Specific operational considerations are given in Table 25–2.

Oscillators

High-frequency oscillators (Fig. 25–4) operate with a "to and fro" application of pressure on the airway opening using either pistons or microprocessor gas controllers.[1, 2, 8] Although simple pistons provide a basic sinusoidal pressure wave form, microprocessor flow controllers can "shape" the inspiratory and expiratory pattern in a variety of

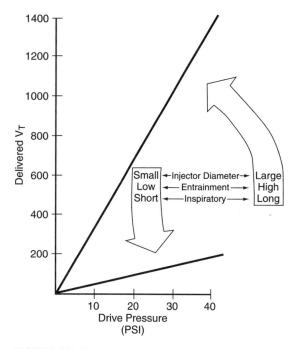

FIGURE 25–3
Relationship between jet drive pressure and ultimately delivered tidal volume (V_T) as a function of several system features. (Reprinted with permission from Tobin M: Principles and Practice of Mechanical Ventilation. New York: McGraw-Hill, 1994.)

ways. Fresh gas is supplied with the ventilator circuit as a "bias flow," and mean airway pressure is adjusted by the relationship between fresh gas inflow and any positive or negative pressure placed on the gas outflow from the bias flow circuit. With oscillators, clinicians usually have the capability to set oscillator frequency, oscillator displacement (volume), inspiratory to expiratory time, and bias flow. The actual delivered fresh gas volume to the lung depends on oscillator displacement volume as it interacts with both the magnitude and the location of the bias flow.[8] In general, the magnitude of the bias flow should be adequate to replenish the oscillator displacement volume, and the bias flow location should be as deep as possible in the airways to minimize dead space. Factors such as endotracheal tube size and inspiratory time that affect jetted volumes also affect oscillator delivered volumes.[8] Also, like jets, pressures in the proximal airway may not be reflective of alveolar

pressures when using high-frequency oscillation.[7, 9–11] Intrinsic PEEP also can develop with high-frequency oscillators, but it probably occurs less than with jets because of the active expiratory phase.[6, 12]

Because delivered volumes are very difficult to monitor with these systems, ventilation parameters often are set using pressure measurements, visual inspection of chest motion, and arterial blood gases.[13] Specific operational considerations are given in Table 25–2.

MECHANISM OF GAS TRANSPORT

Jet or oscillator tidal breaths are usually small and may approach (or even be smaller than) anatomic dead space. For effective CO_2 and O_2 transfer to take place between alveoli and the environment under these circumstances, mechanisms other than conventional bulk flow transport (i.e., **nonconvective gas transport**) must be invoked.[14] This is because the traditional relationship between effective alveolar ventilation (VA) and the frequency (f), tidal volume (V_T), and dead-space volume (V_D) (i.e., VA = f × [V_T − V_D]) becomes meaningless when V_T is less than V_D.

At least five different mechanisms exist to explain gas transport under these seemingly "unphysiologic" conditions[2, 3, 15–20]:

1. Conventional *bulk flow* (i.e., **convective gas transport**) is responsible for gas delivery into the major airways with any high-frequency system. As a consequence, alveoli in close proximity to these airways still can be ventilated principally by this mechanism.[14, 17, 18]

2. If the gas-flow profile during one phase of the ventilatory cycle is parabolic and during the other phase is square, a net flow of gas can occur in one direction through the center of the airway and in the other direction via the periphery *(coaxial flow).* Measurements in models of the human tracheobronchial tree have demonstrated such asymmetric flow profiles, but they are quite complex and depend heavily on airway geometry (especially bifurcations) and gas velocity during different phases of the ventilatory cycle.[14, 15, 17]

TABLE 25–2. High-Frequency Ventilation Operational Considerations

	INFANT JETS	ADULT JETS	INFANT OSCILLATORS	ADULT OSCILLATORS
Initial recommended frequency	7 HZ (IMV background rate of 2)	5 HZ	15 HZ	3–5 HZ
Initial tidal volume parameters	Jet drive pressure to produce 90% of CMV peak pressure; I time 0.02 sec	Jet drive pressure of 25–35 psi; I:E = 1:2–1:1	Amplitude to create chest vibration visually; I:E = 1:1	Amplitude to create chest vibration visually; I:E = 1:2–1:1
To change effective VA	Alter drive pressure*; alter inspiratory time†; alter frequency‡	Alter drive pressure*; alter inspiratory time †; alter frequency‡	Alter pressure amplitudes*; alter inspiratory time †; alter frequency‡	Alter pressure amplitudes*; alter inspiratory time †; alter frequency‡
To change mean P_{AW} (for $\dot{V}/\dot{Q}$ effects on PaO_2)	Alter applied PEEP; alter inspiratory time†	Alter applied PEEP (if available); alter inspiratory time†	Alter bias flow pressures; alter inspiratory time†	Alter bias flow pressures; alter inspiratory time†

CMV, continuous mandatory ventilation; I, inspiratory; I:E, inspiratory: expiratory; IMV, intermittent mandatory ventilation; PaO_2, arterial oxygen pressure; P_{AW}, airway pressure; PEEP, positive end-expiratory pressure; VA, alveolar ventilation; $\dot{V}/\dot{Q}$, ventilation–perfusion.
* ↑ Pressure = ↑ tidal volume = ↑ V_A.
† ↑ Inspiratory time = ↑ tidal volume = ↑ V_A *unless* air trapping develops, in which case tidal volume may ↓.
‡ Frequency response may be variable— ↑ frequency may increase total ventilation *but* ↑ frequency can ↓ tidal volume through shorter inspiratory time and pulse attenuation through narrow endotracheal tubes.

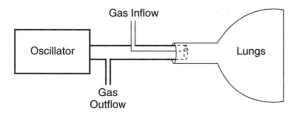

FIGURE 25–4
Schematic diagram of a high-frequency oscillator (HFO) for delivering high-frequency ventilation. Airway pressure oscillations are produced by a piston or membrane or microprocessor flow controller at a selected rate and displacement. Fresh gas inflow occurs through a bias flow. Gas outflow and circuit pressure are regulated by adjusting bias flow and/or pressure near the exhalation port. (Reprinted with permission from Tobin M: Principles and Practice of Mechanical Ventilation. New York: McGraw-Hill, 1994.)

3. *Taylor dispersion* is a complex physical concept that describes gas dispersion along the front of a high-velocity gas flow. The dispersion characteristics are different depending on whether flow is turbulent or laminar. Dispersion also is affected by bifurcations in the airway and the development of flow eddies. Net gas transport occurs as a result of this dispersion of gas molecules beyond the bulk flow front.[14, 16]

4. *Molecular diffusion* is responsible for gas mixing within alveolar units during conventional ventilation. Molecular diffusion is also likely to serve this role during HFV as well. It is unclear whether augmented molecular diffusion serves any additional role during HFV.

5. *Pendelluft* is the phenomenon of intraunit gas mixing due to impedance differences. This intraunit mixing also can involve airway gas and thus produce effective alveolar ventilation. Pendelluft may be particularly pronounced when HFV is used in a lung with heterogeneous impedances.[14]

The relative importance of each of these mechanisms is not clear. In fact, because these mechanics are not mutually exclusive, all may be operative simultaneously and to varying degrees depending on HFV parameters as well as the effects of lung disease on regional mechanics (Fig. 25–5).

Predicting gas exchange as a function of ventilator parameters when these nonconvective flow mechanisms are operative during HFV can be difficult. In general, as nonconvective flow mechanisms become more important, alveolar ventilation becomes increasingly a function of $f \times V_T^2$. The proportionality constant in this relationship is quite small and thus, during nonconvective flow HFV, the $f \times V_T$ product needs to be quite high for effective alveolar ventilation. This is why typical HFV "output" is generally severalfold higher than conventional minute ventilation output from standard ventilators using convective gas transport principles (see Table 25–1). Moreover, because during HFV, VA is affected more by V_T than frequency, tidal displacement affects CO_2 clearance more than frequency. Indeed, increases in frequency, if it produces more air trapping and consequent V_T reduction, can actually reduce effective VA.

Alveolar capillary gas transport during HFV depends on matching effective ventilation with perfusion ($\dot{V}/\dot{Q}$), just as it does with conventional ventilatory strategies. Thus, the alveolar–arterial oxygen difference during HFV remains largely dependent on mean alveolar pressure (and functional residual capacity [FRC]), just as it does with conventional strategies.[1, 13, 21] Although mean airway pressure usually reflects mean alveolar pressure, standing waves and the interaction of inspiratory to expiratory timing on high resistance tubing can affect this relationship.[7, 22] Note that mean airway (alveolar) pressure during HFV can be manipulated by a variety of different maneuvers (see Table 25–2).

APPLICATIONS

As noted previously, there are two theoretical advantages to HFV. The strongest clinical data supporting these advantages come from studies in neonatal and pediatric populations[13, 23–29] (Table 25–3). In these populations, jet breathing frequencies in the range of 250 to 600 breaths per minute or oscillatory frequencies of 500 to 1000 breaths per minute produce adequate gas exchange and often a lower incidence of chronic lung disease in survivors. Several of

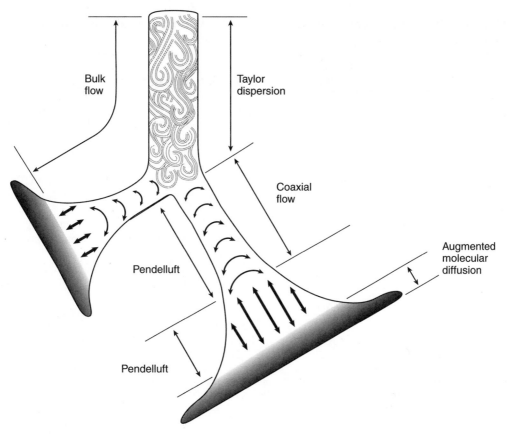

FIGURE 25–5
Modes of gas transport during high-frequency ventilation (HFV) and a tentative sketch of
their zones of dominance. These modes of transport are not mutually exclusive and may
interact extensively depending on HFV settings and disease effects on lung mechanics.
(Reprinted with permission from Chang HK: Mechanisms of gas transport during
ventilation by high frequency oscillation. J Appl Physiol Respir Environ Exercise Physiol
56:553–563, 1984.)

these studies emphasize the need for HFV
to have adequate volume recruitment for
successful application. One study even suggests a mortality benefit to HFV in patients
with pulmonary interstitial emphysema.[29]
In contrast, the largest randomized trial of
HFV (the NIH HIFI trial in 673 premature
infants) showed no improvement in respiratory function or outcome and, indeed, there
was an increased incidence of intraventricular hemorrhage in the HFV group. The
study design of the HIFI trial, however, often has been criticized.[31]

Adult experience with HFV has been limited because devices with adequate ventilation capabilities for adults are few (Table
25–4). Jet devices, however, have been
shown to provide reasonable gas transport

with lower peak airway pressures in adult
respiratory failure.[32–34] Moreover, an oscillator with the capabilities to support gas exchange in the adult has been described recently.[35] However, to date there has been no
reported improvement in outcome and no
reduction in complications with HFV in
adult respiratory failure.

There do appear to be several potential
specific applications for HFV other than
support of respiratory failure in the adult.
First, the reduced peak pressure and faster
rate can alter ventilation distribution and
improve gas exchange in patients with very
large pulmonary air leaks. However, no data
are available demonstrating improved survival in such patients using HFV, and most
clinicians would argue that routine bron-

TABLE 25–3. Published Randomized Controlled Neonatal/Pediatric High-Frequency Ventilation (HFV)

STUDY	HFV DEVICE	PATIENT POPULATION	MAJOR RESULTS/OUTCOME
Kinsella et al[23]	HFO	205 PPHN	When combined with inhaled nitric oxide, improved oxygenation with HFO compared with CV
Gerstman et al[24]	HFO	125 RDS	When used with a lung-recruitment strategy, HFO improved PaO_2 and lowered incidence of chronic lung disease compared with CV
Clark et al[25]	HFO	79 RDS	HFO had fewer treatment failures than CV
Clark et al[26]	HFO	83 RDS	HFO had lower incidence of chronic lung disease than CV
Keszler et al[28]	HFJV	130 RDS	HFJV had lower incidence of chronic lung disease than CV; proper lung recruitment improved oxygenation
Keszler et al[29]	HFJV	144 PIE	HFJV resolved PIE faster than CV; HFJV improved survival when treatment failure cross-over permitted
HIFI[30]	HFO	673 RDS	No difference between HFO and CV except for increase IVH in HFO
Carlo et al[27]	HFJV	42 RDS	No difference between HFJV and CV

CV, conventional ventilation; HFJV, high-frequency jet ventilation; HFO, high-frequency oscillation; HIFI, High Frequency Intervention Trial; IVH, intraventricular hemorrhage; PIE, pulmonary interstitial emphysema; PaO_2, partial pressure of oxygen; PPHN, persistent pulmonary hypertension of the newborn; RDS, respiratory distress syndrome.

chopleural fistulas can be ventilated adequately with conventional mechanical ventilation. Second, although cardiac function generally is not affected by HFV compared with conventional ventilation at a given mean airway pressure, synchronizing the HFV pressures with cardiac systole appears to benefit stroke volume in patients with severe cardiac dysfunction.[36] This is an interesting illustration of how intrathoracic pressure swings, if timed to cardiac systole and diastole, can function as a "ventricular assist" device. Third, reduced thoracoabdominal motion during anesthesia with the use of HFV has been useful in extracorporeal shock-wave lithotripsy by minimizing stone motion and, thus, procedure time.[37] Finally, the open system provided by the jet ventilator (i.e., a system without a need for an exhalation valve or tight-fitting endotracheal tube) offers additional advantages in two areas: (1) this system allows airway surgical procedures (e.g., bronchoscopy or laryngoscopy) to be performed with adequate ventilatory support and low airway pressures[38]; and (2) transtracheal jet venti-

lation in emergency situations can be used by trained individuals.[39]

COMPLICATIONS

There are potential problems that are of particular concern when using HFV. Adequate humidification can be difficult to achieve when using high gas flows and delivered minute volumes.[5] Appropriate systems to provide heat and humidity therefore are needed along with frequent assessment of airway function and sputum consistency. The high gas velocity of HFV also may cause direct physical airway damage. This, along with inadequate humidification, is thought to be responsible for the necrotizing tracheobronchitis that is observed in some neonates on HFV.[13] There is also a theoretical concern that the high gas flows of HFV can cause shearing at the interface of different lung regions having different impedances. This may be a cause of barotrauma to both airways and alveoli. Air trapping also can develop during HFV because of the large deliv-

TABLE 25–4. Published Adult High-Frequency Ventilation (HFV) Studies

STUDY	HFV DEVICE	PATIENT POPULATION	STUDY DESIGN	MAJOR RESULT OUTCOME
Carlon et al[33]	HFJV	300 Respiratory failure	Randomized, controlled	↓ Peak P_{AW}; Comparable PaO_2, $PaCO_2$, mean P_{AW}, outcome to CV
MacIntyre et al[32]	HFJV	58 Respiratory failure	Crossover	↓ Peak P_{AW}; Comparable PaO_2, $PaCO_2$, mean P_{AW} to CV
Gluck et al[34]	HFJV	90 ARDS	Crossover	↑ PaO_2/FiO_2, ↓ $PaCO_2$, ↓ Peak P_{AW}, ↓ PEEP need compared with CV; 15% pneumothorax, 15% mucus desiccation in HFJV
Fort et al[35]	HFO	18 ARDS	Crossover	Comparable PaO_2/FiO_2 compared with CV

ARDS, adult respiratory distress syndrome; CV, conventional ventilation; FiO_2, inspired oxygen concentration; HFJV, high-frequency jet ventilation; HFO, high-frequency oscillation; $PaCO_2$, alveolar partial pressure of carbon dioxide; PaO_2, partial pressure of oxyen; P_{AW}, airway pressure; PEEP, positive end-expiratory pressure.

ered volumes and short expiratory times.[6, 12] Indeed, air trapping is one of the mechanisms of alveolar recruitment during HFV (an intrinsic PEEP effect). However, excessive air trapping during HFV can produce similar effects to undesired air trapping during conventional ventilation (i.e., hyperinflation, reduced cardiac output, and other manifestations of increased intrathoracic pressure). The potential for intraventricular hemorrhage in neonates during HFV may be related to the reduced cardiac output resulting from excessive air trapping.[30]

CONCLUSIONS

HFV is an interesting alternative approach to mechanical ventilatory support that may offer benefits in terms of improved gas exchange and lower maximal alveolar distending pressures. Clinical data demonstrating improved outcome exist for neonatal and some forms of pediatric respiratory failure. No such data, however, exist for adults as yet. Moreover, there are important complications that can develop, and an extensive "learning curve" is required for operators to become skilled at delivering proper support in a safe fashion. As of this writing,

therefore, HFV should be limited to specific applications (e.g., selected neonates, adult airway surgical procedures) only and to centers skilled in its use. Considerably more data are required before extensive application, especially in the adult, is warranted.

REFERENCES

1. Froese AB, Bryan AC: High frequency ventilation. Am Rev Respir Dis 135:1363–1374, 1987.
2. Drazen JM, Kamm RD, Slutsky AS: High-frequency ventilation. Physiol Rev 64:505–543, 1984.
3. Slutsky AS, Kamm RD, Rossing TH, et al: Effects of frequency, tidal volume, and lung volume on CO_2 elimination in dogs by high frequency (2–30 Hz), low tidal volume ventilation. J Clin Invest 68:1475–1484, 1981.
4. Bunnell JB: High frequency hardware. Med Instrumentation 19:208–216, 1985.
5. Carlon GC, Miodownik S, Ray C, Kahn RC: Technical aspects and clinical implications of high frequency jet ventilation with a solonoid valve. Crit Care Med 9:47–50, 1981.
6. Beamer WC, Donald PS, Roger RL, et al: High frequency jet ventilation produces auto-PEEP. Crit Care Med 12:734–737, 1984.
7. Spahn DR, Bush EH, Schmid ER, et al: Resonant amplification and flow/pressure characteristics in high frequency ventilation. Med Biol Eng Comput 26:355–359, 1988.
8. Fredburg JJ, Glass GM, Boynton BR, Frantz ID:

Factors influencing mechanical performance of neonatal high frequency ventilators. J Appl Physiol 62:2485–2490, 1987.

9. All JL, Frantz ID III, Fredberg JJ: Heterogeneity of mean alveolar pressure during high-frequency oscillations. J Appl Physiol 62:223–228, 1987.

10. Fredberg JJ, Keefe DH, Glass GM, et al: Alveolar pressure nonhemogeneity during small amplitude high-frequency oscillation. J Appl Physiol 57:788–800, 1984.

11. Smith DW, Frankel LR, Ariagno RL: Dissociation of mean airway pressure and lung volume during high-frequency oscillatory ventilation. Crit Care Med 16:531–535, 1988.

12. Bancalari A, Gerhardt T, Bancalari E, et al: Gas trapping with high-frequency ventilation: jet versus oscillatory ventilation. J Pediatr 110:617–622, 1987.

13. Coghill CH, Haywood JL, Chatburn RL, et al: Neonatal and pediatric high-frequency ventilation: principles and practice. Respir Care 36:596–612, 1991.

14. Chang HK: Mechanisms of gas transport during ventilation by high frequency oscillation. J Appl Physiol Respir Environ Exerc Physiol 56:553–563, 1984.

15. Brusasco V, Knopp TJ, Rehder K: Gas transport during high-frequency ventilation. J Appl Physiol Respir Environ Exerc Physiol 55:472–478, 1983.

16. Fredberg JJ: Augmented diffusion in the airways can support pulmonary gas exchange. J Appl Physiol Respir Environ Exerc Physiol 49:323–338, 1980.

17. Isabey D, Hart A, Chang HK: Alveolar ventilation during high-frequency oscillation: core dead space concept. J Appl Physiol Respir Environ Exerc Physiol 56:700–707, 1984.

18. Sherer PW, Haselton FR: Convective exchange in oscillatory flow through bronchial-tree models. J Appl Physiol Respir Environ Exerc Physiol 53:1023–1033, 1982.

19. Permutt S, Mitzner W, Weinmann G: Model of gas transport during high-frequency ventilation. J Appl Physiol 58:1956–1970, 1985.

20. Vengas JG, Hales CA, Strieder DJ: A general dimensionless equation of gas transport by high-frequency ventilation. J Appl Physiol 60:1025–1030, 1986.

21. Walsh MC, Carlo WA: Sustained inflation during high frequency oscillatory ventilation improves pulmonary mechanics and oxygenation. J Appl Physiol 65:368–372, 1988.

22. Simon BA, Weinmann GC, Mitzner W: Mean airway pressure and alveolar pressure during high-frequency ventilation. J Appl Physiol 57:1069–1078, 1984.

23. Kinsella JP, Truog WE, Welsh WF, et al: Randomized multicenter trial of inhaled nitric oxide and high frequency oscillatory ventilatory in severe PPHN. J Pediatr 131:55–62, 1988.

24. Gerstman DR, Minton SD, Stoddard RA, et al: The Provo multicenter early HFOV trial. Pediatrics 98:1044–1057, 1996.

25. Clark RH, Yoder BA, Sells MS: Prospective randomized comparison of HFO and conventional ventilation in candidates for ECMO. J Pediatr 124:447–454, 1994.

26. Clark RH, Gerstmann DR, Null DM, deLemos RA: Prospective randomized comparison of HFO and conventional ventilation in RDS. Pediatrics 89:5–12, 1992.

27. Carlo WA, Siner B, Chatburn RL, et al: Early randomized intervention with high-frequency jet ventilation in respiratory distress syndrome. J Pediatr 117:765–770, 1990.

28. Keszler M, Modanlo HD, Brudno DS, et al: Multicenter controlled trial of HFJV in a preterm infant with uncomplicated respiratory distress syndrome. Pediatrics 100:593–599, 1997.

29. Keszler M, Donn SM, Bucciarelli RL, et al: Multicenter controlled trial comparing HFJV and conventional mechanical ventilation in newborn infants with PIE. J Pediatr 119:85–93, 1991.

30. The HIFI Study Group: High-frequency oscillatory ventilation compared with conventional mechanical ventilation in the treatment of respiratory failure in preterm infants. N Engl J Med 320:88–93, 1989.

31. Froese AB: HFOV for adult respiratory distress: let's get it right this time˙ Crit Care Med 25:906–908, 1997.

32. MacIntyre NR, Follett JV, Deitz JL, et al: Jet ventilation at 100 BPM in adult respiratory failure. Am Rev Respir Dis 134:897–901, 1986.

33. Carlon GC, Howland WS, Ray C, et al. High-frequency ventilation: a prospective randomized evaluation. Chest 84:551–559, 1983.

34. Gluck E, Heard S, Petel C, et al. Use of ultra high frequency ventilator in patients with ARDS. Chest 103:1413–1420, 1993.

35. Fort P, Farmer C, Westerman J, et al: HFO ventilator for ARDS—a pilot study. Crit Care Med 25:937–947, 1997.

36. Pinsky MR, Marquez J, Martin D, Klain M: Ventricular assist by cardiac cycle-specific increases in intrathoracic pressures. Chest 91:709–715, 1987.

37. Carlson CA, Boysen PG, Nabber MJ, et al: Conventional vs. high frequency jet ventilation for extracorporeal shock wave lithotripsy. Anesthesiology 63:A530, 1985.

38. MacIntyre NR, Ramage JE, Follett JV: Jet ventilation in support of fiberoptic bronchoscopy. Crit Care Med 15:303–307, 1987.

39. Klain M, Smith RB: High frequency percutaneous transtracheal jet ventilation. Crit Care Med 5:280–285, 1977.

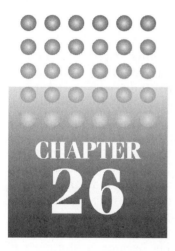

CHAPTER 26

Extracorporeal Techniques for Cardiopulmonary Support

Michael A. Gentile, RRT
Ira M. Cheifetz, MD

HISTORY OF EXTRACORPOREAL LIFE SUPPORT

PATIENT SELECTION AND CRITERIA FOR EXTRACORPOREAL LIFE SUPPORT

TYPES OF EXTRACORPOREAL LIFE SUPPORT
Venoarterial Extracorporeal Life Support
Venovenous Extracorporeal Life Support

COMPLICATIONS ASSOCIATED WITH EXTRACORPOREAL LIFE SUPPORT

PATIENT MANAGEMENT DURING EXTRACORPOREAL LIFE SUPPORT
Ventilator and Respiratory Care
Anticoagulation
Sedation and Analgesia
Nutrition

REFERENCES

KEY WORDS

extracorporeal membrane
oxygenation
intravascular oxygenation

venoarterial bypass
venovenous bypass

Extracorporeal life support (ECLS) or **extracorporeal membrane oxygenation** (ECMO) is an invasive and complex form of cardiopulmonary bypass for patients with severe reversible cardiac and/or pulmonary failure when maximum conventional therapy is not effective. This technique once was used exclusively in the operating room for short-term support during cardiothoracic surgery. The use of ECLS allows for blood circulation and gas exchange outside the body while theoretically resting the heart and lungs. The advantages of extracorporeal techniques are providing adequate gas exchange with less ventilatory support, including a lower inspired oxygen concentration (FiO_2) and reduced airway pressures. Potential complications include clot formation, extensive bleeding due to systemic anticoagulation, including cerebral hemorrhage, and technical failure.

HISTORY OF EXTRACORPOREAL LIFE SUPPORT

The technology used during ECLS is not new. Extracorporeal circulation first was devised as a tool for cardiac surgery. As early as 1936, John Gibbon was attempting to research and develop a roller pump that could sustain life during surgical procedures of the heart and great vessels.[1] In 1944, Kolff and Beck reported the oxygenation of venous blood during dialysis.[2] As the technology of open heart surgery was advanced in the 1950s, so was the use of cardiopulmonary bypass. The first membrane oxygenator was developed by Clowes and associates in 1956.[3] This was a substantial technical advancement, but it could not support life for more than a few hours. Common complications of cardiopulmonary bypass at that time were thrombocytopenia, coagulopathy, hemolysis, and renal and lung dysfunction. Soon it was discovered that the silicone rubber used in these initial membrane oxygenators had uncommon gas transfer characteristics and was unreliable.[4]

The 1960s were a time of intensive laboratory research to prolong the time that cardiopulmonary bypass could be performed and to improve the membrane lungs. An oxygenator constructed of dimethpolysiloxane similar to the one that currently is commonly used was developed in 1963.[5] With such a device, it was possible to perform extended bypass procedures in animals up to 1 week.[6] Several premature neonates were supported with ECLS, but all died of intraventricular hemorrhage.[7-9] The first successful human ECLS case was reported in 1972, in which a 24-year-old male with multiple trauma injuries was supported for 75 hours.[10]

In 1974, the National Institutes of Health sponsored a multicenter, randomized trial that compared venoarterial ECLS with conventional therapy in adult patients with respiratory failure. The results failed to show an improvement in outcome. Both ECLS and conventional therapies demonstrated a dismal survival rate, with no significant difference (9.5% survival rate in ECLS patients and 8.3% in the conventional therapy group).[11]

Meanwhile, the neonatal population was being treated successfully by Bartlett.[12] Throughout the 1980s, more centers started to use ECLS technology for neonates with reversible lung disease who were failing conventional support. In the past decade, ECLS has moved into the intensive care unit (ICU) and has become a standard of care for days and even weeks in the support of patients of many age groups with severe cardiopulmonary dysfunction. Currently there are more than 100 centers throughout the world that have provided ECLS for more than 17,500 patients since 1986.[13] In the 1990s, other therapies have become available and have reduced the number of patients requiring ECLS.[14] Some of these alternative approaches are high-frequency ventilation, surfactant administration, inhaled nitric oxide, and liquid ventilation.

PATIENT SELECTION AND CRITERIA FOR EXTRACORPOREAL LIFE SUPPORT

Although criteria for ECLS varies from center to center and patient to patient, there are several recommendations on which most agree. In the ICU, several diagnoses commonly are associated with ECLS. These are detailed in Tables 26–1 through 26–4.

The general guidelines for neonatal ECLS include a disease process that is deemed reversible, gestational age older than 36 weeks, weight greater than 2 kg, mechanical ventilation for no more than 7 to 10 days before ECLS, no significant immunosuppression, absence of intraventricular hemorrhage, no severe neurologic dysfunction, and no significant chromosomal abnormality. However, many centers perform ECLS on patients with trisomy 21.

For all age groups, ECLS usually is considered after failure of other available therapies (e.g., surfactant, high-frequency ventilation, inhaled nitric oxide, permissive hypercapnea, and liquid ventilation). Addi-

TABLE 26–1. Neonatal Extracorporeal Life Support Diagnoses and Survival Rates

DIAGNOSIS	NO. OF CASES	SURVIVAL RATE (%)
Meconium aspiration syndrome	4671	94
Respiratory distress syndrome	1291	84
Congenital diaphragmatic hernia	2751	59
Sepsis or pneumonia	2032	76
Persistent pulmonary hypertension	1796	82
Air leak syndrome	60	67
Other	609	75
Total	13,210	80

Data from ELSO: Neonatal ECLS Registry. Ann Arbor, MI: Extracorporeal Life Support Organization, January 1998.

tionally, a persistent air leak is a possible indication for ECLS. Some centers use an oxygen index (OI) greater than 40 (Fig. 26–1) and an alveolar–arterial oxygen difference (A–aDO$_2$) greater than 500 × 4 hours (see Fig. 26–1) as ECLS criteria, but other centers use lower cutoffs. These criteria are based on the mortality risk without ECLS. A pre-ECLS OI of between 25 and 40 has been associated with a 50% mortality rate on conventional therapy. If the OI is greater than 40, the chance of mortality historically has been 80%.[15]

TABLE 26–2. Pediatric Extracorporeal Life Support Diagnoses and Survival Rates

DIAGNOSIS	NO. OF CASES	SURVIVAL RATE (%)
Bacterial pneumonia	140	48
Viral pneumonia	449	56
Aspiration	121	63
Adult respiratory distress syndrome	162	52
Others	635	52
Total	1507	53

Data from ELSO: Pediatric Registry. Ann Arbor, MI: Extracorporeal Life Support Organization, 1998.

TABLE 26–3. Cardiac Extracorporeal Life Support Diagnoses and Survival Rates

DIAGNOSIS	NO. OF CASES	SURVIVAL RATE (%)
Cardiac surgery	1752	40
Cardiac transplant	128	39
Myocarditis	66	56
Myocardiopathy	102	52
Other	249	46
Total	2297	42

Data from ELSO: Cardiac ECLS Registry. Ann Arbor, MI: Extracorporeal Life Support Organization, 1998.

For cardiac patients, ECLS criteria include severe and reversible cardiac dysfunction for which maximum therapy has failed. Most cardiac ECLS is performed in the postoperative period, when the patient cannot be weaned from cardiopulmonary bypass or assistance is needed for poor ventricular performance.[16, 17] Patients with severe myocarditis also may be supported with ECLS until the condition resolves or until transplantation is possible.[17] Additionally, ECLS is an option for patients with complicated posttransplant courses.

The use of ECLS to support patients after surgery for congenital heart disease has been increasing because improvements in myocardial and cerebral protection, surgical

TABLE 26–4. Adult Extracorporeal Life Support Diagnoses and Survival Rates

DIAGNOSIS	NO. OF CASES	SURVIVAL RATE (%)
Bacterial pneumonia	54	35
Viral pneumonia	54	63
Aspiration	17	59
Adult respiratory distress syndrome	130	58
Cardiac	167	21
Others	125	48
Total	547	47

Data from ELSO: Adult ECLS Registry. Ann Arbor, MI: Extracorporeal Life Support Organization, 1998.

Oxygenation Index

$$OI = \frac{(FiO_2)\,(P_{AW}) \times 100}{PaO_2}$$

Alveolar–Arterial Oxygen Gradient

$$A - aDO_2 = ([FiO_2\,(P\text{-}47)\,PaCO_2])\,PaO_2$$
$$P = \text{Atmospheric Pressure}$$
$$PaCO_2 = PaCO_2$$

FIGURE 26–1
Alveolar-arterial oxygen difference $(A - aDO_2)$ and oxygen index (OI) calculations.

techniques, and perioperative care have led to the recommendation of early neonatal repair for most congenital heart lesions.

TYPES OF EXTRACORPOREAL LIFE SUPPORT

Venoarterial Extracorporeal Life Support

Venoarterial bypass ECLS (Fig. 26–2) is complete cardiopulmonary bypass that supports both cardiac and pulmonary functions. The system consists of six components: an extracorporeal circuit, a blood-circulating pump, a membrane oxygenator, a heat exchanger, monitoring and safety devices, and patient cannulas.[17] The extracorporeal circuit consists of a series of super tygon tubes and access adapters to circulate venous blood from the patient through the blood-circulating pump and membrane lung back to the patient. The membrane lung is a hollow-fiber silicone oxygenator highly permeable to carbon dioxide (CO_2) and oxygen (O_2) gas exchange. The surface area of the lung, selected according to patient size, and the flow of ventilating gases across the membrane determine the rate of gas exchange. The blood pump provides the driving pressure from the patient's venous circulation across the membrane lung and back to the arterial circulation.

Two types of extracorporeal pumps commonly are used, the rollerhead displacement pump and the centrifugal pump.[17] The circuit cardiac output is a function of blood volume and the speed of pump revolutions.

A heat exchanger placed proximal to the patient's arterial return warms the circulating blood volume to body temperature to help prevent hypothermia from ambient cooling of extracorporeal blood volumes. Appropriately sized cannulas access the circuit to the patient. Specific monitors within the circuit provide information on circuit safety, function, and performance.

Neonatal and pediatric venoarterial extracorporeal support generally accesses the right atrium for venous return via cannulation of the internal jugular vein. The common carotid artery on both neonatal and pediatric patients is cannulated for blood return to the body. Adult patients typically require alteration of this technique, either by direct transthoracic access to the atrium and aorta or by femoral access.[16] Venoarterial ECLS is almost complete cardiopulmonary bypass, draining venous return from the right atrium, circulating the blood through the extracorporeal circuit, and then returning the blood to the aortic arch. Because it is very effective, the patient can be supported for several days to several weeks.[16]

The major advantage of venoarterial ECLS is complete control over the patient's cardiac output and gas exchange. The disadvantages of venoarterial ECLS are that ligation of a major artery is required and there is the possibility of air or clots embolizing to the central nervous system. In larger patients, some centers have successfully started to reconnect the artery after ECLS is discontinued. The major risk to this procedure is again air emboli.[18]

Venovenous Extracorporeal Life Support

Venovenous bypass ECLS (Fig. 26–3) takes only a portion (e.g., 30–60%) of the cardiac output from the venous circulation, passes it through a membrane oxygenator, and returns it to the major veins.[19] Venovenous ECLS is reserved for patients with adequate cardiac output. If cardiac insufficiency develops, the patient must be supported by inotropic support or surgically converted to venoarterial ECLS. Venove-

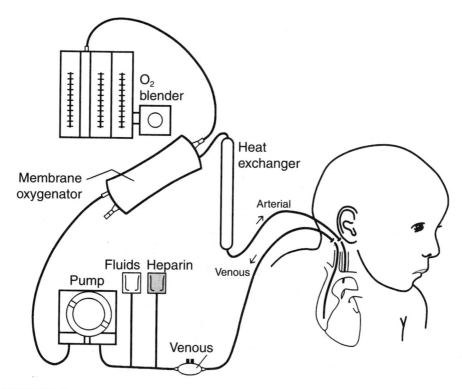

FIGURE 26-2
Venoarterial extracorporeal life support (ECLS). (Reprinted with permission from
Dantzker, DR, MacIntyre, NR, Bakow, ED: Comprehensive Respiratory Care. Philadelphia:
WB Saunders, 1995, p 473.)

nous ECLS accesses venous return in neonatal patients and some pediatric patients
by placement of a double-lumen cannula
into the right atrium through the internal
jugular vein (see Fig. 26–2). Venous return
circulates from the right atrium through the
extracorporeal circuit and returns to the
right atrium.[20] Cannula outflow is placed
proximal to the tricuspid valve to minimize
recirculation of the oxygenated blood from
the extracorporeal system.

In neonatal and pediatric patients, this
technique is gaining popularity for patients
who previously were considered for venoarterial ECLS. Interest in this technique is
increasing because no arterial ligation or
repair is needed and all debris, clots, and
air are routed to the pulmonary circulation
and not to the cerebral or systemic circulation.[16] The major disadvantage to venovenous ECLS is that it does not provide any
cardiac support.

A novel experimental variation of veno-

venous ECLS is the use of the intravascular
oxygenation device. This technique oxygen-
ates venous blood with a membrane oxygenator surgically inserted inside the great
veins.

COMPLICATIONS ASSOCIATED WITH EXTRACORPOREAL LIFE SUPPORT

Complications of ECLS usually are related
to anticoagulation, pre-existing hypoxic or
hypotensive injury to organ function, and
technical and mechanical complications
within the ECLS circuit. Hemorrhage is the
most common (22–76%) and potentially disastrous complication of ECLS.[13, 17, 21] Bleeding can occur in one of three sites: the brain,
at operative sites, or the gastrointestinal
tract. The most devastating of these occurs
in the brain. Proper patient selection (e.g.,
> 2 kg body weight, > 36 weeks gestational
age, and normal head ultrasound results)

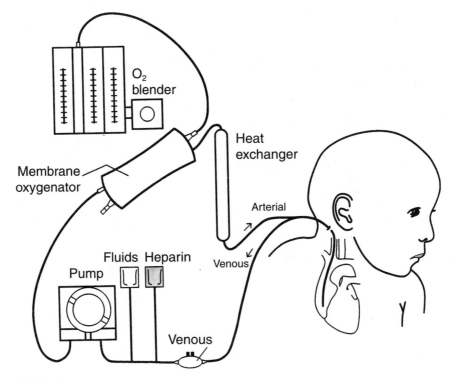

FIGURE 26–3
Double lumen venovenous extracorporeal life support. (Reprinted with permission from
Dantzker DR, MacIntyre NR, Bakow ED: Comprehensive Respiratory Care. Philadelphia:
WB Saunders, 1995, p 474.)

and measurements of serum lactate can help minimize the probability of intracranial hemorrhage. Serum lactates greater than 10 mmol/L have been associated with an increased risk of intracranial bleeding.[22] Maintaining activated clotting times (ACTs) between 180 and 220 seconds also can decrease the incidence of bleeding complications. Seizures during ECLS are associated with fluid and electrolyte abnormalities often seen at the time of cannulation and during the early hours of ECLS. Other problems, including renal failure due to the nonpulsatile flow of ECLS, hemolysis, hypotension, hypertension, pneumothorax, infection, and cardiac arrhythmias, should be recognized early and treated appropriately.[13]

Mechanical and technical complications of ECLS are rare but equally potentially hazardous. The most common complication (29%) of ECLS is clot formation in the circuit.[13] The incidence of clots increases in linear fashion to the length of time on ECLS. Other mechanical complications commonly reported are oxygenator failure, tubing rupture, pump failure, cannulation kinks, heat exchanger malfunction, air in the circuitry, and cracks in the connectors.[13] Meliones and colleagues found a significant association between a calculated "complication score" and a chance of survival, with nonsurvivors having more complications during ECLS.[23]

PATIENT MANAGEMENT DURING EXTRACORPOREAL LIFE SUPPORT

Ventilator and Respiratory Care

The main intent of ECLS is cardiopulmonary support without the intragenic complications known to be associated with high ventilation pressures and oxygen toxicity. With these intentions in mind, ventilatory support may be reduced significantly during ECLS. Maintaining positive end-expiratory pressure (PEEP) levels of 8 to 10 cm H_2O and a low tidal volume or peak inspiratory pressure maintains lung expansion while minimizing barotrauma. Measurement of dynamic lung compliance may be helpful in the assessment of recovery. A dynamic compliance of 0.8 ml/cm H_2O/kg or greater has predicted successful discontinuation of ECLS.[24] Chest physiotherapy, endotracheal suctioning, and bronchoscopy may be performed to remove retained pulmonary secretions. Instillation of surfactant also may be beneficial in decreasing the length of ECLS support.

Anticoagulation

Continuous heparin infusion is adjusted to keep the ACTs between 180 and 220 seconds. If ACT levels are less than 180 seconds, the risk of clot formation in the circuit increases. The ACT level is influenced by blood product administration as well as other substances that are injected into the circuit. The ACTs must be adjusted if hemorrhage or clotting **(blood coagulation)** in the circuit presents problems.

Sedation and Analgesia

A patient receiving ECLS does not need to be treated continuously with neuromuscular blockade with the exception of the initial catheter placement and other surgical procedures. Maintaining muscle function allows for periodic neurologic examinations, observation for seizures, and the potential for mobilizing third-spaced fluids. Commonly used medications for ECLS sedation include morphine, fentanyl, diazepam (Valium), lorazepam (Ativan), and midazolam (Versed). The patients should be sedated only to the point that they are comfortable and not at risk for moving the cannulas.

Nutrition

Nutritional support for ECLS patients must be tailored to the specific caloric and supplement requirements of each patient. It is common practice to start parenteral nutrition within 24 hours of initiation of ECLS. Total parental nutrition may be infused directly into the ECLS circuit. Some centers have reported using enteral feeds via nasogastric tubes without complications.[25]

CONCLUSION

Although the number of patients being treated with ECLS has decreased, there continue to be new investigations on how to best use this technology.[14, 22, 25] New and novel techniques such as inhaled nitric oxide, high-frequency oscillatory ventilation, surfactant, and liquid ventilation have surfaced and may further reduce the number of patients placed on ECLS. In the meantime, the number of cardiac cases may continue to increase as the trend toward performing corrective cardiac surgery in younger patients continues.[26] It is hoped that research will continue to make ECLS safer, resulting in improved overall survival rates. Proper patient selection and early intervention may be the keys to successful treatment of the most critically ill patients with ECLS.

REFERENCES

1. Gibbon JH Jr: Artificial maintenance of circulation during experimental occlusion of the pulmonary artery. Arch Surg 34:1105–1112, 1937.
2. Kolff WJ, Beck HT: Artificial kidney: a dialyzer with a great area. Acta Med Scand 117:121–124, 1944.
3. Clowes GHA Jr, Hopkins AL, Neville WE: An artificial lung dependent upon diffusion of oxygen and carbon dioxide through plastic membranes. J Thorac Surg 32:630–637, 1956.
4. Kammermeyer K: Silicone rubber as a selective barrier. Industrial Chemical Engineering 49:1685, 1957.
5. Kolobow T, Bowman RL: Construction and elimination of an alveolar membrane heart-lung. Trans Am Soc Artif Intern Organs 9:238, 1963.
6. Kolobow T, Zapol WM, Pierce J: High survival and minimal blood damage in lambs exposed to long term venovenous pumping with a polyurethane chamber roller pump with and without a membrane oxygenator. Trans Am Soc Artif Intern Organs 15:172–177, 1969.
7. Dorson WJ, Baker E, Melvin L, et al: A perfusion

system for infants. Trans Am Soc Artif Intern Organs 15:155–160, 1969.

8. White JJ, Andrews HG, Risemberg H, et al: Prolonged respiratory support in newborn infants with a membrane oxygenator. Surgery 70:288–296, 1971.

9. Rashkind WJ, Freeman A, Klein D, et al: Evaluation of a disposable plastic, low volume, pumpless oxygenator as a lung substitute. J Pediatr 66:94–102, 1965.

10. Hill JD, O'Brien TG, Murray JJ, et al: Extracorporeal oxygenation for acute post-traumatic respiratory failure (shock-lung syndrome): use of the Bramson Membrane Lung. N Engl J Med 286:629–634, 1972.

11. Blake LH: Goals and progress of the NHLI collaborative ECMO study. In: Zapol W, Qvist J (eds): Artificial Lungs for Acute Respiratory Failure. New York: Academic Press, 1976, pp 513–524.

12. Bartlett RH, Gazzaniga AB: Extracorporeal circulation for cardiopulmonary failure. Curr Probl Surg 15:1–7, 1978.

13. ELSO: ECLS Registry. Ann Arbor, MI: Extracorporeal Life Support Organization, January 1998.

14. Wilson JM, Bower LK, Thompson JE, et al: ECMO in evolution: the impact of changing patient demographics and alternative therapies on ECMO. J Pediatr Surg 31:1116–1123, 1996.

15. Ortega M, Ramos A, Atkinson J, et al: Oxygenation index can predict outcomes in neonates who are candidates for extracorporeal membrane oxygenation. Pediatr Res 22:462A, 1987.

16. Bartlett RH: Extracorporeal life support for cardiopulmonary failure. Curr Probl Surg 27:621–705, 1990.

17. Kanter KR, Pennington G, Weber TR, et al: Extracorporeal membrane oxygenation for postoperative cardiac support in children. J Thorac Cardiovasc Surg 93:27–35, 1987.

18. Lupinetti FM, Bove EL, Minich, et al: Intermediate-term survival and functional results after arterial repair for transposition of the great arteries. J Thorac Cardiovasc Surg 103:421–427, 1992.

19. Ostu T, Merz SI, Holtquist KA, et al: Laboratory evaluation of a double lumen catheter for venovenous neonatal ECMO. Trans Am Soc Artif Intern Organs 35:647–650, 1989.

20. Anderson HL, Ostu T, Shapman R, et al: Venovenous extracorporeal life support in neonates using a double lumen catheter. Trans Am Soc Artif Intern Organs 35:650–653, 1989.

21. Klein MD, Shaheen KW, Whittlesey GC, et al: Extracorporeal membrane oxygenation for the support of children after repair of congenital heart disease. J Thorac Cardiovasc Surg 100:498–505, 1990.

22. Grayck EN, Meliones JN, Kern FH, et al: Elevated serum lactate correlates with intracranial hemorrhage in neonates treated with extracorporeal life support. Pediatrics 96:914–917, 1995.

23. Meliones JN, Custer JR, Snedecor S, et al: Extracorporeal life support for cardiac assist in pediatric patients: review of the ELSO Registry data. Circulation 84:168–172, 1991.

24. Lotze A, Taylor J, Short BL: The use of lung compliance as a parameter for improvement in lung function in newborns with respiratory failure requiring ECMO. Crit Care 15:226–229, 1987.

25. Pettignano R, Heard M, Davis R, et al: Total enteral nutrition versus total parental nutrition during pediatric extracorporeal membrane oxygenation. Crit Care Med 26:358–363, 1998.

26. Groh MA, Meliones JN, Bove EL, et al: Repair of tetralogy of Fallot in infancy: effect of pulmonary artery size on outcome. Circulation 84:206–212, 1991.

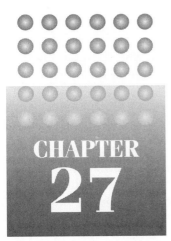

CHAPTER 27

Liquid Ventilation

David S. Foley, MD
Ronald B. Hirschl, MD, FACS

HISTORICAL ASPECTS
PHYSIOLOGY OF PERFLUOROCARBON VENTILATION
TOTAL LIQUID VENTILATION
Laboratory Studies
Clinical Studies

Current Limitations of Total Liquid Ventilation
PARTIAL LIQUID VENTILATION
Laboratory Studies
Clinical Studies
REFERENCES

KEY WORDS

acute respiratory distress syndrome
partial liquid ventilation

perfluorocarbons
respiratory distress syndrome
total liquid ventilation

Acute respiratory distress syndrome (ARDS) is characterized by a severe pulmonary inflammatory response to a variety of insults, leading to interstitial edema, intra-alveolar hemorrhage and exudate, decreased pulmonary compliance, decreased ventilation–perfusion matching, and progressive hypoxemic respiratory failure. This condition affects an estimated 150,000 people per year in the United States.[1] Significant advancements in supportive therapy for patients with ARDS have been made in the past 20 years, including positive end-expiratory pressure (PEEP), inverse-ratio ventilation, permissive hypercapnia, and extracorporeal life support (ECLS). Although these therapies have increased the level of supportive care available to patients

with respiratory failure, ARDS remains a highly lethal condition, with a mortality rate of approximately 50% in the non-neonatal population.[1-3] New strategies for the treatment of severe lung injury are in demand.

Liquid ventilation is an alternative technique for the management of respiratory failure that uses fluorinated organic liquids **(perfluorocarbons)** as a respiratory medium. Perfluorocarbons are an attractive choice for use in gas exchange because of both their high solubilities for the respiratory gases and their low surface tensions.[4] The two most extensively studied liquid ventilation techniques include **total liquid ventilation** (TLV), in which specialized mechanical liquid ventilators deliver perfluo-

433

rocarbon tidal volumes to the lungs, and **partial liquid ventilation** (PLV), in which conventional ventilators supply gas tidal volumes to lungs filled partially with perfluorocarbon.[5] Although liquid ventilation is still investigational, there is growing evidence in laboratory and clinical studies to suggest that it may be effective as a supportive and therapeutic technique for patients with severe lung injury. Following is a description of the history and methods of liquid ventilation, as well as a summary of the laboratory and early clinical evidence to support its development as a new therapy for severe respiratory failure.

HISTORICAL ASPECTS

The concept of instilling liquids into the respiratory tree has existed since the 1920s, when saline was used to lavage the airways of toxic gas inhalation victims.[6] Specifically, intrapulmonary saline has been used extensively in the past 50 years to study respiratory structure–function relationships. The saline-filled lung eliminates the gas–liquid interface in the alveoli and has led to numerous studies of the relative effects of structural and surface active forces on alveolar stability and function.[7-11] Although intrapulmonary saline was used early in the 20th century for both lavage therapy and physiologic studies, use of liquid as an alternative medium for gas exchange was not investigated seriously until 1962. Kylstra and Tissing studied spontaneously breathing dogs immersed in hyperbarically oxygenated saline solutions and were able to achieve adequate levels of arterial oxygenation.[12] Hypercarbia and acidosis developed rapidly in these animals, however, and they did not survive beyond the experimental period. The failure of adequate carbon dioxide (CO_2) clearance was attributed to the low solubility of CO_2 in saline and to the drainage limitations of this relatively dense liquid compared with air. Repeating the experiment with a mechanical-assist device yielded similar results.[13] Although the experiments of Kylstra and colleagues demonstrated the possibility of gas exchange using

a liquid medium, the use of saline for this purpose thus was shown to be limited.

Efforts subsequently were directed toward finding a liquid for supporting gas exchange with both a high solubility for the respiratory gases and a low surface tension. Initially, silicone and vegetable oils were evaluated, but these were found to be too toxic for use in vivo.[14] Interest then turned to the use of perfluorocarbons for liquid ventilation. First produced as a byproduct of reactions used during the Manhattan Project during World War II, these liquids were noted to be clear, odorless, biologically inert, and thermally stable. Most importantly, they were shown to have remarkably low surface tensions (15–18 dynes/cm at 25°C), and high solubilities for both oxygen (45–55 ml O_2/100 ml liquid at 25°C) and carbon dioxide (140–200 ml CO_2/100 ml liquid at 25°C).[15-17] In 1966, Clark and Gollan[18] successfully oxygenated spontaneously breathing mice submerged in perfluorocarbon liquid under normobaric conditions for periods of 4 hours. In addition, they were able to demonstrate survival to gas breathing for weeks after the experiment.[18] By establishing an acceptable medium for gas exchange, this study provided the basis for the development of liquid ventilation in its current forms.

Although the Clark experiment demonstrated the effective oxygenation and survival of animals breathing perfluorocarbons, the relatively high densities and low CO_2 diffusion coefficients of these liquids imposed limitations on spontaneously breathing models, with carbon dioxide clearance and acidosis remaining problematic.[18] In the early 1970s, demand-regulated mechanical liquid ventilators were developed by Moscowitz and Shaffer, in an effort to improve expiratory flow and limit the work of liquid breathing.[19-22] These devices improved the efficiency of carbon dioxide clearance and allowed the development of stable models for the study of liquid ventilation. Variations on these original devices subsequently have been used to study TLV in a number of animal models, ranging in size from premature lambs to adult sheep.[23-31] Studies have been performed exploring the possibility of using inhaled perfluorocarbons as a means of preventing decompression sickness during deep water diving.[32, 33] Liquid ventilation has been used to support premature animal models for the study of both extrauterine development and the neonatal **respiratory distress syndrome** (RDS).[23–27] The findings of improved oxygenation and pulmonary compliance, decreased inflation pressures, and homogenous alveolar inflation in the lungs of total liquid-ventilated models of prematurity provided the first evidence of a possible therapeutic role for liquid ventilation in neonatal respiratory failure. In addition, these findings created interest in the study of TLV for the treatment of ARDS, a condition marked by similar worsening of lung compliance, ventilation–perfusion mismatching, hypoxemia, and risk for ventilator-induced lung injury. Studies have been performed in adult animal models of ARDS, with encouraging results.[28–30] The toxicology of perfluorocarbon inhalation has been investigated extensively, revealing no significant adverse pulmonary or systemic effects.[34–38] Absorption and elimination patterns also have been characterized partially for perfluorocarbons, revealing a small percentage of systemic absorption after liquid ventilation and primary clearance by evaporation from the lung.[39, 40] The first clinical result of this animal research occurred in 1990, when Greenspan and colleagues[41, 42] reported a trial of liquid ventilation in three premature infants with severe RDS using short periods of TLV with a simple gravity-assisted mechanism. Although all three of these moribund infants eventually died, they exhibited trends toward increased pulmonary compliance and improved oxygenation during the short trials.[41, 42]

Although TLV techniques had developed to the point of reproducible results in animal studies, the ventilators used in these studies to support gas exchange for periods longer than the 3 to 5 minutes reported in the Greenspan trial were relatively large and complex, with excessive perfluorocarbon priming volumes. These limitations slowed the movement of liquid ventilation to the clinical setting. A major development in this regard occurred with the evolution of PLV. Although the concept of a transition from total liquid to gas ventilation via a period of partial liquid ventilation had been explored by Shaffer, the technique was investigated specifically by Fuhrman and colleagues in 1991.[43] By gas-ventilating healthy piglets with perfluorocarbon-filled lungs, Fuhrman and colleagues were able to achieve equivalent gas exchange to conventionally ventilated controls for a period of 1 hour without the use of a complex and expensive mechanical liquid ventilator. Over the past decade, PLV has been studied in animal models of neonatal RDS, as well as in adult models of ARDS and gastric acid aspiration.[44–48] These studies demonstrated that PLV was well tolerated and provided enhanced oxygenation and pulmonary compliance in injured animal models. On the basis of these results, human trials of PLV were conducted on neonatal, pediatric, and adult patients maintained with ECLS for severe respiratory failure.[49–51] Although these studies involved a small number of patients, increases in gas exchange and compliance were demonstrated. In addition, the relative safety of the technique was shown across a wide range of age and development. Further trials have followed, with encouraging results.[52–57] Randomized, controlled multicenter human trials of PLV currently are being performed, while attempts to create a total liquid ventilator that is more efficient and suitable for clinical use continue in the laboratory.

PHYSIOLOGY OF PERFLUOROCARBON VENTILATION

Perfluorocarbons (PFC) are derived from common organic compounds by the replacement of carbon-bound hydrogen atoms with fluorine. The derivation of perfluorocarbons can be accomplished through a highly exothermic vapor-phase method using fluorine gas or through the less exothermic, somewhat more stable cobalt trifluoride technique.[58] More recently, these compounds have been produced by electrochemical fluorination, as first described by Simons in 1950.[59] In this process, hydrocarbons are fluorinated by electrolysis in combination with anhydrous hydrofluoric acid, at significantly lower temperatures than in the previously mentioned techniques. The result is a more homogenous product with less carbon–carbon bond cleavage. Using this approach, a wide variety of perfluorocarbon compounds has been produced for use in liquid ventilation research.

Perfluorocarbons used for liquid ventilation are colorless, odorless liquids with unique physical properties, as described by Sargent and Seffl in 1970.[58] These compounds are nearly twice as dense as their hydrocarbon counterparts, with slightly lower kinematic viscosities (ratio of viscosity to density). Their peripheral fluorine atoms are relatively inert, leading to weak intermolecular forces and remarkably low surface tensions. In addition, these fluorine atoms provide a shield for the intramolecular carbon–carbon bonds of perfluorocarbons, making them both thermally stable and chemically nonreactive. Perfluorocarbons containing an iodine or bromine atom, of which the frequently used perflubron (Liquivent, Alliance Pharmaceutical Corp., San Diego, CA) is an example, are both radiopaque and light sensitive.[60] Perfluorocarbons are essentially insoluble in water and alcohol-based solutions and have varying degrees of solubility for hydrocarbons. In contrast, the solubilities of the respiratory gases in perfluorocarbons are significantly greater than their corresponding solubilities in water or nonpolar solvents. For example, the solubility of oxygen in perfluorocarbon liquids is approximately 20 times that in water (45–55 ml O_2/100 ml liquid at 25°C), and carbon dioxide is roughly three times as soluble in perfluorocarbons as is oxygen (140–210 ml CO_2/100 ml liquid at 25°C).[58] Some of the important physical properties of the perfluorocarbons used in liquid ventilation research are shown in Table 27–1.

The unique physical characteristics of perfluorocarbons are crucial to their efficacy as an alternative gas exchange medium during respiratory failure. Because of the remarkably high solubilities of the respiratory gases in perfluorocarbons, these liquids have the potential to support gas exchange under normobaric conditions.[21] The densities of perfluorocarbons facilitate their distribution to the dependent regions of the lung, resulting in the recruitment of segments that tend to be collapsed or filled with inflammatory exudate during severe pulmonary inflammation.[3, 29] In addition, fluid-filled lungs exhibit a redistribution of pulmonary blood flow, with relative equilibration of flow between dependent and nondependent regions.[61–63] During lung injury, albumin leak and lung water content are reduced during liquid ventilation when compared with gas ventilation.[63, 64] In the setting of severe respiratory failure, these effects would theoretically improve ventilation–perfusion matching, resulting in enhanced arterial oxygenation.

Alveolar recruitment and stability are partially maintained by the surfactant-induced reduction of surface tension in small airways, a process that is hindered by the relative deficiency of surfactant in both neonatal RDS and adult ARDS.[2, 4, 8] Because a fluid-filled lung has no gas–liquid interface, surface tension is reduced to insignificant levels, and conditions favoring alveolar collapse are reduced.[8, 9] In addition, because of their low surface tensions, perfluorocarbons may increase alveolar stability by acting as an artificial surfactant, and they do not appear to reduce endogenous surfactant production or activity in animal studies.[60, 65] These effects would lead to an increase in both pulmonary compliance and functional residual capacity during acute lung injury, which has been demonstrated for PLV in oleic acid-injured sheep using body plethysmography.[66]

Another potential benefit of using the dense perfluorocarbon liquids as a therapy for respiratory failure relates to their lavage effect. Patients with severe pulmonary inflammation typically have large amounts of exudate in their airways, containing mucus, hemorrhage, inflammatory cells and mediators, and denuded mucosal cells. This exudate contributes to hypoventilation and ventilation–perfusion mismatching.[3] When trapped in the distal airways, it also may magnify the inflammatory response, leading to increased parenchymal damage. Because of their relative densities, perfluorocarbon

TABLE 27–1. Properties of Perfluorocarbon Liquids*

PROPERTY	FC-77	RM-101	FC-75	PERFLUORODECALIN	PERFLUBRON
Boiling point (°C)	97	101	102	142	142
Density at 25°C (g/cc)	1.78	1.77	1.78	1.95	1.93
Kinematic viscosity (centistrokes at 25°C)	.80	.82	.82	2.90	1.10
Vapor pressure (torr at 25°C)	85	64	63	14	11
Surface tension (dynes/cm at 25°C)	15	15	15	15	18
O_2 solubility at 25°C (ml gas/100 ml liq.)	50	52	52	49	53
CO_2 solubility at 37°C (ml gas/100 ml liq.)	198	160	160	140	210

*Industrial PFCs, FC77, and FC75 from 3M Corp., St. Paul, MN; RM101 from Miteni, Milan, Italy; perfluorodecalin from Green Gross Corp. of Japan and Air Products and Chemicals, Inc., Allentown, PA; perflubron (perfluoroocylbromide) from Alliance Pharmaceutical Corp., San Diego, CA.
From Shaffer TH, Wolfson MR, Clark LC: Liquid ventilation (state of the art review). Pediatr Pulmonol 14:102–109, 1992.

liquids facilitate exudate clearance, through airway lavage during TLV or through the simple displacement of dependent exudate during PLV. Removal of this inflammatory debris may be beneficial in limiting the progression of lung injury during severe respiratory failure. Because perfluorocarbons are poor solvents for water-based solutions, they allow the relatively easy separation and removal of this exudate as it is returned to the ventilator during TLV or suctioned from the trachea during PLV.

Laboratory and clinical studies on the uptake, distribution, elimination, and toxicology of the relatively inert perfluorocarbon liquids indicate that they are absorbed in small quantities during TLV, a process that reaches a steady state after 15 to 30 minutes of liquid breathing.[39, 42] Once in the blood stream, these compounds deposit preferentially in tissues with high lipid contents and are cleared most quickly from lipid-poor tissues with high vascularity, such as muscle. They do not appear to undergo biotransformation after absorption.[39] Their principal route of elimination from the body is through evaporation from the lung, with rates of elimination proportional to the vapor pressure of the particular liquid used.[34, 39] Expired gas samples from human neonates, obtained during and up to 12 hours after TLV therapy for respiratory distress, demonstrated peak perfluorocarbon levels after 15 minutes of liquid breathing,

with decline to control levels at 8 hours post-therapy.[42] Tissue and blood samples from the same infants exhibited declines in perfluorocarbon levels toward control values at 2.5 months post-therapy, with lipid-rich tissues containing the highest concentrations of perfluorocarbons at all sample intervals. Serum perfluorocarbon levels obtained during and after 5 to 7 days of PLV in adult patients have demonstrated peak serum concentrations 24 hours after the last PFC dose (0.26 ± 0.005 mg/dl), declining to 0.18 ± 0.06 mg/dl by 48 hours post-therapy.[67] Chest radiography of adult and neonatal patients has demonstrated significant clearance of perfluorocarbon from the lungs at 5 to 7 days after PLV, although residual amounts have been visualized at 2 to 20 weeks in follow-up of survivors.[68, 69] Despite the detection of trace quantities of perfluorocarbons in various canine and primate tissues for up to 3 years after liquid breathing, hematologic and biochemical analyses have revealed no evidence of systemic toxicity, with transient elevations in white blood cell counts and alkaline phosphatase levels being the only abnormalities noted.[37, 38] In addition, the 3-year survival and clinically normal appearance of these animals support the premise that perfluorocarbons are largely nontoxic. These compounds have even been used intravenously as experimental blood substitutes, with one group reporting survival in rats after nearly complete exchange transfusion of red blood cells with perfluorocarbon FC-43 (3M Corp., St. Paul, MN).[70]

The pulmonary effects of perfluorocarbons on breathing have been studied on both functional and histologic levels in healthy animals. Pulmonary function studies performed in dogs after one hour of liquid ventilation with perfluorocarbon Caroxin-F (Allied Chemical Corp., Morristown, NJ) showed moderate decreases in lung volume, compliance, and arterial oxygen tension (PaO_2) on return to gas breathing, compared with prestudy levels.[34] These abnormalities reversed within 72 hours and remained normal for a follow-up period of 6 months. Similarly, dogs ventilated with perfluorocarbon FX-80 (3M Corp., St. Paul, MN) have survived to air breathing with only transient requirements for supplemental oxygen.[35] Immediate histologic evaluation of previously normal hamster lungs after survival from perfluorocarbon ventilation demonstrated a moderate inflammatory response, with the presence of interstitial edema, intra-alveolar exudate, and polymorphonuclear phagocytes.[71] Within 24 hours of recovery to gas ventilation, the predominant inflammatory cells in the lung were vacuolated macrophages, which appear to be the primary cellular scavenger of perfluorocarbons.[37, 71] Lung tissue macrophage numbers have been shown to gradually decrease over time after perfluorocarbon ventilation and are present in very small numbers at 18 months and 3 years in follow-up of previously liquid-ventilated dogs.[36, 37] In addition, their presence has not been associated with fibrosis or alveolar distortion.[37] Overall, the results of these studies suggest that perfluorocarbons have no significant adverse short- or long-term effects when used in living systems for ventilatory purposes.

TOTAL LIQUID VENTILATION

Total liquid ventilation refers to the process of instilling and removing tidal volumes of perfluorocarbon liquid from the lungs for the purpose of gas exchange. The concept is similar to air breathing and gas ventilation, and centers around the tidal regeneration

of warmed perfluorocarbon that has a high oxygen and low carbon dioxide content. Because of the need for delivering regenerated tidal volumes of liquid in TLV, the process involves the use of specialized mechanical liquid ventilators, which have undergone a number of adaptations over the past 25 years. Because of the flow and diffusional limitations of perfluorocarbons, TLV usually is performed at low respiratory rates (3–9 breaths/min) and with relatively high tidal volumes (14–25 ml/kg).[26–28, 72] Despite its limited clinical use at this point, TLV has several theoretical advantages over conventional gas ventilation with respect to the treatment of severe respiratory failure, as mentioned previously, and has been studied more extensively in animal models than its hybrid counterpart, PLV.

The development of liquid ventilators for the study of TLV in animal models has been a steady process, beginning with spontaneously breathing animals, and evolving from gravitational assistance to more sophisticated methods over the past 25 years. Efforts have centered on improving carbon dioxide clearance, limiting the work of liquid breathing, and simplifying ventilator design for animal experimentation and eventual clinical usage. Moskowitz is credited with the development of the first true mechanical ventilator for liquid breathing, as described in 1970 (Fig. 27–1).[19] This device was a demand-regulated ventilator, which sensed intratracheal pressure changes created by the animal's spontaneous respiratory efforts and activated rubber diaphragms to assist with the delivery and removal of tidal volumes of perfluorocarbon liquid. It consisted of both inspiratory and expiratory limbs and had check valves to direct flow to the desired locations, with expired fluid going to a bubble oxygenator and then recirculating from the oxygenator to the inspiratory limb for the next inspiration. The bubble oxygenator reservoir also was equipped with a heater to keep inspired fluid at desired temperatures during experimentation, thereby eliminating the hypothermia seen during liquid ventilation with room temperature perfluorocarbon in earlier studies.[18] Shaffer and colleagues modified the demand-regulated liquid ventilator by replac-

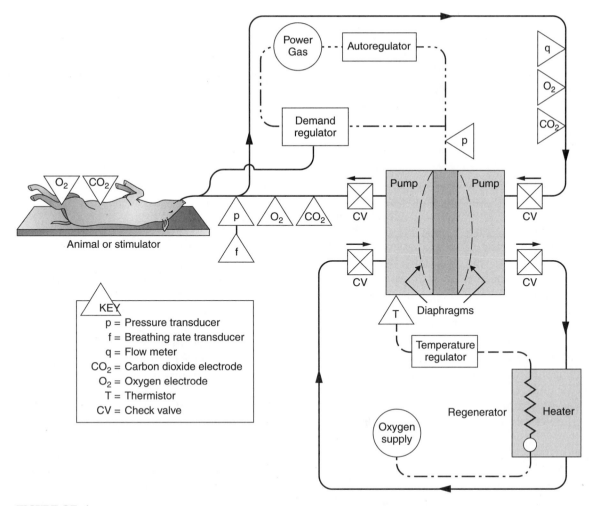

FIGURE 27–1
Schematic representation of the original demand-regulated liquid breathing system, as described by Moskowitz. (From Moskowitz GD: A mechnical respirator for control of liquid breathing. Fed Proc 29:1751–1752, 1970.)

ing the rubber diaphragm pumps with bellows and subsequently roller pumps, which have been used extensively to study TLV in healthy adult canine models and in premature animal models of RDS.[20-22] These studies helped to demonstrate that improved carbon dioxide clearance could be obtained through the mechanically assisted tidal movement of perfluorocarbons in the lungs.

The advent of ECLS led to the development of a second generation of liquid ventilators, which were based on a modified ECLS circuit. This type of ventilator, first described by Curtis and associates in 1990, consisted of a closed circuit inspiratory and expiratory line, with tidal volumes driven by an occlusive roller pump, and fluid oxy-

genation accomplished via a membrane oxygenator.[72] Two pneumatic valves were installed in the system, one to direct flow to the inspiratory or expiratory limb and one that opened to allow siphon drainage to a reservoir during expiration. Thus, inspiratory flow was assisted by a roller pump and expiration by gravity. This system was simplified by Hirschl and colleagues, who eliminated the need for an inspiratory/expiratory valve by stopping the roller pump during expiration, and has been used successfully in a number of studies on healthy infant and injured adult animal models.[29-31, 72] However, expiratory flow in this system was assisted only by gravity, which did not provide optimal control over expiration.

In our laboratory, Meinhardt and colleagues subsequently explored the use of piston-driven liquid ventilation and found enhanced expiratory flow compared with roller pump techniques.[73] On the basis of this observation, a double-piston pump ventilator was developed and used successfully in both healthy and oleic acid–injured rabbits.[74] This finding, combined with the development of more sophisticated computer programming, led to the design of a third type of liquid ventilator that currently is being studied in an adult animal model of respiratory failure[74a] (Fig. 27–2). The Alliance ventilator, also of the double-piston pump variety, controls both piston movement and pneumatic valve position with computer software. Oxygenation is achieved by a bubble oxygenator reservoir, which draws "oxygen-poor" perfluorocarbon from the expiratory piston during inspiration and delivers oxygenated perfluorocarbon to the inspiratory piston during expiration to start the next ventilatory cycle. The more advanced computer programming built into this system allows control of ventilatory parameters, such as inspiratory and expiratory flow rates, tidal volumes, and end-expiratory pressure, via a touch-sensitive computer screen at the front of the device. The current system supports adult animal models of up to 25 kg and is only slightly larger than most conventional gas ventilators. As such, this ventilator currently appears to have the best combination of necessary features for successful TLV and adequate simplicity for clinical use.

Laboratory Studies

The use of TLV to improve pulmonary function in respiratory failure has been studied in various premature, infant, and adult animal models of severe lung injury. Richman and colleagues have reported significant increases in arterial oxygenation and pulmonary compliance in oleic acid-injured adult cats after perfluorocarbon lavage.[26] Shaffer and associates reported both a 50% improvement in arterial oxygenation and a fivefold increase in lung compliance when ventilating premature lambs with a modification of the aforementioned demand-regulated ventilator, compared with gas ventilation control values taken before and after the liquid ventilation procedure.[27] These results were duplicated in a similar study from the same institution using TLV in a meconium aspiration model of premature lambs.[75] The authors also studied the postmortem distribution of pulmonary blood flow in these animals with radioactive carbon microspheres after in vivo injection, finding a trend toward more homogenous pulmonary blood flow during TLV, which has been reported in other experiments on liquid-filled lungs.[59, 61] The encouraging results with respect to models of neonatal RDS led to the use of TLV in adult animal models of severe lung injury. Hirschl and associates evaluated TLV in young adult sheep, after lung injury by oleic acid infusion into the right atrium and saline pulmonary lavage. These animals typically received a severe lung injury and were maintained on venovenous ECLS during the experiment. During TLV for 2.5 hours, these animals demonstrated significant reduc-

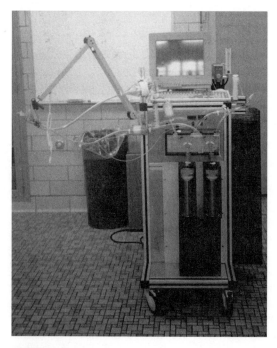

FIGURE 27–2
The current Alliance prototype double-piston liquid ventilator. (Courtesy of Alliance Pharmaceutical Corp., San Diego, CA.)

tions in physiologic shunt (Qps/Qt) and required ECLS flow rates, as well as significant increases in pulmonary compliance when compared with gas-ventilated controls (Fig. 27–3A and B).[28] In addition, gross examination of the lungs of animals treated with TLV and control animals at the end of the experiment demonstrated much less consolidation and atelectasis in the TLV group (Fig. 27–4). A corollary study from the same institution obtained computed tomographic (CT) images of the lungs of oleic acid–injured sheep after gas ventilation or TLV and found uniform distribution of perfluorocarbon and uniform lung expansion in the TLV group, whereas the gas-ventilated lungs showed a consistent pattern of dependent atelectasis and consolidation (Fig. 27–5).[29] Overall, the aforementioned research has demonstrated improved oxygenation and pulmonary compliance during TLV in both infant and adult animal models of severe respiratory failure when compared with conventional techniques. Given the homogenous inflation and distribution of pulmonary blood flow in the lungs of these animals, the studies also provide support for the concept that TLV improves pulmonary

compliance by eliminating surface tension and recruiting dependent alveoli and improves oxygenation by increasing ventilation–perfusion matching in severely injured lungs.

Although animal models of lung injury have demonstrated the potential for the use of TLV as a supportive measure in the setting of severe respiratory failure, there is also evidence that this technique may have a protective effect on injured lungs. The lungs of oleic acid–injured sheep were shown to have much less dependent atelectasis and hemorrhage on gross examination after TLV, as previously mentioned.[28] In addition, histologic examination of these lungs revealed a significant decrease in intra-alveolar hemorrhage, edema, and inflammatory infiltrate when compared with those of gas-ventilated controls (Fig. 27–6). The mechanisms for this apparent decrease in the pulmonary inflammatory response to injury are uncertain at this point. It has been suggested that this protection may be the result of a lavage effect in the airways, with the removal of inflammatory exudate and mediators from alveoli decreasing the magnitude of the inflammatory response.[28] The

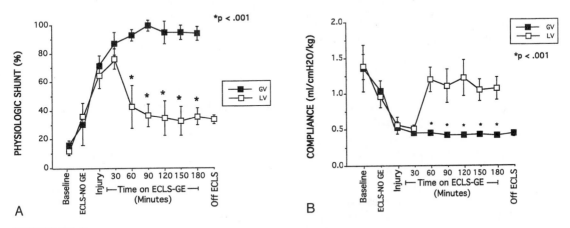

FIGURE 27–3

(A) Calculated pulmonary physiologic shunt at baseline; on extracorporeal life support but without membrane lung gas exchange (ECLS-NO GE); after lung injury; for 3 hours while on extracorporeal life support with membrane lung gas exchange (ECLS-GE); and after discontinuation of extracorporeal life support (Off ECLS). Sheep underwent gas ventilation (GV) or liquid ventilation (LV) while on ECLS and after discontinuation of ECLS, although all sheep underwent GV for the first 30 minutes while on ECLS-GE (*p < 0.01). (B) Pulmonary compliance with inflation to 20 ml/kg gas or perfluorocarbon in the same animals (*p < 0.01). (From Hirschl RB, Parent A, Tooley R, et al: Liquid ventilation improves pulmonary function, gas exchange, and lung injury in a model of respiratory failure. Ann Surg 221:79–88, 1995.)

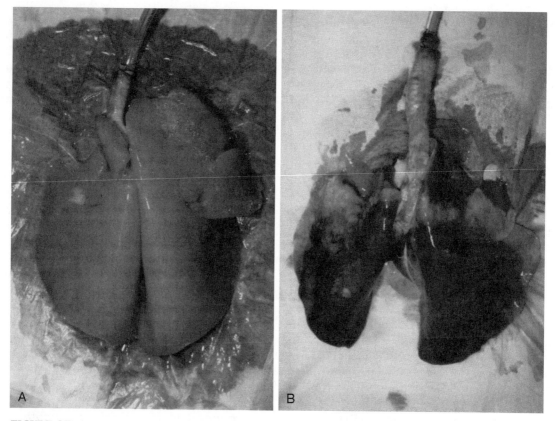

FIGURE 27–4

Posterior (dependent) view of representative noninflated lungs after completion of the protocol and at the time of autopsy in a total liquid-ventilated (LV) *(A)* and a gas-ventilated (GV) *(B)* sheep. Substantial reduction in pulmonary consolidation, atelectasis, and hemorrhage in the LV lungs is noted. (From Hirschl RB, Parent A, Tooley R, et al: Liquid ventilation improves pulmonary function, gas exchange, and lung injury in a model of respiratory failure. Ann Surg 221:79–88, 1995.)

increase in both pulmonary compliance and functional residual capacity (FRC) seen during TLV also may provide a protective effect by allowing inflation of the lungs at lower airway pressures and maintaining alveoli in an inflated, rather than a continuously collapsed or cyclic collapsed/inflated, state. There is even evidence to suggest that perfluorocarbons exert a direct anti-inflammatory effect on tissues. In vitro experiments studying the reperfusion of ischemic myocardium with perfluorocarbons have demonstrated a decrease in the inflammatory infiltrate seen at the site of injury.[76] Perfluorocarbon liquids also have been shown, in vitro, to reduce cytokine production and reactive oxygen species after phagocytic stimulation with lipopolysaccharides and to reduce the neutrophil-mediated

injury of lung epithelial cells.[77, 78] The relative importance and specific mechanisms of these anti-inflammatory effects remain undetermined. However, the possibility of a direct therapeutic role for TLV in the setting of severe lung injury is both exciting and unique and warrants further investigation.

Clinical Studies

Clinical experience with TLV is limited, at this point, to one study of short duration on three premature infants with severe RDS. Greenspan and associates performed TLV for two separate 3- to 5-minute intervals on three moribund infants, all less than 1 kg in weight, with severe RDS refractory to both high-frequency jet ventilation and sur-

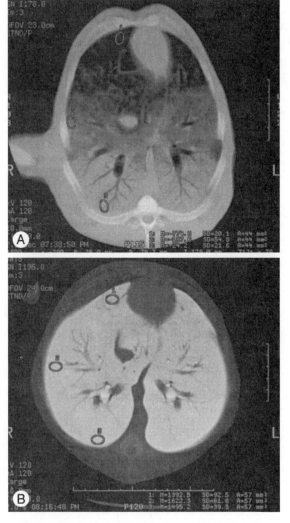

FIGURE 27–5
Representative computed tomography (CT) scans at a level 1 cm above the diaphragm in: (A) a gas-ventilated sheep after lung inflation of 20 ml/kg of gas; (B) a total liquid-ventilated sheep after lung inflation with 20 ml/kg of perfluorocarbon. The 1-cm diameter region of interest shows the technique used to evaluate CT attenuation in nondependent (anterior), middle, and dependent (posterior) regions of both lungs. (From Hirschl RB, Overbeck M, Parent A, et al: Liquid ventilation provides uniform distribution of perfluorocarbon in the setting of respiratory failure. Surgery 116:159–168, 1994.)

factant therapy.[41] The ventilator used was a simple gravity-assisted device, with oxygen bubbled into a reservoir between breaths. All three of the infants studied exhibited increased pulmonary compliance during the

liquid breathing trials, and two of the three showed improved oxygenation. Although all three infants died within 24 hours of the trial, they showed no hemodynamic deterioration during liquid breathing and no complications that could be attributed to the therapy. These results cannot be considered conclusive, based on the small patient sample size and the brevity of the treatment. However, the fact that these moribund infants were able to tolerate the trial is an encouraging precedent with respect to the further application of this technique in the clinical setting.

Current Limitations of Total Liquid Ventilation

Although laboratory and clinical evidence has developed to support the use of TLV in both neonatal and adult respiratory failure, there are problems created by the mechanics of total liquid breathing in lungs that have evolved for the purpose of gas ventilation. Although expiration during air breathing and conventional gas ventilation is largely a passive process, the dramatically higher densities of perfluorocarbons do not allow their effective passive expiratory flow. As a result, potential alveolar ventilation is limited, and spontaneously breathing animals face a dramatically increased work of breathing, rapidly developing hypercarbia and respiratory acidosis.[18] Although the development of mechanical assistance for liquid ventilation has decreased the work of breathing and improved carbon dioxide clearance, effective ventilation is still relatively limited by the flow and diffusional properties of perfluorocarbons.[79–83] Dawson and Elliott have shown that the maximal flow of a gas or liquid medium from the lung is limited to the minimum wave speed of that medium in the respiratory tree and is inversely proportional to its density.[79] Because the densities of perfluorocarbons greatly exceed those of air, the maximal flow possible during expiration of perfluorocarbons from the lungs is much lower. In addition, the diffusion of carbon dioxide into perfluorocarbons is approximately 2500 times slower than into air, which imposes further

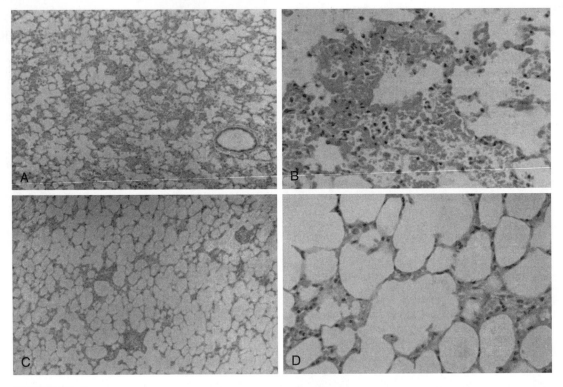

FIGURE 27–6

10× (A and C) and 40× (B and D) views of a biopsy from the lower (dependent) region of the injured lung after completion of the protocol in a representative (A and B), gas-ventilated (GV) and (C and D), total liquid-ventilated (LV) sheep. Reductions in pulmonary vascular congestion, alveolar hemorrhage, alveolar proteinaceous fluid accumulation, and inflammatory infiltration are noted in the LV specimen (From Hirschl RB, Parent A, Tooley R, et al: Liquid ventilation improves pulmonary function, gas exchange, and lung injury in a model of respiratory failure. Ann Surg 221:79–88, 1995.)

limitations on carbon dioxide clearance.[82] Koen and colleagues characterized the maximal flow of perfluorocarbon FC-80 from the lungs of anesthetized cats during liquid breathing and also described the relationship between respiratory rate and diffusional dead space in the lung.[83] They demonstrated that maximal expiratory flow, and hence maximal minute ventilation, is 20 times lower during liquid ventilation compared with gas ventilation (Fig. 27–7A). They also showed that diffusional dead space was inversely proportional to the time that the perfluorocarbons remained in the lungs with each breath and, therefore, was coupled directly to respiratory rate. On the basis of these experiments, the authors were able to calculate maximal alveolar ventilation and carbon dioxide clearance during liquid breathing. They concluded

that carbon dioxide clearance reached its maximum level at a respiratory rate between 3 and 5 breaths per minute, with lower rates limited by low minute ventilation and higher rates limited by excessive diffusional dead space (see Fig. 27–7B). This study provided the physiologic basis for the relatively low respiratory rates and high tidal volumes used in most animal studies on TLV. However, such low respiratory rates make carbon dioxide clearance a limiting variable during TLV.

Preliminary work from our laboratory indicates that flow limitation during liquid expiration becomes more dramatic as lung volumes at end inspiration are reduced.[73] These data suggest the possibility that expiratory flow may be enhanced, during each breath, by tapering from high to low flow rates as more volume is exhaled from the

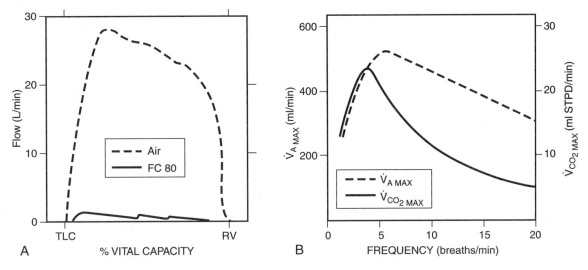

FIGURE 27-7
(A) Typical expiratory flow vs. percent vital capacity curves for anesthetized cats during air (dashed line) and perfluorocarbon (solid line) breathing. (B) Maximal alveolar ventilation (VA_{MAX}) and CO_2 elimination (V_{CO_2} max) as a function of breathing frequency during perfluorocarbon breathing in cats. (From Koen PA, Wolfson MR, Shaffer TH: Fluorocarbon ventilation: maximal expiratory flows and CO_2 elimination. Pediatr Res 24:291–295, 1988.)

lungs. Expiratory flow enhancement would allow for increased respiratory rates, which may be associated with enhanced carbon dioxide clearance. Alternatively, an improvement in the efficiency of expiratory flow may allow the application of an inspiratory dwell period, with more time for each tidal volume to remain in the lungs, thereby reducing the diffusional dead space for each respiratory rate. Ongoing studies are exploring this possibility.

Another proposed physiologic limitation of TLV relates to the cardiovascular effects imposed on a subject with liquid-filled lungs. Once carbon dioxide clearance in healthy animals was increased to acceptable levels by the use of mechanical liquid ventilators, it became apparent that the acidosis seen in earlier experiments included a distinct metabolic component.[60] Lowe and associates examined the hemodynamic and metabolic profiles of cats during gas ventilation and TLV, finding a 48% decrease in cardiac output and associated lactic acidosis during the liquid ventilation portion of the experiment.[84] They attributed this cardiovascular compromise to an increase in pulmonary vascular resistance.[85] Although it is apparent that hemodynamic alterations can occur during TLV, Curtis and colleagues have shown in piglets that a normal cardiac output and acid base balance can be achieved during liquid breathing through intravascular volume expansion.[86] The results of this study suggest that TLV has a similar effect to PEEP on cardiac output and that careful attention to both volume status and functional residual capacity will be important to minimize cardiovascular compromise during the clinical use of this technique.

A final problem that has prevented TLV from reaching the point of substantial clinical trials relates to the complexity and cost of this technique in its current forms. The mechanical ventilators that have been used successfully in animal studies of TLV have been large and complex. Although the developers of these devices have used them efficiently in animal studies, there is concern that the currently developed liquid ventilators would not be transferred easily to the intensive care unit (ICU) setting, where patients rarely have one-to-one ventilator supervision. In addition, most of these devices have had separate inspiratory and expiratory limbs, which has led to the need for large volumes of perfluorocarbon liquid simply to prime the ventilators in larger animal models. Simplification of ventilator design, automation, and reduction of priming volume are important steps in the movement of TLV to the clinical setting.

PARTIAL LIQUID VENTILATION

Partial liquid ventilation refers to the process of gas ventilating perfluorocarbon-filled lungs. This concept was developed from Shaffer's observation that there was generally a smooth transition from total liquid breathing to gas ventilation during animal experiments, when significant amounts of perfluorocarbon were still present in the respiratory tree.[86] This fact, coupled with the desire to simplify the process of liquid ventilation for clinical use, led to the idea that adequate gas exchange could be obtained by superimposing gas ventilation on lungs filled to FRC with perfluorocarbon. Fuhrman and colleagues were the first to specifically report success with this technique, achieving equivalent gas exchange and pulmonary compliance when compared with gas-ventilated control animals during 1 hour of PLV in healthy piglets.[43] Perfluorocarbon dosing in early clinical trials has consisted of initial administration in 5 to 10-ml/kg aliquots, with repeat dosing at intervals ranging from 30 minutes to 3 hours. Initial dosing continues, as tolerated by hemodynamic stability and adequate gas tidal volumes, until either a weight-adjusted estimated FRC is reached (30 ml/kg) or a sustained perfluorocarbon meniscus is present in the endotracheal tube during transient ventilator disconnection (zero PEEP).[50, 52-54] Daily redosing has been based on overall clinical status, inadequate dependent lung filling on lateral chest radiography, and loss of the perfluorocarbon meniscus. In patients with respiratory failure, PLV with perfluorocarbon liquid theoretically would provide some of the benefits of TLV through the recruitment of dependent airways, redistribution of pulmonary blood flow, and lowering of alveolar surface tension. As in TLV, the perfluorocarbons would be able to participate in the gas exchange process because of their high oxygen and carbon dioxide content. These benefits would occur without the need for a complex liquid ventilator, and the problem of liquid flow limitation would be eliminated by the delivery of gas tidal volumes, which would assist with carbon dioxide clearance.

Laboratory Studies

The use of PLV in respiratory failure has been studied in both infant and adult animal models. Leach and associates evaluated PLV for 1 hour in premature lambs with RDS, after delivery by cesarean section. Using a liquid FRC of 30 ml/kg and gas tidal volumes of 15 ml/kg, these animals were found to have fourfold increases in arterial oxygenation, threefold increases in pulmonary compliance, and significant reductions in arterial carbon dioxide levels when compared with gas-ventilated control animals.[44] Similar results have been reported using PLV in saline-lavaged, surfactant-deficient rabbits, with improvement in oxygenation and compliance being proportional to perfluorocarbon dosage in one of these studies.[45, 46] A subsequent evaluation of PLV in piglets after induction of lung injury by gastric acid aspiration showed an increase in arterial oxygenation when compared with gas-ventilated controls, which became statistically significant as the injury matured over the 6-hour experimental period.[47]

Curtis and colleagues have evaluated PLV in an oleic acid–injured adult canine model of ARDS.[87] These animals exhibited a dose-dependent increase in arterial oxygenation, with dogs receiving the largest dose of perfluorocarbon (60 ml/kg) showing the highest oxygen levels. In contrast, although overall pulmonary compliance was improved during PLV, maximum improvement was seen after a perfluorocarbon dose of 40 ml/kg, with further dosing resulting in a decrease in compliance. Hirschl and associates studied PLV for 2.5 hours in young adult sheep maintained on venovenous ECLS after lung injury by oleic acid infusion and saline lavage.[48] Using a smaller perfluorocarbon FRC (35 ml/kg) than the maximal dose used in the Curtis study, the investigators demonstrated an improvement in gas exchange and pulmonary function during PLV, as manifested by decreased physiologic shunt (Qps/Qt) and slightly improved pulmonary compliance when compared with gas-ventilated controls. A separate study from the same institution evaluated oxygen dynamics during PLV in similarly injured sheep and found dose-related increases in oxygen delivery and mixed venous oxygen saturation, which peaked at a perfluorocarbon fill of 40 ml/kg (Fig. 27–8).[88] Further PFC dosing resulted in minimal improvement in oxygenation, with impaired cardiac output levels contributing to decreased oxygen delivery beyond this point.

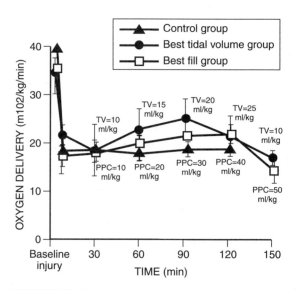

FIGURE 27–8

Oxygen delivery in adult sheep at baseline, after lung injury, and for 150 minutes during conventional gas ventilation (control group), partial liquid ventilation (PLV) with 10 ml/kg incremental increases in perflubron dose from 10 to 50 ml/kg (best fill, BF group), or PLV with 5 ml/kg incremental increases in gas tidal volume from 10 to 30 ml/kg (best tidal volume, BTV group). Values are mean ± SEM (BF: $p = 0.047$ by repeated-measures analysis of variance [ANOVA]; $p = 0.12$ and 0.44 at 90 and 120 minutes when comparison of BF and control data was performed post hoc; BTV: $p = 0.14$ by repeated-measures ANOVA; $p = 0.18$ and 0.88 at 90 and 120 minutes when comparison of BTV and control data was performed post hoc). (From Parent AC, Overbeck MC, Hirschl RB: Oxygen dynamics during partial liquid ventilation in a sheep model of severe respiratory failure. Surgery 121:320–327, 1997.)

The results of these studies show that arterial oxygenation is improved during PLV in various models of both neonatal and adult respiratory failure to levels comparable with those achieved during TLV. In addition, carbon dioxide clearance appears to be facilitated during PLV, which is likely a result of the improved efficiency of gas ventilation in the setting of perfluorocarbon-induced alveolar recruitment. The results with respect to pulmonary compliance are less consistent and may result from gas ventilation being superimposed on liquid-filled lungs during PLV. As would be predicted by their high densities, perfluorocarbons have been shown to distribute predominantly to the dependent region of the lungs during PLV in sheep.[89] Because compliance measurements during PLV studies have been determined by volume and pressure changes after infusion of gas into the lungs, there may be a point during perfluorocarbon dosing at which the beneficial effect of this liquid on compliance is offset by the fact that there is less space in the lungs for gas instillation, especially as tidal volumes approach total lung capacity (TLC). In addition, although perfluorocarbons may act as an artificial surfactant because of their low surface tensions, the alveolar gas–liquid interface is not eliminated completely during PLV, so improvement in compliance would not be expected to be as dramatic as is seen during TLV. The cumulative laboratory work on PLV suggests that both pulmonary compliance and oxygen delivery enhancement are dose dependent, with maximal improvements in these parameters achieved at a perfluorocarbon dose near FRC.

As in TLV, there is some early evidence to suggest that PLV may exert a protective effect on the lungs in animal models of respiratory failure. The lungs of oleic acid–injured sheep have been examined by histologic survey after 2.5 hours of PLV and compared with those of gas-ventilated controls.[48] As in a similar study from the same institution on TLV, the PLV animals exhibited much less intra-alveolar hemorrhage, edema, and inflammatory infiltrate. A randomized controlled study by Quintel and associates examined pulmonary histology and morphometrics in oleic acid–injured sheep and found decreased diffuse alveolar damage scores, alveolar septal thickness, and pulmonary capillary diameters, as well as increased alveolar inflation in the lungs of sheep randomized to PLV (Fig. 27–9).[90] In contrast, an earlier report found no histologic difference between the lungs of dogs randomized to PLV or gas ventilation after oleic acid injury.[87] The discrepancy in these results may relate to the lower perfluorocarbon doses used in the former studies, which also reported more consistent increases in pulmonary compliance and may have avoided the overdistension of nondependent airways. The protective effects of PLV may relate to the recruitment of dependent alveoli at lower inflation pressures, a lavage effect of the perfluorocarbon liquid and/or a direct anti-inflammatory effect of the PFC itself. Lipopolysaccharide-stimulated macrophages have been shown to have less expression of the inflammatory cytokines tumor neurosis factor-α, interleukin-1, and interleukin-6, as well as diminished nitric oxide (NO) and hydrogen peroxide (H_2O_2) production after in vitro exposure to perfluorocarbon.[77, 91, 92] In vitro studies also have demonstrated reductions in neutrophil activation and chemotaxis after perfluorocarbon exposure, as well as a perfluorocarbon-associated protection of lung epithelial cells from neutrophil-mediated injury.[78, 93]

Cobra venom factor lung-injured animals demonstrate reductions in neutrophil infiltration and albumin leak during PLV when compared with gas ventilation.[64, 94] Although the specific mechanisms by which PLV protects injured lungs have not been described fully, the potential of an active therapeutic role for this technique in the setting of respiratory failure suggests exciting possibilities and warrants further study.

Clinical Studies

The first clinical report of the use of PLV for respiratory failure occurred in 1995.[49] Hirschl and associates used PLV as an adjunctive therapy to ECLS on 19 patients (10 adults, 4 children, and 5 neonates) with severe respiratory failure from a variety of causes. Although this study did not include a control group, patients undergoing PLV had significant decreases in alveolar–arterial oxygen gradients (A–a DO_2) and significant increases in pulmonary compliance during short periods of ECLS discontinuation, compared with pretreatment values. These patients exhibited no hemodynamic compromise during PLV, and associated complications were limited to nine pneumofluorothoraces, six of which had existed before the onset of treatment. The overall

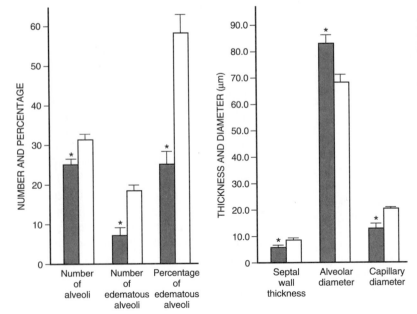

FIGURE 27–9
Morphometric analysis of biopsy samples from the lungs of sheep after injury by oleic acid infusion to the right atrium. Solid bars represent sheep randomized to 2.5 hours of partial liquid ventilation (PLV), whereas open bars represent sheep randomized to gas ventilation over the same time period (∗ = statistically significant difference). (From Quintel M, Heine M, Hirschl R, et al: Effects of partial liquid ventilation on lung injury in a model of acute respiratory failure. Crit Care Med 26:833–843, 1998.)

survival rate was 58%. A multicenter, non-controlled trial investigating the use of PLV in 10 premature infants (24–34 weeks' gestation) with surfactant-refractory RDS reported a 138% increase in PaO_2 and a 61% increase in pulmonary compliance over 1 to 3 days of therapy.[55] The overall survival rate of the infants to term was 80%, an encouraging number given the poor physiologic status of these patients before the trial. Significant complications potentially attributed to the use of PLV included intracranial hemorrhage (two patients) and pneumothorax (one patient). These results have been repeated in other small studies on infants with respiratory failure of enough severity to warrant ECLS.[56, 57] With evidence that surfactant deficiency may play a role in the ventilation–perfusion mismatching seen in infants with congenital diaphragmatic hernia (CDH),[95] a study has examined the use of PLV in four patients maintained on ECLS for this disorder, showing significantly improved PaO_2 levels and lung compliance during short periods of ECLS discontinuation, with trends toward improvement in CO_2 clearance and arterial oxygen content.[96] A multicenter, noncontrolled phase I/II trial evaluating 96 hours of PLV in nine adults with severe ARDS demonstrated a significant reduction in A–a DO_2 by 48 hours of therapy, from 430 ± 27 to 229 ± 17 mm Hg (Fig. 27–10).[52] Weight-adjusted pulmonary compliance was unchanged during the study. Severe complications potentially resulting from the therapy were limited to two cases of transient hypoxia and one case of hyperbilirubinemia, and the survival rate to the 28-day outcome end point was 78%. A similar trial in 10 children with ARDS also demonstrated reductions in A–aDO_2, with an overall survival rate to the 28-day outcome end point of 80%.[53] Significant complications included the development of pneumothoraces in three patients. A subsequent phase II randomized, controlled multicenter trial of PLV in 90 adult patients with ARDS reinforced the safety of this technique when employed over an average of 80 hours. Although no differences in overall 28-day ventilation parameters, mortality, or the number of ventilator-free days were observed, trends toward improvement in 28-day mor-

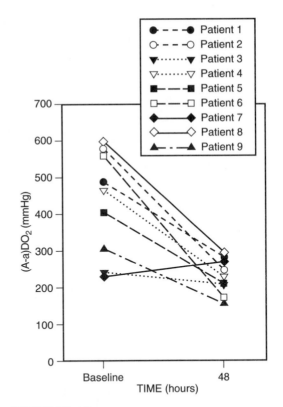

FIGURE 27–10

(A-a)DO2 for 9 adult patients at baseline and 48 hours after the institution of partial liquid ventilation therapy for acute respiratory distress syndrome (ARDS)(p = 0.013 by ANOVA). (From Hirschl RB, Conrad S, Kaiser R, et al: Partial liquid ventilation in adult patients with ARDS: a multicenter phase I/II trial. Ann Surg 228:692–700, 1998).

tality and ventilator-free days in patients younger than age 55 with acute lung injury (ALI) or ARDS were noted.[54] The results of these studies have demonstrated the safety and potential benefits of PLV with respect to acute lung injury, across a wide range of age and pathology. The extent to which this technique will become clinically useful in the setting of severe respiratory failure depends on the conclusion of ongoing larger prospective, randomized controlled studies that compare PLV with conventional therapies.

CONCLUSION

Liquid ventilation has developed from a scientific curiosity to the doorstep of clinical utility over the past 30 years. TLV has been hindered in its evolution to clinical application by the complexity of the devices needed for its employment and by the mechanical problems created by the tidal flow of dense perfluorocarbon liquids in an elastic respiratory tree. Nonetheless, this technique has shown great promise in animal models of severe respiratory failure and may offer some supportive and therapeutic advantages over PLV with respect to an enhanced lavage effect and its complete elimination of the gas–liquid interface in the lung. Future efforts are needed with respect to simplification of the mechanical liquid ventilator, which would both facilitate clinical usage and lower the cost of treatment. In addition, improvements in expiratory flow techniques would be valuable to improve carbon dioxide clearance to levels comparable to those seen in established modes of respiratory support. PLV has been studied extensively in animal models of respiratory failure, as well as in several clinical trials, with encouraging results. This relatively simple therapy appears to have many of the advantages of TLV with respect to oxygenation and lung recruitment, and it may provide enhanced carbon dioxide clearance and lung protection. The efficacy of this technique in the clinical setting, as well as the optimal PFC dosing schedule, will be determined by the completion of randomized, controlled clinical trials. If results of these trials confirm the earlier reports of improved pulmonary function in the setting of severe lung injury, PLV should become a much more commonly used therapy for neonatal, pediatric, and adult patients with respiratory failure.

REFERENCES

1. Andreadis W, Petty TL: Adult respiratory distress syndrome: problems and progress. Am Rev Respir Dis 132:1344–1346, 1985.
2. Bartlett RH, Morris AH, Fairly HB, et al: A prospective study of acute hypoxemic respiratory failure. Chest 89:684–689, 1986.
3. Gattinoni L, D'Andrea L, Pelosi P, et al: Regional effects and mechanism of positive end expiratory pressure in early adult respiratory distress syndrome. Am Rev Respir Dis 136:730–736, 1987.
4. Wolfson MR, Shaffer TH: Liquid ventilation during early development:theory, physiologic processes and application. J Appl Physiol 13: 1–12, 1990.
5. Gauger PG, Pranikoff T, Schreiner RJ, et al: Initial experience with partial liquid ventilation in pediatric patients with the acute respiratory distress syndrome. Crit Care Med 24:22, 1996.
6. Winternitz MC, Smith GH: Preliminary studies in intratracheal therapy. In: Winternitz MC (ed): Pathology of War Gas Poisoning. New Haven: Yale University Press, 1920, pp 144–160.
7. Neergaard DV: Neue Auffassungen uber einer grundbegriff der atemmechanic. Die retraktionskraft der lunge, abhangug van der oberflachenspannung in den alveolen. Z Gesamte Exp Med 66:373–394, 1929.
8. Clements JA: Surface tension in lung extracts. Proc Soc Exp Biol Med 10:170–172, 1957.
9. Avery ME, Mead J: Surface properties in relation to atelectasis and hyaline membrane disease. Am J Dis Child 97:517–523, 1959.
10. Clements JA, Tierney DF: Alveolar stability associated with altered surface tension. In Clements JA (ed): Handbook of Physiology: Respiration. Bethesda: American Physiological Society, 1964, pp 1565–1583.
11. Mead J, Whittenberger JL, Radford EP: Surface tension as a factor in pulmonary volume-pressure hysteresis. J Appl Physiol 10:191–196, 1957.
12. Kylstra JA, Tissing MO: Fluid breathing. In Boerema I, Brummelkamp WH, Meyne NG (eds): Clinical Applications of Hyperbaric Oxygen. Amsterdam, Elsevier, 1964, pp 371–379.
13. Kylstra JA, Pagenelli CV, Lanphier EH: Pulmonary gas exchange in dogs ventilated with a hyperbarically oxygenated liquid. J Appl Physiol 21:177–184, 1966.
14. Clark LC: Introduction to federation proceedings. Fed Proc 29:698, 1970.
15. Kylstra JA, Schoenfish WH: Alveolar surface tension in the perfluorocarbon-filled lung. J Appl Physiol 33:32–35, 1972.
16. Tham MK, Walker RD, Modell JH: Physical properties of and gas solubilities in selected fluorinated ethers. J Chem Eng Data 18:385–386, 1973.
17. Zander R: O_2-Loslichkeit in fluorocarbonen. Res Exp Med 164:97–109, 1974.
18. Clark LC, Gollan F: Survival of mammals breathing organic liquids equilibrated with oxygen at atmospheric pressures. Science 152:1755–1756, 1966.
19. Moskowitz GD: A mechanical respirator for control of liquid breathing. Fed Proc 29:1751–1752, 1970.
20. Moskowitz GD, Shaffer TH, Dubin SE: Liquid breathing trials and animal studies with a demand-regulated breathing system. Med Instrum 9:28–33, 1973.
21. Shaffer TH, Moskowitz GD: Demand-controlled liquid ventilation of the lungs. J Appl Physiol 36:208–213, 1974.
22. Shaffer TH, Moskowitz GD: An electromechanical demand-regulated liquid breathing system. IEEE Trans Biomed Eng 22:24–28, 1975.
23. Wolfson MR, Tran N, Bhutani VK, et al: A new

experimental approach for the study of cardiopulmonary physiology during early development. J Appl Physiol 65:1436–1443, 1988.

24. Wolfson MR, Durrant JD, Tran NN, et al: The effect of age and oxygenation on the brainstem auditory evoked potential in the immature lamb. In: Jones ET (ed): Fetal and Neonatal Development. Ithaca: Perinatology Press, 1988, pp 229–234.

25. Wolfson MR, Tran N, Bhutani VK, et al: Age related changes in cardiovascular and metabolic function. Fed Proc 44:466, 1985.

26. Richman PS, Wolfson MR, Shaffer TH: Lung lavage with oxygenated perfluorochemical liquid in acute lung injury. Crit Care Med 21:768–776, 1993.

27. Shaffer TH, Douglas PR, Lowe CA, et al: The effects of liquid ventilation on cardiopulmonary function in preterm lambs. Pediatr Res 17:303–306, 1983.

28. Hirschl RB, Parent AP, Tooley R, et al: Liquid ventilation improves pulmonary function, gas exchange and lung injury in a model of respiratory failure. Ann Surg 221:79–88, 1995.

29. Hirschl RB, Overbeck M, Parent A, et al: Liquid ventilation provides uniform distribution of perfluorocarbon in the setting of respiratory failure. Surgery 116:159–168, 1994.

30. Hirschl RB, Tooley R, Parent A, et al: Evaluation of gas exchange, pulmonary compliance and lung injury during total followed by partial liquid ventilation in the acute respiratory distress syndrome. Crit Care Med 24:1001–1008, 1996.

31. Hirschl RB, Mey SI, Montoya JP, et al: Development and application of a simplified liquid ventilator. Crit Care Med 23:157–163, 1995.

32. Gollan F, Clark LC: Prevention of bends by breathing an organic liquid. Trans Assoc Am Physicians 29:102–109, 1967.

33. Harris DJ, Coggin RR, Roby J, et al: Liquid ventilation in dogs: an apparatus for normobaric and hyperbaric studies. J Appl Physiol 54:1141–1148, 1983.

34. Saga S, Modell JH, Calderwood HW: Pulmonary function after ventilation with fluorocarbon liquid P-12F(Caroxin-F). J Appl Physiol 34:160–169, 1973.

35. Modell JH, Newby EJ, Ruiz BC: Long term survival of dogs after breathing oxygenated fluorocarbon liquid. Fed Proc 29:1731–1736, 1970.

36. Modell JH, Hood CI, Kuck EJ, et al: Oxygenation by ventilation with fluorocarbon liquid(FX-80). Anesthesiology 34:312–320, 1971.

37. Calderwood HW, Ruiz BC, Tham MK, et al: Residual levels and biochemical changes after ventilation with a perfluorinated liquid. J Appl Physiol 39:603–607, 1975.

38. Modell JH, Calderwood HW, Ruiz BC, et al: Liquid ventilation of primates. Chest 69:67–81, 1976.

39. Holaday DA, Fiserova-Bergerova V, Modell JH: Uptake, distribution and excretion of fluorocarbon FX-80 (Perfluorobutyl perfluorotetrahydrofuran) during liquid breathing in the dog. Anesthesiology 13:387–394, 1972.

40. Shaffer TH, Wolfson MR, Greenspan JS, et al: Liquid ventilation: uptake, biodistribution and elimination of perfluorocarbon liquid (PFC). Pediatr Res 31:223A, 1992.

41. Greenspan JS, Wolfson MR, Rubenstein SD, et al: Liquid ventilation of human preterm neonates. J Pediatr 117:106–111, 1990.

42. Wolfson MR, Clark LC, Hoffman RE, et al: Liquid ventilation in neonates: uptake, distribution and elimination of the liquid. Pediatr Res 27:37A, 1990.

43. Fuhrman BP, Paczan PR, De Francisis M: Perfluorocarbon-associated gas exchange. Crit Care Med 19:712–722, 1991.

44. Leach CL, Fuhrman BP, Morin FC III: Perfluorocarbon-associated gas exchange in respiratory distress syndrome: a prospective, randomized controlled study. Crit Care Med 21:1270–1278, 1993.

45. Tutuncu AS, Faithfull NS, Lachman B: Comparison of ventilatory support with intratracheal perfluorocarbon administration and conventional mechanical ventilation in animals with acute respiratory failure. Am Rev Respir Dis 148:785–792, 1993.

46. Tutuncu AS, Faithfull NS, Lachman B: Intratracheal perflurocarbon combined with mechanical ventilation in experimental respiratory distress syndrome: dose dependent improvement of gas exchange: Crit Care Med 21:962–969, 1993.

47. Nesti FD, Fuhrman BP, Steinhorn DM, et al: Perfluorocarbon-associated gas exchange in gastric acid aspiration. Crit Care Med 22:1445–1452, 1994.

48. Hirschl RB, Tooley R, Parent AC, et al: Improvement in gas exchange, pulmonary function and lung injury with partial liquid ventilation. Chest 108:500–508, 1995.

49. Hirschl RB, Pranikoff T, Gauger P, et al: Liquid ventilation in adults, children and neonates. Lancet 346:1201–1202, 1995.

50. Hirschl RB, Pranikoff T, Wise C, et al: Initial experience with partial liquid ventilation in adult patients with the acute respiratory distress syndrome. JAMA 275:383–389, 1996.

51. Gauger PG, Pranikoff TP, Schreiner RJ, et al: Initial experience with partial liquid ventilation in pediatric patients with the acute respiratory distress syndrome. Crit Care Med 24:16–22, 1996.

52. Hirschl RB, Conrad S, Kaiser R, et al: Partial liquid ventilation in adult patients with ARDS: a multicenter phase I/II trial. Ann Surg 228:692–700, 1998.

53. Toro-Figueroa LO, Melinoes JN, Curtis SE, et al: Perflubron partial liquid ventilation (PLV) in children with ARDS: a safety and efficacy pilot study. Crit Care Med 24:150A, 1996.

54. Bartlett R, Croce M, Hirschl R, et al: A phase II randomized controlled trial of partial liquid ventilation (PLV) in patients with acute hypoxemic respiratory failure (AHRF). Crit Care Med 25:A35(1), 1997. Presented at the 26th SCCM symposium, 1996, San Diego, CA.

55. Leach CL, Greenspan JS, Rubenstein SD, et al: Partial liquid ventilation with perflubron in in-

fants with severe respiratory distress syndrome. N Engl J Med 335:761–767, 1996.

56. Gross GW, Greenspan JS, Fox WW, et al: Use of liquid ventilation with perflubron during extracorporeal membrane oxygenation: chest radiographic appearances. Radiology 194:717–720, 1995.

57. Greenspan JS, Fox WW, Rubenstein SD, et al: Partial liquid ventilation in critically ill infants receiving extracorporeal life support. Pediatrics 99:E2, 1997.

58. Sargent JW, Seffl RJ: Properties of perfluorinated liquids. Fed Proc 29:1699–1703, 1970.

59. Simons JH (ed): Fluorine Chemistry, vol. I, II, V. New York: Academic Press, 1950.

60. Shaffer TH, Wolfson MR, Clark LC: Liquid ventilation (state of the art review). Pediatr Pulmonol 14:102–109, 1992.

61. West JB, Dolley CT, Matthews CME, et al: Distribution of blood flow and ventilation in the saline-filled lung. J Appl Physiol 20:1107–1117, 1965.

62. Lowe CA, Shaffer TH: Redistribution of pulmonary blood flow in the fluorocarbon-filled lung. Fed Proc 40;587A, 1981.

63. Gauger PG, Overbeck MC, Koeppe RA, et al: Distribution of pulmonary blood flow and total lung water during partial liquid ventilation in acute lung injury. Surgery 122:313–323, 1997.

64. Colton DM, Till GO, Johnson KJ, et al: Partial liquid ventilation decreases albumin leak in the setting of acute lung injury. J Crit Care 13:136–139, 1998.

65. Leach CL, Holm B, Morin FC: Partial liquid ventilation in premature neonates with respiratory distress syndrome: efficacy and compatibility with exogenous surfactant. J Pediatr 126:412–420, 1995.

66. Gauger PG, Overbeck MC, Chambers SD, et al: Partial liquid ventilation improves gas exchange and increases EELV in acute lung injury. J Appl Physiol 84:1566–1572, 1998.

67. Reickert CA, Pranikoff T, Overbeck MC, et al: The pulmonary and systemic distribution and elimination of perflubron from adult patients treated with partial liquid ventilation. Crit Care Med (submitted).

68. Gross GW, Greenspan JS, Fox WW, et al: Use of liquid ventilation with perflubron during extracorporeal membrane oxygenation: chest radiographic appearances. Radiology 194:717–720, 1995.

69. Kazerooni EA, Pranikoff TP, Cascade PN, et al: Partial liquid ventilation with perflubron during extracorporeal life support in adults: chest radiographic appearances. Radiology 198:137–142, 1996.

70. Geyer RP: Whole animal perfusion with fluorocarbon dispersions. Fed Proc 29:1758–1763, 1970.

71. Patel MM, Szanto P, Yates B, et al: Survival and histopathologic changes in lungs of hamsters following synthetic liquid breathing. Fed Proc 29:1740–1745, 1970.

72. Curtis SE, Fuhrman BP, Howland DF: Airway and alveolar pressures during perfluorocarbon breathing in infant lambs. J Appl Physiol 68:2322–2328, 1990.

73. Meinhardt JP, Sawada S, Quintel M, Hirschl RB: Comparison of static airway pressures during total liquid ventilation while applying different expiratory modes and time patterns. Anesthesiology (submitted).

74. Meinhardt JP, Quintel M, Hirschl RB: Development and application of a double piston configured total liquid ventilation device. Crit Care Med (submitted).

74a. Sekins KM, Nugent L, Mazzoni M, et al: Recent innovations in total liquid ventilation system and component design. Biomed Instrument Technol 33:277–284, 1999.

75. Shaffer TH, Lowe CA, Bhutani VK, et al: Liquid ventilation: effects on pulmonary function in distressed meconium-stained lambs. Pediatr Res 18:47–52, 1984.

76. Schaer GL, Buddenmeier KJ, Kelly RF, et al: Perfluorochemical emulsions in myocardial ischemia and infarction: how beneficial and by what mechanism? Presented at the Fifth International Symposium on Blood Substitutes, March 17–20, 1993, San Diego, CA.

77. Smith TM, Steinhorn DM, Thusu K, et al: A liquid perfluorochemical decreases the in vivo production of reactive oxygen species by alveolar macrophages. Crit Care Med 23:1533–1538, 1995.

78. Varani J, Hirschl RB, Dame M, et al: Perfluorocarbon protects lung epithelial cells from neutrophil-mediated injury in an in vitro model of liquid ventilation therapy. Shock 6:339–344, 1996.

79. Dawson SV, Elliott EA: Wave-speed limitation in expiratory flow: a unifying concept. J Appl Physiol 43:498–515, 1977.

80. Dawson SV, Elliott EA: Use of the choke point in the prediction of flow limitation in elastic tubes. Fed Proc 39:2765–2770, 1980.

81. Dawson SV, Elliott EA: Test of the wave-speed theory of flow limitation in elastic tubes. J Appl Physiol 43:516–522, 1977.

82. Schoenfisch WH, Kylstra KA: Maximum expiratory flow and estimated CO_2 elimination in liquid-ventilated dogs lungs. J Appl Physiol 35:117–121, 1973.

83. Koen PA, Wolfson MR, Shaffer TH: Fluorocarbon ventilation: maximal expiratory flow and CO_2 elimination. Pediatr Res 24:291–295, 1988.

84. Lowe CA, Tuma RF, Sivieri EM, et al: Liquid ventilation: cardiopulmonary adjustments with secondary hyperlactatemia and acidosis. J Appl Physiol 47:1051–1056, 1979.

85. Lowe CA, Shaffer TH: Pulmonary vascular resistance in the fluorocarbon-filled lung. J Appl Physiol 60:154–159, 1986.

86. Curtis SE, Fuhrman BP, Howland DF, et al: Cardiac output during liquid (perfluorocarbon) breathing in newborn piglets. Crit Care Med 19:225–230, 1991.

87. Curtis SE, Peek JT, Kelly DR: Partial liquid breathing with perflubron improves arterial oxygenation in acute canine lung injury. Am J Physiol 75:2696–2702, 1993.

88. Parent AC, Overbeck MC, Hirschl RB: Oxygen dy-

namics during partial liquid ventilation in a sheep model of severe respiratory failure. Surgery 121:320–327, 1997.

89. Quintel M, Hirschl RB, Roth H, et al: Computed tomographic assessment of perflubron and gas distribution during partial liquid ventilation for acute respiratory failure. Am J Respir Crit Care Med 158:249–255, 1998.

90. Quintel M, Heine M, Hirschl R, et al: Effects of partial liquid ventilation on lung injury in a model of acute respiratory failure. Crit Care Med 26:833–843, 1998.

91. Thomassen MJ, Buhrow LT, Wiedemann HP: Perflubron decreases inflammatory cytokine production by human alveolar macrophages. Crit Care Med 25: 2045–2047, 1997.

92. Steinhorn DM, Smith TM, Fuhrman BP, et al: Perflubron decreases nitric oxide (NO) production by alveolar macrophages (AM) in vitro. Pediatr Res 37:314A, 1995.

93. Rossman JE, Caty MG, Rich GA, et al: Neutrophil activation and chemotaxis after in vitro treatment with perfluorocarbon. J Pediatr Surg 31:1147–1151, 1996.

94. Colton DM, Hirschl RB, Johnson KJ, et al: Neutrophil infiltration is reduced during partial liquid ventilation in the setting of lung injury. Surg Forum 45:668–670, 1994.

95. Wilcox D, Glick P, Karamanoukian H, et al: Pathophysiology of congenital diaphragmatic hernia V: effect of exogenous surfactant therapy on gas exchange and lung mechanics in the lamb congenital diaphragmatic hernia model. J Pediatr Surg 124:289–293, 1994.

96. Pranikoff T, Gauger P, Hirschl RB: Partial liquid ventilation in newborn patients with congenital diaphagmatic hernia. J Pediatr Surg 31:613–618, 1996.

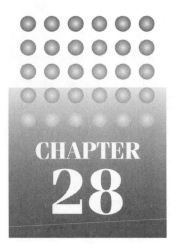

CHAPTER 28

Heliox and Inhaled Nitric Oxide

Dean Hess, PhD, RRT

HELIOX
Physics and Physiology
Clinical Applications
Delivery Systems
INHALED NITRIC OXIDE
Biology of Nitric Oxide
Nitric Oxide in Exhaled Gas
Selective Pulmonary
    Vasodilation

Clinical Applications
Toxicity and Complications
    of Inhaled Nitric Oxide
Delivery Systems for
    Inhaled Nitric Oxide
Monitoring of Nitric Oxide
    and Nitrogen Dioxide
REFERENCES

KEY WORDS

Bernoulli's principle
density
Graham's law

helium
laminar flow
peroxynitrite

Reynolds' number
turbulent flow

Gas mixtures of air and oxygen are usually administered to produce the desired inspired oxygen concentration (FiO_2). However, there may be clinical circumstances in which it is desirable to substitute helium for air. In recent years, there also has been increasing clinical interest in providing very low concentrations of nitric oxide in the inspired gas of some patients. In this chapter, clinical applications of **helium** and **nitric oxide** are discussed.

HELIOX

Physics and Physiology

The physical properties of helium are different from those of air or oxygen.[1] The densi-

ties of helium, air, and oxygen are 0.18, 1.29, and 1.43 kg/m³, respectively. The viscosities of helium, air, and oxygen are 201.8, 188.5, and 211.4 poise, respectively. The **density** and viscosity of heliox (80% helium/20% oxygen) are 0.43 kg/m³ and 203.6 poise, respectively. Note that the density of helium is lower than that for air or oxygen, but its viscosity is higher than air and lower than oxygen. Being an inert gas, helium is nonreactive with body tissues. It is also relatively insoluble in body fluids.

The effect of heliox on gas flow depends on whether the flow is laminar or turbulent. According to Poiseuille's law, **laminar flow** is affected by the radius of the conducting tube (r), the pressure gradient (ΔP), the viscosity of the gas (η), and the length of the conducting tube (l):

$$\dot{V} \cong (\pi\ r^4\ \Delta P)/(8\ \eta\ l)$$

For **turbulent flow**, Poiseuille's law predicts that flow is affected by the radius of the conducting tube (r), the pressure gradient (ΔP), the density of the gas (ρ), and the length of the conducting tube (l):

$$\dot{V}^2 \cong (4\ \pi\ r^5\ \Delta P)/(\rho\ l)$$

Note that turbulent flow is density dependent, whereas laminar flow is density independent. In other words, use of heliox would be expected to have a greater effect on turbulent flow. In fact, heliox might adversely affect laminar flow because it has a greater viscosity than air.

Whether flow is laminar or turbulent is determined by the **Reynolds' number** (Re):

$$Re \cong inertial\ forces/viscous\ forces$$
$$\cong (v\ r\ \rho)/(\eta)$$

where v is velocity of gas movement, r is the radius of the conducting tube, ρ is density, and η is viscosity. A low Reynolds' number causes flow to be laminar. Because of its lower density and higher viscosity, heliox produces a lower Reynolds' number and a greater tendency for laminar flow. Laminar flow is desirable because it is more energy efficient than turbulent flow. According to the Reynolds' number, gas flow tends to be laminar in small peripheral airways of the lungs and turbulent in larger central airways. Therefore, heliox might be expected to have limited benefit for diseases affecting small airways (e.g., emphysema), whereas it might be useful for diseases affecting larger airways (e.g., asthma or postextubation stridor).

For gas flow through an orifice (i.e., axial acceleration), flow has only a weak dependence on the Reynolds' number and is affected by density:

$$\dot{V} \cong \Delta P/\rho$$

In other words, flow through an orifice (e.g.,

constricted airway), increases if the density of the gas decreases (e.g., heliox).[2, 3]

Bernoulli's principle and **Graham's law** are also important relative to heliox therapy. Bernoulli's principle states that the pressure required to produce flow is affected by the mass of the gas:

$$(P_1 - P_2) = (\tfrac{1}{2})(m)(v_2{}^2 - v_1{}^2)$$

where $(P_1 - P_2)$, is the pressure required to produce flow $(v_2{}^2 - v_1{}^2)$, is the difference in velocity between P_1 and P_2, and m is the mass of the gas. In other words, less pressure is required to produce flow with heliox than air or oxygen. Graham's law states that the rate of diffusion is inversely related to the square root of gas density. Thus, heliox diffuses at a rate 1.8 times greater than oxygen. This explains why the flow of heliox through an oxygen flowmeter is 1.8 times greater than the indicated flow.

Clinical Applications

A common use of heliox is to reduce resistance with upper airway obstruction.[4–7] An example of this application is postextubation stridor, most of the evidence for which comes from anecdotal reports. In a double-blind, randomized, controlled, crossover trial, 13 children with postextubation stridor breathed heliox versus oxygen-enriched air.[8] There was a 38% reduction in respiratory distress with heliox breathing, but no significant effect with oxygen-enriched air.

There also have been reports of the use of heliox for the treatment of asthma.[9–16] In spontaneously breathing asthmatic patients, heliox has been reported to decrease arterial partial pressure of carbon dioxide ($PaCO_2$), increase peak flow, and decrease pulsus paradoxus. The reduction in pulsus paradoxus may be particularly important because it reflects a reduction in inspiratory muscle work (Fig. 28–1).[12] Heliox also has been used with intubated and mechanically ventilated asthmatic patients, in whom it has been reported to produce a reduction in $PaCO_2$ with a lower peak airway pressure.[14]

In two case series, an improvement in

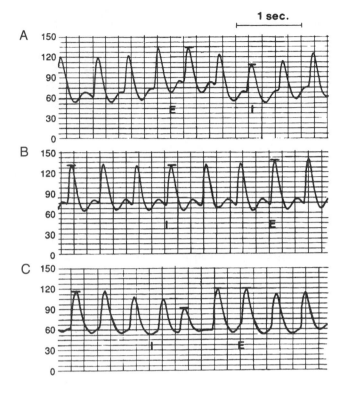

FIGURE 28–1
Radial artery pressure tracings from a patient with severe asthma before (A), during (B), and after (C) the administration of heliox. Note the reduction in degree of pulsus paradoxus with heliox. (From Manthous CA, Hall JB, Caputo MA, et al: Heliox improves pulsus paradoxus and peak expiratory flow in nonintubated patients with severe asthma. Am J Respir Crit Care Med 151:310–314, 1995. © American Lung Association.

oxygenation and dynamic compliance was reported with heliox breathing after cardiac surgery.[17, 18] These reports were uncontrolled and the mechanism is unclear— particularly because relatively low concentrations of helium were used (≤ 40%). In an experimental model, it also has been reported that heliox facilitates the resolution of pneumothorax. However, there has been no clinical confirmation of this effect.[19]

Delivery Systems

For spontaneously breathing patients, heliox is administered by face mask with a reservoir bag (Fig. 28–2).[1] A Y-piece is attached to the mask to allow concurrent delivery of aerosolized medications. Sufficient flow to keep the reservoir bag inflated is required. This is often at least 12 to 15 L/min and requires 3 to 6 cylinders per day.

Heliox administration via mechanical ventilation can be problematic.[1] Ventilators are designed to deliver a mixture of air and oxygen. The different density and viscosity of helium can affect the delivered tidal volume and the measurement of exhaled tidal

volume (Fig. 28–3).[20] For some ventilators (e.g., Puritan-Bennett 7200, Puritan-Bennett, Carlsbad, CA), no reliable tidal volume is delivered with heliox. For other ventilators, there may be a much higher delivered tidal volume than desired. This problem can be circumvented partially by using pressure ventilation rather than volume ventilation. Unlike flow sensors, pressure sensors are not affected by a different gas composition.

The effect of heliox on the ability of the ventilator to correctly monitor flow and tidal volume depends on the method that is used for this measurement. Monitoring devices that are density dependent are inaccurate in the presence of heliox. Devices that use the principle of thermal conductivity also are affected. However, devices that are affected by gas viscosity rather than gas density are affected to a lesser degree because the viscosity of helium is only slightly different from that of air or oxygen. Screen pneumotachometers, such as those used in the Servo 900 and 300 ventilators (Siemens, Danvers, MA), are affected by viscosity rather than density.[21] Thus, the flow sensors in these ventilators are affected to a lesser degree than occurs in other ventilators. The

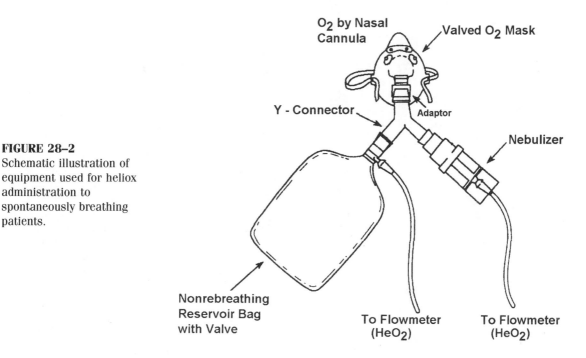

FIGURE 28–2
Schematic illustration of equipment used for heliox administration to spontaneously breathing patients.

O₂ by Nasal Cannula

Valved O₂ Mask

Y - Connector

Adaptor

Nebulizer

Nonrebreathing Reservoir Bag with Valve

To Flowmeter (HeO₂)

To Flowmeter (HeO₂)

accuracy of commonly used bedside respirometers is also affected by heliox. Regardless of the ventilator, extreme caution must be exercised with the delivery of heliox. This should not be attempted unless the clinicians providing this therapy are familiar with the performance of the ventilator with heliox. Unless a volume displacement spirometer is used, exhaled tidal volumes are suspect and likely incorrect. Also, many ventilators waste gas as part of the normal pneumatic function of the device, resulting in gas loss and necessitating frequent cylinder changes.

The FiO_2 requirement of the patient limits the helium concentration that can be administered. If an FiO_2 greater than 0.40 is required, the limited concentration of helium is unlikely to produce clinical benefit. Several studies have reported improved aerosol penetration and deposition in the lungs with the nebulizer powered with heliox rather than air.[22, 23] Heliox can affect nebulizer function, resulting in a smaller particle size, reduced output, and longer nebulization time.[24]

INHALED NITRIC OXIDE

Nitric oxide (NO) is a ubiquitous, highly reactive, gaseous, diatomic radical[25] that is important physiologically at very low concentrations (Table 28–1). Atmospheric concentrations of NO usually range between 10 and 100 ppb and concentrations of 400 to 1000 ppm routinely are inhaled by people who smoke cigarettes.[26, 27] Because it is considered an occupational and environmental pollutant, the Occupational Safety and Health Administration (OSHA) developed exposure limits for NO exposure in the workplace.[28] NO is an important messenger molecule, and many cell types have shown the capacity to produce NO. The action of common nitrosovasodilators (e.g., sodium nitroprusside and nitroglycerin) is a result of their release of NO. NO is present in low concentration in the hospital compressed gas supply, and this may produce physiologic effects in patients breathing this gas.[29, 30] Since the mid 1980s, clinical and academic interest in NO moved from environmental and public health to cellular biology and physiology. Because it is a vasodilator, there is much clinical interest in the use of inhaled NO in the treatment of diseases characterized by pulmonary hypertension and hypoxemia. Although inhaled NO has not yet been approved by the U.S. Food and Drug Administration (FDA) for general use, several large multicenter randomized placebo-controlled studies have been conducted

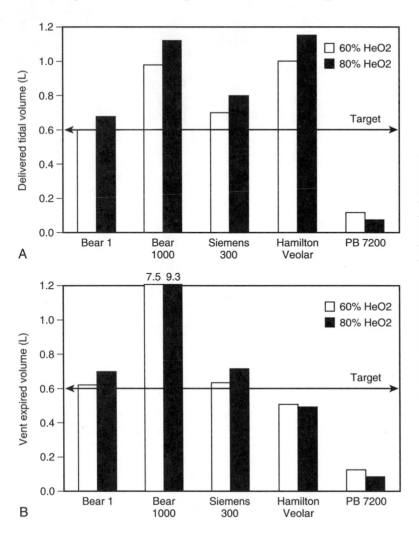

FIGURE 28–3

(A) Delivered tidal volume for five mechanical ventilators with heliox; target tidal volume in each case was 0.6 L. (B) Measured expired tidal volume for five mechanical ventilators with heliox; target tidal volume in each case was 0.6 L. (Data from McArthur CD, Adams AB, Suzuki S: Effect of helium/oxygen mixtures on delivered and expired tidal volume during mechanical ventilation. Am J Respir Crit Care Med 153:A370, 1996.)

or are under way to evaluate the safety and efficacy of inhaled NO.

Biology of Nitric Oxide

L-Arginine is the substrate for NO synthesis in biologic systems (Fig. 28–4).[25] NO is produced in the presence of NO synthase (NOS). It is lipophilic and readily diffuses across cell membranes to adjacent cells, thus serving as a local messenger molecule. NO typically diffuses from its cell of origin to a neighboring cell, where it binds with guanylate cyclase. Activation of guanylate cyclase results in the production of cyclic guanosine 3′,5′-monophosphate (cGMP) from guanosine triphosphate (GTP), which produces a biologic effect within the cell (e.g., smooth muscle relaxation). The time

TABLE 28–1. Concentration of Nitric Oxide and Nitrogen Dioxide Usually Are Expressed in Concentrations of Parts per Million (ppm) or Parts per Billion (ppb)

% = 1/100
ppm = 1/1,000,000
10,000 ppm = 1%
1000 ppb = 1 ppm

between NO production and guanylate cyclase activation is very short because of a half-life of less than 5 seconds for NO in physiologic systems. Inhibitors of guanylate cyclase (e.g., methylene blue) and inhibitors of NOS decrease cGMP levels, whereas inhibitors of phosphodiesterase (e.g., zapri-

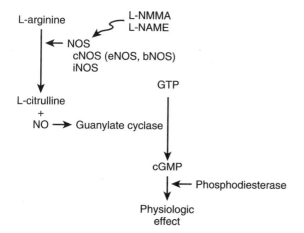

FIGURE 28–4

Biologic pathway for endogenous production of nitric oxide (NO). bNOS, neuronal type constitutive nitric oxide synthase; cGMP, cyclic guanosine 3′,5′-monophosphate; cNOS, constitutive nitric oxide synthase; eNOS, endothelial nitric oxide synthase; GTP, guanosine triphosphate; iNOS, inducible nitric oxide synthase; L-NAME, L-NG-arginine methyl ester; L-NMMA, L-NG-monomethyl arginine; NOS, nitric oxide synthase.

nast or dipyridamole) increase cGMP levels.[31, 32] NO also has cGMP-independent effects. Laboratory studies suggest that inhaled NO has important effects in reducing some forms of lung and tissue injury, including the ability to scavenge oxygen-free radicals, reduce oxygen toxicity, and inhibit platelet and leukocyte aggregation.[25] Early and continued therapy with inhaled NO may be beneficial if these effects are clinically relevant. The cGMP-independent effect of inhaled NO on hemoglobin function may be important in individuals with sickle cell disease.[33]

NOS isoforms are classified as constitutive (cNOS) or inducible (iNOS or type II).[25] cNOS is always present within cells, whereas iNOS is expressed only after induction by stimuli such as cytokines, microbes, or microbial products. There are two forms of cNOS, an endothelial type (eNOS or type III) and a neuronal type (bNOS or type I). Inhibitors of NOS include L-NG-monomethyl arginine (L-NMMA) and L-NG-arginine methyl ester (L-NAME). There is currently much ongoing research into the role of NO in endotoxemia and sepsis. Studies have

shown that NOS inhibitors reverse hypotension during sepsis; however, the clinical benefit of this remains to be determined.

NO is metabolized and excreted via a number of pathways.[25] In oxygen mixtures, it is oxidized to NO_2 and converted to nitric and nitrous acids in aqueous solutions. NO_2 may remain in the lungs for prolonged periods of time because it reacts with water to produce nitric acid and undergoes irreversible reactive absorption by pulmonary epithelial lining fluid.[34] In aqueous solutions, nitric oxide also reacts rapidly with superoxide (O_2^-) to form **peroxynitrite** (**OONO⁻**), which is a strong oxidant that catalyzes membrane lipid peroxidation. NO forms complexes with transitional metal complexes, including those in metalloproteins such as hemoglobin. In tissues, nitrosation of iron-containing enzymes and iron-sulfur proteins of target cells may be responsible for the cytotoxic action of NO generated by activated macrophages. S-Nitrosothiols are formed in plasma and have been identified in human airway lining fluid and in the plasma of healthy subjects and patients inhaling NO mixtures.[35] NO is converted to nitrates and nitrites in plasma and is excreted primarily by the kidney. In the circulation, NO combines extremely rapidly with hemoglobin to form nitrosyl-hemoglobin and then methemoglobin.

Nitric Oxide in Exhaled Gas

Nitric oxide is present in exhaled gas.[36] Measurable levels of NO (7–130 ppb) are present in the nasopharynx. In the paranasal sinuses, NO levels are much higher (approximately 10 ppm), and it has been suggested that the bacteriostatic effects of NO may be responsible for maintaining the sterility of the sinuses.[37] NO in the nasopharynx is inhaled, and much of that is absorbed. When the trachea is intubated, NO levels are reduced in inhaled and exhaled gas.[38] Such reductions of endogenously produced inhaled NO may be associated with small reductions of arterial oxygen pressure (PaO_2), suggesting that inhaled endogenous NO might have a role in the normal regulation of ventilation–perfusion ($\dot{V}/\dot{Q}$). Exhaled levels of NO are increased in inflammatory conditions such as asthma and bronchiectasis[39-44] and may be the result of increased iNOS activity of neutrophils and macrophages.[45-48] Exhaled NO also has been reported to be increased with the hepatopulmonary syndrome.[49] Inhaled steroid therapy appears to decrease exhaled NO levels in asthmatics and patients with bronchiectasis.[40, 41] Levels of exhaled NO have been reported to be decreased in those who are smokers or hypertensive.[50, 51] In experimental animals, exhaled NO has been reported to be increased by sepsis[52] and the administration of positive end-expiratory pressure (PEEP),[53] nitroglycerin, or nitroprusside.[54] The analysis of exhaled NO concentration is complicated because exhaled levels may vary with changes of ventilatory pattern, pulmonary blood flow, and diffusing capacity.[55]

Selective Pulmonary Vasodilation

The term *selective pulmonary vasodilation* is used to indicate two physiologic phenomena (Fig. 28–5).[56] First, selective pulmonary vasodilators reduce pulmonary vascular resistance without affecting systemic vascular resistance. Second, a selective pulmonary vasodilator affects vascular resistance only

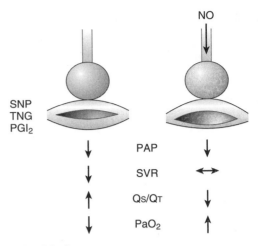

FIGURE 28–6
Physiologic effects of intravenous vasodilators *(left)* compared with the inhaled vasodilator nitric oxide (NO) *(right)*. PAP, pulmonary artery pressure; PGI_2, epoprostenol (prostacyclin); Qs/QT, intrapulmonary shunt fraction; SNP, sodium nitroprusside; SVR, systemic vascular resistance; TNG, nitroglycerin.

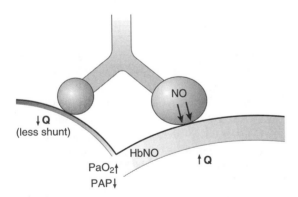

FIGURE 28–5
Because of selective pulmonary vasodilation, inhaled nitric oxide (NO) redistributes pulmonary blood flow from unventilated lung units to ventilated lung units. Inhaled nitric oxide does not produce systemic vasodilation because it is rapidly bound to hemoglobin (Hb). PAP, pulmonary artery pressure.

near ventilated alveoli. Inspired vasodilators are delivered to those lung units that are ventilated. NO is not a selective pulmonary vasodilator per se but becomes one when inhaled. Inhaled NO selectively improves blood flow to ventilated alveoli, which produces a reduction in intrapulmonary shunt and improved oxygenation.[56] The selective pulmonary vasodilation demonstrated by inhaled NO is due in large part to high affinity of hemoglobin for NO, which is approximately 10^6 times as great as the affinity of hemoglobin for O_2. In contrast to inhaled NO, intravenous vasodilators (e.g., sodium nitroprusside, nitroglycerin, prostacyclin) are not selective. Although intravenous vasodilators lower pulmonary artery pressure, they also lower systemic blood pressure (Fig. 28–6). Moreover, these agents increase blood flow to both ventilated and unventilated lung units, resulting in an increased intrapulmonary shunt and a lower PaO_2.[57]

Clinical Applications

Although the use of inhaled nitric oxide is currently investigational, it has been reported for a variety of indications.

Nitric Oxide for Acute Respiratory Distress Syndrome

Acute respiratory distress syndrome (ARDS) is characterized by acute, noncardiogenic respiratory failure, hypoxemia, and bilateral pulmonary consolidations. Regardless of the etiology, a diffuse injury of the alveolar epithelium and endothelium results in intrapulmonary shunt, deadspace ventilation, decreased lung compliance, and pulmonary hypertension. Acute pulmonary hypertension is characteristic of severe ARDS and is independent of cardiac output, hypoxemia, and left atrial hypertension.[58, 59] The etiology of the pulmonary hypertension of ARDS is complex and may be the result of thrombotic vascular occlusion or vascular compression by consolidated areas of the lung. Vasoconstrictor inflammatory mediators and local hypoxia induce a dynamic component of vasoconstriction that may be reversible with pharmacologic treatment. Pulmonary hypertension in ARDS fosters the development of pulmonary edema and increases right ventricular afterload.

Rossaint and associates[60] first reported the use of inhaled NO in 10 patients with ARDS. Inhaled NO reduced pulmonary ar-

tery pressure, increased PaO_2, and decreased shunt. This occurred with no change in systemic arterial blood pressure or any apparent toxicity. This study was followed by others with similar results in both adult and pediatric patients.[61, 62] Bigatello and colleagues[63] showed that during prolonged inhalation of 2 to 20 ppm NO, the mean pulmonary artery pressure was always lower with NO than without NO, the PaO_2 was always higher with NO than without NO, and the mean systemic arterial pressure was not affected by inhaled NO (Fig. 28–7). The inspired NO concentration was reduced in each patient over time, suggesting that tachyphylaxis (severe reaction to a drug) to NO did not occur. Over the first 5 years of experience in 88 patients with severe ARDS at the Massachusetts General Hospital, approximately 60% of the patients had a clinically meaningful response to NO inhalation (i.e., a $\geq 20\%$ improvement of the PaO_2 and/or pulmonary artery pressures),[64] and an initial favorable response to NO was sustained over the first 48 hours of NO inhalation.

In a phase II trial, 177 patients with nonseptic ARDS were enrolled in a multicenter placebo-controlled double-blinded study.[65]

FIGURE 28–7

Individual responses to inhaled nitric oxide (NO) of patients with acute respiratory distress syndrome (ARDS). MAP, mean arterial pressure; MPAP, mean pulmonary artery pressure; $\dot{Q}VA/\dot{Q}T$, venous admixture. (From Bigatello LM, Hurford WE, Kacmarek RM, et al: Prolonged inhalation of low concentrations of nitric oxide in patients with severe adult respiratory distress syndrome: effects on pulmonary hemodynamics and oxygenation. Anesthesiology 80:761–770, 1994.)

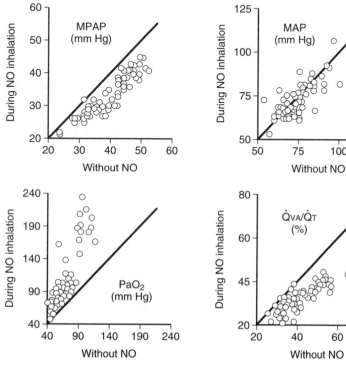

Patients were assigned randomly to receive 0, 1.25, 5, 20, 40, or 80 ppm of inhaled NO. There was a 60% positive response to NO ($\geq$ 20% increase in PaO_2) compared with 24% with placebo. The intensity of mechanical ventilation was lower for patients breathing NO compared with placebo over the first week of therapy. In a subgroup of patients without organ system failure, inhaled NO at 5 ppm was associated with an increased number of days alive and ventilator free through day 28 after initiation of therapy (62% vs. 44%). A phase III trial has been completed comparing 5 ppm of inhaled NO to placebo, but as of this writing the results are unavailable. In contrast to this, a phase III study conducted in Europe (263 patients) reported a mortality rate at 30 days of 45% for patients receiving NO and 38% for patients receiving conventional therapy.[66] There are important differences between the design of these studies. The European study was not blinded, and only patients who were respondents (25% improvement in PaO_2) were randomized. This design excludes the possibility that inhaled NO may have benefits beyond an improvement in oxygenation that might affect outcome. For example, there is evidence that inhaled NO might have beneficial anti-inflammatory effects[67] that might not be reflected in immediate improvement in oxygenation or pulmonary hypertension.

The best dose of inhaled NO for patients with ARDS is not known. However, current evidence suggests that the appropriate dose is low.[68-71] Gerlach and associates reported that the physiologic effects of NO inhalation may be achieved in some patients with ARDS using a very low concentration ($\leq$ 1 ppm).[68] The maximum increase of the PaO_2 occurred between 1 and 10 ppm NO, whereas the maximum pulmonary vasodilation occurred between 10 and 100 ppm NO (Fig. 28–8). The results of the phase II clinical study of inhaled NO for ARDS suggest that the best outcomes occur at 5 ppm.[65]

Variable responses to inhaled NO have been observed and may be related to several physiologic factors. Patients with the greatest degree of pulmonary hypertension respond best to NO inhalation. A favorable response to inhaled NO also has been related to the degree of alveolar recruitment.[72, 73] From the first 5 years of experience with inhaled NO at the Massachusetts General Hospital, the only independent predictor of poor response to inhaled NO was the presence of septic shock.[64] This observation confirms the findings of others who have reported a limited response rate in septic patients with ARDS.[74] The massive release of endogenous NO that contributes to the hypotension of septic shock may impair the pulmonary vasodilator response to exogenous NO. In a lipopolysaccharide (LPS)-induced rat model of acute lung injury, the pulmonary vasodilator response to inhaled NO was impaired, and there was decreased cGMP release into the lung perfusate. This was attributed partly to an increased activity of pulmonary phosphodiesterase.[75]

Nitric Oxide for Hypoxemic Respiratory Failure of the Newborn

Since the early 1990s, several case series have reported the use of inhaled NO for persistent pulmonary hypertension of the newborn (PPHN).[76-91] In addition, a multicenter, randomized, double-blinded study of inhaled NO for PPHN has been conducted.[92] In that study, 58 full-term infants with PPHN were assigned to a control (no NO) or NO (80 ppm) with conventional time-cycled, pressure-limited ventilation. Thirty infants received NO, 53% of whom had a twofold increase in PaO_2. The improvement in PaO_2 was sustained over the treatment duration of 2 to 8.5 days. In the NO group, there was a 40% requirement for extracorporeal life support (ECLS), which was significantly lower than the control group, which had a 71% occurrence. The results of this study establish a role for inhaled NO in term infants with PPHN.

Other causes of hypoxemic respiratory failure in newborns include pneumonia, sepsis, meconium aspiration, and respiratory distress syndrome. A large randomized study conducted by the Neonatal Inhaled Nitric Oxide Study Group compared the use of inhaled NO to conventional therapy in 235 term infants with hypoxemic respiratory failure.[93] The 121 infants randomized

FIGURE 28-8
Dose response of inhaled nitric oxide (NO) for PaO_2 and mean pulmonary artery pressure. ED_{50}, median effective dose; P_{PA}, mean pulmonary artery pressure. (From Gerlach H, Rossaint R, Pappert D., et al: Time-course and dose-response of nitric oxide inhalation for systemic oxygenation and pulmonary hypertension in patients with adult respiratory distress syndrome. Eur J Clin Invest 23:499–502, 1993.)

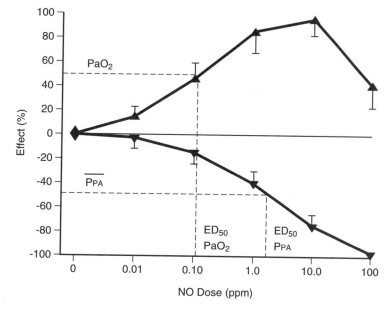

to control therapy were treated with standard treatment strategies, including conventional mechanical ventilation, high-frequency ventilation, and surfactant therapy. The other 114 infants received inhaled NO in addition to standard therapy. The NO group had a 46% incidence of mortality or need for ECLS at 120 days, which was significantly lower than the control group (67% incidence of mortality or need for ECLS). The ECLS requirement was 39% in the NO group and 55% in the control group. Some of the infants did not have an initial response to 20 ppm NO and had no additional response at a dose of 80 ppm. Toxicity was similar in each group. This large and rigorous study established a role for inhaled NO in this patient population.

In some centers, the use of NO has become an important adjunct in the treatment and evaluation of pulmonary hypertension associated with congenital heart disease.[94–97] Inhaled NO has been used to manage pulmonary hypertension in the perioperative period[98–100] and to evaluate pulmonary vascular reactivity in patients with congenital heart disease.[96, 101–103]

Other Applications

Inhaled NO is being investigated as treatment for a number of other indications, in-

cluding primary pulmonary hypertension,[104–106] bronchospasm,[107–109] sickle cell disease,[33] cardiothoracic surgery,[98, 110, 111] and heart or lung transplantation.[112–127]

Toxicity and Complications of Inhaled Nitric Oxide

NO has many effects—some lifesaving, some potentially toxic. With the investigational use of inhaled NO, the issue of iatrogenic toxicity has become clinically important. Inhaled NO has been administered to thousands of patients in hundreds of hospitals around the world as part of investigational protocols since 1991. The toxicity of inhaled NO appears to be low when the drug is used by clinicians familiar with its use. However, a number of potential toxicities and complications should be appreciated by those using this treatment modality.[128]

Direct Toxicity

In very high concentrations, inhaled NO may have direct toxic effects on the lungs. In a patient who died after iatrogenic poisoning with NO (concentration not specified) from a contaminated nitrous oxide cylinder, the lungs at autopsy were edematous and solid.[129] In farmers exposed to high levels of the oxides of nitrogen, silo filler's disease develops, which is characterized by dyspnea, hypoxemia, and pulmonary edema.[130] It should be appreciated, however, that the NO concentrations in these instances are extremely high—much greater than that used therapeutically or stored in therapeutic NO cylinders. NO concentrations as great as 1000 ppm may be present in cigarette smoke,[26, 27] which does not produce acute mortality. Inhalation of 15 to 20 ppm NO for 15 minutes has been reported to produce a small decrease in PaO_2 (mean 7 mm Hg) and an increase in airway resistance in healthy adult volunteers.[131] Breathing 1 ppm NO has produced a small decrease in specific airway conductance in healthy volunteers[132] and 80 ppm inhaled NO decreased airway conductance in subjects with chronic obstructive pulmonary disease (COPD).[133] Whether these effects have any relevance to the administration of inhaled NO to patients with acute respiratory failure is unknown. To date, none of these toxic effects have been reported in patients receiving therapeutic doses of inhaled NO during acute respiratory failure.

Nitrogen Dioxide Production

Nitrogen dioxide (NO_2) is produced spontaneously from NO and O_2. The conversion rate of NO to NO_2 is determined by the O_2 concentration, the square of the NO concentration, and the residence time of NO with O_2.[134] OSHA has set safety limits for NO_2 at 5 ppm,[28] but airway reactivity and parenchymal lung injury have been reported with inhalation of 2 ppm NO_2 or less.[135–141] Although antioxidants present in lung fluids protect healthy individuals from the effects of breathing 2 ppm NO_2,[142] it is prudent to keep the inhaled NO_2 concentration as low as possible because its effects in an injured lung are unknown. There is a potential for conversion of NO to NO_2 in the lungs, although a relatively long residence time is required to produce 2 ppm NO_2 at the NO concentrations typically used in the treatment of ARDS.[134]

Methemoglobinemia

Methemoglobin (metHb) is produced when the iron in heme is oxidized from Fe^{+2} to Fe^{+3}. In the oxidized form, iron cannot bind to O_2 and the affinity of the other heme groups for O_2 increases (i.e., shifts the oxyhemoglobin dissociation curve to the left). Normal methemoglobin is less than 2%, and levels of less than 5% do not require treatment. The normal metHb blood level may be due, in part, to metabolism of endogenous NO. Methemoglobin reductase within erythrocytes converts endogenously produced methemoglobin to normal hemoglobin. Production of methemoglobin after NO exposure has been known for years.[143–147] Methemoglobinemia is uncommon at the NO doses used for therapeutic inhalation ($\leq$ 20 ppm). There have been a few cases of methemoglobinemia reported in association with inhaled NO therapy, generally with high doses of inhaled NO (e.g., 80 ppm).[148, 149] In patients with decreased metHb reductase (e.g., newborns and those with a hereditary deficiency), methemoglobinemia may be more likely. The usual treatment of methemoglobinemia is infusion of methylene blue, which increases NADH metHb reductase. Methemoglobinemia also can be treated with ascorbic acid (vitamin C). Because methylene blue may inhibit the effect of guanylate cyclase, there is concern that methylene blue treatment might counteract the effects of inhaled NO.[150, 151] However, the importance of this effect has been questioned.[152, 153]

Production of Peroxynitrite

In biological systems, NO reacts with O_2^- to produce peroxynitrite: NO + O_2^- → $ONOO^-$.[154, 155] Peroxynitrite is unstable at physiologic pH because it protonates to peroxynitrous acid, which decomposes with a half-life less than 1 second to NO_2 and the hydroxyl radical. The toxicity of O_2^- may be related to its reactivity with NO to produce $ONOO^-$. Superoxide dismutase may prevent the production of $ONOO^-$ by decreasing the availability of O_2^- to react with NO. Many important toxicities of peroxynitrite have been reported.[154] In an autopsy study, high levels of nitrotyrosine were reported in the lungs of patients who died with acute respiratory failure, suggesting peroxynitrite production in human acute lung injury.[156, 157] In contrast, there was little evidence of peroxynitrite formation in the lungs of control subjects who died without acute lung injury. The peroxynitrite in this study was the result of endogenous NO production (the patients were *not* breathing inhaled NO). Virtually nothing is known about the potential intracellular toxicity of inhaled NO at the doses used therapeutically.

Paradoxical Response

Some patients fail to respond to inhaled NO, although this is not necessarily seen as an adverse effect. In patients with ARDS, approximately 40% do not have an initial improvement in PaO_2/FiO_2 or pulmonary vascular resistance of at least 20%. A paradoxical response to inhaled NO in a newborn infant has been reported, in whom there was a worsening of arterial oxygenation and arterial blood pressure with NO doses of 7 and 15 ppm.[158] Worsening of hypoxemia in patients with COPD who received inhaled NO also has been reported[159, 160] and has been attributed to impaired $\dot{V}/\dot{Q}$ matching. This suggests that inhaled NO should be used cautiously in patients in whom hypoxemia is due to $\dot{V}/\dot{Q}$ imbalance rather than shunt.[161]

Platelet Inhibition

Inhibition of platelet adhesion, aggregation, and agglutination has been reported with inhaled NO. When healthy volunteers were exposed to 30 ppm inhaled NO for 15 minutes, bleeding time increased by 33%.[162] In patients with ARDS, platelet aggregation and agglutination were decreased significantly with inhaled NO.[163] However, the antithrombotic effect was not associated with a change in bleeding time. Although it is prudent to consider coagulopathy when deciding to use inhaled NO, the clinical importance of this effect remains unclear. An increased incidence of bleeding diathesis has not been noted in prospective randomized trials of NO inhalation.

Increased Left Ventricular Filling Pressure

Several studies have examined the effects of inhaled NO in patients with left ventricular dysfunction.[164–166] At high doses (40–80 ppm), inhaled NO has been reported to decrease pulmonary vascular resistance and increase pulmonary capillary wedge pressure in some patients with severe left ventricular dysfunction. Presumably, the acute reduction of right ventricular afterload may produce an increase in pulmonary venous return to the left heart. This would increase left ventricular filling pressure and might worsen pulmonary edema. Although this effect may be dose related, inhaled NO should be avoided in patients with severe left ventricular dysfunction (pulmonary capillary wedge pressure ≥ 25 mm Hg). Treatment of the left ventricular dysfunction (e.g., diuretics, inotropes) often corrects the associated pulmonary dysfunction so that a selective pulmonary vasodilator is not necessary.

Rebound Hypoxemia and Pulmonary Hypertension

Withdrawal of inhaled NO has been found to be problematic for some patients. Rossaint and associates reported a decrease in arterial oxygenation and an increase in pulmonary artery pressure (PAP) with daily trials of NO withdrawal (Fig. 28–9).[60] Others have reported worsening hypoxemia and pulmonary hypertension when inhaled NO was discontinued.[167–169] In some cases, the degree of hypoxemia and pulmonary hypertension is greater after discontinuation of NO than at baseline, leading to hemodynamic instability. In a review of 88 patients with ARDS treated with inhaled NO, rebound developed in 5 patients (6%) when inhaled NO was discontinued.[64] All were on high levels of ventilatory support and required vasopressor therapy for septic shock. Reinstitution of NO inhalation promptly corrected the hemodynamic instability, and NO withdrawal was postponed until the patient was less severely ill. The reasons for this rebound effect are not entirely known, but they may relate to feedback inhibition of NOS activity. The following guidelines

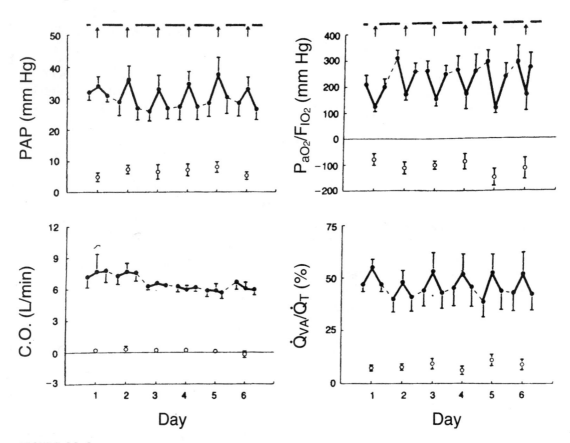

FIGURE 28–9

Response to daily trials of withdraw of inhaled nitric oxide (NO). Note that the pulmonary artery pressure and arterial oxygenation worsens when NO is withdrawn, as indicated by the arrows. C.O., cardiac output; PAP, pulmonary artery pressure; QVA/QT, venous admixture. (From Rossaint R, Falke KJ, Lopez F, et al: Inhaled nitric oxide for the adult respiratory distress syndrome. N Engl J Med 328:399–405, 1993. Copyright Massachusetts Medical Society.)

may help avoid the deleterious effects of rebound during withdrawal of inhaled NO. First use the lowest effective NO dose (5 ppm or less). Second, do not withdraw inhaled NO until the patient's clinical status has improved sufficiently (e.g., FiO_2 = 0.40, PEEP = 5 cm H_2O, hemodynamic stability). Third, increase the FiO_2 to 0.60–0.70 before withdrawal of inhaled NO,[78] and prepare to support the patient's hemodynamics if necessary. Discontinuation of inhaled NO has been well tolerated under these conditions.

Delivery Systems for Inhaled Nitric Oxide

Various delivery systems have been constructed for investigational use in pa-

tients.[56, 134, 170–187] A pipeline delivery system for NO also has been described.[188] Because investigators have used different delivery systems and analysis methods, it is difficult to compare the actual dose administered in various studies. Following are important considerations when building a system for delivery of inhaled NO:

- Dependable and safe system: Complex systems will more likely permit errors that could compromise ventilation, oxygenation, or delivery of the correct NO dose. The function of NO delivery systems must be thoroughly evaluated in the laboratory before patient use.
- Precise and stable NO dose delivery: A precise and stable dose must be delivered to avoid complications associated with in-

haled NO. The dose should not vary with changes in ventilatory pattern or FiO_2.

- Limit NO_2 production: The level of inhaled NO_2 must be kept as low as possible.
- NO and NO_2 monitoring: Inhaled NO must be monitored to ensure that the correct dose is delivered, and inhaled NO_2 must be monitored because of its potentially injurious effects.
- Maintain proper ventilator function: Care must be taken to ensure that adapting the ventilator to deliver NO does not affect its function. The alarm systems should not be affected. The addition of NO lowers the FiO_2, and for that reason, it should be monitored after the site of NO titration into the system (note that it is impossible to deliver 100% O_2 during inhaled NO therapy). There is concern regarding the effect of NO on the internal components of ventilators, blenders, and flowmeters that are exposed to NO. However, damage or malfunction of equipment related to NO exposure has not been reported.

Injection Systems

A simple method to deliver NO is continuous administration into the inspiratory limb of the ventilator circuit. The mean NO concentration delivered to the patient is estimated from the NO flow and the minute ventilation:

$$\text{desired (NO)} = \text{NO flow} \times \text{source (NO)}/\dot{V}_E$$

However, such systems are not recommended for use with adult ventilators, which have phasic flow (i.e., flow only during inspiration). With such systems, the inspiratory circuit fills with NO during expiration and a large bolus of NO is delivered to the patient with the beginning of each breath. The degree of underestimation of the calculated dose with this delivery system is a function of the expiratory time. When expiratory time is short, the delivered NO concentration is lower because of less time for filling the inspiratory limb with NO. This method results in an inspired NO concentration that may be more than double the calculated dose. NO delivery using this method is affected by the inspiratory flow

waveform, by the minute ventilation, and by the site at which NO is titrated into the circuit. Continuous injection does not deliver a stable dose with ventilatory modes such as pressure support ventilation (PSV) or synchronized intermittent mandatory ventilation (SIMV), in which tidal volume and inspiratory time vary from breath to breath (Fig. 28–10). Injection of additional gas into the circuit augments tidal volume during either volume or pressure control ventilation, and triggering of the ventilator is compromised for systems that continuously inject flow into the system. To deliver a more stable NO concentration with continuous injection into the inspiratory limb, mixing chambers can be used. However, mixing chambers adversely affect circuit compression volume.

Systems that inject a continuous flow of NO into the inspiratory circuit are of particular concern during clinical use because the inspiratory circuit fills with O_2-deficient gas during the expiratory phase. The patient may receive a hypoxic gas mixture during the subsequent breath. For example, using an 800-ppm NO source and an NO flow of 300 ml/min (to produce an average NO of 20 ppm with a $\dot{V}_E$ of 12 L/min), the total NO flow during a 5-second period (respiratory rate 12/min) is 25 ml. At a tidal volume of 300 ml, this results in a reduction in FiO_2 of 8%. If the expiratory time is 30 seconds (near apnea) and the subsequent tidal volume is 300 ml, then the FiO_2 is reduced by 50%.

NO may be injected into the ventilator circuit only during the inspiratory phase. This method has been accomplished by using a nebulizer drive mechanism that operates during inspiration. The gas supply to the nebulizer contains the NO required to achieve the desired patient dose after mixing with gas delivered from the ventilator. Because the gas flow from the nebulizer is constant during inspiration, this method delivers a constant NO dose only with constant flow ventilation. It does not work well with varying inspiratory flow patterns such as pressure control (see Fig. 28–10). This system also augments tidal volume delivery from the ventilator and decreases the FiO_2. The major benefit of this method is that

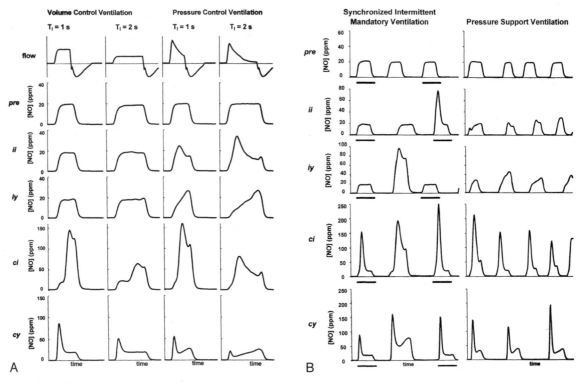

FIGURE 28–10

Nitric oxide (NO) delivery using five delivery systems (pre, premixing system; ii, inspiratory injection of NO into the circuit; iy, inspiratory injection of NO at the Y-piece; ci, continuous injection of NO into the circuit; cy, continuous injection of NO at the Y-piece). Note that only the premixing system delivers a constant NO concentration regardless of the inspiratory flow pattern. (A) Volume control ventilation vs. pressure control ventilation. (B) Synchronized intermittent mandatory ventilation vs. pressure support ventilation. (From Imanaka H, Hess D, Kirmse M, et al: Inaccuracies of nitric oxide delivery systems during adult mechanical ventilation. Anesthesiology 86:676–688, 1997.)

it minimizes NO_2 generation because the residence of NO in an O_2-containing gas mixture is minimized. However, it does not allow precise control of the inspired NO concentration and is only available with a few ventilator systems. For this method to be acceptable, flow from the ventilator must be measured continuously and precisely, and the injected dose of NO must be titrated precisely so that the delivered NO and inspiratory flow waveform are not affected. A case of severe methemoglobinemia (67% metHb) has been reported using this delivery system.[189] This was attributed to very high delivered NO concentrations resulting from a fixed NO injection with variable inspiratory times and tidal volumes during pressure support ventilation. Because of the relatively slow response time of NO ana-

lyzers, these variable high doses were not detected.

If NO is continuously added at the Y-piece, the inspiratory circuit does not fill with NO during the expiratory phase. Instead, the NO bleeds out the expiratory limb of the ventilator during expiration. However, it is not possible to measure the inspired NO concentration with this method, and the dose can be approximated only by mathematical calculation. This system suffers many of the same limitations of NO titration into the inspiratory circuit, such as augmentation of tidal volume, reduction in FiO_2, decreased ability to trigger the ventilator, and changes in delivered NO dose with changes in inspiratory flow and minute ventilation. For this system, NO is injected into the Y-piece during the inspiratory phase. This system functions well when inspiratory flow and minute ventilation are constant. However, when inspiratory flow is not constant (e.g., pressure control ventilation) or minute ventilation varies (e.g., SIMV or PSV), the delivered NO concentration is variable and unpredictable. Like the system that continuously injects NO into the inspiratory circuit, FiO_2 and tidal volume are augmented by the NO gas flow.

Another method that has been used is the administration of a constant flow of NO delivered through the endotracheal tube into the trachea. Problems associated with this method are similar to titration at the Y-piece. In addition, this method is dangerous. During apnea, O_2-free NO gas continues to flow into the trachea and quickly produces hypoxia.

Premixing System

Many articles have described systems to administer inhaled NO to adult mechanically ventilated patients by premixing the NO with N_2 (or air) and introducing the mixture proximal to the gas inlet of the ventilator.[56, 170, 190] These systems typically add the $O_2/N_2/NO$ gas mixture to the low flow inlet of the Servo 900C ventilator or the high pressure air or O_2 inlet of a ventilator such as the Nellcor Puritan-Bennett 7200 (Puritan-Bennett, Carlsbad, CA). A system to accomplish this using the Puritan-Bennett 7200 ventilator has been described (Fig. 28–

11). Using an air/O_2 blender, NO (e.g., 800 ppm) is added to the O_2 inlet of the blender, and N_2 or air is added to the air inlet of the blender. The choice of air or N_2 as the diluent is determined by the extent of NO_2 generation. NO must be mixed with N_2 with high delivered NO doses (> 20 ppm), high FiO_2 (e.g., > 0.90), or low minute ventilation.[134] The gas mixture leaving the blender is delivered to the high pressure air inlet of the ventilator. The final NO concentration delivered to the patient is determined by the FiO_2 settings on the external blender and the ventilator. Although nomograms have been developed to determine the correct blender setting to achieve the desired NO concentration, this always must be confirmed by direct measurement. FiO_2 also must be analyzed because of the effect of NO/N_2 dilution on delivered FiO_2.

Air/O_2 blenders do not always deliver a precise NO concentration. This is particularly problematic when two or more blenders are used in series, which can result in flow from one of the blenders that is less than that required for accurate gas mixing (blenders usually require 15 L/min to be accurate). Although multiple blenders in series can be used to deliver the desired dose, such systems may be superfluous and unnecessarily complex. By their design, it is not possible to stop flow completely from either gas in the blender. In other words, NO is delivered with the blender set at 0.21 (as much as 2 ppm). This creates the illu-

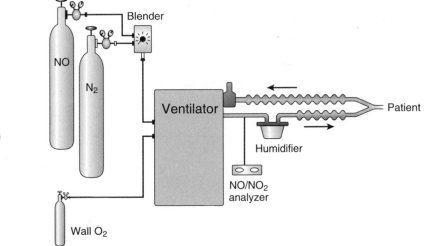

FIGURE 28–11
Schematic drawing of the premixing nitric oxide (NO) delivery system.

sion that NO therapy has been discontinued, which can result in rebound hypoxemia and pulmonary hypertension when the NO delivery system is disconnected from the ventilator. Because most of the NO_2 in the delivery system is produced in the high-pressure hoses, the high-pressure hoses in the NO delivery system should be kept as short as possible to limit NO_2 production.

Premixing before the ventilator is used has the advantage that the NO dose is constant throughout inspiration and is not affected by changes in minute ventilation or flow waveform,[64] but there is a greater NO_2 production with ventilators that have large internal volumes.[134] A soda lime canister placed in the inspiratory limb of the ventilator has been used to absorb NO_2. However, commercially available preparations vary in their ability to remove NO_2, soda lime can absorb NO as well as NO_2, and the canister has the potential to affect ventilator function.[190–193] Although there is a potential for damage to the blender and ventilator because of the NO with this system, this has not been reported. One potential disadvantage of this system is that the NO dose changes when the ventilator FiO_2 setting is changed. However, it is easy to compensate for this by adjusting the setting on the external blender. Another potential issue with this system is the effect of nebulized medications. Depending on how this is accomplished, the nebulizer may affect the delivered NO dose (even for systems that power the nebulizer from the ventilator).

Pediatric Mechanical Ventilation

For continuous-flow ventilators such as those used in pediatrics (including high-frequency oscillators), NO can be titrated into the inspiratory limb of the ventilator circuit (Fig. 28–12).[62, 190] Ideally NO should be titrated into the system near the ventilator outlet for adequate mixing before reaching the patient, and FiO_2 should be analyzed distal to this point of NO introduction into the system. NO_2 generation should be relatively low because the residence time in the system is short. The expected NO can be calculated as:

$$[NO] = (NO \text{ flow} \times \text{source } [NO]) / (NO \text{ flow} + \text{ventilator flow})$$

However, this should be considered an approximation, and the actual delivered NO should be measured. Once the NO is established, the dose should remain constant, provided that the total flow through the system does not change. Gas streaming can occur when NO is infused into a continuous flow of gas.[177, 179] Because of this effect, the highest NO concentration is closest to the tubing wall nearest to the infusion port, and the lowest concentration is between the tubing axis and the tubing further wall. Gas mixing is greater with corrugated tubing than smooth tubing. Gas mixing is virtually complete 12 inches (30 cm) from the point of NO infusion. Thus, it is prudent to infuse NO at least 12 inches (30 cm) from the point of monitoring to avoid dosing errors.

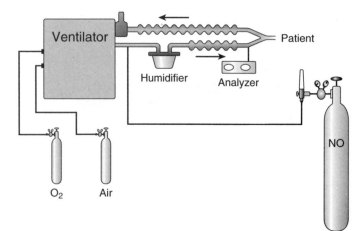

FIGURE 28–12
Schematic drawing of a delivery system for nitric oxide (NO) delivery using a continuous flow pediatric ventilator.

Inhaled NO with high-frequency oscillatory ventilation by titration into the continuous gas stream proximal to the humidifier (injection upstream from the humidifier) is important for best mixing. However, NO delivery by high-frequency jet ventilation is unreliable and should be avoided.[175] The jet ventilator is used in tandem with a conventional ventilator. During jet ventilation, there is no entrainment of NO from the conventional ventilator circuit. When conditions are such that the conventional ventilator interrupts the jet ventilator, large and unreliable concentrations of NO are delivered. Thus, NO should not be delivered by jet ventilation until reliable methods are designed to accomplish this. This is likely to be problematic because of the difficulty of measuring NO distal to the point of gas injection into the airway (i.e., the trachea).

I-NOvent Delivery System

The I-NOvent Delivery System (Datex Ohmeda, Madison, WI) is a universal NO delivery system designed for use with most conventional critical care ventilators.[194, 195] It can be used with either phasic-flow ventilators (e.g., adults) or continuous-flow ventilators (e.g., neonates). In its typical configuration, the delivery system is mounted on a transport cart that holds two NO therapy gas cylinders (Fig. 28–13). The system is configured for 0 to 80 ppm using an 800-ppm cylinder. An integral battery provides 30 minutes of uninterrupted NO delivery in the absence of an external power source. An injection module is inserted into the inspiratory circuit at the outlet of the ventilator. The injection module consists of a hot film flow sensor and a gas injection tube. Flow in the ventilator circuit is measured precisely, and NO is injected proportional to that flow to provide the desired NO dose. This design allows a precise and constant NO concentration in the inspired gas for any ventilatory pattern. NO flows through either a high or a low flow controller. The high and low flow controllers ensure that the delivered NO concentration is accurate over a wide range of ventilator flows and desired NO concentrations. Further, resi-

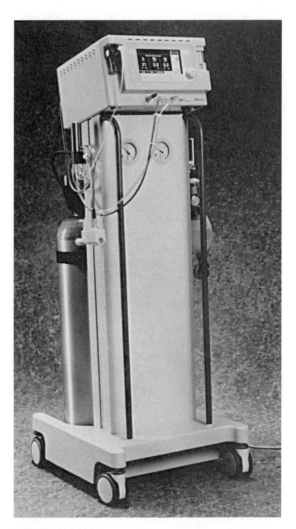

FIGURE 28–13
Ohmeda INOvent Nitric Oxide Delivery System. (Courtesy of Datex Ohmeda, Madison, WI.)

dence time is short and thus NO_2 generation is minimal.

The I-NOvent Delivery System includes gas monitoring of O_2, NO, and NO_2. Gas is sampled downstream from the point of injection near the Y-piece in the inspiratory circuit. Gas concentrations are measured using electrochemical cells that can be calibrated at regular intervals by the user. A number of gas delivery alarms can be set by the user: high NO, low NO, high NO_2, high O_2, and low O_2. Additional alarms include those for loss of source gas pressure, weak or failed electrochemical cells, calibration required, delivery system failures, and monitoring failures. The I-NOvent Delivery System uses a dual-channel design. One channel controls NO delivery, and the other controls monitoring. This design permits NO delivery independent of monitoring, which is an important safety feature. Further, the monitoring system can be calibrated without interruption of NO delivery. A manual NO delivery system is provided by the I-NOvent Delivery System. With an oxygen flow to the manual ventilator set at 15 L/min, I-NOvent injects gas to provide an NO concentration of 20 ppm. As with any manual ventilator system for NO, the bag should be squeezed three to five times to clear residual NO_2 before it is attached to the patient.

Scavenging Issues

There are concerns regarding contamination of the environment with NO and NO_2, and the potential for adverse effects on health care providers.[196] The OSHA exposure limits for NO (a time-weighted average of 25 ppm for 8 hours in the workplace) is higher than the typical NO dose ($\leq$ 20 ppm). In ICU environments that have more than 6 air exchanges/hour, ambient NO levels should remain very low. Ambient NO levels are very low during NO administration (< 0.25 ppm), with or without scavenging (Fig. 28–14).[56, 190] If scavenging is used, it should be constructed so that it does not affect the function of the ventilator or expiratory resistance. Scavenging gases from

the expiratory port of the ventilator does not completely eliminate ambient contamination because the ventilator may internally leak gas (containing NO) as part of its normal operation. Scavenging typically has been achieved by aspiration of expired gases into the hospital vacuum system. Alternatively, expired gas can be passed through a canister of potassium permanganate and charcoal to remove both NO and NO_2.

Monitoring of Nitric Oxide and Nitrogen Dioxide

Although the theoretical dilutions to achieve the desired NO concentration can be estimated, analysis is mandatory to avoid complications resulting from inaccurate dosing. Also, NO_2 should be measured because it may be generated in NO delivery systems and is toxic.

Chemiluminescence techniques measure gas concentrations by stimulated photoemission.[197–199] The sample gas reacts with ozone (O_3) to produce NO_2 with an electron in an excited state (NO_2*). A photon is released in the 600- to 3000-nm wavelength range when the excited electron of NO_2* decays to its basal energy level. This is measured by a photomultiplier tube that proportionately converts the intensity of luminescence into an electrical signal for display. Only a small percentage of NO is converted to NO_2*, and most of it is converted to an

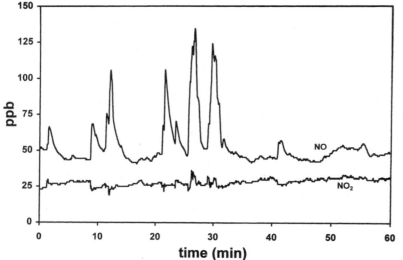

FIGURE 28–14
Ambient nitric oxide (NO) levels with 100 ppm delivered into a patient room at a flow of 8 L/min. Note that the ambient levels remain very low.

unexcited NO_2. The ozone concentration in the reaction chamber exceeds the NO concentration by several orders of magnitude to ensure that NO_2^* production depends only on the NO concentration. NO_2 is measured indirectly by first converting NO_2 to NO and then measuring the total NO concentration. The conversion of NO_2 to NO requires a high-efficiency converter. Thermal catalytic converters are made of high-grade stainless steel and operate at 600° to 800°C. Chemical converters typically use molybdenum or carbon to achieve NO_2 conversion at lower temperatures. Chemical converters tend to be more stable and less subject to interference from other gas species but gradually are consumed by the reaction and must be replenished periodically. The reaction chamber is operated at a subatmospheric pressure to minimize the effects of variations in background gas composition. The NO_2 concentration is the difference between the total nitrogen oxides measured (NOx) and the NO concentration.

The accuracy of chemiluminescence analyzers is subject to quenching. Quenching is the conversion of NO_2^* within the converter to NO_2 by random collisions with other gas molecules. The degree of quenching is determined by the composition of the background gas. The gases O_2, CO_2, and H_2O are known to quench NO_2^* photoemissions to a greater extent than N_2, resulting in a false reduction of the measured NO concentration.[200] Water vapor produces the greatest quenching on a percent basis. O_2 causes less quenching of the NO signal but may have a profound impact on accuracy because it is present in high concentrations. An O_2 concentration near 100% reduces the NO signal by 7% to 15% and the NOx signal by 15% to 26% with a stainless steel reaction chamber. Quenching takes place in all analyzers but is most problematic with stainless steel chambers. With the stainless steel chamber, NO_2 quenching exceeds NO quenching, producing low or negative NO_2 concentrations. Therefore, NO_2 measurements at high oxygen concentrations are unreliable and should be corrected for the known quenching of the analyzer. Although quenching also occurs with molybdenum converters,

the NO and NOx signals are affected equally.

Electrochemical techniques for detection of NO and NO_2 are based on the principle that these gases react with electrolyte solutions.[197, 198, 201–204] Electrons are liberated or consumed, generating a current between two polarized electrodes in proportion to the concentration of NO or NO_2 in the sample gas. Electrochemical analyzers are similar to polarographic electrodes. These cells contain a semipermeable membrane and three electrodes submerged in an electrolyte. Although the electrolyte composition, the electrode configuration, and the type of diffusion barrier differ among manufacturers, these analyzers all share the same principles. The diffusion barrier allows limited passage of sample gas into the electrolyte bath. NO then reacts with the electrolyte solution at the sensing electrode. The electrolyte solution is a highly conductive concentrated acid or alkali solution and is constrained in a material (plastic or glass mesh) that prevents movement of the electrolyte. The counter electrode is further from the membrane and is exposed to much lower concentrations of NO and NO_2. The reference electrode provides a bias voltage by applying an external potential so that the sensing electrode is kept at the correct operating voltage. The sensor is connected to a low impedance circuit that measures current flow (proportional to the NO/NO_2 concentration of the sample gas) by measuring voltage across a resistance. The accuracy of electrochemical analyzers has been found acceptable in the range used clinically. Temperature can affect the background zero current in electrochemical sensors and cause zero current drift. However, this is not an important issue in the temperature range of 20° to 40°C. The accuracy of some electrochemical analyzers is affected by pressure, which is an important consideration in mechanical ventilation systems. The effects of pressure on the analyzer can be reduced by using a sidestream sampling technique that exposes the cell to the same pressure at all times.

REFERENCES

1. Manthous CA, Morgan S, Pohlman A, et al: Heliox in the treatment of airflow obstruction: a

critical review of the literature. Respir Care 42:1034–1042, 1997.

2. Eisenkraft JB, Barker SJ: Helium and gas flow. Anesth Analg 76:452–453, 1993.

3. Papamoschou D: Theoretical validation of the respiratory benefits of helium-oxygen mixtures. Respir Physiol 99:183–190, 1995.

4. Skrinskas GJ, Hyland RH, Hutcheon MA: Using helium–oxygen mixtures in the management of acute upper airway obstruction. Can Med Assoc J 128:555–558, 1983.

5. Lu TS, Ohmura A, Wong KC, et al: Helium-oxygen in treatment of upper airway obstruction. Anesthesiology 45:678–680, 1976.

6. Curtis JL, Mahlmeister M, Fink JB, et al: Helium–oxygen gas therapy: use and availability for the emergency treatment of inoperable airway obstruction. Chest 90:455–457, 1986.

7. Boorstein JM, Boorstein SM, Humphries GN, et al: Using helium–oxygen mixtures in the emergency management of acute upper airway obstruction. Ann Emerg Med 18:688–690, 1989.

8. Kemper KJ, Ritz RH, Benson MS, et al: Helium-oxygen mixture in the treatment of postextubation stridor in pediatric trauma patients. Crit Care Med 19:356–359, 1991.

9. Martin-Barbaz F, Barnoud D, Carpendier F, et al: Use of helium and oxygen mixtures in status asthmaticus. Rev Pneumol Clin 43:186–189, 1987.

10. Shiue ST, Gluck EH: The use of helium–oxygen mixtures in the support of patients with status asthmaticus and respiratory acidosis. J Asthma 26:177–180, 1989.

11. Kass JE, Castriotta RJ: Heliox therapy in acute severe asthma. Chest 107:757–760, 1995.

12. Manthous CA, Hall JB, Caputo MA, et al: Heliox improves pulsus paradoxus and peak expiratory flow in nonintubated patients with severe asthma. Am J Respir Crit Care Med 151:310–314, 1995.

13. Kudukis TM, Manthous CA, Schmidt GA, et al: Inhaled helium–oxygen revisited: effect of helium–oxygen during the treatment of status asthmaticus in children. J Pediatr 130:217–224, 1997.

14. Gluck EH, Onorato DJ, Castriotta R: Helium-oxygen mixtures in intubated patients with status asthmaticus and respiratory acidosis. Chest 98:693–698, 1990.

15. Carter ER, Webb CR, Moffitt DR: Evaluation of heliox in children hospitalized with acute severe asthma: a randomized crossover trial. Chest 109:1256–1261, 1996.

16. Austan F: Heliox inhalation in status asthmaticus and respiratory acidemia: a brief report. Heart Lung 25:155–157, 1996.

17. Yahagi N, Kumon K, Haruna M, et al: Helium/oxygen breathing improves hypoxemia after cardiac surgery. Artif Organs 21:24–27, 1997.

18. Yahagi N, Kumon K, Tanigami H, et al: Helium/oxygen breathing improved hypoxemia after cardiac surgery: case reports. Anesth Analg 80:1042–1045, 1995.

19. Barr J, Lushkov G, Starinsky R, et al: Heliox therapy for pneumothorax: new indication for an old remedy. Ann Emerg Med 30:159–162, 1997.

20. McArthur CD, Adams AB, Suzuki S: Effect of helium/oxygen mixtures on delivered and expired tidal volume during mechanical ventilation. Am J Respir Crit Care Med 153:A370, 1996.

21. Kirmse M, Hess D, Imanaka H, et al: Accurate tidal volume delivery during mechanical ventilation with helium/oxygen mixtures. Respir Care 41:954, 1996.

22. Svartengren M, Anderson M, Philipson K, et al: Human lung deposition of particles suspended in air or in helium/oxygen mixture. Exp Lung Res 15:575–585, 1989.

23. Anderson M, Svartengren M, Bylin G, et al: Deposition in asthmatics of particles inhaled in air or in helium–oxygen. Am Rev Respir Dis 147:524–528, 1993.

24. Acosta FL, Camargo CA, Ritz RH, et al: Effect of heliox on nebulizer function. Chest 112:11S, 1997.

25. Hurford WE: The biological basis for inhaled nitric oxide. Respir Care Clin North Am 3:357–369, 1997.

26. Dupuy PM, Lancon JP, Francoise M, et al: Inhaled cigarette smoke selectively reverses human hypoxic vasoconstriction. Intensive Care Med 21:941–944, 1995.

27. Norman V, Keith CH: Nitrogen oxides in tobacco smoke. Durham: Liggett and Myers Tobacco Co, 1965.

28. Anonymous: NIOSH recommendations for occupational safety and health standards, 1988. MMWR Morb Mortal Wkly Rep 37:1–29, 1988.

29. Lee KH, Tan PS, Rico P, et al: Low levels of nitric oxide as contaminant in hospital compressed air: physiologic significance? Crit Care Med 25:1143–1146, 1997.

30. Pinsky MR, Genc F, Lee KH, et al: Contamination of hospital compressed air with nitric oxide: unwitting replacement therapy. Chest 111:1759–1763, 1997.

31. al-Alaiyan S, al-Omran A, Dyer D: The use of phosphodiesterase inhibitor (dipyridamole) to wean from inhaled nitric oxide. Intensive Care Med 22:1093–1095, 1996.

32. Ichinose F, Adrie C, Hurford WE, et al: Prolonged pulmonary vasodilator action of inhaled nitric oxide by zaprinast in awake lambs. J Appl Physiol 78:1288–1295, 1995.

33. Head CA, Brugnara C, Martinez-Ruiz R, et al: Low concentrations of nitric oxide increase oxygen affinity of sickle erythrocytes in vitro and in vivo. J Clin Invest 100:1193–1198, 1997.

34. Postlethwait EM, Langford SD, Bidani A: Kinetics of NO_2 air space absorption in isolated rat lungs. J Appl Physiol 1973:1939–1945, 1992.

35. Stamler JS, Jaraki O, Osborne J, et al: Nitric oxide circulates in mammalian plasma primarily as an S-nitroso adduct of serum albumin. Proc Natl Acad Sci USA 89:7674–7677, 1992.

36. Lundberg JO, Weitzberg E, Lundberg JM, et al: Nitric oxide in exhaled air. Eur Respir J 9:2671–2680, 1996.

37. Lundberg JO, Farkas-Szallasi T, Weitzberg E, et al: High nitric oxide production in human paranasal sinuses. Nat Med 1:370–373, 1995.
38. Gerlach H, Rossaint R, Pappert D, et al: Autoinhalation of nitric oxide after endogenous synthesis in nasopharynx. Lancet 343:518–519, 1994.
39. Alving K, Fornhem C, Lundberg JM: Pulmonary effects of endogenous and exogenous nitric oxide in the pig: relation to cigarette smoke inhalation. Br J Pharmacol 110:739–746, 1993.
40. Kharitonov SA, Yates D, Robbins RA, et al: Increased nitric oxide in exhaled air of asthmatic patients. Lancet 343:133–135, 1994.
41. Kharitonov SA, O'Connor BJ, Evans DJ, et al: Allergen-induced late asthmatic reactions are associated with elevation of exhaled nitric oxide. Am J Respir Crit Care Med 151:1894–1899, 1995.
42. Kharitonov SA, Wells AU, O'Connor BJ, et al: Elevated levels of exhaled nitric oxide in bronchiectasis. Am J Respir Crit Care Med 151:1889–1893, 1995.
43. Persson MG, Zetterstrom O, Agrenius V, et al: Single-breath nitric oxide measurements in asthmatic patients and smokers. Lancet 343:146–147, 1994.
44. Alving K, Weitzberg E, Lundberg JM: Increased amount of nitric oxide in exhaled air of asthmatics. Eur Respir J 6:1368–1370, 1993.
45. Massaro AF, Mehta S, Lilly CM, et al: Elevated nitric oxide concentrations in isolated lower airway gas of asthmatic subjects. Am J Respir Crit Care Med 153:1510–1514, 1996.
46. Tsujino I, Miyamoto K, Nishimura M, et al. Production of nitric oxide (NO) in intrathoracic airways of normal humans. Am J Respir Crit Care Med 154:1370–1374, 1996.
47. Kharitonov SA, Chung KF, Evans D, et al: Increased exhaled nitric oxide in asthma is mainly derived from the lower respiratory tract. Am J Respir Crit Care Med 153:1773–1780, 1996.
48. Silkoff PE, McClean PA, Slutsky AS, et al: Marked flow-dependence of exhaled nitric oxide using a new technique to exclude nasal nitric oxide. Am J Respir Crit Care Med 155:260–267, 1997.
49. Cremona G, Higenbottam TW, Mayoral V, et al: Elevated exhaled nitric oxide in patients with hepatopulmonary syndrome. Eur Respir J 8:1883–1885, 1995.
50. Persson MG, Agvald P, Gustafsson LE: Detection of nitric oxide in exhaled air during administration of nitroglycerin in vivo. Br J Pharmacol 111:825–828, 1994.
51. Schilling J, Holzer P, Guggenbach M, et al: Reduced endogenous nitric oxide in the exhaled air of smokers and hypertensives. Eur Respir J 7:467–471, 1994.
52. Stewart TE, Valenza F, Ribeiro SP, et al: Increased nitric oxide in exhaled gas as an early marker of lung inflammation in a model of sepsis. Am J Respir Crit Care Med 151:713–718, 1995.
53. Persson MG, Lonnqvist PA, Gustafsson LE: Positive end-expiratory pressure ventilation elicits increases in endogenously formed nitric oxide as detected in air exhaled by rabbits. Anesthesiology 82:969–974, 1995.
54. Husain M, Adrie C, Ichinose F, et al: Exhaled nitric oxide as a marker for organic nitrate tolerance. Circulation 89:2498–2502, 1994.
55. Hyde RW, Geigel EJ, Olszowka AJ, et al: Determination of production of nitric oxide by lower airways of humans—theory. J Appl Physiol 82:1290–1296, 1997.
56. Hess D, Bigatello L, Kacmarek RM, et al: Use of inhaled nitric oxide in patients with acute respiratory distress syndrome. Respir Care 41:424–446, 1996.
57. Wood G: Effect of antihypertensive agents on the arterial partial pressure of oxygen and venous admixture after cardiac surgery. Crit Care Med 25:1807–1812, 1997.
58. Zapol WM, Jones R: Vascular components of ARDS: clinical pulmonary hemodynamics and morphology. Am Rev Respir Dis 136:471–474, 1987.
59. Zapol WM, Snider MT: Pulmonary hypertension in severe acute respiratory failure. N Engl J Med 296:476–480, 1977.
60. Rossaint R, Falke KJ, Lopez F, et al: Inhaled nitric oxide for the adult respiratory distress syndrome. N Engl J Med 328:399–405, 1993.
61. Bigatello LM, Hurford WE, Hess D: Use of inhaled nitric oxide for ARDS. Respir Care Clin North Am 3:437–458, 1997.
62. Betit P: Nitric oxide administration during pediatric mechanical ventilation. Respir Care Clin North Am 2:587–605, 1996.
63. Bigatello LM, Hurford WE, Kacmarek RM, et al: Prolonged inhalation of low concentrations of nitric oxide in patients with severe adult respiratory distress syndrome: effects on pulmonary hemodynamics and oxygenation. Anesthesiology 80:761–770, 1994.
64. Manktelow C, Bigatello LM, Hess D, et al: Physiologic determinants of the response to inhaled nitric oxide in patients with acute respiratory distress syndrome. Anesthesiology 87:297–307, 1997.
65. Dellinger RP, Zimmerman JL, Taylor RW, et al: Inhaled nitric oxide in patients with acute respiratory distress syndrome: results of a randomized phase II trial. Crit Care Med 26:15–23, 1998.
66. Lundin S, Mang H, Smithies M, et al: Inhalation of nitric oxide in acute lung injury: preliminary results of a European multicenter study. Intensive Care Med 23:S2, 1997.
67. Chollet-Martin S, Gatecel C, Kermarrec N, et al: Alveolar neutrophil functions and cytokine levels in patients with the adult respiratory distress syndrome during nitric oxide inhalation. Am J Respir Crit Care Med 153:985–990, 1996.
68. Gerlach H, Rossaint R, Pappert D, et al: Time-course and dose-response of nitric oxide inhalation for systemic oxygenation and pulmonary hypertension in patients with adult respiratory distress syndrome. Eur J Clin Invest 23:499–502, 1993.

69. Demirakca S, Dotsch J, Knothe C, et al: Inhaled nitric oxide in neonatal and pediatric acute respiratory distress syndrome: dose response, prolonged inhalation, and weaning. Crit Care Med 24:1913–1919, 1996.

70. Lowson SM, Rich GF, McArdle PA, et al: The response of varying concentrations of inhaled nitric oxide in patients with acute respiratory distress syndrome. Anesth Analg 82:574–581, 1996.

71. Nakagawa TA, Morris A, Gomez RJ, et al: Dose response to inhaled nitric oxide in pediatric patients with pulmonary hypertension and acute respiratory distress syndrome. J Pediatr 131:63–69, 1997.

72. Putensen C, Rasanen J, Lopez FA, et al: Continuous positive airway pressure modulates effect of inhaled nitric oxide on the ventilation-perfusion distributions in canine lung injury. Chest 106:1563–1569, 1994.

73. Puybasset L, Rouby JJ, Mourgeon E, et al: Factors influencing cardiopulmonary effects of inhaled nitric oxide in acute respiratory failure. Am J Respir Crit Care Med 152:318–328, 1995.

74. Krafft P, Fridrich P, Fitzgerald RD, et al: Effectiveness of nitric oxide inhalation in septic ARDS. Chest 109:486–493, 1996.

75. Holzmann A, Bloch KD, Sanchez LS, et al: Hyporesponsiveness to inhaled nitric oxide in isolated, perfused lungs from endotoxin-challenged rats. Am J Physiol 271:L981–L986, 1996.

76. Abman SH, Kinsella JP, Schaffer MS, et al: Inhaled nitric oxide in the management of a premature newborn with severe respiratory distress and pulmonary hypertension. Pediatrics 92:606–609, 1993.

77. Abman SH, Kinsella JP: Inhaled nitric oxide for persistent pulmonary hypertension of the newborn: the physiology matters. Pediatrics 96:1153–1155, 1995.

78. Aly H, Sahni R, Wung JT: Weaning strategy with inhaled nitric oxide treatment in persistent pulmonary hypertension of the newborn. Arch Dis Child 76:F118–F122, 1997.

79. Buhrer C, Merker G, Falke K, et al: Dose-response to inhaled nitric oxide in acute hypoxemic respiratory failure of newborn infants: a preliminary report. Pediatr Pulmonol 19:291–298, 1995.

80. Day RW, Lynch JM, White KS, et al: Acute response to inhaled nitric oxide in newborns with respiratory failure and pulmonary hypertension. Pediatrics 98:698–705, 1996.

81. Fineman JR, Zwass MS: Inhaled nitric oxide therapy for persistent pulmonary hypertension of the newborn. Acta Paediatrica Japonica 37:425–430, 1995.

82. Goldman AP, Tasker RC, Haworth SG, et al: Four patterns of response to inhaled nitric oxide for persistent pulmonary hypertension of the newborn. Pediatrics 98:706–713, 1996.

83. Hoffman GM, Ross GA, Day SE, et al: Inhaled nitric oxide reduces the utilization of extracorporeal membrane oxygenation in persistent pulmonary hypertension of the newborn. Crit Care Med 25:352–359, 1997.

84. Kinsella JP, Shaffer E, Neish SR, et al: Low-dose inhalational nitric oxide in persistent pulmonary hypertension of the newborn. Lancet 340:8819–8820, 1992.

85. Kinsella JP, Neish SR, Ivy DD, et al: Clinical responses to prolonged treatment of persistent pulmonary hypertension of the newborn with low doses of inhaled nitric oxide. J. Pediatr 123:103–108, 1993.

86. Kinsella JP, Abman SH: Clinical pathophysiology of persistent pulmonary hypertension of the newborn and the role of inhaled nitric oxide therapy. J Perinatol 16:S24–S27, 1996.

87. Kinsella JP, Truog WE, Walsh WF, et al: Randomized, multicenter trial of inhaled nitric oxide and high-frequency oscillatory ventilation in severe, persistent pulmonary hypertension of the newborn. J Pediatr 131:55–62, 1997.

88. Muller W, Kachel W, Lasch P, et al: Inhaled nitric oxide for avoidance of extracorporeal membrane oxygenation in the treatment of severe persistent pulmonary hypertension of the newborn. Intensive Care Med 22:71–76, 1996.

89. Roberts JD, Polaner DM, Lang P, et al: Inhaled nitric oxide in persistent pulmonary hypertension of the newborn. Lancet 340:818–819, 1992.

90. Roberts JD Jr: Inhaled nitric oxide for treatment of pulmonary artery hypertension in the newborn and infant. Crit Care Med 21:S374–S376, 1993.

91. Turbow R, Waffarn F, Yang L, et al: Variable oxygenation response to inhaled nitric oxide in severe persistent pulmonary hypertension of the newborn. Acta Paediatr 84:1305–1308, 1995.

92. Roberts JD Jr, Fineman JR, Morin FC, et al: Inhaled nitric oxide and persistent pulmonary hypertension of the newborn: the Inhaled Nitric Oxide Study Group. N Engl J Med 336:605–610, 1997.

93. Anonymous: Inhaled nitric oxide in full-term and nearly full-term infants with hypoxic respiratory failure: the Neonatal Inhaled Nitric Oxide Study Group. N Engl J Med 336:597–604, 1997.

94. Okamoto K, Sato T, Kurose M, et al: Successful use of inhaled nitric oxide for treatment of severe hypoxemia in an infant with total anomalous pulmonary venous return. Anesthesiology 81:256–259, 1994.

95. Morris GN, Lowson SM, Rich GF: Transient effects of inhaled nitric oxide for prolonged postoperative treatment of hypoxemia after surgical correction of total anomalous pulmonary venous return. J Cardiovasc Vasc Anesth 9:713–716, 1995.

96. Roberts JD Jr, Lang P, Bigatello LM, et al: Inhaled nitric oxide in congenital heart disease. Circulation 87:447–453, 1993.

97. Matsui J, Yahagi N, Kumon K, et al: Effects of inhaled nitric oxide on postoperative pulmonary circulation in patients with congenital heart disease. Artif Organs 21:17–20, 1997.

98. Wessel DL: Inhaled nitric oxide for the treatment of pulmonary hypertension before and after cardiopulmonary bypass. Crit Care Med 21:S344–S345, 1993.

99. Journois D, Pouard P, Mauriat P, et al: Inhaled nitric oxide as a therapy for pulmonary hypertension after operations for congenital heart defects. J Thorac Cardiovasc Surg 107:1129–1135, 1994.

100. Beghetti M, Habre W, Friedli B, et al: Continuous low dose inhaled nitric oxide for treatment of severe pulmonary hypertension after cardiac surgery in paediatric patients. Br Heart J 73:65–68, 1995.

101. Berner M, Beghetti M, Spahr-Schopfer I, et al: Inhaled nitric oxide to test the vasodilator capacity of the pulmonary vascular bed in children with long-standing pulmonary hypertension and congenital heart disease. Am J Cardiol 77:532–535, 1996.

102. Winberg P, Lundell BP, Gustafsson LE: Effect of inhaled nitric oxide on raised pulmonary vascular resistance in children with congenital heart disease. Br Heart J 71:282–286, 1994.

103. Atz AM, Adatia I, Jonas RA, et al: Inhaled nitric oxide in children with pulmonary hypertension and congenital mitral stenosis. Am J Cardiol 77:316–319, 1996.

104. Sitbon O, Brenot F, Denjean A, et al: Inhaled nitric oxide as a screening vasodilator agent in primary pulmonary hypertension: a dose-response study and comparison with prostacyclin. Am J Respir Crit Care Med 151:384–389, 1995.

105. Channick RN, Newhart JW, Johnson FW, et al: Pulsed delivery of inhaled nitric oxide to patients with primary pulmonary hypertension: an ambulatory delivery system and initial clinical tests. Chest 109:1545–1549, 1996.

106. Snell GI, Salamonsen RF, Bergin P, et al: Inhaled nitric oxide used as a bridge to heart–lung transplantation in a patient with end-stage pulmonary hypertension. Am J Respir Crit Care Med 151:1263–1266, 1995.

107. Brown RH, Zerhouni EA, Hirshman CA: Reversal of bronchoconstriction by inhaled nitric oxide: histamine versus methacholine. Am J Respir Crit Care Med 150:233–237, 1994.

108. Kacmarek RM, Ripple R, Cockrill BA, et al: Inhaled nitric oxide: a bronchodilator in mild asthmatics with methacholine-induced bronchospasm. Am J Respir Crit Care Med 153:128–135, 1996.

109. Sanna A, Kurtansky A, Veriter C, et al: Bronchodilator effect of inhaled nitric oxide in healthy men. Am J Respir Crit Care Med 150:1702–1704, 1994.

110. Bichel T, Spahr-Schopfer I, Berner M, et al: Successful weaning from cardiopulmonary bypass after cardiac surgery using inhaled nitric oxide. Paediatr Anaesth 7:335–339, 1997.

111. Fullerton DA, McIntyre RC Jr: Inhaled nitric oxide: therapeutic applications in cardiothoracic surgery. Ann Thorac Surg 61:1856–1864, 1996.

112. Adatia I, Lillehei C, Arnold JH, et al: Inhaled nitric oxide in the treatment of postoperative graft dysfunction after lung transplantation. Ann Thorac Surg 57:1311–1318, 1994.

113. Adatia I, Perry S, Landzberg M, et al: Inhaled nitric oxide and hemodynamic evaluation of patients with pulmonary hypertension before transplantation. J Am Coll Cardiol 25:1656–1664, 1995.

114. Auler JJO, Carmona MJ, Bocchi EA, et al: Low doses of inhaled nitric oxide in heart transplant recipients. J Heart Lung Transplant 15:443–450, 1996.

115. Bacha EA, Herve P, Murakami S, et al: Lasting beneficial effect of short-term inhaled nitric oxide on graft function after lung transplantation. J Thorac Cardiovasc Surg 112:590–598, 1996.

116. Bacha EA, Sellak H, Murakami S, et al: Inhaled nitric oxide attenuates reperfusion injury in non-heartbeating-donor lung transplantation. Transplantation 63:1380–1386, 1997.

117. Barzaghi N, Olivei M, Minzioni G, et al: ECMO and inhaled nitric oxide for cardiopulmonary failure after heart retransplantation. Ann Thorac Surg 63:533–535, 1997.

118. Foubert L, Latimer R, Oduro A, et al: Use of inhaled nitric oxide to reduce pulmonary hypertension after heart transplantation. J Cardiovasc Vasc Anesth 7:506–507, 1993.

119. George SJ, Boscoe MJ: Inhaled nitric oxide for right ventricular dysfunction following cardiac transplantation. Br J Clin Pract 51:53–55, 1997.

120. Kieler-Jensen N, Ricksten SE, Stenqvist O, et al: Inhaled nitric oxide in the evaluation of heart transplant candidates with elevated pulmonary vascular resistance. J Heart Lung Transplant 13:366–375, 1994.

121. Kieler-Jensen N, Lundin S, Ricksten SE: Vasodilator therapy after heart transplantation: effects of inhaled nitric oxide and intravenous prostacyclin, prostaglandin E$_1$, and sodium nitroprusside. J Heart Lung Transplant 14:436–443, 1995.

122. Lindberg L, Kimblad PO, Sjoberg T, et al: Inhaled nitric oxide reveals and attenuates endothelial dysfunction after lung transplantation. Ann Thorac Surg 62:1639–1643, 1996.

123. Macdonald P, Mundy J, Rogers P, et al: Successful treatment of life-threatening acute reperfusion injury after lung transplantation with inhaled nitric oxide. J Thorac Cardiovasc Surg 110:861–863, 1995.

124. Murakami S, Bacha EA, Herve P, et al: Prevention of reperfusion injury by inhaled nitric oxide in lungs harvested from non-heart-beating donors: Paris-Sud University Lung Transplantation Group. Ann Thorac Surg 62:1632–1638, 1996.

125. Murakami S, Bacha EA, Mazmanian GM, et al: Effects of various timings and concentrations of inhaled nitric oxide in lung ischemia-reperfusion. Am J Respir Crit Care Med 156:454–458, 1997.

126. Murakami S, Bacha EA, Herve P, et al: Inhaled nitric oxide and pentoxifylline in rat lung transplantation from non–heart-beating donors. J Thorac Cardiovasc Surg 113:821–829, 1997.

127. Williams TJ, Salamonsen RF, Snell G, et al: Preliminary experience with inhaled nitric oxide for acute pulmonary hypertension after heart transplantation. J Heart Lung Transplant 14:419–423, 1995.

128. Hess D, Bigatello L, Hurford WE: Toxicity and complications of inhaled nitric oxide. Respir Care Clin North Am 3:487–503, 1997.

129. Clutton-Brock J: Two cases of poisoning by contamination of nitrous oxide with higher oxides of nitrogen during anaesthesia. Br J Anaesth 39:388–392, 1967.

130. Zwemer FL, Pratt DS, May JJ: Silo Filler's disease in New York State. Am Rev Respir Dis 146:650–653, 1992.

131. von Nieding G, Wagner JM, Krekeler H: Investigation of the acute effects of nitrogen monoxide on lung function in man. Proceedings of the Third International Clean Air Congress, Dusseldorf, 1973. Verlag des Vereins Deutcher Ingenieure.

132. Kagawa J: Respiratory effects of 2-hr exposure to 1.0 ppm nitric oxide in normal subjects. Environ Res 22:485–490, 1982.

133. Frostell C, Hogman M, Hedenstrom H, et al: Is nitric oxide inhalation beneficial for the asthmatic patient? Am Rev Respir Dis 147:A515, 1993.

134. Nishimura M, Hess D, Kacmarek RM, et al: Nitrogen dioxide production during mechanical ventilation with nitric oxide in adults: effects of ventilator internal volume, air versus nitrogen dilution, minute ventilation, and inspired oxygen fraction. Anesthesiology 82:1246–1254, 1995.

135. Bauer MA, Utell MJ, Morrow PE, et al: Inhalation of 0.30 ppm nitrogen dioxide potentiates exercise-induced bronchospasm in asthmatics. Am Rev Respir Dis 134:1203–1208, 1986.

136. Frampton MW, Morrow PE, Cos C, et al: Effects of nitrogen dioxide exposure on pulmonary function and airway reactivity in normal humans. Am Rev Respir Dis 143:522–527, 1991.

137. Hazucha MJ, Folinsbee LJ, Seal E, et al: Lung function responses of healthy women after sequential exposures to NO_2 and O_3. Am J Respir Crit Care Med 150:642–647, 1994.

138. Kleinman MT, Bailey RM, Linn WS, et al: Effect of 0.2 ppm nitrogen dioxide on pulmonary function and response to bronchoprovocation in asthmatics. J Toxicol Environ Health 12:815–826, 1983.

139. Orehek J, Massari JP, Gayard P, et al: Effects of short-term, low level nitrogen dioxide exposure on bronchial sensitivity of asthmatic patients. J Clin Invest 74:301–307, 1976.

140. Blomberg A, Krishna MT, Bocchino V, et al: The inflammatory effects of 2 ppm NO_2 on the airways of healthy subjects. Am J Respir Crit Care Med 156:418–424, 1997.

141. Studnicka M, Hacki E, Pischinger J, et al: Traffic-related NO_2 and the prevalence of asthma and respiratory symptoms in seven year olds. Eur Respir J 10:2275–2278, 1997.

142. Kelly FJ, Blomberg A, Frew A, et al: Antioxidant kinetics in lung lavage fluid following exposure of humans to nitrogen dioxide. Am J Respir Crit Care Med 154:1700–1705, 1996.

143. Azoulay E, Lachia L, Blayo MC, et al: Methemoglobinemia induced by nitric oxide in whole blood: quantitative relationship. Toxicol Eur Res 1:7–12, 1978.

144. Chien JC: Reactions of nitric oxide with methemoglobin. J Am Chem Soc 91:2166–2168, 1969.

145. Iwamoto J, Krasney JA, Morin FC: Methemoglobin production by nitric oxide in fresh sheep blood. Respir Physiol 1994:273–283, 1994.

146. Toothill C: The chemistry of the in-vivo reaction between hemoglobin and various oxides of nitrogen. Br J Anaesth 39:405–412, 1967.

147. Young JD, Sear JW, Valvini EM: Kinetics of methaemoglobin and serum nitrogen oxide production during inhalation of nitric oxide in volunteers. Br J Anaesth 76:652–656, 1996.

148. Wessel DL, Adatia I, Thompson JE, et al: Delivery and monitoring of inhaled nitric oxide in patients with pulmonary hypertension. Crit Care Med 22:930–938, 1994.

149. Hovenga S, Koenders ME, van der Werf TS, et al: Methaemoglobinaemia after inhalation of nitric oxide for treatment of hydrochlorothiazide-induced pulmonary edema. Lancet 348:1035–1036, 1996.

150. Keaney J, John F, Puyana J-C, et al: Methylene blue reverses endotoxin-induced hypotension. Circ Res 74:1121–1125, 1994.

151. Martin W, Villani GM, Jothiananan D, et al: Selective blockade of endothelium-dependent and glyceryl trinitrate-induced relaxation by hemoglobin and by methylene blue in the rabbit aorta. J Pharmacol Exp Ther 232:708–716, 1985.

152. Mayer B, Brunner F, Schmidt K: Inhibition of nitric oxide synthase by methylene blue. Biochem Pharm 45:367–374, 1993.

153. Young JD, Dyar OJ, Xiong L, et al: Effect of methylene blue on the vasodilator action of inhaled nitric oxide in hypoxic sheep. Br J Anaesth 73:511–516, 1994.

154. Freeman B: Free radical chemistry of nitric oxide: looking at the dark side. Chest 105:79S–84S, 1994.

155. Stamler JS, Singel DJ, Loscalzo J: Biochemisty of nitric oxide and its redox-activated forms. Science 258:1989–1992, 1993.

156. Stamler JS, Osborne JA, Jaraki O, et al: Adverse vascular effects of homocysteine are modulated by endothelium-derived relaxing factor and related oxides of nitrogen. J Clin Invest 91:308–318, 1993.

157. Kooy NW, Royall JA, Ye YZ, et al: Evidence for in vivo peroxynitrite production in human acute lung injury. Am J Respir Crit Care Med 151:1250–1254, 1995.

158. Oriot D, Boussemart T, Berthier M, et al: Paradoxical effect of inhaled nitric oxide in a newborn with pulmonary hypertension. Lancet 342:364–365, 1993.

159. Barbera JA, Roger N, Roca J, et al: Worsening of pulmonary gas exchange with nitric oxide inhalation in chronic obstructive pulmonary disease. Lancet 347:436–440, 1996.

160. Katayama Y, Higenbottam TW, Diaz DAMJ, et al: Inhaled nitric oxide and arterial oxygen tension in patients with chronic obstructive pulmonary disease and severe pulmonary hypertension. Thorax 52:120–124, 1997.

161. Hopkins SR, Johnson EC, Richardson RS, et al: Effects of inhaled nitric oxide on gas exchange in lungs with shunt or poorly ventilated areas. Am J Respir Crit Care Med 156:484–491, 1997.

162. Hogman M, Frostell C, Arnberg H, et al: Bleeding time prolongation and NO inhalation. Lancet 341:1664–1665, 1993.

163. Samama CM, Diaby M, Fellahi JL, et al: Inhibition of platelet aggregation by inhaled nitric oxide in patients with acute respiratory distress syndrome. Anesthesiology 83:56–65, 1995.

164. Bocchi EA, Bacal F, Auler JO Jr, et al: Inhaled nitric oxide leading to pulmonary edema in stable severe heart failure. Am J Cardiol 74:70–72, 1994.

165. Loh E, Stamler JS, Hare JM, et al: Cardiovascular effects of inhaled nitric oxide in patients with left ventricular dysfunction. Circulation 90:2780–2785, 1994.

166. Semigran MJ, Cockrill BA, Kacmarek R, et al: Hemodynamic effects of inhaled nitric oxide in heart failure. J Am Coll Cardiol 24:982–988, 1994.

167. Lavoie A, Hall JB, Olson DM, et al: Life-threatening effects of discontinuing inhaled nitric oxide in severe respiratory failure. Am J Respir Crit Care Med 153:1985–1987, 1996.

168. Miller OI, Tang SF, Keech A, et al: Rebound pulmonary hypertension on withdrawal from inhaled nitric oxide. Lancet 346:51–52, 1995.

169. Atz AM, Adatia I, Wessel DL: Rebound pulmonary hypertension after inhalation of nitric oxide. Ann Thorac Surg 62:1759–1764, 1996.

170. Hess D, Kacmarek RM, Ritz R, et al: Inhaled nitric oxide delivery systems: a role for respiratory therapists. Respir Care 40:702–705, 1995.

171. Betit P, Adatia I, Benjamin P, et al: Inhaled nitric oxide: evaluation of a continuous titration delivery technique for infant mechanical and manual ventilation. Respir Care 40:706–715, 1995.

172. De Jaegere AP, Jacobs FI, Laheij NG, et al: Variation of inhaled nitric oxide concentration with the use of a continuous flow ventilator. Crit Care Med 25:995–1002, 1997.

173. Fernandez R, Artigas A, Blanch L: Ventilatory factors affecting inhaled nitric oxide concentrations during continuous-flow administration. J Crit Care 11:138–143, 1996.

174. Imanaka H, Hess D, Kirmse M, et al: Inaccuracies of nitric oxide delivery systems during adult mechanical ventilation. Anesthesiology 86:676–688, 1997.

175. Mortimer TW, Math MCM, Fajardo CA: Inhaled nitric oxide delivery with high-frequency jet ventilation: a bench study. Respir Care 41:895–902, 1996.

176. Putensen C, Rasanen J, Thomson S, et al: Method of delivering constant nitric oxide concentrations during full and partial ventilatory support. J Clin Monit 11:23–31, 1995.

177. Skimming JW, Cassin S, Blanch PB: Nitric oxide administration using constant-flow ventilation. Chest 108:1065–1072, 1995.

178. Stenqvist O, Kjelltoft R, Lundin S: Evaluation of a new system for ventilatory administration of nitric oxide. Acta Anaesthesiol Scand 37:687–691, 1993.

179. Skimming JW, Blanch PB, Banner MJ: Behavior of nitric oxide infused at constant flow rates directly into a breathing circuit during controlled mechanical ventilation. Crit Care Med 25:1410–1416, 1997.

180. Dube L, Francoeur M, Troncy E, et al: Comparison of two administration techniques of inhaled nitric oxide on nitrogen dioxide production. Can J Anaesth 42:922–927, 1995.

181. Foubert L, Mareels K, Fredholm M, et al: A study of mixing conditions during nitric oxide administration using simultaneous fast response chemiluminescence and capnograpy. Br J Anaesth 78:436–438, 1997.

182. Losa M, Tibballs J, Carter B, et al: Generation of nitrogen dioxide during nitric oxide therapy and mechanical ventilation of children with a Servo 900C ventilator. Intensive Care Med 23:450–455, 1997.

183. Westfelt UN, Lundin S, Stenqvist O: Nitric oxide administration after the ventilator: evaluation of mixing conditions. Acta Anaesthesiol Scand 41:266–273, 1997.

184. Westfelt UN, Lundin S, Stenqvist O: Safety aspects of delivery and monitoring of nitric oxide during mechanical ventilation. Acta Anaesthesiol Scand 41:302–310, 1997.

185. Sydow M, Bristow F, Zinserling J, et al: Flow-proportional administration of nitric oxide with a new delivery system: inspiratory nitric oxide concentration fluctuation during different flow conditions. Chest 112:496–504, 1997.

186. Sydow M, Bristow F, Zinserling J, et al: Variation of nitric oxide concentration during inspiration. Crit Care Med 25:365–371, 1997.

187. Mourgeon E, Gallart L, Umamaheswara Rao GS, et al: Distribution of inhaled nitric oxide during sequential and continuous administration into the inspiratory limb of the ventilator. Intensive Care Med 23:849–858, 1997.

188. Whiteley SM, Cohen AT, Laycock D, et al: Nitric oxide: description of a pipeline delivery system. Anaesthesia 52:561–566, 1997.

189. Hovenga S, Koenders MEF, van der Werf TS, et al: Methemoglobinemia after inhalation of nitric oxide for treatment of hydrochlorothiazide-induced pulmonary edema. Lancet 348:1035–1036, 1996.

190. Hess D, Ritz R, Branson RD: Delivery systems for inhaled nitric oxide. Respir Care Clin North Am 3:371–410, 1997.

191. Ishibe T, Sato T, Hayashi T, et al: Absorption of nitrogen dioxide and nitric oxide by soda lime. Br J Anaesth 75:330–333, 1995.

192. Pickett JA, Moors AH, Latimer RD, et al: The role of soda lime during administration of inhaled nitric oxide. Br J Anaesth 72:683–685, 1994.

193. Weimann J, Hagenah JU, Motsch J: Reduction

in nitrogen dioxide concentration by soda lime preparations during simulated nitric oxide inhalation. Br J Anaesth 79:641–644, 1997.

194. Young JD, Roberts M, Gale LB: Laboratory evaluation of the INOvent nitric oxide delivery device. Br J Anaesth 79:398–401, 1997.

195. Kirme M, Hess D: Delivery of inhaled nitric oxide using the Ohmeda INOvent delivery system. Chest 113:1650–1657, 1998.

196. Dhillon JS, Kronick JB, Singh NC, et al: A portable nitric oxide scavenging system designed for use on neonatal transport. Crit Care Med 24:1068–1071, 1996.

197. Body SC, Hartigan PM, Shernan SK, et al: Nitric oxide delivery, measurement and clinical application. J Cardiothorac Vasc Anesthesia 9:748–763, 1995.

198. Body SC, Hartigan PM: Manufacture and measurement of nitrogen oxides. Respir Care Clin North Am 3:411–434, 1997.

199. Nishimura M, Imanaka H, Uchiyama A, et al: Nitric oxide (NO) measurement accuracy. J Clin Monit 13:241–248, 1977.

200. van der Mark TW, Kort E, Meijer RJ, et al: Water vapour and carbon dioxide decrease nitric oxide readings. Eur Respir J 10:2120–2123, 1997.

201. Nelin LD, Christman NT, Morrisey JF, et al: Electrochemical nitric oxide and nitrogen dioxide analyzer for use with inhaled nitric oxide. J Appl Physiol 81:1423–1429, 1996.

202. Betit P, Grenier B, Thompson JE, et al: Evaluation of four analyzers used to monitor nitric oxide and nitrogen dioxide concentrations during inhaled nitric oxide administration. Respir Care 41:817–825, 1996.

203. Strauss JM, Krohn S, Sumpelmann R, et al: Evaluation of two electrochemical monitors for measurement of inhaled nitric oxide. Anaesthesia 51:151–154, 1996.

204. Purtz EP, Hess D, Kacmarek RM: Evaluation of electrochemical nitric oxide and nitrogen dioxide analyzers suitable for use during mechanical ventilation. J Clin Monit 13:25–34, 1997.

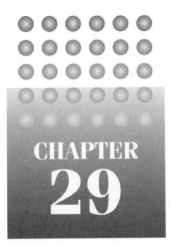

Noninvasive Ventilation

Richard G. Wunderink, MD
S. Gregory Jennings, MD

RATIONALE FOR NONINVASIVE POSITIVE PRESSURE VENTILATION

INDICATIONS FOR NONINVASIVE POSITIVE PRESSURE VENTILATION
Acute Exacerbations of Chronic Obstructive Pulmonary Disease
Other Indications

CONTRAINDICATIONS TO NONINVASIVE POSITIVE PRESSURE VENTILATION

EFFECTIVENESS OF NONINVASIVE POSITIVE PRESSURE VENTILATION

TECHNICAL APPLICATION OF NONINVASIVE POSITIVE PRESSURE VENTILATION
Mask Type
Ventilator Settings
Ventilators
Monitoring
Weaning

COMPLICATIONS OF NONINVASIVE POSITIVE PRESSURE VENTILATION
REFERENCES

KEY WORDS

chronic obstructive pulmonary disease
noninvasive ventilation

positive pressure ventilation
postextubation stridor
respiratory insufficiency

Noninvasive ventilation can be defined loosely as the provision of assisted ventilation without the use of an endotracheal tube or tracheostomy. Although many ways exist to provide this type of ventilation using either negative or positive pressure,[1] this chapter is limited a discussion of noninvasive **positive pressure ventilation** (NPPV). NPPV usually is accomplished with the use of a mask that covers either the mouth and nose or the nose only. Because maintenance of positive pressure during inspiration with the use of these masks actually does constitute assisted ventilation, mask continuous positive airway pressure (CPAP) technically fits into the category of NPPV. However, mask CPAP is discussed only in terms of contrast with other forms of NPPV. The discussion, therefore, centers mainly on provision of positive pressure above the baseline CPAP during inspiration. The chapter also focuses on the use of NPPV in the acutely ill patient. Although many of the principles of NPPV also can be applied in the chronic ventilator setting, the additional complexities of care for these patients precludes a full discussion in this chapter.

RATIONALE FOR NONINVASIVE POSITIVE PRESSURE VENTILATION

The driving force behind the use of NPPV is an attempt to avoid the complications associated with the act of endotracheal intubation and complications of prolonged endotracheal intubation.[2] Some of these potential benefits of NPPV are listed in Table 29–1. Although many of these theoretical advantages have not been realized in clinical practice, the benefits of avoiding endotracheal intubation generally are so accepted that this alone has been used as the end point for many studies of NPPV.

The physiologic rationale for NPPV is to provide inspiratory assistance, essentially unloading the respiratory muscles while avoiding the adverse consequences of endotracheal intubation. Brochard and associ-

TABLE 29–1. Potential Benefits and Risks of Noninvasive Positive Pressure Ventilation (NPPV)

POTENTIAL BENEFITS
Avoidance of endotracheal intubation
Decreased duration of ventilation
Decreased incidence of pneumonia
Decreased incidence of sinusitis
Improved ability to communicate
Ability to eat and drink
Preservation of effective cough
    (nasal NPPV only)
Decreased need for sedation/paralysis
POTENTIAL RISKS
Facial skin necrosis
Increased aspiration risk
Increased duration of ventilation in patients
    who fail NPPV
Difficulty providing adequate calories enterally
Decreased ability to cough (full face mask)
Increased myocardial ischemia

ates found significant reductions in the pressure–time product and diaphragmatic electromyogram (EMG) activity with NPPV in patients with **chronic obstructive pulmonary disease** (COPD).[3] Use of NPPV in patients who are purely hypoxemic without significant excess work of breathing, such as patients with pulmonary embolism, has less justification. Although NPPV can be provided in either intermittent mandatory ventilation (IMV) or continuous mechanical ventilation (CMV) modes, NPPV is not as effective in patients whose respiratory drive is compromised. In most hypoventilating patients in which NPPV is successful, such as patients with COPD and carbon dioxide (CO_2) narcosis, return of an intact respiratory drive rapidly occurs. Mask CPAP alone is beneficial in reversing auto-positive end-expiratory pressure (PEEP) and dynamic hyperinflation in patients with COPD. The addition of pressure support to PEEP with NPPV appears to have additive effects in reducing work of breathing.[4]

INDICATIONS FOR NONINVASIVE POSITIVE PRESSURE VENTILATION

The indications for NPPV are almost as numerous as those for invasive mechanical ventilation (Table 29–2). In general, NPPV tends to be more successful in patients with obstructive airway disease as opposed to other types of **respiratory insufficiency**.[1,5] Probably the most important determinant of success is that the underlying disorder should be rapidly reversible. The benefit of NPPV is to support the patient until other therapeutic maneuvers decrease the work of breathing such that further support is not needed. The need to provide NPPV over a prolonged period of days will decrease the margin of benefit over endotracheal intubation.

Acute Exacerbations of Chronic Obstructive Pulmonary Disease

The greatest experimental validity for the use of NPPV is for acute exacerbations of COPD (Table 29–3). Three randomized con-

TABLE 29–2. Causes of Acute Respiratory Failure in Reported Noninvasive Positive Pressure Ventilation (NPPV) Use

Acute exacerbation of chronic obstructive
    pulmonary disease (COPD)
Adult respiratory distress syndrome (ARDS)
Asthma
Cardiogenic pulmonary edema
Community-acquired pneumonia
Cystic fibrosis (CF)
Hypoventilation syndromes
    Obstructive sleep apnea (OSA)
    Obesity hypoventilation syndrome
    Congestive heart failure with Cheyne-Stokes
      respirations
Lung cancer
Near-drowning
Neuromuscular disease
Pneumocystis carinii pneumonia (PCP)
Postoperative respiratory insufficiency
Postextubation stridor
Pulmonary embolus
Restrictive lung disease
Trauma
Upper airway obstruction

trol trials of NPPV versus conventional management have been performed in patients with COPD.[6–8] A consistent trend in all the studies was successful avoidance of endotracheal intubation with the use of NPPV. In a multicenter study of NPPV via nasal mask, Brochard and colleagues found that only 26% of patients with COPD initially treated with NPPV eventually required intubation, compared with 74% of controls.[7] Kramer and associates found a similar significant reduction in intubation rates.[8] The benefit of NPPV for avoidance of intubation was so marked that the number needed to treat (NNT) to show a difference from standard therapy was only three patients. A tendency toward lower mortality in NPPV patients than in those randomized to invasive ventilation also was seen.[6, 7] Brochard and colleagues[7] found a shorter length of hospital stay and demonstrated a lower complication rate in NPPV patients (relative risk 0.42). The evidence appears clear from these randomized studies, as well as a wealth of observational studies, that

initial use of NPPV as opposed to intubation with traditional ventilation results in lower mortality and morbidity in patients with COPD exacerbations.[1, 9]

Criticisms of these randomized trials, however, deserve mention.[9] Brochard and colleagues actually randomized only 31% of the patients with COPD who were treated.[7] Only 69% of those received beta-agonist bronchodilators at the time of randomization. The duration of ventilation was somewhat excessive in the control group. Kramer and associates[8] found similar rates of avoidance of endotracheal intubation, yet the control group had a much shorter duration of ventilation. For that reason, the mean duration of ventilation in the NPPV patients in that study actually exceeded that of controls.[8] Of perhaps more concern was the significantly longer duration of ventilation (25 days) in patients in whom ventilation failed in the study by Brochard and colleagues[7] and an excessive mortality in failure patients found by Guerin and colleagues.[10] The latter finding may be one of the greatest potential risks of NPPV.

The mechanism of benefit is probably multifactorial and varies slightly from patient to patient. Relief of excess work of breathing due to acute bronchospasm is probably the most general benefit. More effective ventilation than that achieved spontaneously in patients with acute exacerbations of chronic bronchitis may reverse some CO_2 narcosis, and therefore intubation could be avoided. Reversal of dynamic airway trapping by providing small amounts of CPAP may decrease the dynamic hyperinflation that put the inspiratory respiratory muscles at a mechanical disadvantage.[4] Whether patients with true respiratory muscle fatigue, manifested by paradoxical abdominal respirations, can be managed with NPPV alone is unclear.

The real issue for NPPV in acute exacerbations of COPD is appropriate patient selection. As noted previously, Brochard and colleagues could randomize only 31% of patients with exacerbations of COPD who could potentially benefit from NPPV.[7] In addition, nearly one quarter of the control patients required intubation within the first hour after randomization despite an exclu-

TABLE 29–3. Results of Randomized Controlled Trials of Noninvasive Positive Pressure Ventilation

DISEASE	INTERVENTION	OUTCOME	NPPV	CONTROL	RRR	ARR	NNT	P
COPD[6]	Nasal/volume	Mortality	3/30 (0.10)	9/30 (0.30)	66.7%	0.20	5	0.11
COPD[7]	Nasal/PS	Mortality	4/43 (0.09)	12/42 (0.29)	69.0%	0.20	5	0.02
Mixed[8]	Nasal/BiPAP	Mortality	1/16 (0.06)	2/15 (0.13)	53.8%	0.07	14	0.60
Mixed: No COPD[13]	Face/PS	Mortality	7/21 (0.33)	10/20 (0.50)	34.0%	0.17	6	0.46
$pCO_2 > 45$*	Face/PS	Mortality	1/11 (0.09)	4/6 (0.67)	86.6%	0.58	2	0.06
$pCO_2 \le 45$*	Face/PS	Mortality	6/10 (0.60)	6/14 (0.43)	−34%	−0.17	6	0.76
Pulmonary edema[13]	Nasal/BiPAP	Mortality	1/14 (0.07)	2/13 (0.15)†	46.7%	0.08	14	0.60
COPD[7]	Nasal/PS	Intubation	11/43 (0.26)	31/42 (0.74)	64.9%	0.48	2	0.001
Mixed[8]	Nasal/BiPAP	Intubation	5/16 (0.31)	11/15 (0.73)	57.5%	0.42	3	0.05
COPD*	Nasal/BiPAP	Intubation	1/11 (0.09)	8/12 (0.67)	86.6%	0.58	2	0.017
Mixed: No COPD[13]	Face/PS	Intubation	13/21 (0.62)	14/20 (0.70)	11.4%	0.08	14	0.88
$pCO_2 > 45$*	Face/PS	Intubation	4/11 (0.36)	6/6 (1.00)	64.0%	0.64	2	0.02
$pCO_2 \le 45$*	Face/PS	Intubation	9/10 (0.90)	8/14 (0.57)	−57.9%	−0.33	3	0.17
Pulmonary edema[13]	Nasal/BiPAP	Intubation	1/14 (0.07)	1/13 (0.08)	12.5%	0.01	100	1.0
COPD[7]	Nasal/PS	Complications	7/43 (0.16)	20/42 (0.48)	66.7%	0.32	3	0.001
Pulmonary edema[13]	Nasal/BiPap	Myocardial infarction	10/14 (0.71)	4/13 (0.31)	−43%	−0.40	3	0.06

Modified from Wunderink RG, Hill NS: Continuous and periodic applications of noninvasive ventilation in respiratory failure. Respir Care 42:394–402, 1997.

*Subgroup analysis.

†Control was nasal continuous positive airway pressure (CPAP); ARR, absolute risk reduction; BiPAP, bilevel airway pressure; COPD, chronic obstructive pulmonary disease; NPPV, noninvasive positive pressure ventilation; NNT, number needed to treat; PCO₂, partial pressure of carbon dioxide; PS, pressure support; RRR, relative risk reduction.

sion criteria of "need for immediate intubation." NPPV probably is instituted optimally in patients who have severe respiratory insufficiency that has not yet progressed to true respiratory failure. A subjective assessment of this distinction was not very accurate in the study by Brochard and colleagues.[7] Defining these patients by blood gases also appears to be ineffective. Meduri and associates found that patients who had acute respiratory insufficiency had no better response to NPPV than did patients who had acute respiratory failure as defined by arterial blood gas values and a subjective impression of the need for immediate intubation.[11] If all acute exacerbations of COPD were treated with NPPV, the excess cost of NPPV compared with nonventilatory management would be astronomical. Further research is needed to clearly define prospectively which patients may benefit from NPPV in acute exacerbations of COPD.[9]

Other Indications

The appropriateness of NPPV for other indications for mechanical ventilation is less clear (see Table 29–3). Two randomized studies generally found no reduction in intubation using NPPV in patients without COPD.[8, 12] In a subgroup of patients without COPD but with elevated CO_2 levels, a trend toward decreased mortality with NPPV emerged, but the duration of ventilation between NPPV and control groups did not differ.[12] Other related variables (hospital stay, intensive care unit [ICU] stay) also showed no difference between patients with initial NPPV and controls. Although there may be benefit to patients without COPD with high CO_2 levels, prospective randomized trials are necessary to demonstrate efficacy for NPPV in this subgroup.[1, 9]

These two studies clearly were compromised by the heterogeneity of the populations studied. Only one randomized study has been completed for a homogeneous group of patients without COPD. Mehta and associates[13] found a significant improvement in vital signs and various parameters of ventilation in patients with cardiogenic pulmonary edema who were randomized to nasal NPPV. However, the group with

NPPV also had a significantly higher incidence of myocardial infarction (71%) than did patients randomized to nasal CPAP (31%) and to historic controls. No difference in intubation rates, length of stay, or mortality was noted between CPAP patients and NPPV patients.

Further randomized controlled studies definitely are needed before strong recommendations for use of NPPV can be made for patients with forms of respiratory failure other than COPD. Several comments can be made regarding findings of observational studies of NPPV in a variety of these disorders.

Atelectasis

NPPV has been used extensively for the treatment of atelectasis, especially in the postoperative patient.[2, 14] Success probably is predicated on the mechanism of atelectasis. If caused by splinting or generalized weakness, NPPV may be efficacious; the real issue is whether NPPV is different from mask CPAP or intermittent positive pressure breathing (IPPB). Mask CPAP has been demonstrated to be effective in reversing and/or preventing atelectasis in postoperative patients. IPPB also has demonstrated benefit in cooperative patients with neuromuscular disorders, such as kyphoscoliosis. In contrast, if atelectasis is the result of retained secretions, full face mask NPPV has the potential to be deleterious because it interferes with expectoration. An air bronchogram in the atelectatic segment on chest radiograph suggests the absence of a large mucus plug.

Postextubation Stridor

Postextubation stridor may be an important indication for NPPV, especially if it is caused by laryngeal edema.[5] The onset of stridor immediately after extubation is likely the result of vocal cord edema and probably is treated best by immediate reintubation. However, if stridor occurs 30 minutes or more postextubation, the mechanism is more likely laryngeal edema. Because even an edematous larynx can be distended by positive airway pressure,

NPPV with CPAP may be able to overcome the increased resistance to airflow similar to the well-documented benefit of CPAP in obstructive sleep apnea. Postextubation laryngeal edema usually can be relieved relatively quickly with the use of racemic epinephrine, corticosteroids, and/or diuresis, and thus is an example of a rapidly reversible condition amenable to NPPV.

A more provocative possibility for the use of NPPV is to accelerate the weaning process itself. Approximately 50% of patients who extubate themselves do not require reintubation. Many of these patients were being weaned actively at the time of self-extubation. This suggests that clinicians may be more conservative than warranted in weaning some patients. The possibility of converting to NPPV in patients who are clinically borderline for extubation may allow for earlier extubation.

Asthma

Given the high morbidity of intubation in asthmatic patients, successful management with NPPV would be highly desirable. Acute asthma attacks have been treated successfully with NPPV.[15] However, probably more than any other disorder, use of NPPV in status asthmaticus requires a cooperative patient. If claustrophobia and anxiety can be overcome, NPPV may be able to decrease significantly the work of breathing of asthmatic patients. Additional potential benefits include CPAP to overcome auto-PEEP and more effective delivery of beta-adrenergic bronchodilators when nebulized through the ventilator circuit.

Hypoventilation Syndromes

Occasionally, patients with chronic hypoventilation syndromes, such as the obesity/hypoventilation syndrome or obstructive sleep apnea, are admitted to the ICU for exacerbations resulting from some intercurrent problem. Logically, increasing the level of inspiratory pressure support may stabilize the patient while the underlying cause for worsening is treated. The literature on NPPV is not clear regarding the benefit in this patient population.

"Do Not Intubate" Patients

Several studies have described the use of NPPV in patients who have refused intubation.[2] Once again, routine use of NPPV in this patient population markedly increases the cost of care in patients whose condition is often terminal. The indication for use of NPPV should be similar to that of patients willing to undergo full resuscitation, with the main criterion being the ability to quickly reverse the underlying cause of respiratory insufficiency.[1]

Other Indications

Case reports or cohort studies have been published with the use of NPPV for a large number of other indications.[2] In general, NPPV appears to be of potential benefit in two groups of patients. The first is those with acute causes of respiratory insufficiency who may require only a short period of ventilatory support until the underlying problem can be corrected. For this reason, adult respiratory distress syndrome (ARDS) appears to be an unlikely indication. The second group is patients with borderline respiratory insufficiency who require only low-level or intermittent support until definitive therapy can be provided. Use of NPPV as a bridge to lung transplant in cystic fibrosis patients is an example of the latter. This second indication blurs the distinction between use of NPPV in the acute care setting and the use of chronic outpatient NPPV.

CONTRAINDICATIONS TO NONINVASIVE POSITIVE PRESSURE VENTILATION

Only a few absolute contraindications to NPPV exist. These include cardiopulmonary arrest or hemodynamic instability, apnea or the need for immediate intubation, facial burns, facial or cranial trauma, uncontrolled vomiting or gastrointestinal bleeding, and the need for airway protection.

An uncooperative patient also represents a near-absolute contraindication. Although extreme anxiety makes use of NPPV difficult, a few patients can be managed successfully with NPPV with significant coaching and reassurance and the judicious use of sedation.

Because NPPV does provide positive intrathoracic pressure, hypotension secondary to decreased preload can develop in hypovolemic patients with the application of NPPV, similar to initiation of invasive ventilation. This hypotension does respond fairly readily to volume infusion. Mehta and associates[13] found greater hypotension with NPPV than with nasal CPAP in patients with acute pulmonary edema. Therefore, cardiogenic shock and probably septic shock should be relative contraindications.

Contraindications based on diagnosis are less helpful to discriminate between patients who will or will not respond to NPPV. Because of the severe hypoxemia, high minute ventilation, decreased compliance, and prolonged course in typical patients, patients with ARDS are unlikely to respond to NPPV. Similarly, patients with an acute process superimposed on chronic fibrotic lung disease are less likely to be managed optimally with NPPV. Use of NPPV in massively obese patients whose problem is not mainly secondary to upper airway obstruction also has been associated with frequent failure.

Several studies have suggested that patients with high severity of illness scores are less likely to respond to NPPV.[7, 9, 16] Therefore, the acutely, severely ill patient with multiple-organ dysfunction also is an unlikely candidate for NPPV.

Overall, the percentage of patients who appear to be appropriate candidates for a trial of NPPV is approximately 23%,[5] with a slightly higher percentage in a pure COPD population.[7]

EFFECTIVENESS OF NONINVASIVE POSITIVE PRESSURE VENTILATION

The efficacy of NPPV found in the aforementioned studies may not translate directly into clinical practice; that is, the effectiveness of NPPV in general practice may not be the same as in an experimental setting with a narrowly defined population. NPPV is much more operator dependent than traditional mechanical ventilation. Bott and colleagues, in a small study of patients with COPD, found a significant variation in mortality between centers with the use of NPPV.[6] This finding suggests that factors other than patient diagnosis are important in outcome. The factors that may be important for effectiveness are listed in Table 29–4.

The comfort level of the respiratory care practitioner (RCP) in providing NPPV is critical to its success. It is the RCP who is in frequent attendance at the bedside of the patient on NPPV, not the physician. NPPV may require more of the RCP's time than traditional intubation and mechanical ventilation, especially at the onset. When NPPV first is introduced to an institution, the initial step is to convince RCPs that NPPV can work. Later, the major issue is defining which manipulations are important to provide for patient ventilator synchrony because the variability from patient to patient is much greater than with intubation and mechanical ventilation. To address these problems, several centers have started with a dedicated team to provide NPPV.[5, 14] As the success of NPPV is demonstrated by the specialized team, more of the RCPs are trained, and ultimately, NPPV can be provided as a standard part of respiratory care services. If this approach is not taken, a significant educational effort clearly is required to train RCPs to provide NPPV. As RCP training programs incorporate NPPV into their curriculum, increasing

TABLE 29–4. Factors Important in the Effectiveness of Noninvasive Positive Pressure Ventilation

Patient selection
Acceptance and comfort level of respiratory care
    practitioners
Patient anxiety; cooperativeness
Patient/ventilator synchrony
Technical aspects
    Mask
    Ventilator mode
    Ventilator settings
    Monitoring

familiarity with the technique will reduce apprehension involving its use. In the meantime, a variety of educational programs, including tapes and hands-on workshops, are available to gain skill in providing NPPV.

Patient-ventilator synchrony is probably the second most important factor in the success of NPPV. As with traditional mechanical ventilation, if inappropriately applied, the patient work of breathing on NPPV actually may exceed that of spontaneous breathing. Of the various components to patient-ventilator synchrony, patient anxiety is one of the important issues. Tachypneic, dyspneic patients often need to be convinced that the use of a tight-fitting mask actually will improve their breathing. Therefore, the first several minutes of provision of NPPV are often crucial to its success. Communication, reassurance, and coaching by the physician or RCP at the bedside is a very important component of the efficacy of NPPV. Other components of patient-ventilator synchrony are discussed in the next section. However, the attitude of the RCP and the patient cannot be overemphasized in discussing the efficacy of NPPV.

TECHNICAL APPLICATION OF NONINVASIVE POSITIVE PRESSURE VENTILATION

Mask Type

An important component of the success of NPPV is the interface between the ventilator and the patient. Selection of the type and size of mask and securing the mask are critically important when patients are ventilated without intubation. NPPV has been delivered via both nasal masks and full face masks. Because successful application of NPPV has been accomplished with both, which type is preferable is unclear. A consistent finding is that no single mask optimally manages all patients. Conversely, familiarity with the mask and the proper means of fitting is one of the operator variables critical to the success of NPPV. Therefore, familiarity with and access to a variety of masks are desirable.

Nasal masks are the most frequently used interface for NPPV. Although several different types are available, the typical mask is a triangular plastic device with a soft material around the flanges to obtain an air seal and a circular port for tube connection. Alternatively, a mask currently is available that seals only the distal portion of the nose, with ventilation administered through soft rubber tubes inserted into the nostrils. Nasal masks offer the advantages of allowing for oral feedings while lowering the risk of aspiration and facilitating the clearing of oral secretions. In addition, the feeling of claustrophobia is lower with nasal masks, and they are much easier to fit in edentulous or bearded patients. The potential for rebreathing CO_2 also is reduced greatly because nasal masks have 60% less dead space than face masks and the patient can exhale through the mouth if necessary.

However, nasal masks have serious limitations. Because a significant portion ($\geq$ 50%) of total airway resistance occurs in the nasal passages, the actual amount of pressure support delivered to the lower respiratory tract may be less than the displayed level of pressure support. Difficulty in adequately ventilating patients who also have narrowed or collapsed airways, common with acute respiratory failure or immediately after major thoracoabdominal surgery, may result, and these patients may require the use of a face mask or intubation. Even higher total airway resistance may occur in patients who have underlying nasal obstruction either for anatomic reasons or acute rhinosinusitis.

Another important consideration in nasal NPPV is the ability of the patient to forgo mouth breathing. Once again, a significant decrement in the amount of actual pressure support received by the lower respiratory tract occurs when the patient continues to breathe through the mouth instead of the nose. This can be alleviated partially with the use of a chin strap. However, increasing the complexity of the apparatus may counteract its reported benefits.

In contrast, full face masks have a significant problem with provision of a tight enough seal at the skin to avoid complications. Full face masks are particularly problematic in patients who are edentulous, in whom the mask tends to slide up off the chin and to actually rest in the oral cavity. Presence of a heavy beard also may make a tight seal difficult. A minimal amount of leak around the mask is tolerable and can be accommodated by the ventilatory settings if flow triggering is available. However, a large leak increases the risk of complications such as eye irritation, and increases the possibility of nasal skin necrosis secondary to attempts to tighten the mask. In addition, full face masks have difficulty delivering the pressure to the lower respiratory tract in patients who have a large tongue that may obstruct the oral pharynx. Not only does this make passage of airflow through the mouth difficult, but the posterior displacement of the tongue may even prevent the benefit of airflow through the nose. Patients with a full face mask have significantly more difficulty coughing and expectorating than do those with a nasal mask, and retained secretions are a problem. If the patient is producing a large volume of secretions, NPPV via a full face mask needs to be interrupted to allow the patient to expectorate on a regular basis.

Mouthpiece or lip seal devices have been introduced for patients with neuromuscular disease undergoing chronic noninvasive ventilation. Their use in cooperative patients with acute respiratory insufficiency has not been assessed.

Ventilator Settings

Although NPPV has been provided in a variety of ventilator modes, most studies have used pressure-assisted ventilation rather than volume cycle ventilators. However, successful NPPV has been accomplished with volume cycle ventilation.[6, 17] Patients tend to tolerate pressure-cycled ventilation somewhat better,[17] and the risk of barotrauma and degree of air leak are likely to be less than with volume cycle ventilation.

The need for CPAP is variable. Many investigators routinely use CPAP to partially compensate for small air leaks. The most successful use of NPPV has been in patients with acute exacerbations of COPD. In these situations, CPAP provided by NPPV relieves the autoPEEP and air trapping common in these patients to the same degree that extrinsic PEEP in intubated patients relieves this problem. In addition, CPAP tends to keep the oropharynx from collapsing before the onset of inspiration and therefore allows better triggering of the ventilator by the patient. However, in a few patients, CPAP may result in dynamic hyperinflation.

Ventilators

The resurgence of interest in NPPV in the acute care setting followed the development of home ventilators,[2] mainly to provide CPAP for patients with obstructive sleep apnea. In the late 1980s, the first portable pressure-targeted ventilators were introduced, called bilevel CPAP or bilevel pressure ventilators. These ventilators quickly became the standard for CPAP and NPPV in the noncritical care setting. The types of ventilators used for NPPV have ranged from custom models designed specifically for NPPV to portable ventilators designed for home CPAP or NPPV use to standard ICU-type ventilators. Several researchers have compared portable models with standard ICU ventilators.[18] In general, peak flows are comparable and sometimes higher with portable pressure-targeted ventilators, certainly enough to satisfy patient demand with reasonable inspiratory pressure settings. However, Lofaso and associates noted that use of one of the most common types (BiPAP) without the addition of a nonrebreathing isolation valve may increase work of breathing by 50% due to CO_2 rebreathing.[19] Setting PEEP at 4 cm H_2O or greater eliminates the CO_2 rebreathing problem, and the potential for rebreathing in the dead space of a full face mask can be eliminated by using a nasal mask, although this has not been proved. Inspiratory trigger times, inspiratory trigger pressures, expiratory delay times, and the incidence of supraplateau expiratory pressures were comparable to those associated with common ICU ventilators.

These values are far from ideal, however,

because high expiratory resistance may occur as a result of small exhalation ports, and a wide variation in expiratory delay times from cycle to cycle using the same device has been noted. Active exhalation often begins using accessory muscles before the ventilator cycles to exhalation, producing an overshoot above the peak inspiratory pressure. This overshoot can be marked in patients with COPD because their inspiratory flow rates are relatively high at the end of inspiration. Correction of this problem is only possible with models that have adjustable end-expiratory triggers that can be tailored to each patient's inspiratory pattern. Kacmarek has suggested that the major concerns regarding routine use of portable pressure-targeted ventilators in the ICU are the ability to provide high inspired oxygen concentration (FiO_2) levels and the lack of alarms or monitors.[18]

Monitoring

Monitoring a patient on NPPV is crucial and probably accounts for the greatest variance in success of NPPV.[1, 2] Initiation of NPPV appears to be somewhat more time intensive for the respiratory therapist; however, this time appears to be vital for success. In addition to monitoring for leaks around the mask, monitoring of the amount of ventilation actually provided is important.

A necessary component of monitoring is physically examining the patient for synchrony with mechanical ventilation. Patients in whom attempts at NPPV are unsuccessful often have an asynchronous respiratory pattern. Not only is the amount of air leak and potential autoPEEP increased but also added work of breathing may occur as the patient actively exhales against the ventilator during the inspiratory cycle. Although asynchrony also occurs in patients who are intubated and mechanically ventilated, the number of interventions available to increase synchrony is fewer with NPPV. In addition, the degree of accessory muscle use can be assessed only at the bedside. If the patient continues to require accessory inspiratory muscle use or if he or she develops paradoxical abdominal respirations, the probability of a successful treatment with NPPV alone is reduced significantly.

Conversion of the rapid shallow breathing pattern of patients in respiratory distress to a slower deeper pattern is associated with a successful course of NPPV. The degree of reduction in respiratory rate is proportional to both underlying minute ventilation and the amount of pressure or volume support that is chosen for NPPV settings. Titration up of the level of pressure support may be associated with a better outcome if a greater tidal volume results. In general, provision of an exhaled tidal volume that is in the 5- to 6-ml/kg or greater range usually is associated with successful NPPV. Although respiratory rates of 20 or less usually suggest adequate NPPV, the ability to breathe at higher rates in patients who are hypercatabolic or on lower levels of pressure support also has been associated with successful outcomes.[8]

Improvement in respiratory parameters usually occurs within the first hour.[20] Meduri and associates found that significant reduction in the degree of CO_2 retention[20] within the first hour in patients with hypercarbic respiratory failure was associated with successful NPPV.[11] In other studies using nasal NPPV in a COPD population, similar overall success rates were reported despite no significant decrease in the degree of hypercarbia.[8] Although these contrasting results in patients with persistent hypercarbia may reflect differences between nasal and mask CPAP, the converse finding of significant decrease in hypercarbia within the first hour of NPPV is a reliable predictor of successful NPPV.

Weaning

There has been no systematic study of weaning from NPPV. In general, researchers have used two approaches to weaning—a progressive reduction in the level of pressure delivered with pressure cycle ventilation or progressively increasing periods of time off NPPV, similar to T-piece trials for patients who have undergone intuba-

tion. Several theoretical advantages to intermittent trials off NPPV exist. For patients ventilated with a full face mask, these periods off NPPV allow time for expectoration and/or intake of oral nutrition and fluids. Another important theoretical consideration is to provide a period of time for reperfusion of areas of skin that have been pressure points with the use of either type of mask, thus reducing the risk of pressure necrosis.

As with intubation and mechanical ventilation, reversal of the underlying process causing respiratory failure is the most important factor in successful discontinuation of ventilation. With a rapidly reversible problem, simple discontinuation of NPPV is the most expeditious way to wean. NPPV then can be reinstituted if the patient's condition worsens.

COMPLICATIONS OF NONINVASIVE POSITIVE PRESSURE VENTILATION

Although the main rationale for use of NPPV is to decrease complications associated with endotracheal intubation, NPPV has its own set of complications.[16] The most common problems with NPPV are associated with the interface between ventilator and patient. Pressure necrosis over the bridge of the nose remains the most common complication of both types of mask. This can be alleviated somewhat by the use of a cushion for areas in which pressure is applied over a bony surface, such as the nasal bridge, forehead, and chin. This also may cut down on the amount of injury induced by chafing of the skin during small movements of the mask. However, the major intervention to reduce facial skin necrosis is to avoid an excessive tension on the headgear straps holding the mask in place. The degree of tension on the harness should easily allow placement of a finger between the harness and the face. Use of ventilators that allow for leak compensation, appropriate fitting of a mask, and tolerance of a small air leak in a patient who is synchronizing well with the ventilator also make this complication less common.

Masks should always be of a clear, soft

material so that secretions can be observed without removing the seal, and irritation can be minimized. However, the skin needs to be inspected daily for necrosis, skin rashes, and abrasions. Nasal, sinus, or ear pain is common at the initiation of NPPV. If NPPV is begun at high peak inspiratory pressure (15–20 cm H_2O), the patient often cannot tolerate the initial discomfort, and traditional mechanical ventilation may be the only alternative. If NPPV is started at low pressure (5–10 cm H_2O), the patient typically becomes accustomed to the noise and discomfort, and pressure can be increased slowly to the level desired. Nasal congestion and dryness usually can be alleviated with a combination of decongestants and emollients or humidification of the inspired air using passover-type humidifiers, if necessary. Oral dryness often responds to adjustment of straps to reduce air leakage from the mouth. Eye dryness and irritation may occur when there is air leakage around the nasal bridge; mask adjustment generally solves the problem, but switching to another mask type may be required.

Pneumothorax is rare but its occurrence is possible at high pressures, particularly in patients with bullous lung disease and air trapping. Another rare complication may occur with the use of pressure-cycled NPPV in patients with large air leaks around the mask. If the air leak is so large that the off-cycle mechanism for pressure support is not triggered, the patient essentially receives CPAP at the set level of pressure support. This results in significant hyperinflation and air trapping.

The most serious complication associated with NPPV—especially with the use of a face mask—is aspiration. Although patients with decreased mentation are not good candidates for NPPV because of the high risk of aspiration, other patients also may experience temporary difficulty in clearing secretions while they are being ventilated. Clinicians must closely monitor the ability of the patient to clear secretions and not hesitate to intubate for this indication. Guerin and colleagues found that the highest incidence of ventilator-associated pneumonia (and the highest mortality) was in the group of patients in whom NPPV failed and who required intubation.[10]

Gastric insufflation has been frequently reported as a complication of NPPV. Although the usual ventilatory pressures used for NPPV do not exceed the tension in the normal lower esophageal sphincter, a variety of conditions and medications used in critically ill patients may affect sphincter tone. With increased gastric pressures, the risks of vomiting and aspiration increase significantly. The risk of aspiration may counteract the purported benefit of NPPV in decreasing the incidence of ventilator-associated pneumonia.

NPPV has become an important component in the armamentarium of the critical care physician. In centers that have developed the needed expertise and support structures, NPPV can be used routinely to manage patients with acute exacerbations of COPD, with a high rate of success. Although the use of NPPV for other indications is less well proved, selective use in patients, on the basis of an understanding of the physiologic benefits of NPPV and the patients' underlying respiratory problem, may offer a legitimate alternative to endotracheal intubation for mechanical ventilatory support. A significant amount of additional research is needed to define further the appropriate use of NPPV.

REFERENCES

1. Bach JR, Brougher P, Hess DR, et al: Consensus conference: noninvasive positive pressure ventilation. Respir Care 42:364–369, 1997.
2. Meduri GU: Noninvasive positive-pressure ventilation in patients with acute respiratory failure. Clin Chest Med 17:513–553, 1996.
3. Brochard L, Isabey D, Piquet J, et al: Reversal of acute exacerbations of chronic obstructive lung disease by inspiratory assistance with a face mask. N Engl J Med 323:1523–1530, 1990.
4. Appendini L, Patessio A, Zanaboni S, et al: Physiologic effects of positive end-expiratory pressure and mask pressure support during exacerbations of chronic obstructive pulmonary disease. Am J Respir Crit Care Med 149:1069–1076, 1994.
5. Meduri GU, Turner RE, Abou-Shala N, et al: Noninvasive positive pressure ventilation via face mask: first-line intervention in patients with acute hypercapnic and hypoxemic respiratory failure. Chest 109:179–193, 1996.

6. Bott J, Carroll MP, Conway JH, et al: Randomized controlled trial of nasal ventilation in acute ventilatory failure due to chronic obstructive airways disease. Lancet 341:1555–1558, 1993.

7. Brochard L, Mancebo J, Wysocki M, et al: Noninvasive ventilation for acute exacerbations of chronic obstructive pulmonary disease. N Engl J Med 333:817–822, 1995.

8. Kramer N, Meyer TJ, Meharg J, et al: Randomized, prospective trial of noninvasive positive pressure ventilation in acute respiratory failure. Am J Respir Crit Care Med 151:1799–1806, 1995.

9. Wunderink RG, Hill NS: Continuous and periodic applications of noninvasive ventilation in respiratory failure. Respir Care 42:394–402, 1997.

10. Guerin C, Girard R, Chemorin C, et al: Facial mask noninvasive mechanical ventilation reduces the incidence of nosocomial pneumonia: a prospective epidemiological survey from a single ICU. Intensive Care Med 23:1024–1032, 1997.

11. Meduri GU, Abou-Shala N, Fox RC, et al: Noninvasive face mask mechanical ventilation in patients with acute hypercapnic respiratory failure. Chest 100:445–454, 1991.

12. Wysocki M, Tric L, Wolff MA, et al: Noninvasive pressure support ventilation in patients with acute respiratory failure: a randomized comparison with conventional therapy. Chest 107:761–768, 1995.

13. Mehta S, Jay GD, Woolard RH, et al: Randomized, prospective trial of bilevel versus continuous positive airway pressure in acute pulmonary edema. Crit Care Med 25:620–628, 1997.

14. Pennock BE, Crawshaw L, Kaplan PD: Noninvasive nasal mask ventilation for acute respiratory failure. Chest 105:441–444, 1994.

15. Meduri GU, Cook TR, Turner RE, et al: Noninvasive positive pressure ventilation in status asthmaticus. Chest 110:767–774, 1996.

16. Hill NS: Complications of noninvasive positive pressure ventilation. Respir Care 42:432–442, 1997.

17. Vitacca M, Rubini F, Foglio K, et al: Non-invasive modalities of positive pressure ventilation improve the outcome of acute exacerbations in COLD patients. Intensive Care Med 19:450–455, 1993.

18. Kacmarek RM: Characteristics of pressure-targeted ventilators used for noninvasive positive pressure ventilation. Respir Care 42:380–388, 1997.

19. Lofaso F, Brochard L, Touchard D, et al: Evaluation of carbon dioxide rebreathing during pressure support ventilation with airway management system (BiPAP) devices. Chest 108:772–778, 1995.

20. Hess D: Noninvasive positive pressure ventilation: predictors of success and failure for adult acute care applications. Respir Care 42:424–431, 1997.

Case Studies in Mechanical Ventilation

Neil MacIntyre, MD

A series of questions pertaining to each case study follows the case study text and the illustrations. The numbered answers to the questions begin on page 504.

CASE STUDY 1. PARENCHYMAL LUNG INJURY (Reference Chapter 18)

MJ, a 46-year-old man without a prior history of cardiopulmonary disease, is brought to the hospital after a massive exposure to chlorine gas in a workplace accident. He is intubated in the Emergency Room and presents to the intensive care unit unresponsive and on a mechanical ventilator. His chest x-ray shows bilateral infiltrates and his arterial blood gases with an FiO_2 of 0.6 are PO_2 51, PCO_2 42, and pH 7.35.

Figure 1

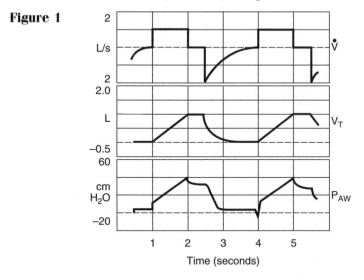

Time (seconds)

Questions

Figure 1 shows his ventilator graphics. (1) What mode of support is he receiving? _____ (2) What is the peak airway pressure (Ppeak)? _____ (3) What is the plateau airway pressure (Pplat)? _____ (4) What is the baseline airway pressure (PEEP)? _____ (5) What is the inspiratory flow (V')? _____ (6) What is the delivered tidal volume (V_T)? _____ (7) Calculate static compliance (V_T/Pplat–PEEP). _____ (8) Calculate inspiratory airway resistance (Ppeak–Pplat/V'). _____

Figure 2

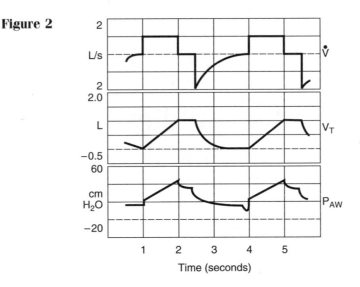

In Figure 2 PEEP has been increased and the PO_2 has improved to 81. (9) What is the PEEP setting now? _____ (10) What is the plateau pressure now? _____ (11) What is the compliance now? _____ (12) Does this represent alveolar recruitment? _____ (13) Why or why not? _____

Figure 3

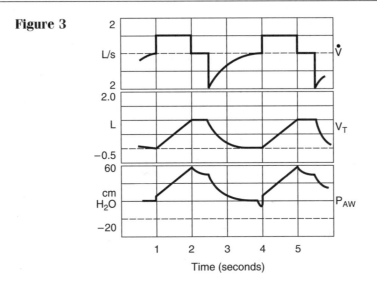

In Figure 3 PEEP has been further increased and the PO_2 has gone to 71. (14) What is the PEEP setting now? _____ (15) What is the plateau pressure now?_____ (16) What is the compliance now? _____ (17) Does this represent alveolar recruitment? _____ (18) Why or why not? _____

The PEEP is returned to Figure 2 levels and the PO_2 to 85. PCO_2 remains 42 and pH remains 7.35. (19) Should anything else be done at this time and why or why not? _____

CASE STUDY 2. PARENCHYMAL LUNG INJURY (Reference Chapter 18)

PD is a 65-year-old woman with febrile neutropenia and progressive bilateral pulmonary infiltrates on chest x-ray. She is on a ventilator with an FiO_2 of 1.0. The PO_2 is 54, the PCO_2 is 62, and the pH is 7.17.

Figure 4

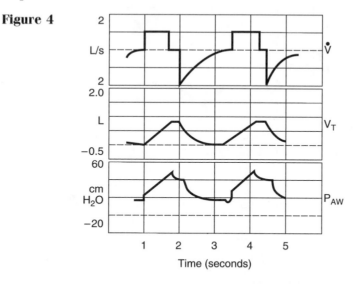

Questions

Figure 4 shows her ventilator graphics. (20) What is the mode? _____ (21) What is the peak airway pressure (Ppeak)? _____ (22) What is the plateau airway pressure (Pplat)? _____ (23) What is the baseline airway pressure (PEEP)? _____ (24) What is the inspiratory flow (V')? _____ (25) What is the delivered tidal volume (V_T)? _____ (26) What is the static compliance (V_T/Pplat–PEEP)? _____

Figure 5

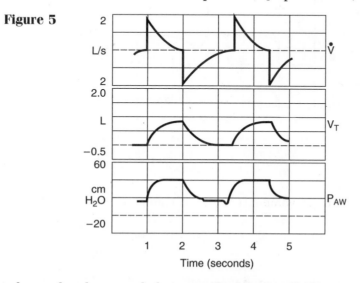

(27) What change has been made between Figures 4 and 5? _____ (28) How was the inspiratory pressure set to give the same V_T as that in Figure 4? _____ (29) What considerations were made in setting the inspiratory time to match ventilation of Figure 4? _____ (30) What is the static compliance now? _____ (31) Is this different from what is shown in Figure 4? _____ (32) Would you have expected them to be different? _____

Figure 6

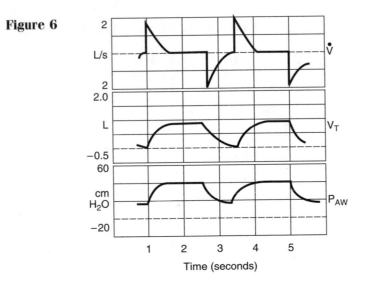

The blood gases remain essentially unchanged. (33) What change has been made between Figures 5 and 6? _____ (34) Did mean airway pressure change? _____
(35) Why or why not? _____
(36) Did air trapping develop? _____ (37) Give two graphical signs why or why not. A. _____ B. _____
(38) If you performed an expiratory hold maneuver, what would you observe? _____
_____

Figure 7

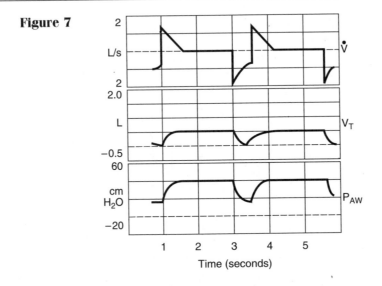

Blood gases show some improvement. (39) What change has been made between Figures 6 and 7? _____
_____ (40) Did mean airway pressure change? _____ (41) Did air trapping develop? _____ (42) Give two graphical signs why or why not. A. _____ B. _____
(43) What is the calculated static compliance now? _____
(44) Why is this different from that in Figure 6? _____
_____

(45) If you assume that true static compliance did not change between Figures 6 and 7, can you calculate the intrinsic PEEP that developed? _____

_____
_____

(46) If you performed an expiratory hold maneuver, what would you observe? _____
_____

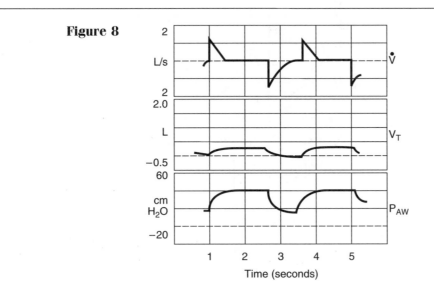

Figure 8

Time (seconds)

You return to the settings of Figure 6 and arterial blood gases improve. Two hours later, the patient becomes hypotensive and develops the graphics shown in Figure 8. (47) What ventilator parameter has been most affected? _____ (48) What is the compliance now? _____ (49) What are the most important diagnoses to consider? _____ (50) Had this been volume-targeted ventilation and assuming that alarms were not activated, what would have happened to Pplat? _____ (51) What would have happened to V_T? _____

CASE STUDY 3. ACUTE AIRFLOW OBSTRUCTION (Reference Chapter 19)

BF is a 39-year-old woman with severe asthma who presents to the emergency room with a respiratory arrest. She is resuscitated, intubated, and placed on a mechanical ventilator. Her initial blood gases on 100% O_2 are PO_2 102, PCO_2 38, and pH 7.42.

Figure 9

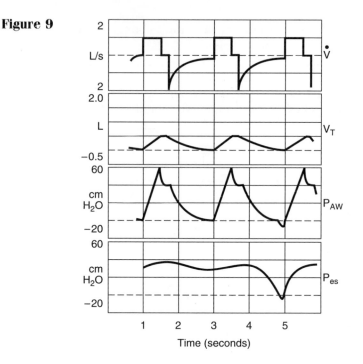

Questions

Her initial ventilator graphics are displayed in Figure 9. (52) What mode of support is she receiving? _____ (53) What is the peak airway pressure (Ppeak)? _____ (54) What is the plateau airway pressure (Pplat)? _____ (55) What is the baseline airway pressure (PEEP)? _____ (56) What is the inspiratory flow (V')? _____ (57) What is the delivered tidal volume (V_T)? _____

(58) Calculate static compliance (V_T/Pplat–PEEP). _____ (59) Calculate inspiratory airway resistance (Ppeak–Pplat/V'). _____ (60) Is air trapping present? _____ (61) Why or why not? _____

(62) Using the esophageal pressure tracing during the assisted breath, what level of intrinsic PEEP is present? _____ (63) Is this air trapping/intrinsic PEEP contributing to the increased plateau pressure? _____

(64) If this pressure is taken into account, what is the true inspiratory change in intra-alveolar (plateau-PEEP) pressure? _____

(65) What is true respiratory system compliance? _____

(66) Name four actions that could be taken to reduce air trapping/intrinsic PEEP in this patient?   A. _____   B. _____   C. _____   D. _____ (67) What additional step could be taken to improve triggering of the assisted breath?

CASE STUDY 4. ACUTE EXACERBATION OF CHRONIC AIRWAY OBSTRUCTION (Reference Chapter 19)

LT is a 66-year-old man with COPD who is intubated in the Emergency Room for respiratory failure. His initial blood gases on an FiO_2 of 0.5 are PO_2 98, PcO_2 78, and pH 7.08.

Figure 10

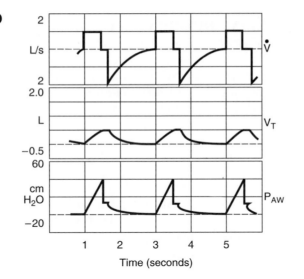

Time (seconds)

Questions

His ventilator graphics are shown in Figure 10. (68) Is air trapping present? _____
(69) Why or why not? _____ (70) What would happen with an
expiratory hold maneuver? _____ (71) What would happen to this expiratory
hold maneuver if the patient made inspiratory/expiratory efforts? _____
(72) Calculate static compliance (V_T/Pplat–PEEP). _____ (73) Calculate inspiratory
airway resistance (Ppeak–Pplat/V'). _____ (74) What change would you make at this
time? _____ (75) What two parameters would you monitor as you did
this? A. _____ B. _____

Figure 11

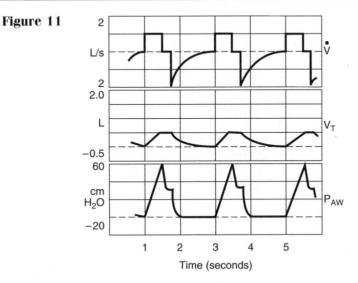

Time (seconds)

The next day, blood gases have improved and you have returned to the settings of Figure
10. However, later that day, the patient becomes hypotensive and the graphics in Figure 11
appear. (76) What is the static compliance? _____
(77) What diagnoses must be considered immediately? _____
(78) Had this been pressure-targeted ventilation and assuming that no alarms were activated, what would have happened to Pplat? _____
(79) What would have happened to V_T? _____

CASE STUDY 5. RECOVERING RESPIRATORY FAILURE/WEANING AND PARTIAL SUPPORT (Reference Chapters 9 and 20)

JR is a 54-year-old man with mild COPD who is intubated for respiratory failure following bilateral pneumonia. After four days of antibiotics and mechanical ventilatory support, his chest x-ray is clearing, PEEP has been reduced to 5, and FiO_2 is 0.4. He is awake and making efforts to breathe.

Questions

(80) What assessments are most likely to determine his potential for ventilator discontinuation? _____ (81) How often should these assessments be performed if he is deemed unfit for discontinuation today? _____

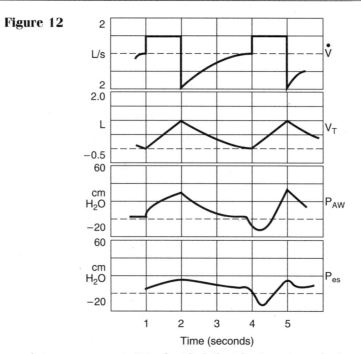

Figure 12

Time (seconds)

After appropriate assessment, it is decided that he is not ready for ventilator discontinuation. He is then placed on a substantial level of volume-targeted ventilation as displayed in Figure 12. (82) What are two obvious sources of imposed loading in Figure 12?

A. _____

B. _____

(83) What can be done?

A. _____

B. _____

Figure 13

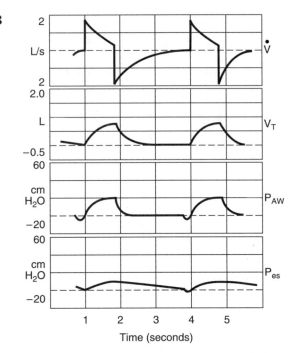

You choose another mode of assisted ventilation for this patient (Fig. 13). (84) What is this mode? _____ (85) How does pressure support differ from pressure assist? _____

(86) Does this mode appear synchronous with ventilatory efforts? _____
(87) Why is it or why is it not better than the volume-targeted breaths of Figure 12? _____

(88) What new mode has been introduced that may be helpful under these circumstances?

Figure 14

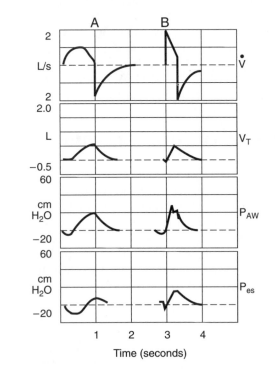

In an effort to improve flow synchrony, you adjust the pressure rate of rise setting in Figure 14. (89) Did you make the rise time faster or slower in breath A? _____ (90) Did you make the rise time faster or slower in breath B? _____ (91) Which rate of rise (Figure 13, Figure 14A,14B) seems most synchronous with the patient? _____

Figure 15

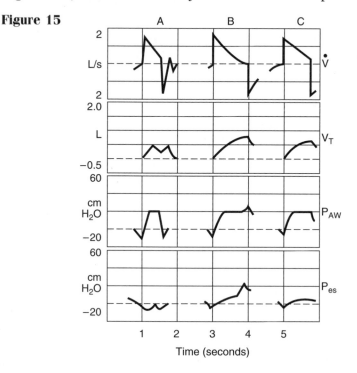

You set the optimal pressure rate of rise settings and maintain support until the next morning. The patient, however, again is deemed not ready for discontinuation and you return him to pressure support. Later that morning the patient seems to have difficulty synchronizing breath termination. You switch to pressure assist in an effort to control inspiratory time and improve cycle synchrony. In Figure 15 are three different inspiratory time settings. (92) Which setting is too long and forces the patient to actively force the breath off? _____ (93) Which setting is too short and leaves the patient demanding more gas at end inspiration? _____ (94) Which breath has the proper inspiratory time? _____

CASE STUDY 6. PARTIAL VENTILATORY SUPPORT AND LOAD SHARING
(Reference Chapter 9)

PH, a 42-year-old alcoholic man, is recovering from respiratory failure caused by aspiration pneumonia. You insert an esophageal balloon to assess load distribution between patient and ventilator. As you adjust the level of pressure support, you see three different patterns displayed on the pressure–time graphics as ventilatory loads are borne entirely by the ventilator, as ventilatory loads are shared between ventilator and patient, and as ventilatory loads are borne entirely by the patient (Figure 16). In these displays, load is characterized as a shaded pressure–time product (PTP).

Figure 16

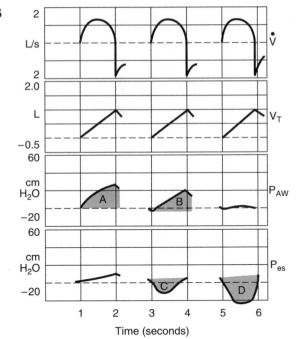

Time (seconds)

Questions

(95) Which shaded PTP represents ventilator load during total ventilatory support? _____ (96) Which shaded PTP represents ventilator load during partial (shared) support? _____ (97) Which shaded PTP represents patient load during an unassisted and unsupported breath? _____ (98) Which shaded PTP represents patient load during partial (shared) support? _____

(99) If flow and volume are equal during the three breaths in Figure 16, should PTP in *A* be equal to PTP in *D*? _____ (100) Why or why not? _____
(101) Should the sum of PTP in *B* plus PTP in *C* = PTP in *A* or *D*? _____

ANSWERS

Case Study 1

1. VACV
2. 40
3. 30
4. 5
5. 1 L/sec
6. 1000 ml
7. 1000/25 = 40
8. 10/1 = 10
9. 15
10. 35
11. 1000/20 = 50
12. Yes
13. Improved compliance
14. 20
15. 50
16. 1000/30 = 33 (rounded)
17. No
18. Worsening compliance and increased Pplat suggest overdistension
19. Pplat of 35 is still excessive; reduce V_T, accept higher CO_2

Case Study 2

20. VACV
21. 50
22. 40
23. 15
24. 1 L/sec
25. 750 ml
26. 750/25 = 30
27. Change to PACV
28. Match Pplat
29. Adequate to match V_T during VACV, short pause, adequate T_e
30. 750/25 = 30
31. No
32. No; same lung disease
33. Longer T_i with I:E reversal
34. Yes
35. Longer time of inspiratory pressure
36. No
37. A. No change V_T
    B. Adequate T_e
38. No change in baseline pressure
39. Longer T_i
40. Yes
41. Yes
42. A. V_T decreased
    B. Inadequate T_e with flow not returning to zero
43. 500/25 = 20
44. Intrinsic PEEP not included in the calculation of Pplat–PEEP
45. Yes; Static compliance = V_T/Pplat − total PEEP (applied plus intrinsic). Thus with a V_T of 500, a static compliance of 30 (Fig. 6), and a Pplat of 40, total PEEP must be 24 (compliance = V_T/Pplat–total PEEP; 30 = 500/40–24) and intrinsic PEEP (total-applied) is 24 − 15 = 9
46. Increase in baseline pressure
47. V_T
48. 250/25 = 10
49. Pneumothorax, airway obstruction
50. Increased
51. Not changed

Case Study 3

52. VACV
53. 60
54. 40
55. 0
56. 1 L/sec
57. 500
58. 500/40 = 12.5
59. 20/1 = 20
60. Yes
61. Inadequate expiratory time such that flow does not return to zero
62. 30
63. Yes
64. 40 − 30 = 10
65. 500/10 = 50
66. A. Reduce V_T
    B. Reduce T_i
    C. Reduce frequency
    D. Use a low-density gas (heliox)
67. Apply PEEP to equilibrate circuit PEEP with intrinsic PEEP

Case Study 4

68. No
69. Expiratory flow returns to zero
70. No change in baseline pressure

71. Baseline pressure would be falsely reduced or elevated
72. $500/10 = 50$
73. $30/1 = 30$
74. Increase frequency and/or V_T
75. A. Pplat; keep below 30–35
    B. Expiratory flow tracing to assess adequacy of T_e
76. $500/30 = 17$ (rounded)
77. Pneumothorax, airway obstruction
78. Nothing
79. Decreased

Case Study 5

80. f/V_T, mental status, discomfort after 1- to 2-hour discontinuation assessment
81. Daily
82. A. Insensitive trigger
    B. Inadequate flow delivery
83. A. Increase sensitivity or change to flow trigger
    B. Increase set flow or change to pressure-targeted mode
84. PSV

85. Pressure support terminates on flow reduction (T_i can vary), whereas pressure assist has a clinician-set T_i
86. Yes
87. Adjustable flow responds to patient effort
88. Proportional assist ventilation (PAV); it also adjusts to patient effort
89. Slower
90. Faster
91. Figure 13
92. B
93. A
94. C

Case Study 6

95. A
96. B
97. D
98. C
99. Yes
100. Same respiratory system mechanical properties and ventilatory pattern
101. Yes

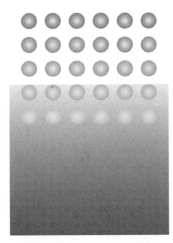

Glossary

Abdominal pressure Pressure within the abdominal space. This is often used as a reference to intrathoracic pressures in order to calculate transdiaphragmatic pressures. This pressure is commonly measured in either the gastric space or the urinary bladder.

Absolute humidity The amount of water vapor present in a gas mixture. Typically expressed in mg H_2O/L.

Active heat and moisture exchanger A device that combines a passive humidifier and a heated humidifier to reduce water usage and increase moisture output.

Acute respiratory distress syndrome (ARDS) A severe pulmonary inflammatory response to a variety of insults, resulting in capillary leak, interstitial edema, intra-alveolar hemorrhage and exudate, decreased pulmonary compliance, decreased ventilation-perfusion matching, and progressive hypoxemic respiratory failure.

Active expiration Expiration assisted by the ventilatory muscles.

Adaptive support ventilation A mode of ventilatory support in which the ventilator can choose ventilator settings following the input of patient weight and % minute volume. The ventilator operates in the pressure control and pressure support modes and can change I:E during mandatory breaths.

Air trapping See *Intrinsic PEEP*. This is sometimes also called "occult" PEEP.

Airway anatomy The anatomic structures in the head, neck, and thorax through which ventilation occurs.

Airway pressure Pressure in the airways of the lung, often assumed to be identical to ventilator circuit problems.

Airway pressure release ventilation (APRV) A respiratory support pattern that provides a moderately high level of continuous airway pressure that is interspersed with brief deflation (release) periods. Spontaneous breaths can occur throughout the ventilatory cycle.

Alarm A visual and/or auditory signal that occurs when a monitored parameter has exceeded a set limit.

Alarm event Any condition or occurrence that triggers an alarm and requires clinician awareness or action.

Alternate care sites Sites of care for mechanically ventilated patients that are outside the acute care hospital. Examples include long-term facilities, skilled nursing facilities, and the home.

American Heart Association device classification system The system by which devices used during cardiopulmonary resuscitation are classified based on usefulness and possibility of doing harm. This system includes the following: *Class I*–A therapeutic option that is usually indicated, is always acceptable, and is considered useful and effective. *Class II*–A therapeutic option that is acceptable, is of uncertain efficacy, and may be controversial. *Class IIa*–A therapeutic option for which the weight of evidence is in favor of its usefulness and efficacy. *Class IIb*–A therapeutic option that is not well established by evidence but may be helpful and probably is not harmful. *Class III*–A therapeutic option that is inappropriate, is without scientific supporting data, and may be harmful.

Antibiotics Chemical agents that kill micro-organisms or inhibit their growth.

APACHE An acronym for the Acute Physiologic and Chronic Health Evaluation Score. It represents a simple scoring system used to predict outcome.

ARDS An acronym for the acute respiratory distress syndrome. This syndrome is characterized by an acute lung injury producing a noncardiogenic edema, bilateral chest x-ray infiltrates and severe hypoxemia.

Aspiration Describes the introduction of oral, nasal, pharyngeal, or gastric contents into the lung.

Assessments for ventilator withdrawal A series of clinical observations and physiologic measurements designed to determine the potential for patients to be withdrawn from mechanical ventilation.

Assisted expiration Expiratory flow generated by a negative change in transrespiratory pressure due to an external agent (such as a drop in airway pressure below baseline.)

Assisted inspiration Inspiratory flow generated by a positive change in transrespiratory pressure due to an external agent (such as a rise in airway pressure above baseline).

Assisted ventilation The process of providing a positive pressure breath in response to a patient's inspiratory effort.

AutoPEEP See *Intrinsic PEEP.*

Bag valve resuscitator Consists of a self-inflating bag, oxygen reservoir, and non-rebreathing valve. The operator ventilates the patient by squeezing the self-inflating bag, which forces air into the non-rebreathing valve and to the patient. The self-inflating bag is typically made of a resilient material such as rubber, silicon, or polyvi-

nylchloride. Most self-inflating bags have a volume of around 2.0L for adults.

Barotrauma/volutrauma Injury to the lung due to excessive pressure and/or volume in the lung.

Barrier device A flexible sheet that typically contains a valve and/or filter separating the rescuer from the patient.

Basic airway management Procedures to maintain a patent airway without the use of an endotracheal tube.

Bernoulli's principle The physical principle of a lowered pressure around a moving fluid or gas.

Broncho-alveolar lavage The procedure whereby distal regions of the lung are washed with fluid for the purpose of obtaining samples for diagnosis.

Bronchodilator A drug that expands the lumina of the air passages of the lungs.

Bubble humidifier A humidifier that imparts heat and moisture to gas as it is released under the surface of the water and "bubbles" to the surface.

Calcium chloride A hygroscopic chemical substance that enhances the heat- and moisture-exchanging capabilities of the passive humidifier.

Cardiopulmonary interactions The interactions of changes in intrathoracic pressures and volumes on cardiovascular function.

Cascade humidifier A type of bubble humidifier that uses an underwater grid to increase the gas/liquid interface and increase humidity.

Chronic obstruction pulmonary disease (COPD) A disease process involving chronic inflammation of the airways. Variants include chronic bronchitis (disease predominance in the large airways) and emphysema (disease predominance in the smaller airways and alveolar regions).

Closed circuit suction catheter A suction catheter designed to be used in-line with the ventilator circuit so that the ventilator does not need to be disconnected. Closed circuit suctioning has been associated with fewer complications than traditional suctioning techniques.

Closed-loop control A control scheme in which the actual output of a system is measured and compared with the desired output. If there is a difference caused by external disturbances, the actual output is modified to bring it closer to the desired output.

Colorimetric CO_2 detector A device which detects the presence of carbon dioxide in expired gas and indicates the presence of CO_2 by changing color (usually yellow to purple).

Compliance The relative ease at which a body or tissue stretches or deforms.

Compressible volume The volume of gas that distends the ventilator circuit during delivery of a positive pressure breath. This volume is considered "lost," as it is not delivered to the patient.

Compressor A device that is designed to compress a gas (usually air).

Condensation Water that collects in the ventilator circuit as gas cools when the amount of water vapor present exceeds the carrying capacity of the gas.

Constant positive airway pressure (CPAP) A therapeutic modality that maintains a constant transrespiratory pressure. CPAP is not a ventilatory mode because it does not generate a tidal volume.

Control circuit: The ventilator subsystem responsible for controlling the drive mechanism and/or the output control valves.

Control variable The variable (either pressure, volume, flow, or time) that the ventilator manipulates to cause inspiration. This variable is identified by the fact that its behavior remains consistent despite changes in ventilatory load.

Convective gas transport Gas transport that moves O_2 and CO_2 in discrete volumes ("bulk flow").

Cricoid pressure Pushing down on the cricoid membrane, thereby collapsing the esophagus against the cervical vertebrae. Cricoid pressure has been shown to prevent gastric insufflation during mask ventilation.

Cricothyroidotomy The procedure whereby an airway is obtained through the crycothyroid membrane into the trachea.

Cuff pressure The pressure exerted by the tracheal tube cuff on the airway mucosa.

Cycle To end a mechanically supported inspiration.

Cycle time The duration of the delivery of gas under positive pressure during inspiration until a cycle criterion is met.

Cycle synchrony Dead space. The process of matching the ventilator breath termination to the termination of the patient's effort during interactive breaths.

Dead volume Volume of medication in a nebulizer that cannot be aerosolized due to device construction.

Demand valve A valving system in a mechanical ventilator that responds to a patient effort.

Density The quality of being compact or dense.

Dual control Modes of ventilation whereby two or more variables may control breath delivery depending upon certain circumstances.

End-expiratory pressure (EEP) The baseline transrespiratory pressure that exists at the end of the expiratory time. This pressure is often positive (PEEP).

End-expiratory valve A mechanical valve that regulates pressure during the expiratory phase.

Endotracheal tube An artificial airway passed through the nose or mouth past the vocal cords and into the trachea.

End points Measurements used to determine safety and efficiency.

Engineering assessment Techniques to assess the mechanical performance of a device.

Esophageal obturator airway Artificial airway inserted in the esophagus. The device occludes the esophagus so that delivered ventilation enters the lung.

Esophageal pressure Pressure measured in the midesophagus and taken to represent pleural pressure.

Expiratory flow time The time during which expiratory flow occurs.

Expiratory phase (expiration) The part of the ventilatory cycle from the beginning of expiratory flow to the beginning of inspiratory flow.

Expiratory pause time The time during the expiratory phase when no flow is occurring.

Expiratory time The duration of the expiratory phase.

Expired air resuscitation Rescue breathing during cardiopulmonary resuscitation in which the rescuer's exhaled gas provides ventilation for the victim. Types of expired air resuscitation include mouth-to-mouth and mouth-to-mask ventilation.

External compressor A device external to the ventilator used to supply pneumatic source power.

Extracorporeal membrane oxygenation (ECMO) A technique whereby blood is taken from a vein, passed through a device that adds oxygen, and then returned to the patient either into one of the great veins or the arterial circuit.

Flow Rate of gas delivery in and out of the lung.

Flow synchrony Matching of ventilator flow deliver to patient efforts during interactive breaths.

Food and Drug Administration US government agency charged with ensuring safety and efficacy of medical devices.

Gas consumption Gas consumed by a ventilator that does not participate in ventilation of the patient. The gas is used to control ventilator function and is wasted.

Gastric insufflation Forcing air into the stomach during positive pressure ventilation in an uninstrumented airway.

Gauge pressure Pressure measured relative to atmospheric pressure.

Gravitational sedimentation Deposition of aerosol due to weight of the particle in a stagnant air stream.

Graham's law The rapidity of diffusion of two gases varies inversely with the square root of their densities.

Heat and moisture exchanger A passive humidifier that uses only physical means of heat and moisture exchange.

Heat and moisture exchanging filter A passive humidifier that uses physical means of heat and moisture exchange and includes a breathing circuit filter.

Heated wire circuit A ventilator circuit that contains electric wires that heat the gas as it travels down the circuit. These devices help eliminate or minimize condensate.

Helium (He) A gas that is much less dense than air and/or oxygen and thus requires less pressure to effect flow through given resistance.

High flow humidifier A humidification device used to add moisture to inspired gases and flows used during mechanical ventilation.

High frequency ventilation (HFV) Ventilatory support characterized by frequencies greater than physiologic breaths per minute.

HME booster A device that adds moisture to inspired gas between the passive humidifier and the patient.

Hygroscopic heat and moisture exchanger A passive humidifier in which both physical and chemical means of heat and moisture exchange are used.

Hygroscopic heat and moisture exchanging filter A passive humidifier in which both physical and chemical means of heat and moisture exchange are used; it incorporates a breathing circuit filter.

Hyperbaric oxygen therapy (HBO) The administration of oxygen at high levels of pressure (greater than atmospheric; i.e., at sea level atmospheric pressure is 760 mm Hg). During hyperbaric exposure, plasma-dissolved oxygen increases approximately 2 vol % for every atmosphere increase in inspired oxygen. Typical applications of HBO include decompression sickness, gas gangrene, carbon monoxide poisoning, cyanide poisoning, and circulatory disorders.

Independent lung ventilation (ILV) A method by which the gas flow to each lung is effectively separated mechanically by either two small endotracheal tubes (ETT) or one specifically designed double-lumen ETT for the purpose of differential ventilation of each lung, with different ventilation parameters.

Indirect calorimetry A technique that measures oxygen consumption and CO_2 production to predict nutritional needs and quantify metabolic activity.

Inertial impaction The process of removing large aerosol particles from a carrier gas due to greater inertia. Larger particles travel in a straight trajectory and impact against objects in their path.

Inspiratory/expiratory timing The ratio of inspiratory time to expiratory time (I:E ratio).

Inspiratory phase (inspiration) The part of the ventilatory cycle from the beginning of inspiratory flow to the beginning of expiratory flow. Any inspiratory pause is included in the inspiratory phase.

Inspiratory flow time The time during the inspiratory phase when flow is being delivered.

Inspiratory pause time Inspiratory pause is a brief pause (0.5 to 2 seconds) at end-inspiration during which pressure is held constant and flow is zero. Under those conditions, airway pressure is equal to end inspiratory alveolar pressure. The pause may also improve gas mixing.

Inspiratory time Inspiratory time (expressed in seconds) is the duration of inspiration during mechanical ventilation. As inspiratory time increases, mean airway pressure increases and the I:E ratio becomes higher.

Inspired gas concentrations The partial pressures of oxygen, nitrogen, and other therapeutic gases such as helium or nitric oxide that may be in the inspired gas mixture.

Internal compressor A device inside the ventilator used to convert either pneumatic or electric source power into inspiratory pressure.

Intravascular oxygenation A technique whereby blood oxygenation devices are inserted into the vasculature.

Intrinsic PEEP End-expiratory pressure in the lung as a consequence of excessive minute ventilation, an inadequately set expiratory time or airway obstruction preventing lung emptying. Intrinsic PEEP is sometimes referred to as air trapping, auto-PEEP, and occult PEEP.

Jets Ventilatory devices used in a technique to deliver HFV.

Laminar flow Flow through a tube that flows parallel to the tube walls in concentric layers with linear velocities that increase toward the center of the tube.

Laryngeal mask airway A device used to direct gas delivery into the larynx without an endotracial tube.

Laryngoscope Device designed to permit visualization of the larynx and airways through the mouth.

Lithium chloride A hygroscopic chemical substance that enhances the heat- and moisture-exchanging capabilities of the passive humidifier.

Limit To set a maximum value for pressure, volume, or flow during mechanically supported inspiration (or expiration); the preset maximum value for pressure, volume, or flow during an assisted inspiration (or expiration). Inspiration (or expiration) does not terminate because the limit value has been met.

Lung protective strategies Mechanical ventilation strategies designed to limit/reduce overdistension and under-recruitment of the lung so as to minimize iatrogenic lung injury.

Mandatory breath A mechanical breath that is initiated and terminated by the ventilator rather than by the patient's ventilatory drive.

Mass median aerodynamic diameter (MMAD) The particle diameter around which the mass of particle diameters is equally distributed.

Mean airway pressure The average pressure that exists at the airway opening over the ventilatory period. It is usually measured as gauge pressure. Mean airway pressure is mathematically equivalent to the area under the time-pressure curve (from the beginning of one breath to the beginning of the next breath) divided by the ventilatory period.

Mechanical ventilation The technique of providing by means of a machine either some or all of the work of breathing for a patient.

Mechanical ventilation outcome Descriptions of the important results from using mechanical ventilation. Generally recognized important outcomes are mortality, length of stay on the ventilator, and iatrogenic complications.

Metered dose inhaler A device in which a pressurized canister is used to deliver a precise dose of aerosolized medication.

Minimal occlusive technique The technique for maintaining the endotracheal tube cuff in which a volume of gas is used in the cuff sufficient to allow a small air leak at end-inspiration.

Minimal seal technique The technique for maintaining the endotracheal tube cuff in which uses a volume of gas is used in the cuff sufficient to prevent a leak at end-inspiration.

Minute ventilation (MV) The total amount of gas moving in or out of the lungs during 1 minute.

Monitor A routine repetitive or continuous measurement of a parameter.

Moisture output The amount of moisture delivered to the patient from a passive humidifier expressed in mg H_2O/L.

Mucociliary escalator The cilia and mucus layer that propel mucus and foreign bodies up the respiratory tree to be swallowed or expectorated.

Muscle fatigue A condition of muscle dysfunction that is recoverable by rest.

Muscle overload A condition in which the load on the muscles is excessive and may cause fatigue.

Myopathy Any disease of muscle.

Non-convective gas transport Movement of O_2 and CO_2 by mechanisms other than bulk flow movement of discrete tidal volumes.

Noninvasive ventilation Techniques of assisting or controlling ventilation using devices that do not require endotracheal tube placement.

Obstructive lung disease Disease characterized by airway narrowing.

Open-loop control A control scheme in which the output of a system is determined by the initial setting of the controller with no corrections made to accommodate disturbances in the output caused by external factors.

Oro- and nasopharyngeal airways Devices inserted into the mouth or the nose to help maintain airway patency.

Oscillators A technique to deliver HFV utilizing oscillating piston or membrane.

Overdistension The process of providing excessive volume to lung regions, thereby causing a "stretch" injury.

Oxidant injury An injury that can occur to living tissue when excessive oxygen concentrations are used. The mediators of oxygen injury are a variety of free radicals generated in the presence of high oxygen concentrations.

Oxygen (O) A chemical element. It constitutes about 20 percent of atmospheric air and is the essential agent in the respiration of plants and animals. Although noninflammable, it is necessary to support combustion.

Oxygen delivery system A device used to deliver oxygen concentrations above ambient air to the lungs through the upper airway.

Oxygen powered breathing device A device that consists of a demand valve that can be manually or patient triggered. The OPD is connected to a 50-psig source of gas and connects to the patient via a standard 15/22 mm connector. During manual activation of the demand valve, the operator depresses the actuator, allowing flow to travel to the patient.

Oxygen toxicity The pathologic response of the body and its tissues resulting from long-term exposure to high partial pressure of oxygen; pulmonary manifestations include cellular changes causing congestion, inflammation, and edema.

Paralysis Loss or impairment of motor function in part due to a lesion of the neural or muscular mechanism; also, by analogy, impairment of sensory function.

Parenchymal lung injury Lung injury resulting from processes affecting the alveolar capillary interface, the interstitium, or the vasculature.

Partial liquid ventilation The achievement of gas exchange through the use of oxygen soluble (often perfluorocarbon) liquid in the functional residual capacity of the lung.

Partial ventilatory support Mechanical ventilatory support in which the patient and the ventilator share the ventilatory load.

Passive expiration Expiration not assisted by the ventilatory muscles.

Passover humidifier A humidifier that imparts heat and moisture to gas flowing over the surface of the water. Also, a humidifier that collects the patient's expired heat and moisture and returns it on inspiration.

PEEP Acronym for positive end-expiratory pressure.

Perfluorocarbons Perfluorocarbons are colorless, odorless, and inert liquids produced by the fluorination of common organic hydrocarbons. These liquids have gained popularity as an alternative respiratory medium because of their high solubilities for the respiratory gases and their low surface tensions.

Permissive hypercapnia Ventilatory support strategy that accepts hypercapnia as a trade-off to excessive lung distension.

Peroxynitritic A substance produced by nitric oxide that is potentially toxic.

Phase One of four significant events that occur during a ventilatory cycle: (1) the change from expiratory time to inspiratory time, (2) inspiratory time, (3) the change from inspiratory time to expiratory time, and (4) expiratory time.

Phase variable A variable (such as pressure, volume, flow, or time) that is measured and used to initiate some phase of the ventilatory cycle.

Phase variable value The magnitude of a phase variable.

Pleural pressure Pressure inside the pleural space (between the lungs and chest wall) often reflected as esophageal pressure.

Pneumonia Infection in lung parenchyma.

Positive pressure ventilation Use of positive airway pressure to support ventilation.

Postextubation stridor The sound that occurs in an extubated patient from flow through an upper airway narrowed by inflammation from an endotracheal tube.

Pressure gradients The difference in pressure across a resistance or a compliance structure.

Pressure-time product A quantification of ventilation load that is obtained by integrating pressure over time. (See *work* below for an alternative load expression).

Pressure-volume plots Graphical display of applied pressure over volume. The area of the plot is work.

Proportional assist ventilation (PAV) An interactive ventilatory support mode that provides patient-triggered breaths in which flow and volume delivery are controlled by clinician-set "gains" placed on sensed patient effort. With PAV, increases in patient effort result in increased flow, volume, and airway pressure.

Protected specimen brush This is a small brush at the end of a long catheter designed to sample distal airways for microorganisms. It has an outer sheath to "protect" it from contamination from upper airway microorganisms.

Pulmonary artery hypertension High pressures within the pulmonary vasculature. This is usually caused by an increase in pulmonary vascular resistance secondary to lung disease, and/or hypoxia.

Rainout See *Condensation*.

Relative humidity The amount of water vapor in a gas compared with the maximum amount of water that gas can carry. Relative humidity is expressed as a percent.

Resistance Impedance to flow in a tube or conduit; quantified as ratio of the difference in pressure between the two points along a tube length divided by the volumetric flow of the fluid per unit time.

Respiratory distress syndrome (RDS) A result of surfactant deficiency and/or a pulmonary insult in the neonatal period, this condition is marked by tachypnea, hypoxemia, decreased pulmonary compliance, and alveolar collapse.

Respiratory insufficiency The inability of the body to provide adequate arterial oxygenation.

Respiratory quotient Ratio of CO_2 production to O_2 consumption.

Responsiveness A description of demand valve performance that refers to how fast the valve can respond to a patient demand.

Resting energy expenditure The caloric consumption of a patient.

Reynolds number A dimensionless number that predicts whether flow will be laminar or turbulent based on gas velocity, viscosity, density, and tube diameter. A Reynolds number <2000 indicates laminar flow and >2000 indicates turbulent flow.

Right ventricular dysfunction Dysfunction of the right ventricle induced by high pulmonary vascular resistance (right ventricularor intrinsic heart disease).

Saturated The state of gas that is carrying the maximum possible amount of water vapor. Saturated gas is at 100% relative humidity.

Sedation The allaying of irritability or excitement, especially by administration of a sedative.

Sedation level score Score used to determine the adequacy of sedation based on patient response to stimuli.

Sellick maneuver Technique of providing cricoid pressure named for its inventor.

Sensitivity A measure of the amount of effort that must be generated by a patient to trigger a mechanical ventilator into the inspiratory phase; alternatively, the mechanism used to set or control this level.

Shunting Pulmonary capillary blood completely bypassing ventilated alveoli.

Small-volume nebulizer An aerosol generator that requires a gas source to nebulize liquid medications.

Spacer A device used to improve aerosol delivery by stabilizing particle size and reducing the need for breath/actuation coordination. Can be used in ambulatory and mechanically ventilated patients.

Spontaneous breath Breath that is both patient initiated and patient terminated.

Spontaneous ventilatory drive Inherent ventilatory drive set by the patient's ventilatory control center in the brain.

Suction catheter A thin, hollow plastic tube containing several distal holes used for removal of airway secretions by application of negative pressure.

Surfactant Lung lining fluid that reduces surface tensions.

Sympathomimetics Adrenergic; producing effects resembling those of impulses transmitted by the adrenergic postganglionic fibers of the sympathetic nervous system.

Total liquid ventilation The achievement of gas exchange through the delivery of tidal volumes of perfluorocarbon liquid to the lungs, using a specialized mechanical liquid ventilator.

Total ventilatory support Mechical ventilatory support supplying total unloading of a patient's ventilatory muscles.

Tracheal gas insufflation (TGI) A technique whereby a low flow of fresh gas is delivered to the distal end of the endotracheal tube through a small diameter catheter. This flow can be either continuous (i.e., throughout the ventilatory cycle) or delivered only during exhalation. The primary purpose of TGI is to flush the upper airway with fresh gas during exhalation and thereby to reduce functional dead space.

Tracheal intubation The technique by which a tube is inserted into the trachea in order to supply a patent airway.

Train-of-four A method of monitoring neuromuscular blockade in patients. A sequence of four electrical stimuli are delivered to electrodes placed over a nerve (usually the temporal or radial nerve) and the twitch of the involved muscle group is measured to gauge neuromuscular blockade. If four stimuli are provided and no twitches are present, blockade is deep. If two of four stimuli result in twitches, blockade is usually sufficient.

Transducer A device capable of converting one form of energy into another and commonly used for measurement of physical events; for example, a pressure transducer may convert the physical phenomenon of force per unit area into an analog electrical signal.

Transrespiratory pressure The pressure difference between airway and body surface.

Trigger To initiate the inspiratory phase of an assisted breath.

Turbulent flow Flow characterized by formation of currents and eddies resulting in chaotic movement of gas molecules and a Reynolds number >2000.

Under-recruitment The phenomenon of alveolar collapse that persists because of inadequate expiratory pressure. Linked to lung injury.

Venoarterial bypass Technique for cardiopulmonary bypass (see extracorporeal oxygenation).

Venovenous bypass Technique for cardiopulmonary bypass (see extracorporeal oxygenation).

Ventilator circuit The plastic nondisposable or disposable tubing (22 mm OD for adults) that connects the mechanical ventilator to the artificial airway or mask.

Ventilation distribution The description of how the tidal volume is distributed to the millions of alveolar units.

Ventilation/perfusion (V/Q) relationships Quantification of the relationship of ventilation to perfusion in alveolar capillary units. This is normally 1. Very high V/Q units are effectively dead space. V/Q units of 0 are shunts.

Ventilator dependence Need for mechanical ventilation.

Ventilator discontinuation Discontinuation of mechanical ventilation support from a patient.

Volume Space occupied by matter measured in milliliters or liters.

Volume-assured pressure support A mode of ventilator operation that allows automated adjustment of inspiratory pressure (pressure support) based upon tidal volume.

Weaning Gradual reduction in partial ventilatory support.

Weaning techniques Ventilator strategies that accomplish weaning.

Work A quantification of ventilation load that is obtained by integrating pressure over volume. (See *Pressure time product* above for an alternative load expression.)

Index

Note: Page numbers in *italics* refer to illustrations; page numbers followed by t refer to tables.

A-aDO$_2$. See *Alveolar-arterial oxygen difference (A-aDO$_2$)*.
A/C ventilation. See *Assist/control (A/C) ventilation*.
Absolute humidity, 103–104
  relationship of gas temperature to, water vapor pressure, and, 104t
Acinetobacter spp., pneumonia from, 309, 310t, 319
Active hygroscopic heat and moisture exchangers (active HHMEs), 115–116
Acute lung injury (ALI), 330–331
  diagnostic criteria for, 331t
  mortality from, 338t
Acute Physiology and Chronic Health Evaluation (APACHE), 227
Acute respiratory distress syndrome (ARDS), 330–331
  diagnostic criteria for, 331t
  mortality from, 338t
  nitric oxide for, 461–462
  PLV in, 449
  prone positioning in, clinical effects of, 292–293
    physiologic mechanisms of, 290–291
  studies of ventilator-induced lung injury in patients with, 217–219
Adaptive support ventilation (ASV), 77–79
  classification of, 77–79
  descriptive definition of, 77
  manufacturer terms for, 77
  minimum and maximum values for ventilator variables in, 78t
Adenovirus, pneumonia from, 311
Adhesive tape, securing endotracheal tube by, *91*
Aerosol, delivery of, factors affecting, 117–118
  during mechanical ventilation, 119–125

Aerosol *(Continued)*
  deposition of, in intubated/ventilated patients, factors affecting, 121t
Aerosol generators, types of, 118–119
Aerosol therapy, 116–125
  with antibiotics, 275
  with anti-inflammatory agents, 274
  with antimuscarinics, 273–274
  with DNase, 278
  factors that can affect response to, during mechanical ventilation, 270t
  general therapeutic considerations in, 269–270
  recommendations for, in ventilated patients, 125
  with ribavirin, 276–277
  with surfactant, 278–280
  with sympathomimetics, 272–273
Air embolism, systemic, 214
Air trapping. See also *Intrinsic positive end-expiratory pressure (intrinsic PEEP)*.
  in obstructive airway disease, 341, 344
  monitoring of, 139
Airway(s), anatomy of, 239–241
  examination of, in assessment for intubation, 246–247
  in parenchymal lung injury, 331
  management of, 239–256
Airway maintenance, equipment for, in patient transport, 384
Airway obstruction, acute, case study in, 497–498
  less severe, partial ventilatory support for, 344–345
  pathophysiology of, 341
  requiring total ventilator support, mode selection in, 342–343
  ventilation settings and strategies in, 342–344

Airway obstruction *(Continued)*
  respiratory failure due to, causes of, 340–341
  outcome of, 346
  total support for, goals of mechanical ventilation in providing, 341–342
  simple maneuvers to relieve, 241–242
  upper, heliox for, 455
Airway pressure, changes in, required for triggering CPAP systems, *193*
Airway pressure release ventilation (APRV), 68–69, 197, 401–403
  airway pressure, volume, and flow during, *402*
  classification of, 68–69
  data on, 402–403
  description of/rationale for, 401–402
  descriptive definition of, 68
  for parenchymal lung injury, 337–338
  manufacturer terms for, 68
  other terms for, 68
  pressure, flow, and volume vs time in, *70*
  recommendations for, 403
Alarm conditions, interpreting and responding to, 142
Alarm systems, auto-set parameters in, examples of, 143t
  ventilator, 46–49, 139–143
    classification of, 47t
    cost-effectiveness of, 142–143
    maximizing sensitivity and specificity of, 142
Albuterol, aerosol therapy with, 272–273
Alfentanil, 261
Alveolar-arterial oxygen difference (A-aDO$_2$), as ECLS criterion, *428*
Alveolar capillary gas transport, 161–171
  in context of overall oxygen delivery, 169–171

Alveolar overdistention, 216
  monitoring of, 137–138
Alveolar space, oxygen gradient from,
  to mitochondria, *174*
Alveolar under-recruitment, monitoring
  of, 138–139
Alveoli, anatomy of, 241
  collapsed, changes to, under PEEP,
    167
AMV. See *Assisted mechanical
  ventilation (AMV)*.
Analgesia, in ECLS, 431
Anemic hypoxia, 180
Anesthetic agents, 259–260
Anesthetic gases, in total ventilatory
    support for airway obstruction, 344
4-Anilinopiperidines, 261
Antibiotics, aerosolized, 274–276
    aerosol therapy with, during me-
      chanical ventilation, 275
    clinical utility of, 274–275
    factors affecting delivery of, 275t
    for pneumonia prophylaxis, 320
    for ventilator-associated pneumonia,
      313–316
Anticoagulation, in ECLS, 431
Anti-inflammatory agents, 274
  aerosol therapy with, 274
Antimuscarinics, 273–274
  aerosol therapy with, 272–273
  clinical utility of, 273
APACHE. See *Acute Physiology and
  Chronic Health Evaluation
  (APACHE)*.
APRV. See *Airway pressure release
  ventilation (APRV)*.
Arrhythmias, from endotracheal
  suctioning, 97
Arterial oxygen pressure (PO$_2$), for
  venous blood of different organ
  systems, 180t
Arterial oxygenation, monitoring, during
  oxygen therapy, 182
Artificial airway, care of, 88–94
  respiratory tract/physiologic effects of
    breathing cool, dry gases via,
    106t
Artificial noses. See *Passive humidifiers*.
Aspergillus fumigatus, pneumonia from,
  310t
Aspergillus spp., pneumonia from, 312,
  316
Aspiration, in NPPV, 491
  reducing, pneumonia prevention by,
    319–320
Aspiration pneumonia, nutrition support
    and, 233
Assist/control (A/C) ventilation, 55–59
  classification of, 58–59
  descriptive definition of, 55–58
  for parenchymal lung injury, 334–335
  for total ventilatory support in airway
    obstruction, 342–343
  in ventilator weaning, 351–355

Assist/control (A/C) ventilation
    (Continued)
  manufacturer terms for, 58
  other terms for, 58
  pressure control (PC), pressure, flow,
    and volume vs time in, *61*
  volume control (VC), pressure, flow,
    and volume vs time in, *60*
Assisted breath, 25
Assisted mechanical ventilation (AMV),
    59–60
  classification of, 59–60
  descriptive definition of, 59
  manufacturer terms for, 59
  other terms for, 59
Assister/controller/spontaneous
    breathing, 30
Assister/controllers, 30
Assisters, 30
Asthma, effect of posture and position
    in, 289–290
  heliox for, 455
  NPPV for, 485
  radial artery pressure tracings in, be-
    fore, during, and after heliox ad-
    ministration, *456*
ASV. See *Adaptive support ventilation
  (ASV)*.
ATC. See *Automatic tube compensation
  (ATC)*.
Atelectasis, NPPV for, 485
  in patients with neuromuscular weak-
    ness, effect of position on, 289
Atracurium, 263–264
Auto-positive end-expiratory pressure
  (AutoPEEP). See *Intrinsic positive
  end-expiratory pressure (intrinsic
  PEEP)*.
Automatic tube compensation (ATC),
    79–80
  classification of, 79–80
  descriptive definition of, 79
  manufacturer terms for, 79
  vs. PSV, in overcoming endotracheal
    tube resistance, *79*
AutoMode, 76–77
  classification of, 76–77
  descriptive definition of, 76
  manufacturer terms for, 76
AutoPEEP. See *Intrinsic positive end-
  expiratory pressure (intrinsic
  PEEP)*.

Bag-valve resuscitators, 372–375
  description of, 372–373
  ventilation efficiency of, 373–374
BAL. See *Bronchoalveolar lavage
  (BAL)*.
Barrier devices, emergency ventilation,
  369
Baseline variables, 23
Benzodiazepines, 257–259

Bernoulli's principle, 455
Beta-2 agonists, 270–273
  adverse effects of, *271*
  aerosol therapy with, during mechani-
    cal ventilation, 272–273
  clinical utility of, 271–272
Body weight, in nutritional assessment,
  227
Breath parameters, ventilator, 191t
Breath types, comparison of, 25t
  designed to fully unload ventilatory
    muscles, 194–196
  designed to partially unload ventila-
    tory muscles, 196–198
  for modes of ventilator operation,
    56t–57t
  not affecting ventilatory muscle loads,
    198
Breathing loads, calculation of, from
    pressure/flow/volume
    measurements, 136–137
Bronchi, anatomy of, 241
Bronchial suctioning, 95–96
Bronchoalveolar lavage (BAL), in
    diagnosis of ventilator-associated
    pneumonia, 306–307
  interpreting quantitative culture re-
    sults from, 307–309
Bronchodilator therapy. See also *Aerosol
  therapy*.
  flow volume loops before and after,
    in ventilated patient with COPD,
    122
Bronchodilators, 270–274
  monitoring efficacy of, in aerosol ther-
    apy, 122–125
Bronchoscopes, fiberoptic, 248
Bronchoscopy, in diagnosis of
    ventilator-associated pneumonia,
    306–309
Bubble humidifier, 107, *108*

Calcium chloride, as hygroscopic
    additive for passive humidifier, 112
Calorimetry, indirect, 229–231
Candida spp., pneumonia from, 312
Capnograph, response of, to esophageal
    and endotracheal intubation, *89*
Capnography, in airway management,
  248
Carbohydrates, in nutrition support
    regimen, 231–232
Carbon dioxide, alveolar-capillary
    pressure gradient for, 162–163
  excess production of, overfeeding
    and, 226
Carbon dioxide detector, colorimetric,
  89–90
Carbon monoxide, biochemical effects
    of, 186t
Carbon monoxide poisoning, oxygen
    therapy for, 185–186

Cardiac arrest, lung compliance after, 365–366
Cardiopulomonary resuscitation (CPR), ventilation during, 365–366
Cardiorespiratory interactions, 205–209
    manipulation of, for specific patho-physiologic conditions, 209–210
Cardiorespiratory system, goals of, 205
Cardiovascular system, effects of liquid breathing on, 445
    effects of respiratory support on, 204–210
Cascade humidifier, 107–108
Chemiluminescence, 472
Chest compliance, 149–150
    effect of posture and position on, in healthy subjects, 287
Chest radiography, for determining tube position, 90
Chin lift, 241–242
Chlamydia pneumoniae, pneumonia from, 312
Chlordiazepoxide, 258
Chronic obstructive pulmonary disease (COPD), acute exacerbations of, case study in, 498–499
    NPPV for, 482–484
    effect of posture and position in, 289–290
    NPPV in, 482
    nutritional requirements in, 228–229
Circuit flows, extraneous, monitoring of, 139
Circuit leaks, monitoring of, 139
Cisatracurium, 263–264
Closed circuit suction catheter, 95
Closed-loop control, 10–11
CMV. See Continuous mandatory ventilation (CMV); Cytomegalovirus (CMV).
Coaxial flow, in HFV, 418
Colorimetric carbon dioxide detector, 89–90
Compliance, 148–151
    calculation of, from pressure/flow/volume measurements, 136
    effect of posture and position on, in healthy subjects, 287
    hysteresis and, 149
    in parenchymal lung injury, 331
    lung, after cardiac arrest, 365–366
        normal, elevated, and reduced, pressure and volume control ventilation at, 54
    lung and chest, 149–150
    regional, 150–151
    regional abnormality of, effect of, on distribution of tidal breath, 332
    volume-dependence of, 148–149
Compressed gas regulator/direct ventilator drive mechanism, 35–36, 37
Compressible volume, 45, 86
    effects of, on flow volume loop, 86

Compressors, 34
Conditional variables, 23–26
Conducting airways, anatomy of, 241
Continuous mandatory ventilation (CMV), 53–55
    classification of, 55
    descriptive definition of, 53
    manufacturer terms for, 53–55
    other terms for, 53
    pressure control (PC-CMV), pressure, flow, and volume vs time during, 59
    volume control (VC-CMV), pressure, flow, and volume vs time during, 58
Continuous positive airway pressure (CPAP), 67–68, 181–182, 198, 199
    classification of, 67–68
    delivery systems for, airway pressure changes required to trigger, 193
    descriptive definition of, 67
    in NPPV, 488–489
    in ventilator weaning, 355
    manufacturer terms for, 67
    other terms for, 67
    pressure, flow, and volume vs time in, 69
Control, ventilator, scheme for, 4–46
Control circuit alarms, 48
Control circuits, ventilator, 33
Control variables, 9, 11–14
    criteria for determining, during ventilator-assisted inspiration, 8
Controllers, 30
Convective gas transport, in HFV, 418
COPD. See Chronic obstructive pulmonary disease (COPD).
Corticosteroids, inhaled, 274
Corynebacterium spp., pneumonia from, 310t
CPAP. See Continuous positive airway pressure (CPAP).
CPR. See Cardiopulmonary resuscitation (CPR).
Cricoid pressure, 368
Cricothyroidotomy, 254–255
Cycle dys-synchrony, examples of, 200
    monitoring of, 137
Cycle time, 22
Cycle variables, 22–23
    calculation of, from pressure/flow/volume measurements, 137
Cycling, 22–23, 198–201
Cytomegalovirus (CMV), pneumonia from, 311–312, 316

Dead space, effect of passive humidifier on, 112
Deep sulcus sign, 213
Deoxyribonuclease, recombinant human, aerosolized, 277–278
    aerosol therapy with, during mechanical ventilation, 278

Deoxyribonuclease (Continued)
    clinical utility of, 277–278
Diarrhea, in monitoring response to nutrition support, 233
Diazepam, 257–258
Diet-induced thermogenesis (DIT), 228–229
Differential pressure flowmeters, 134–135
Diffusion impairment, hypoxemia from, 179
DNase. See Deoxyribonuclease.
Double-loop control. See Dual control ventilation.
Doxacurium, 263t, 264
Drive mechanisms, ventilator, 33–36
Drug box, in patient transport, 384
Dual control ventilation, 11, 12, 13
    breath to breath, 74–76
        pressure-limited, flow-cycled, 74–75
            classification of, 74–75
            descriptive definition of, 74
            effect of decreased compliance on, 75
            manufacturer terms for, 74
        pressure-limited, time-cycled, 75–76
            classification of, 76
            descriptive definition of, 75
            effects of improved compliance on, 77
            manufacturer terms for, 75
    within a breath, 72–74
        classification of, 73–74
        descriptive definition of, 72–73
        manufacturer terms for, 73
        other terms for, 73

EAR. See Expired air resuscitation (EAR).
ECLS. See Extracorporeal life support (ECLS).
Efficacy testing, criteria for, 395t
    different perspectives of, 397t
    proposed scheme for, based on risk and cost, 398
    selecting appropriate strategy for, 396–398
    types of, 395–396
    types of end points for, 396t
Elastance, 5–6
Electric motor/direct ventilator drive mechanism, 35, 36
Electric motor/rack and pinion ventilator drive mechanism, 35, 36
Electric motor/rotating crank and piston rod ventilator drive mechanism, 35, 36
Electric power, loss of, ventilator alarm for, 46
Electromagnetic poppet valve, output control by, 36

Emergency ventilation, barrier devices for, 369
techniques of, 366–367
Emphysema, pulmonary interstitial, 212–214
subcutaneous, 214
End-expiratory valves, 88
Endobronchial blockers, 404–405
Endobronchial intubation, 252–253
Endotracheal suctioning, 94–97
complications of, 96–97
use of saline instillation in, 96
Endotracheal tube cuff, for long-term use, features of, 360t
management of, 92–94
monitoring pressure in, 92–94
system for, 93
Endotracheal tubes, 86, 247
changing, 255
double-lumen, 403–405
position of, 88–91
resistance of, imposed work caused by, 199
risk of infection from, 301–302
securing of, 91–94
Enteral feeding, 232–233
Enterobacter spp., pneumonia from, 309, 310t, 319
Escherichia coli, pneumonia from, 309, 310t
Esophageal balloon, 133
in partial support for airway obstruction, 345
"sniff" test for proper placement of, 133
Esophageal detection devices, 90
Esophageal intubation, detection of, 89–90
Esophageal obturator airway, 242, 243
Events, level 1, alarm goals in, 139–140
level 2, alarm goals in, 140–141
level 3, alarm goals in, 141
level 4, alarm goals in, 141–142
levels of, and alarm strategies, 139–142
Exhalation valves, 87–88
Expiration, resistance and, 151–152
Expiratory airway resistance, measurement of, for monitoring bronchodilator efficacy, 122–123
Expiratory flow, vs percent vital capacity, for cats during air and perfluorocarbon breathing, 445
Expiratory flow time, 14, 23
Expiratory hold maneuver, 157
Expiratory loads, imposed, 201
Expiratory pause time, 23
Expired air resuscitation (EAR), 365, 366–368
assessment of, 366–367
description of, 366
Expired gas alarms, 49
Exponential pressure waveforms, 39–40
External compressors, 34

Extracorporeal life support (ECLS), 425–431
adult, diagnoses and survival rates in, 427t
anticoagulation in, 431
cardiac, criteria for, 427–428
diagnoses and survival rates in, 427t
complications of, 429–430
history of, 426
neonatal, criteria for, 426
diagnoses and survival rates in, 427t
nutrition in, 431
patient management during, 430–431
patient selection and criteria for, 426–428
pediatric, diagnoses and survival rates in, 427t
sedation and analgesia in, 431
types of, 428–429
venoarterial bypass, 428, 429
venovenous bypass, 428–429
ventilator and respiratory care in, 430–431

Face masks, full, for NPPV, 488
Fat, in nutrition support regimen, 231–232
FDO₂. See Oxygen concentration, delivered (FDO₂).
Fentanyl, 261
Fiberoptic bronchoscopes, 248
Flow, measurement of, 146–148
Flow alarms, 48
Flow dys-synchrony, manifestations of, 194
monitoring of, 137
Flow pattern, ventilator-delivered, 192–198
Flow resistor, 88
Flow sensors, 134–135
Flow triggering, 18–19, 20
and pressure triggering, comparison of, 19t
Flow waveforms, 41–43
during PAV, 81
ramp, 41–43
rectangular, 41
sinusoidal, 43
Flow-controlled ventilation, 14
Flowmeters, differential pressure, 134–135
"hot-wire," 135
ultrasonic, 135
Fluidic logic components, ventilator control circuit consisting of, 35
Food and Drug Administration (FDA), assessment of mechanical ventilation innovations by, 397
FRC. See Functional residual capacity (FRC).

Frequency settings, in airway obstruction, for total ventilatory support, 335
for total ventilatory support in parenchymal lung injury, 335
Full face masks, for NPPV, 488
Functional residual capacity (FRC), effect of posture and position on, in healthy subjects, 284
in parenchymal lung injury, 331
Fungi, pneumonia from, 312

Gas concentration monitors, 135
Gas temperature, relationship of absolute humidity, water vapor pressure, and, 104t
Gastric colonization, reducing, pneumonia prevention by, 319–320
ventilator-associated pneumonia and, 302
Gastric insufflation, cricoid pressure to prevent, 368
in NPPV, 491
vs. delivered tidal volume, in emergency ventilation, 367
Gastrointestinal tract, assessment of, for enteral nutrition, 228
Graham's law, 455
Gravitation sedimentation, 118
Gravitational effects, 287

Haemophilus influenzae, pneumonia from, 309–310
Haemophilus spp., pneumonia from, 309–310
Haloperidol, 261
Heat and moisture exchanger booster (HME booster), 116
Heat and moisture exchangers (HMEs), 109, 110
Heat and moisture exchanging filter (HMEF), 109–110
Heated humidifiers, 106–108
types of, 107–108
vs. passive humidifiers, for mechanical ventilation, 116t
Helium-oxygen (Heliox), 186, 454–457
clinical applications of, 455–456
delivery systems for, 456–457
mechanical ventilators with, delivered tidal volumes for, 458
physics and physiology of, 454–455
Hemoglobin, oxygen equilibrium curve of, 175–176
Herpes simplex virus (HSV), pneumonia from, 311–312
HFJV. See High-frequency jet ventilation (HFJV).
HFOV. See High-frequency oscillatory ventilation (HFOV).
HFV. See High frequency ventilation (HFV).

HHMEs. See *Hygroscopic heat and moisture exchangers (HHMEs)*.
High altitude, oxygen therapy for, 185
High-frequency jet ventilation (HFJV), 416–417
    cardiovascular effects of, 205
    device for, *417*
    for pulmonary hypertension and right ventricular dysfunction, 210
    for respiratory failure, 210
    relationship between jet drive pressure and delivered tidal volume in, *418*
High-frequency oscillatory ventilation (HFOV), 417–418
    cardiovascular effects of, 205
    device for, *420*
    for respiratory failure, 210
High-frequency ventilation (HFV), 415–423
    adult, published studies of, 423t
    applications of, 420–422
    complications of, 422–423
    conceptual rationale for, *416*
    definitions/rationales in, 415–426
    devices for, 416–418
    mechanism of gas transport in, 418–420, *421*
    neonatal/pediatric, randomized controlled studies of, 422t
    operational considerations in, 419t
    vs. conventional ventilation, 416t
Histologic evaluation, in ventilator-associated pneumonia, 303
Histotoxic hypoxia, 181
HME booster. See *Heat and moisture exchanger booster (HME booster)*.
HMEF. See Heat and moisture exchanging filter (HMEF).
HMEs. See Heat and moisture exchangers (HMEs).
"Hot-wire" flowmeters, 135
HSV. See *Herpes simplex virus (HSV)*.
Humidification, physical properties of, 103–104
    physiologic properties of, 104–106
Humidifiers, bubble, 107, *108*
    cascade, 107–108
    high-flow (heated), 106–108
    types of, 107–108
    passive, 108–113
        characteristics of, 111–113
    passover, 107, *108*
    risk of infection from, 301
    use of, in mechanical ventilation, 113–115
Humidity, 103–104
Hygroscopic heat and moisture exchangers (HHMEs), 115–116
    active, 115–116
Hyperbaric chambers, modifications of mechanical ventilation for, 411–412
Hypercapneic respiratory failure, 341
Hypercapnia, permissive, 217, 331–332, 342

Hypoventilation, hypoxemia from, 177
Hypoventilation syndromes, NPPV for, 485
Hypoxemia, from endotracheal suctioning, 97
    in parenchymal lung injury, 332
    physiologic mechanisms of, 177–179
    rebound, from nitric oxide withdrawal, 465–466
Hypoxemic respiratory failure of newborn, nitric oxide for, 462–463
Hypoxia, tissue, biochemical markers of, 182–183
    causes of, 179–181
Hypoxic drive, blunting of, from oxygen therapy, 183–184
Hypoxic hypoxia, 180
Hysteresis, compliance and, 149

ILV. See *Independent lung ventilation (ILV)*.
Impedance triggering, 21
IMV. See *Intermittent mandatory ventilation (IMV)*.
Independent lung ventilation (ILV), 403–406
    asynchronous, 406
    data on, 406
    description of/rationale for, 403–406
    recommendations for, 406
    synchronized, 405–406
Inertial impaction, 117–118
Infection, device-related, risk of, 300–302
    pulmonary defenses against, 300
Infection control, for prevention of ventilator-associated pneumonia, 317–319
Influenza virus, pneumonia from, 311
Infusion pumps, in patient transport, 384
Inhaler, metered-dose, 119
    reccomendations for use of, 125t
    ventilator circuit adapters for, *119*
I-NOvent Delivery System, 471–472
Input power, ventilator, 3–4
Input power alarms, ventilator, 46–48
Inspiration, resistance and, 151–152
Inspiratory-expiratory time relationship, in airway obstruction, for total ventilatory support, 335
    effects of, on V/Q matching, 167–169
    in parenchymal lung injury, for total ventilatory support, 336–337
Inspiratory flow pattern, effects of, on V/Q matching, 167–169
    effects of changing, on pressure waveform during volume control ventilation, *53*
Inspiratory flow time, 11, 14, 21
Inspiratory pause time, 21
Inspiratory phase, 21
Inspiratory time, in airway obstruction, for total ventilatory support, 343–344

Inspiratory time *(Continued)*
    in parenchymal lung injury, for total ventilatory support, 336–337
Inspired gas alarms, 49
Intermittent mandatory ventilation (IMV), 60–61, 197–198
    classification of, 60–61
    descriptive definition of, 60
    for airway obstruction, 344
    for parenchymal lung injury, 337
    in ventilator weaning, 351–355
    manufacturer terms for, 60
    other terms for, 60
    pressure control (PC-IMV), pressure, flow, and volume vs time in, *62*
    synchronized (SIMV), 61–62
Internal compressors, 35
Intrathoracic pressures, and perfusion, 169
Intrinsic positive end-expiratory pressure (intrinsic PEEP), as function of lung mechanics, *152*
    changes in, after bronchodilator therapy, 123, *124*
    effects of, on airway pressure during positive pressure ventilation, *342*
    on pressure- and volume targeted ventilation, 156–158
    from passive humidifier, 111
    impact of, on triggering, *193*
    in NPPV, 489
    in obstructive airway disease, 341, 344–345
    in parenchymal lung injury, 336–337
    monitoring of, 139
Inverse ratio ventilation (IRV), 169
Ipratropium bromide, aerosol therapy with, 273–274
IRV. See *Inverse ratio ventilation (IRV)*.
Isothermic saturation boundary, 105–106

Jaw thrust, 241–242

Klebsiella pneumoniae, pneumonia from, 309, 310t, 319
Klebsiella spp., pneumonia from, 309, 310t

Laminar flow, 454–455
Laryngeal mask airway, 243, *244*
Laryngoscope, 247
    proper positioning of, *251*
Laryngoscope blades, *248*
Larynx, anatomy of, 240–241
Lateral decubitus position, CT image of chest in, during anesthesia, *285*
Left ventricular afterload, effect of ventilatory manipulations on, 207–209

Left ventricular dysfunction, manipulations of cardiorespiratory interactions for, 210

Left ventricular filling pressure, increased, from inhaled nitric oxide, 465

Left ventricular preload, effect of ventilatory manipulations on, 207–209

Legionella pneumophila, pneumonia from, 310t

Legionella spp., pneumonia from, 312

Light wands, 248, 253

Limit variables, 21–22

Liquid ventilation, 433–450
    historical aspects of, 434–435
    partial (PLV), 446–450
    physiology of, 435–438
    total (TLV), 438–446

Liquid ventilator, demand-regulated, *439*
    double-piston, *440*

Lithium chloride, as hygroscopic additive for passive humidifier, 112

Load sharing, partial support and, case study in, 502–503

Lorazepam, 258t, 259

Low-density gases, in total ventilatory support for airway obstruction, 344. See also *Helium-oxygen (Heliox)*.

Lower airway, anatomy of, 239–241

Lung, effects of right-to-left shunt on gas exchange in, *178*
    four-zone model of, *171*
    three-zone model of, perfusion in, *288*
    two-compartment model of, effects of V/Q mismatch in, *178*

Lung compliance, 149–150
    after cardiac arrest, 365–366
    effect of posture and position on, in healthy subjects, 287
    normal, elevated, and reduced, pressure and volume control ventilation at, *54*

Lung inflation, 148–153
    regional, effect of posture and position on, in ARDS, 291–292
    in healthy subjects, 286–287

Lung injury, acute, 330–331
    diagnostic criteria for, 331t
    mortality from, 338t
    from mechanical ventilation, 212–219
    parenchymal, case studies in, 493–497
    mechanical ventilation for, 330–338
    pathophysiology of, 331–332
    total ventilatory support for, goals of mechanical ventilation to provide, 332–334
    strategies for, 334–337
    ventilation modes in, 334–335
    stretch-induced acute, 214–219, 333–334
    clinical studies of, 217–218

Lung injury *(Continued)*
    experimental studies of, 214–217
    unilateral, effect of "good side down" positioning in, 290t
    effect of posture and position in, 290

Lung mechanics. See *Respiratory mechanics*.

Lung perfusion, distribution of, effect of posture and position on, in ARDS, 291–292
    in healthy subjects, 288–289
    three-zone model of, *288*

Lung volumes, effect of posture and position on, in healthy subjects, 284
    in parenchymal lung injury, 331

Magnetic resonance imaging (MRI), modifications of mechanical ventilation for, 411

Mallampati signs, *246*

Mandatory breaths, 25
    algorithm defining, *26*
    backup, 201
    hierarchical order of characteristics applied to, *30*

Mandatory minute ventilation (MMV), 70–71
    automated ventilator weaning by, 354t
    classification of, 70–71
    descriptive definition of, 70
    manufacturer terms for, 70
    other terms for, 70

Manual triggering, 16

MAP. See *Mean alveolar pressure (MAP)*.

Masks, full face, for NPPV, 488
    for NPPV, 487–488
    for oxygen therapy, 181–182
    nasal, for NPPV, 488

Mass median aerodynamic diameter (MMAD), 117

MDI. See *Metered-dose inhaler (MDI)*.

Mean alveolar pressure (MAP), relationship of PAP and, using various stragies to increase MAP, *169*

Mechanical loads, 153–155

Mechanical ventilation, basic concepts of, 3
    computerized physician order entry screens for, schematic diagram of, *32*
    innovations in, 394–398
    clinical outcome assessment of, 396
    efficacy testing of, 395–398
    engineering and clinical performance assessment of, 395
    physiologic assessment of, 395–396
    long-term, 357–363

Mechanical ventilation *(Continued)*
    strategies of, 361–363
    lung injury from, 212–219
    modifications on conventional, 400–412
    noninvasive. See also *Noninvasive positive pressure ventilation (NPPV)*.
    vs. invasive, for long-term ventilatory support, 359
    pediatric, using inhaled nitric oxide, 470–471

Mechanical ventilators, alarm systems for, 46–49, 139–143
    classification of, 47t
    classification of, 1–49
    outline of system for, 2t
    control scheme for, 4–46
    control subsystems for, 33
    drive mechanisms for, 33–36
    electric, 4, 35
    for long-term use, 359–361
    for NPPV, 489
    hyperbaric chamber-compatible, 411–412
    input power for, 3–4
    alarms for failure of, 46–48
    interactive design features of, 191–201
    MRI-compatible, 411
    pneumatic, 4, 35–36, *37*

Meperidine, 260–261

Metaproterenol, aerosol therapy with, 272–273

Metered-dose inhaler (MDI), 119
    reccomendations for use of, 125t
    ventilator circuit adapters for, *119*

Methemoglobinemia, from nitric oxide inhalation therapy, 464

Midazolam, 258–259

Minimal leak technique, 92

Minimal occlusion technique, 92

Minimal seal technique, 92

Mitochondria, oxygen gradient from alveolar space to, *174*

MMAD. See *Mass median aerodynamic diameter (MMAD)*.

MMV. See *Mandatory minute ventilation (MMV)*.

MO-MA resuscitation. See *Mouth-to-mask (MO-MA) resuscitation*.

MO-MO resuscitation. See *Mouth-to-mouth (MO-MO) resuscitation*.

Molecular diffusion, in HFV, 420

Monitoring, during mechanical ventilation, essential, recommended, and optional variables for, 132t
    intensity of, cost effectiveness of, *138*
    normal and abnormal pattern recognition in, 137–139
    during oxygen therapy, 182–183
    patient's clinical status and, 182

Monitoring (*Continued*)
  in NPPV, 489–490
  of neuromuscular blockade, 265
  of response to nutrition support, 233–234
  of sedation, 261–262
Monitors, flow, 134–135
  gas concentration, 135
  in airway management, 248
  NO and NO_2, 472–473
  patient-ventilator interface, 131–139
  portable, for patient transport, 380
  pressure, 132–134
  pressure/flow/volume, calculations from, 135–137
  ventilator, 131–139
  volume, 134–135
Monoplace hyperbaric chambers, mechanical ventilation in, 411–412
Moraxella catarrhalis, pneumonia from, 310t
Morphine, 260
Motion, equation of, 6
  ventilator classification scheme based on, *24*
Motion triggering, 21
Motors, ventilator, 34–36
Mouth-to-mask (MO-MA) resuscitation, 365, 366–367, 370–372
  assessment of, 370–372
  description of, 370
  device for, *370*
Mouth-to-mouth (MO-MO) resuscitation, 365, 366–367
  disease transmission in, 368–369
MRI. See *Magnetic resonance imaging (MRI)*.
Multiplace hyperbaric chambers, mechanical ventilation in, 412
Mycoplasma pneumoniae, pneumonia from, 312

Narcotics, 260–261
Nasal cannulae, for oxygen therapy, 181
Nasal intubation, 251–252
Nasal masks, for NPPV, 488
Nasopharyngeal airway, 242–243
Nebulizer, small-volume, 118–119
  recommendations for use of, 125t
Needle cricothyroidotomy, 254–255
Neuroleptics, 261
Neuromuscular blockade, monitoring of, 265
Neuromuscular blocking agents, 263–265
  adverse effects of, 264–265
  choice of, 265
Neuromuscular disease, respiratory effects of posture and position in, 289
Nitric oxide (NO), 457–458
  ambient levels of, during NO administration, *472*

Nitric oxide (NO) (*Continued*)
  biology of, 458–459
  endogenous production of, biologic pathway for, 459
  in exhaled gas, 459–460
  inhaled, 186–187, 457–473
    clinical applications of, 460–463
    complications of, 463–466
    delivery systems for, 466–472
    direct toxicity of, 463–464
    dose response of, *463*
    injection systems for, 467–469
    I-NOvent Delivery System for, 471–472
    paradoxical response to, 465
    pediatric mechanical ventilation systems using, 470–471
    premixing systems for, 469–470
    scavenging issues in use of, 472
    withdrawal of, response to, *466*
  monitoring of, 472–473
Nitric oxide synthase (NOS), 458–459
Nitrogen dioxide (NO_2), monitoring of, 472–473
  production of, in nitric oxide inhalation therapy, 464
NO. See *Nitric oxide (NO)*.
Noninvasive positive pressure ventilation (NPPV), 481–491
  causes of acute respiratory failure for use of, 483t
  complications of, 490–491
  contraindications to, 486
  effectiveness of, 486–487
    factors important in, 487t
  indications for, 482–486
  in partial support for airway obstruction, 345
  potential benefits and risks of, 482t
  rationale for, 482
  results of randomized controlled trials of, 484t
  technical application of, 487–490
  vs. invasive, for long-term ventilatory support, 359
Nonrebreathing masks, 181
Nonrebreathing valve (NRV), performance of, 374–375
NOS. See *Nitric oxide synthase (NOS)*.
Nose, anatomy of, 240
NPPV. See *Noninvasive positive pressure ventilation (NPPV)*.
NRV. See *Nonrebreathing valve (NRV)*.
Nutrition, in ECLS, 431
  of mechanically ventilated patient, 224–234
Nutrition support regimen, design of, 231–233
  monitoring response to and patient tolerance of, 233–234
Nutritional assessment, 227–228
Nutritional requirements, 228–229

Obstructive airway disease, effect of posture and position in, 289–290

Obstructive airway disease (*Continued*)
  mechanical ventilation for, 340–346
    partial support modes of, for less severe obstruction and during weaning, 344–345
    total ventilatory support strategies in, 342–344
  requiring mechanical ventilation, mortality for patients with, 345t
OI. See *Oxygen index (OI)*.
Open-loop control, 10
Oral cavity, anatomy of, 239–240
Oral intubation, 250
Oropharyneal airway, 242
Orthopnea, in patients with neuromuscular weakness, effect of position on, 289
Output alarms, 48–49
Output control valve, ventilator, 36–37
Output waveforms, 37–46
  effects of patient circuit on, 43–46
  flow, 41–43
  pressure, 39–41
  volume, 41
Overfeeding, effect of, on mechanically ventilated patient, 226–227
Oxygen, 173–174
  alveolar-capillary pressure gradient for, 162–163
  in venous blood of different organ systems, 180t
  mixed venous, decreased content of, hypoxemia from, 179
    partial pressure of (PVO_2), assessing tissue oxygenation from, 183
  partial pressure of (PO_2), arterial, for venous blood of different organ systems, 180t
  supplemental, 173–187. See also *Oxygen therapy*.
    delivery of, 181–182
    techniques for administration of, 181–183
  supply and consumption of, in various organs, 176t
  tissue, direct measurement of, 183
Oxygen concentration, delivered (FDO_2), in mouth-to-mask resuscitation, 370–372
    using standard inhalation technique, *371*
  in mouth-to-mouth resuscitation, 366–367
  inspired (FiO_2), in airway obstruction, for total ventilatory support, 344
  in parenchymal lung injury, for total ventilatory support, 335–336
  of bag-valve devices, 374
  provided by Venturi masks, 182t
Oxygen consumption, 176
Oxygen delivery, overall, alveolar capillary gas transport in context of, 169–171

Oxygen gradient, from alveolar space to mitochondria, *174*
Oxygen index (OI), as ECLS criterion, *428*
Oxygen pathway, 174–176
Oxygen saturation, mixed venous (PVO_2), assessing tissue oxygenation from, 183
Oxygen therapy, adverse effects of, 183–185
  monitoring during, 182–183
  rationale for, 177–181
  special applications of, 185–187
Oxygen transport, 175–176
Oxygen uptake, 174–175
Oxygenation, arterial, monitoring of, during oxygen therapy, 182
  tissue, monitoring of, during oxygen therapy, 182–183
Oyxgen, pulmonary toxicity of, 184–185
Oxygen-hemoglobin equilibrium curve, 175–176
Oxygen-powered breathing devices, 375–379
  assessment of, 376
  description of, 375–376

Pancuronium, 263
PAP. See *Peak alveolar pressure (PAP)*.
Parainfluenza virus, pneumonia from, 311
Paralyzation, 262–265
Parameters, 6
Parenchymal lung injury, case studies in, 493–497
  causes of, 330–331
  less than total support and weaning in, strategies for, 337–338
  mechanical ventilation strategies for, 330–338
  pathophysiology of, 331–332
  total ventilatory support for, strategies for, 334–337
Parenchymal respiratory failure, outcome of, 338
Partial liquid ventilation (PLV), 446–450
  clinical studies of, 448–449
  laboratory studies of, 446–448
Partial rebreathing masks, 181
Partial ventilatory support, airway pressure flow and pleural pressure patterns in, *351*
  and load sharing, case study in, 502–503
  for less severe airway obstruction, 344–345
  in recovering respiratory failure, case study in, 500–502
  modes of, 352t
  weaning from, 351–355
Passive humidifiers, 108–113

Passive humidifiers *(Continued)*
  additives and, 112
  characteristics of, 111–113
  choosing, 113
  cost of, 112–113
  dead space and, 112
  moisture output of, 111
  resistance of, 111–112
  use of, in mechanical ventilation, 113–115
  vs. heated humidifiers, for mechanical ventilation, 116t
Passover humidifier, 107, *108*
Patient events, alarm goals in, 141–142
Patient history, in assessment for intubation, 243–244
Patient positioning, 283–294
  to relieve airway obstruction, 241
Patient transport, 379–386
  equipment for, 379–380
  physiologic effects and risks of, 384–386
  portable monitor for, 380
  preparation for, 379
  reasons for, 379
  staff required for, 380t
Patient-ventilator interactions, 189–202
  check of, 97–98
  monitors and displays for, 132–139
  patient events affecting, alarm goals in, 141
Patient-ventilator interface, 85–98
Patient-ventilator synchrony, future approaches to improving, 201–202
  in weaning to partial support, 352–353
PAV. See *Pressure assist ventilation (PAV)*; *Proportional assist ventilation (PAV)*.
PCIVR. See Pressure control inverse ratio ventilation (PCIRV).
Peak alveolar pressure (PAP), relationship of MAP and, using various stragies to increase MAP, *169*
PEEP. See *Positive end-expiratory pressure (PEEP)*.
PEEP valves. See *End-expiratory valves*.
Pendelluft, *343*
  in HFV, 420
Percent cycle time, 22
Percent inspiratory time, 22
Percent pause time, 22
Perfluorocarbons, 435–438
  properties of, 437t
Permissive hypercapnia, 217, 331–332, 342
Peroxynitrite, 459
  production of, in nitric oxide inhalation therapy, 464–465
Persistent pulmonary hypertension of the newborn (PPHN), nitric oxide for, 462

Pharynx, anatomy of, 240
Phase variables, 14–23, 25
  criteria for determining, *15*
Physical examination, in assessment for intubation, 245–246
Platelet inhibition, from inhaled nitric oxide, 465
Pleural pressures, regional, effect of posture and position on, in healthy subjects, 284–286
PLV. See *Partial liquid ventilation (PLV)*.
Pneumatic diaphragm, output control by, 37
Pneumatic poppet valve, output control by, 36
Pneumatic power, loss of, ventilator alarm for, 46
Pneumococcus, pneumonia from, 309–310
Pneumocystis carinii, pneumonia from, 316
Pneumomediastinum, 212–214
Pneumonia, aspiration, nutrition support and, 233
  underfeeding and, 226
  ventilator-associated, 296–321
    diagnosis of, 302–306
      bronchoscopic techniques in, 306–309
      diagnostic criteria for, in adults, 304t
    empirical therapy for, 314–315
    epidemiology of, 297
      by ICU type, 298t
    incidence of, 297–298
    microbiology of, 309–311
    morbidity, mortality, and other costs of, 298–299
    pathogenesis of, 299–302
    prevention of, 316–320
      antibiotic prophylaxis for, 320
      by reducing gastric colonization and aspiration, 319–320
      CDC recommendations for, 317t–318t
      infection control for, 317–319
    risk factors for, 297–298, 299t
    specific therapy for, 315–316
    treatment of, 312–316
      host considerations in, 313–314
Pneumoperitoneum, 214
Pneumothorax, 212–214
  deep sulcus sign of, *213*
  in NPPV, 491
PO₂. See *Oxygen, partial pressure of (PO₂)*.
Poiseuille's law, 454–455
Positive end-expiratory pressure (PEEP), 6, 16–17
  changes to collapsed alveoli under, *167*
  definition of, 165
  in airway obstruction, for total ventilatory support, 344

Positive end-expiratory pressure (PEEP)
(*Continued*)
in parenchymal lung injury, 333–334
for total ventilatory support, 335–336
intrinsic, changes in, after bronchodilator therapy, 123, *124*
as function of lung mechanics, *152*
effects of, on pressure- and volume targeted ventilation, 156–158
in obstructive airway disease, 341–342, 344–345
in parenchymal lung injury, 336–337
impact of, on triggering, *193*
monitoring of, 139
rationale for, 165–166
strategies to apply, 166–167
Positive end-expiratory pressure/fraction of inspired oxygen (PEEP/FiO$_2$), algorithm for, in NIH ARDS Network MV protocol, 336t
Postextubation stridor, NPPV for, 485
Postintubation procedures, 253–255
Posture/position. See also *Patient positioning.*
effects of, in respiratory disease, 289–293
on healthy subjects, 284–289
PPHN. See *Persistent pulmonary hypertension of the newborn (PPHN).*
Pressure, measurement of, 146–148
sites of, during mechanical ventilation, *147*
Pressure alarms, 48
Pressure assist ventilation (PAV), for airway obstruction, 344
for parenchymal lung injury, 337
in ventilator weaning, 351
Pressure control breaths, and volume control breaths, comparison of, 55t, 155–156
Pressure control inverse ratio ventilation (PCIRV), 69–70
classification of, 70
descriptive definition of, 69
manufacturer terms for, 69–70
other terms for, 69
Pressure control–synchronized intermittent mandatory ventilation (PC-SIMV), pressure, flow, and volume vs. time during, *64*
Pressure sensors, 132–134
Pressure support breath, and effects of increasing rise time and decreasing cycle criteria, *68*
effects of changing the pressure rise time during, *196*
important components of, *65*
pressure and flow waveforms demonstrating pressure cycling of, *67*
Pressure support ventilation (PSV), 62–67

Pressure support ventilation (PSV)
(*Continued*)
classification of, 63–67
compared with PAV, effect of increasing patient effort during, *407*
comparison of different ventilators for, 66t
descriptive definition of, 62
for airway obstruction, 344
for parenchymal lung injury, 337
in ventilator weaning, 351–355
manufacturer terms for, 63
other terms for, 62–63
pressure, flow, and volume vs. time during, *65*
vs. ATC, in overcoming endotracheal tube resistance, *79*
work shifting using, *154*
Pressure triggering, 16–18
and flow triggering, comparison of, 19t
Pressure waveforms, 39–41
during PAV, *81*
effects of changing inspiratory flow patterns on, during volume control ventilation, *53*
exponential, 39–40
oscillating, 40–41
rectangular, 39
sinusoidal, 40
Pressure control–assist/control (PC-A/C) ventilation, for parenchymal lung injury, 334–335
for total ventilatory support in airway obstruction, 342–343
pressure, flow, and volume vs. time in, *61*
Pressure control–continuous mechanical ventilation (PC-CMV), pressure, flow, and volume vs. time during, *59*
using inspiratory > expiratory time, *71*
Pressure control–intermittent mandatory ventilation (PC-IMV), pressure, flow, and volume vs. time in, *62*
Pressure-controlled ventilation, 13
at normal, elevated, and reduced lung compliance, 54
for long-term support, 361
influence diagram for, *27*
output waveforms for, *7, 38, 40*
vs. volume control, 52–53
Pressure-time product (PTP), 153–155
load shifting as reflected in, *155*
Prone position, clinical effects of, in ARDS, 292–293
CT of chest in, in ARDS, *292*
physiologic effect of, in ARDS, 290–291
Propofol, 259–260
Proportional assist, 8
Proportional assist ventilation (PAV), 80–82, 202

Proportional assist ventilation (PAV)
(*Continued*)
classification of, 80–82
compared with PSV, effect of increasing patient effort during, *407*
data on, 408
description of/rationale for, 406–408
descriptive definition of, 80
effect of increasing patient effort during, *407*
manufacturer terms for, 80
other terms for, 80
pressure, volume, and flow waveforms during, *81*
recommendations for, 408–409
Proportional valve, output control by, 36–37
Protected specimen brush (PSB), 305, 307
interpreting quantitative culture results from, 307–309
Protein, in nutrition support regimen, 231–232
Proteus mirabilis, pneumonia from, 310t
Proteus spp., pneumonia from, 310t
PSB. See *Protected specimen brush (PSB).*
Pseudomonas aeruginosa, pneumonia from, 309, 310t, 319
PSV. See *Pressure support ventilation (PSV).*
PTP. See *Pressure-time product (PTP).*
Pulmonary edema, from mechanical ventilation, experimental studies of, 214–217
Pulmonary hypertension, manipulations of cardiorespiratory interactions for, 209–210
rebound hypoxemia and, from nitric oxide withdrawal, 465–466
Pulmonary interstitial emphysema, 212–214
Pulmonary mechanics, effect of posture and position on, in healthy subjects, 287
Pulmonary oxygen toxicity, 184–185
Pulmonary vascular resistance (PVR), components of, *208*
Pulmonary vasodilation, selective, 460
Pulse oximetry, in airway management, 248
PVO$_2$. See *Oxygen, mixed venous, partial pressure of (PVO$_2$).*

Ramp flow waveforms, 41–43
ascending, 42–43
descending, 43
Ramp volume waveforms, 41
Ramsay scale, modified, 262t
RDS. See *Respiratory distress syndrome (RDS).*
Reactive oxygen species (ROS), biologic sources of, 184t

Rectangular flow waveforms, 41
Rectangular pressure waveforms, 39
REE. See *Resting energy expenditure (REE)*.
Rehabilitation, comprehensive, role of, in long-term ventilator-dependent patient, 363
Relative humidity, 103–104
Remifentanil, 261
Residual volumes, in monitoring response to nutrition support, 233
Resistance, 6, 151–153
    calculation of, from pressure/flow/volume measurements, 136
    effect of posture and position on, in healthy subjects, 287
    expiratory airway, measurement of, for monitoring bronchodilator efficacy, 122–123
    inspiration/expiration and, 151–152
    of natural and artifical airway, 152–153
    of passive humidifier, 111–112
    regional differences in, 153
    volume and, 151
Respiratory center drive, effect of underfeeding on, 225
Respiratory disease, effect of posture and position in, 289–293
Respiratory distress syndrome (RDS), neonatal, TLV for, 442–443
Respiratory failure, due to airflow obstruction, causes of, 340–341
    hypercapneic, 341
    hypoxemic, of the newborn, nitric oxide for, 462–463
    manipulations of cardiorespiratory interactions for, 210
    parenchymal, outcome of, 338
    recovering, case study in, 500–502
Respiratory mechanics, 146–159
    lung inflation and, 148–153
    measurements of, 146–148
    ventilator control and, 4–11
Respiratory muscle function, effect of underfeeding on, 225
Respiratory muscle overload, 341
Respiratory quotient (RQ), 226–227
    in indirect calorimetry, 229–231
Respiratory syncytial virus (RSV), pneumonia from, 311
Resting energy expenditure (REE), 226, 229
    in indirect caolrimetry, 229–231
Reynolds number, 455
Ribavirin, aerosolized, 276–277
    aerosol therapy with, during mechanical ventilation, 276–277
    general considerations for, 276
Right heart, venous return to, factors affecting, 206
Right ventricular afterload, effect of ventilatory manipulations on, 207
Right ventricular dysfunction, manipulations of cardiorespiratory interactions for, 209–210

Right ventricular preload, effect of ventilatory manipulations on, 206–207
Right-to-left shunt, effects of, on gas exchange in two-compartment lung model, 179
    hypoxemia from, 178
Rocuronium, 263t, 264
ROS. See *Reactive oxygen species (ROS)*.
RQ. See *Respiratory quotient (RQ)*.
RSV. See *Respiratory syncytial virus (RSV)*.

Saline, instillation of, in endotracheal suctioning, 96
Saturation, 103
Secretion retention, in patients with neuromuscular weakness, effect of position on, 289
Sedation, 257
    agent of choice for, 262
    in ECLS, 431
    monitoring aspects of, 261–262
Sedation level score, 262
Selective pulmonary vasodilation, 460
Selective ventilation distribution circuit (SVDC), 405
Sellick maneuver, 368
Serratia marcescens, pneumonia from, 310t
SIMV. See *Synchronized intermittent mandatory ventilation (SIMV)*.
Sinusoidal flow waveforms, 43
Sinusoidal pressure waveforms, 40
Sinusoidal volume waveforms, 41
SIRS. See *Systemic inflammatory response syndrome (SIRS)*.
Small-volume nebulizer (SVN), 118–119
    recommendations for use of, 125t
Spacer, 119
Spontaneous breathing parameters, calculation of, from pressure/flow/volume measurements, 137
Spontaneous breaths, 25
    algorithm defining, *26*
    hierarchical order of characteristics applied to, *30*
Spontaneous ventilatory drive, ventilator tracking of, 190–191
Spontaneous ventilatory pattern, determinants and characteristics of, 190
Stagnant hypoxia, 181
Staphylococcus, coagulation-negative, pneumonia from, 310t
Staphylococcus aureus, pneumonia from, 309–310
Static pressure-volume plot, *148*
    approximation of, by slow-flow, single-breath technique, *149*
Stethoscope, in patient transport, 384

Streptococcus, group B, pneumonia from, 310t
Stylets/guides, endotracheal tube, 247–248
Subcutaneous emphysema, 214
Suction catheter, 85, 94–95
    closed circuit, 95
Sufentanil, 261
Supine position, before anesthesia, *285, 286*
    CT images of chest in, after anesthesia, *286*
    in ARDS, *292*
Supported breath, 25
Surfactant, clinical utility of, in adults, 279–280
    in infants, 279
    commonly used preparations of, source and composition of, 279t
    lung injury and, 216
    replacement of, 278–280
SVDC. See *Selective ventilation distribution circuit (SVDC)*.
SVN. See *Small-volume nebulizer (SVN)*.
SVO$_2$. See *Oxygen saturation, mixed venous (SVO$_2$)*.
Sympathomimetics, 270–273
    adverse effects of, *271*
    aerosol therapy with, during mechanical ventilation, 272–273
    clinical utility of, 271–272
Synchronized intermittent mandatory ventilation (SIMV), 61–62
    classification of, 61–62
    descriptive definition of, 61
    manufacturer terms for, 61
    other terms for, 61
    patient work per liter of ventilation in, *195*
    pressure control (PC-SIMV), pressure, flow, and volume vs. time during, *64*
    "window" concept for synchronizing breaths during, *63*
Systemic inflammatory response syndrome (SIRS), 170–171

Tactile orotracheal intubation, 252
Taylor dispersion, in HFV, 420
TEE. See *Total energy expenditure (TEE)*.
TGI. See *Tracheal gas insufflation (TGI)*.
Threshold resistor, *88*
Tidal volume, delivered, in emergency ventilation techniques, *367*
    for mechanical ventilators with heliox, *458*
    relationship between jet drive pressure and, in HFJV, *418*
    vs. gastric insufflation, in emergency ventilation, *367*

Tidal volume settings, for total ventilatory support in airway obstruction, 343
for total ventilatory support in parenchymal lung injury, 335
Time alarms, 48–49
Time triggering, 16
Time-controlled ventilation, 14
Tissue oxygenation, monitoring, during oxygen therapy, 182–183
Total energy expenditure (TEE), 231
Total liquid ventilation (TLV), 438–446
clinical studies of, 442–443
current limitations of, 443–446
laboratory studies of, 440–442, 443, 444
Trachea, anatomy of, 241
Tracheal gas insufflation (TGI), 409–411
data on, 409–410
description of/rationale for, 409
recommendations for, 410–411
Tracheal intubation, 243–256
assessing patient for, 243–247
awake vs. anesthetized, 249
choice of route for, 248–249
patients refusing, NPPV for, 486
performance of, 248–253
preparation for, 249–250
problems with visualization in, 250–251
procedures after, 253–255
selecting equipment for, 247–248
Tracheostomy tubes, changing, 255
for long-term use, design features of, 360t
materials for, 360t
Train-of-four monitoring, 265
Transport ventilators, 376–379
ancillary equipment for, 383–384
assembly and disassembly of, 377
assessment of, 378–379
breathing valve for, 378
description of, 376–377
durability of, 378, 383
ease of operation of, 377, 383
gas consumption of, 383
maintenance of, 378
operational characteristics of, 377, 381–382
portability of, 377, 382
power source for, 377, 382–383
safety of, 377–378, 383
Transrespiratory pressure, 5
Trigger problems, monitoring of, 137
Trigger variables, 15–21
Triggering, 15–21, 191–192
of CPAP systems, airway pressure changes required for, 193
sensitivity and responsiveness of, 192
Turbulent flow, 455

Ultrasonic flowmeters, 135

Underfeeding, effect of, on mechanically ventilated patient, 225–226
Upper airway, anatomy of, 239–241
Upper airway obstruction, heliox for, 455

V/Q matching. See Ventilation-perfusion (V/Q) matching.
V/Q mismatch. See Ventilation-perfusion (V/Q) mismatch.
V/Q relationship. See Ventilation-perfusion (V/Q) relationship.
VAP. See Pneumonia, ventilator-associated.
VAPS. See Volume-assured pressure support (VAPS).
Vecuronium, 263
Venous oxygen, mixed, decreased content of, hypoxemia from, 179
Ventilation distribution, 158–159
effect of posture and position on, in healthy subjects, 287–288
Ventilation modes, 26–29, 51–82
breath types for, 56t–57t
classification of, 27–29
combining, 72
dual control, 72–76
general, 29–33
Ventilation-perfusion (V/Q) matching, 163–165
inspiratory flow pattern and inspiratory-expiratory time relationship effects on, 167–169
intrathoracic pressures and, 169
positive pressure ventilation effects on, 165–169
Ventilation-perfusion (V/Q) mismatch, effects of, in two-compartment lung model, 178
hypoxemia from, 177–178
in parenchymal lung injury, 331–332, 333
Ventilation-perfusion (V/Q) relationship, 175
effect of posture and position on, in healthy subjects, 289
Ventilator(s), for CPR, American Heart Association recommendations for, 365
Ventilator circuit, 85–88
ventilation of, 86–87
Ventilator dependence, 350
category 1, diseases associated with, 358t
management of, 362, 363
outcomes over 1 year in, 358t
weaning success in, 362
category 2, diseases associated with, 359t
management of, 363
causes and outcomes of, 358–359

Ventilator dependence (Continued)
role of comprehensive rehabilitation in, 363
Ventilator discontinuation, 348–355
criteria for considering, 349–350
criteria to predict success of, 349t
importance of strategies of, 349
managing patient not yet ready for, 349t
Ventilator events, alarm goals in, 139–141
Ventilator settings, and lung mechanics, interaction of, 155–159
for NPPV, 488–489
frequency-tidal volume, for total ventilatory support in parenchymal lung injury, 335
Ventilator-to-mask ventilation, 376–379
Ventilatory muscles, breaths designed to fully unload, 194–196
breaths designed to partially unload, 196–198
breaths not affecting, 198
Venturi masks, 181
FiO₂ provided by, 182t
Viruses, pneumonia from, 311
Volume, compliance and, 148–149
excessive, lung injury and, 216
measurement of, 146–148
resistance and, 151
Volume alarms, 48
Volume control breaths, and pressure control breaths, comparison of, 55t, 155–156
Volume control–assist/control (VC-A/C) ventilation, 195
for parenchymal lung injury, 334–335
for total ventilatory support in airway obstruction, 342–343
pressure, flow, and volume vs. time in, 60
Volume control–continuous mechanical ventilation (PC-CMV), pressure, flow, and volume vs. time during, using inspiratory > expiratory time, 72
Volume control–continuous mechanical ventilation (VC-CMV), pressure, flow, and volume vs. time during, 58
Volume-assured pressure support (VAPS), 73–74, 201
automated ventilator weaning by, 354t
possible breath delivery characteristics during, 74
Volume-controlled ventilation, 13–14
at normal, elevated, and reduced lung compliance, 54
effects of changing inspiratory flow pattern on pressure waveform during, 53
for long-term support, 359–361
influence diagram for, 27
output waveforms for, 7, 38

Volume-controlled ventilation
  (Continued)
  vs. pressure control, 52–53
Volume sensors, 134–135
Volume support, automated ventilator
  weaning by, 354t
Volume triggering, 19–21
Volume waveforms, 41
  during PAV, 81
  ramp, 41
  sinusoidal, 41

Water vapor content, 104
Water vapor pressure, relationship of

Water vapor pressure (Continued)
  gas temperature, absolute humidity,
  and, 104t
Waveforms, effects of patient circuit on,
  43–46
  output, 37–46
  flow, 41–43
  pressure, 39–41
  volume, 41
Weaning, from NPPV, 489
  ventilator, 348–355
    aggressiveness of, patient fatigue
    and, 352t
    automated, 354
    importance of strategies of,
    349

Weaning (Continued)
  in recovering respiratory failure,
    case study in, 500–502
  patient loads in, 353
  proposed strategy for, 354–355
  success of, in category 1 ventilator
    dependence, 362
    using different strategies, 354t
  synchrony and load characteristics
    in, 352–353
Weaning units, 363
Wick humidifier, 108, 109
Work (W), 153–155
  patient, configurations of, in various
    forms of partial support, 353
  shifting of, using PSV, 154